Contributing Authors

Mary Anderson, R.N., M.S.N. C.N.S.

Elizabeth Arnold, R.N., M.S.N., C.N.S.

Sara Bishop, Ph.D., R.N.C.

Mary Ann Boyd, Ph.D., D.N.S., A.P.R.N., B.C.

Robin B. Britt, Ed.D., R.N.

Kellie D. Bryant, R.N., M.S., N.P., C.C.E

Mary Cassem, R.N., M.S.

Rita Rudd Cinquemani, R.N., M.S.

Daria M. Close, R.N., M.S.N.

Carol L. Collins, R.N., M.S.

Linda Crossett, R.N., M.S.N., C.S.

Pat Crotwell, R.N., M.S.N.

Deborah Davenport, R.N., M.S.N., C.C.R.N.

Debra Danforth, R.N., M.S., A.R.N.P.

Camille Davis, R.N., M.S.N.

Bonnie Dolson, R.N., M.S.

Judith Driscoll, R.N., M.Ed., M.S.N.

Karen F. Duncan, R.N., M.S.

Laurie K. Erford, R.N., M.S.N.

Jean Flick, R.N., M.S.

Sally E. Fletcher, R.N., M.S.N., A.P.R.N., B.C.

Karen Frith, Ph.D., R.N.

Judy Hammond, Ph.D., R.N.C.

Ray Hargrove-Huttel, Ph.D., R.N.

Erin Jaynes, R.N., M.S.N.

Florence Jemes, R.N., M.S.N., C.S.

Barbara Kearney, Ph.D., R.N.

Kathryn A. Lauchner, Ph.D., R.N.

Robin Lockhart, Ph.D. (c), R.N.

Mary Lou Martin, R.N., M.S.N., C.P.N.P.

Berthine Pam Mc

Jane Mathis, R.N

Susan Morrison, Ph.D., R.N.

Ainslie Nibert, Ph.D., R.N.

Cynthia K. Peterson, R.N., M.S.N.

Patricia Smith, R.N.C., M.S.N.

Kim Tankel, R.N., M.S.N.

Betty Tracy, R.N., M.N.

Katherine Lynn Wieck, Ph.D., R.N.

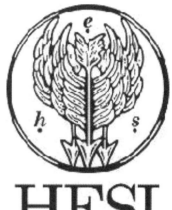

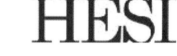

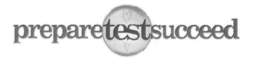

Editors
Donna Boyd
Cynthia Considine
Elizabeth A. Saccoman, B.A.

Art Work and Technical Support
Amber M. Hall, B.B.A.
Sally G. McGee, R.N., B.S.
Antoinette Mundy

For updates/corrections go to
www.hesitest.com and click on "Students"

Health Education Systems, Inc.

2656 South Loop West, Suite 690
Houston, TX 77054

H.E.S.I. NCLEX-RN ® Review Manual   **ISBN 0-9656678-1-2**
Copyright © 2005, Health Education Systems, Inc. All rights reserved.

Editors
Donna Boyd
Cynthia Considine
Elizabeth A. Saccoman, B.A.

Art Work and Technical Support
Adriana Gonzalez, B.B.A.
Sally G. McGee, R.N., B.S.
Antoinette Mundy

TABLE OF CONTENTS

FIGURES

iii

WELCOME

Welcome to the **Health Education Systems, Inc., (HESI)** *NCLEX-RN® Review.*

CONGRATULATIONS! You have chosen an outstanding review course to prepare you for what is very likely the most important test you have ever taken or will ever take.

THREE CHEERS FOR YOU! You have made the wise decision to prepare, in a structured way, for the NCLEX-RN®.

You have already successfully completed a basic nursing program and are well acquainted with your ability to take and pass tests and to perform successfully in the clinical area.

You have the basic knowledge required to pass the licensing exam. However, it is wise to:
1. Organize your knowledge.
2. Review content learned during the years of your basic nursing curriculum.
3. Identify weaknesses in content knowledge so that you can focus your study time appropriately.
4. Develop test-taking skills so you can demonstrate the knowledge you have.
5. Reduce your level of anxiety by increasing your predictability.
6. Know what to expect. Remember: "Knowledge Is Power." You are powerful when you are well prepared and know what to expect.

LICENSING EXAM--NCLEX-RN®

The main purpose of a licensing exam like the NCLEX-RN® is to protect the public.

The NCLEX-RN®:
1. Was developed by the National Council of State Boards of Nursing.
2. Is administered by the State Board of Nurse Examiners.
3. Is designed to test candidates':
   A. Capabilities for safe and effective nursing practice.
   B. "Essential" nursing knowledge.

JOB ANALYSIS STUDIES
"Essential" knowledge is determined by job analysis studies.

> **HESI HINT:** The Council is quite concerned that the licensing exam measure *current, entry level* nursing behaviors. For this reason, job analysis studies are conducted *every three years.* These studies determine how frequently different types of nursing activities are performed, how often they are delegated, and how critical they are to client safety with criticality given more value than frequency.

Job analysis studies indicate that newly-licensed registered nurses are using all five categories of the nursing process and that such use is evenly distributed throughout the five nursing process areas. Therefore, equal attention is given to each part of the nursing process in selecting test items. *(See figure 1-1, The Nursing Process)*

Nursing diagnoses are formulated during the analysis portion of the nursing process. They give form and direction to the nursing process, promote priority setting, and guide nursing actions. *(See figure 1-2, Components of a Nursing Diagnosis)*

To qualify as a nursing diagnosis, the primary responsibility and accountability for recognition and treatment rests with the nurse.

The National Conference of the North American Nursing Diagnosis Association (NANDA) provided the following definition of a nursing diagnosis: "Nursing diagnosis is a clinical judgment about individual, family, or community responses to actual and potential health problems/life processes. Nursing diagnoses provide the basis for selection of nursing interventions to achieve outcomes for which the nurse is accountable." *(See figure 1-3, NANDA-Approved Nursing Diagnoses)*

THE NURSING PROCESS	
CATEGORY	ACTIVITIES ASSOCIATED WITH NURSING PROCESS
ASSESSMENT	• Gather objective and subjective data. • Verify data.
ANALYSIS	• Interpret data. • Collect additional data when necessary. • Identify and communicate nursing diagnoses. • Determine health team's ability to meet client's needs.
PLANNING	• Determine and prioritize goals of care. Include client, significant others, and health team in setting goals. • Develop and modify plan for delivery of client's care.
IMPLEMENTATION	• Organize and manage the client's care. • Perform or assist in performance of client's care. • Counsel and teach client, significant others, and health team. • Provide care specifically directed toward achieving goals.
EVALUATION	• Compare actual outcomes with expected outcomes. • Evaluate compliance with the established regimen or plan. • Record and describe client's response to plan. • Modify plan as indicated, and set priorities.

Figure 1-1

NCLEX-RN® questions regarding nursing diagnosis can take several forms:

1. You may be given the nursing diagnosis in the stem and asked to select an appropriate nursing intervention based on the stated nursing diagnosis.
2. You may be asked to select, from the four choices, an appropriate nursing diagnosis for the described case.
3. You may be asked to choose from 4 nursing diagnoses, the one that should have priority based on the data in the stem.

4. Job analysis studies have identified categories of care provided by nurses called "Client Needs." The test plan is structured according to these categories. *(See figure 1-4, Client Needs)*

> **HESI HINT:** A nursing diagnosis is not a medical diagnosis.
> • **It must be subject to nursing management.**
> • **The etiology may or may not arise from a medical diagnosis.**

COMPONENTS OF A NURSING DIAGNOSIS	
COMPONENT	EXPLANATION
RESPONSE	• Includes potential or actual health response. • Describes measurable outcomes that can be derived. • Cites potential for changes based on nursing actions. • Example: Alteration in comfort, pain.
ETIOLOGY	• Includes potential or actual health response. • Addresses independent, interdependent, and dependent nursing functions. • Example: Related to fractured left ankle.

Figure 1-2

NANDA-Approved Nursing Diagnoses
(For more information see www.nanda.org)

Sleep - Rest	Sexuality - Reproductive	Value - Belief
• Sleep deprivation • Disturbed Sleep patterns • Readiness for enhanced Sleep	• Rape trauma syndrome • Rape trauma syndrome: compound reaction • Rape trauma syndrome: silent reaction • Sexual dysfunction • Ineffective Sexuality patterns	• Impaired religiosity • Readiness for enhanced Religiosity or Spiritual Well-Being • Risk for impaired Religiosity • Spiritual distress • Risk for Spiritual distress

Activity - Exercise	Nutrition - Metabolic
• Activity intolerance • Risk for Activity intolerance • Ineffective Airway clearance • Autonomic dysreflexia • Risk for Autonomic dysreflexia • Ineffective Breathing pattern • Decreased Cardiac output • Risk for delayed Development • Risk for Disuse syndrome • Deficient Diversional activity • Adult Failure to thrive • Fatigue • Impaired Gas exchange • Delayed Growth and development • Risk for disproportionate Growth • Impaired Home maintenance • Disorganized Infant behavior • Risk for disorganized Infant behavior • Readiness for enhanced organized Infant behavior • Impaired bed Mobility • Impaired physical Mobility • Impaired wheelchair Mobility • Sedentary lifestyle • Risk for peripheral Neurovascular dysfunction • Bathing/hygiene Self-care deficit • Dressing/grooming Self-care deficit • Feeding Self-care deficit • Toileting Self-care deficit • Delayed Surgical recovery • Ineffective Tissue perfusion (specify type) • Impaired Transfer ability • Impaired spontaneous Ventilation • Dysfunctional Ventilatory weaning response • Impaired Walking	• Risk for Aspiration • Risk for imbalanced Body temperature • Effective Breastfeeding • Ineffective Breastfeeding • Interrupted Breastfeeding • Impaired Dentition • Readiness for enhanced Fluid balance • Deficient Fluid volume • Excess Fluid volume • Risk for deficient Fluid volume • Risk for excess Fluid volume • Hyperthermia • Hypothermia • Nausea • Readiness for enhanced Nutrition • Imbalanced Nutrition: less than body requirements • Imbalanced Nutrition: more than body requirements • Risk for imbalanced Nutrition: more than body requirements • Ineffective Infant feeding pattern • Impaired Oral mucous membrane • Impaired Skin integrity • Risk for impaired Skin integrity • Impaired Tissue integrity • Ineffective Thermoregulation • Impaired Swallowing

Figure 1-3

NANDA-APPROVED NURSING DIAGNOSES (CONTINUED)

HEALTH PERCEPTION-HEALTH MANAGMENT

- Latex Allergy response
- Risk for latex Allergy response
- Risk for Sudden Infant Death syndrome
- Disturbed Energy field
- Risk for Falls
- Supportive Family role performance
- Health-seeking behaviors (specify)
- Ineffective Health maintenance
- Risk for Infection
- Risk for Injury
- Risk for perioperative-positioning Injury
- Deficient Knowledge (specify)
- Readiness for enhanced Knowledge of (specify)
- Noncompliance
- Risk for Poisoning
- Ineffective Protection
- Risk for Suffocation
- Effective Therapeutic regimen management
- Ineffective Therapeutic regimen management
- Ineffective community Therapeutic regimen management
- Ineffective family Therapeutic regimen management
- Readiness for enhanced Therapeutic regimen management
- Risk for Trauma
- Wandering

ROLE-RELATIONSHIP

- Risk for impaired parent/infant/child Attachment
- Caregiver role strain
- Risk for Caregiver role strain
- Impaired verbal Communication
- Readiness for enhanced Communication
- Parental role Conflict
- Dysfunctional Family processes: alcoholism
- Interrupted Family processes
- Readiness for enhanced Family processes
- Anticipatory Grieving
- Dysfunctional Grieving
- Impaired Parenting
- Risk for impaired Parenting
- Readiness for enhanced Parenting
- Relocation stress syndrome
- Risk for Relocation stress syndrome
- Social Isolation
- Impaired Social Interaction
- Chronic Sorrow
- Risk for other-directed Violence
- Risk for self-directed Violence

SELF-PERCEPTION

- Anxiety
- Death Anxiety
- Disturbed Body image
- Fear
- Hopelessness
- Disturbed personal Identity
- Risk for Loneliness
- Powerlessness
- Risk for Powerlessness
- Disturbed Self-concept
- Readiness for enhanced Self-concept
- Self-esteem Disturbance
- Chronic low Self-esteem
- Situational low Self-esteem
- Risk for situational low Self-esteem
- Self-mutilation
- Risk for Self-mutilation

ELIMINATION

- Bowel Incontinence
- Perceived Constipation
- Constipation
- Risk for Constipation
- Diarrhea
- Functional urinary Incontinence
- Reflex urinary Incontinence
- Stress urinary Incontinence
- Total urinary Incontinence
- Urge urinary Incontinence
- Risk for urge urinary Incontinence
- Altered Urinary elimination
- Readiness for enhanced Urinary elimination
- Impaired Urinary elimination
- Urinary Retention

COGNITIVE-PERCEPTUAL

- Impaired Comfort
- Chronic pain
- Nausea
- Decisional Conflict (specify)
- Acute Confusion
- Chronic Confusion
- Impaired Environmental interpretation syndrome
- Decreased Intracranial adaptive capacity
- Impaired Memory
- Unilateral Neglect
- Acute Pain
- Disturbed Sensory perception
- Disturbed Thought processes

COPING-STRESS TOLERANCE

- Impaired Adjustment
- Compromised family Coping
- Defensive Coping
- Disabled family Coping
- Ineffective Coping
- Ineffective community Coping
- Readiness for enhanced Coping
- Readiness for enhanced community Coping
- Readiness for enhanced family Coping
- Ineffective Denial
- Post-trauma syndrome
- Risk for Post-trauma syndrome
- Risk for Suicide

Figure 1-3 (continued)

CLIENT NEEDS		
CATEGORY OF CLIENT NEEDS	% OF NCLEX-RN®	ACTIVITIES
SAFE, EFFECTIVE ENVIRONMENT • *Management of Care* • *Safety and Infection Control*	13 to 19 % 8 to 14 %	• Coordinate care, Quality assurance, Goal oriented care, Environmental safety • Preparation for treatments and procedures • Safe and effective treatments and procedures
HEALTH PROMOTION & MAINTENANCE	6 to 12 %	• Continued growth and development • Self-care • Integrity of support systems • Prevention and early treatment of health problems
PSYCHOSOCIAL INTEGRITY	6 to 12%	• Promote and support emotional, mental, and social well-being
PHYSIOLOGICAL INTEGRITY • *Basic Care & Comfort* • *Pharmocological & Parenteral Therapies* • *Reduction of Risk Potential* • *Physiological Adaptation*	6 to 12 % 13 to 19 % 13 to 19% 11 to 17 %	• Physiological adaptation • Reduction of risk potential • Activities of daily living • Care r/t medication administration and parental therapies • Provision of basic comfort and care

Based on the results of the 2002 Practice Analysis, the 2004 NCLEX-RN test plan was revised. There was a reduction in the percentage of test items in "Psychosocial Integrity" and "Health Promotion and Maintenance." There was an increase in the percentage of test items allocated to "Management of Care," "Safety and Infection Control," and "Pharmacological and Parenteral Therapies." Consequently, as much as 88% of the test may be dedicated to questions which test SAFE nursing practice and maintenance of PHYSIOLOGICAL INTEGRITY, which might also be regarded as dealing with SAFE practice.

Figure 1-4

HESI HINT: For more information on the NCLEX-RN® test plan and content related to each category/subcategory, go to http://www.ncsbn.org

HESI HINT: Answering NCLEX-RN® questions correctly often depends on setting priorities properly, on making judgments about priorities, and on analyzing the case and formulating a decision about care (or the correct response) based on priorities. Using Maslow's Hierarchy of Needs can help you set priorities. *(See figure 1-5, Maslow's Hierarchy of Needs)*

PRIORITIZING NURSING CARE

Many NCLEX-RN® test items are designed to test your ability to set priorities, for example:

1. Identify the **MOST IMPORTANT** nursing diagnosis.
2. Which nursing intervention is **MOST IMPORTANT**?
3. Which nursing action should be done **FIRST**?
4. Which response is **BEST**?

SETTING PRIORITIES
Texans often say, "Remember the Alamo."

Those taking the NCLEX-RN® should "Remember Maslow."

MASLOW'S HIERARCHY OF NEEDS		
NEED	**DEFINITION**	**NURSING IMPLICATIONS**
PHYSIOLOGIC	Biologic needs for food, shelter, water, sleep, oxygen, sexual expression	The priority biologic need is breathing, i.e., an open airway. Review *Figure 1-4*, the Client Needs activities associated with Physiological Integrity. If you were asked to identify the *most important* action, you would identify needs associated with physiological integrity, e.g., providing an open airway, as the *most important* nursing action.
SAFETY	Avoiding harm; attaining security, order, and physical safety	Review *Figure 1-4*, the activities associated with Safe, Effective Environment. Ensuring that the client's environment is SAFE is a priority, e.g., teaching an older client to remove throw rugs which pose a safety hazard when ambulating would have a greater priority than teaching him/her how to use a walker - *first* priority is *SAFETY*, then coping skills.
LOVE AND BELONGING	Giving and receiving affection; companionship; and identification with a group	Although these needs are important, (*described in Figure 1-4, Client Needs*, activities associated with Psychosocial Integrity) they are less important than physiologic or safety needs. For example, it is more important for a client to have an open airway and a safe environment for ambulating than it is to assist him/her to become part of a support group. However, assisting the client in becoming a part of a support group would have higher priority than assisting him/her in developing self-esteem. The sense of belonging would come *first*, and such a sense might help in developing self-esteem.
ESTEEM AND RECOGNITION	Self-esteem and respect of others; success in work; prestige	
SELF-ACTUALIZATION	Fulfillment of unique potential	It is important to understand the last two needs in Maslow's Hierarchy. They could deal with Client Needs associated with Health Promotion and Maintenance such as continued growth and development and self-care, as well as those associated with Psychosocial Integrity. However, you will probably not be asked to prioritize needs at this level. Remember, it is the goal of the Council to ensure SAFE nursing practice and such practice does not usually deal with the client's self-actualization or aesthetic needs.
AESTHETIC	Search for beauty and spiritual goals	

Figure 1-5

STUDYWARE™ CD

These test items are designed for TEACHING purposes – NOT evaluation. Candidates taking the **HESI NCLEX-RN® Review** receive a CD containing the practice test items. Included on the CD are 6 different exams: Fundamentals, Pediatric, Maternity, Pharmacology, Psychiatric/Mental Health, and Medical/Surgical, as well as a Behavioral Inventory which is a self-study profile to help you get to know yourself better. A 75-question practice exam which follows the NCLEX-RN test blueprint is also included on the CD. Each exam contains excellent rationales and may be taken up to 5 times.

1. The practice test uses the CAT format, i.e., it has the same screen format as the NCLEX-RN®.
2. Because the items presented on the practice test are provided as learning experiences, these test items are not "adaptive," i.e., candidates are required to answer *all* items.
3. At the completion of a practice test, candidates can print their results by clicking the view/print score button.
4. All practice tests have been categorized according to three criteria: Nursing Process, Client Needs, and Clinical Specialty Areas. You will receive a comparison score, which describes how you compare with others who have answered the same items.

HESI HINT: The scoring technique used in this review will enable you to pinpoint your weaknesses and focus your study time so that you can demonstrate your maximum capabilities on the licensure exam.

SAMPLE TEST ITEMS

Sample test items are presented throughout this course.

Class review and discussion of test items are intended to:

1. Provide you with an understanding of the style of questions included in the NCLEX-RN®.
2. Familiarize you with the type of choices or answers available on the exam.
3. Allow you to benefit from "group wisdom" through discussion of the test items.

HESI HINT: The night before taking the NCLEX-RN®, allow only 30 minutes of study time. This 30-minute period should be designated for review of test-taking strategies only. Practice these strategies with various practice test items if you wish (30 minutes only. Do not take an entire test). Spend the night before the exam doing something you ENJOY; something that promotes stress reduction, something that does NOT involve alcohol or other mind-altering drugs. Only YOU can identify the "special something" that will work for you. Remember, YOU CAN BE SUCCESSFUL! After completing this course and your designated study, you will have done what is necessary to pass the exam.

NCLEX-RN® CAT

Computer Adaptive Testing (CAT) will be used for implementation of the NCLEX-RN®.

1. The CAT is administered at a testing center selected by the Council (Council is used as the abbreviation for the NCSBN throughout this book).
2. ETS is responsible for adapting the NCLEX-RN® to the CAT format, processing candidate applications, and transmitting test results to its data center for scoring.
3. The testing centers are located throughout the United States.
4. The Council generates the NCLEX-RN® test items.

THE WAY IT WORKS

1. The NCLEX-RN® consists of 75 to 265 multiple choice or alternative format questions (15 of which are "pilot items") presented on a computer screen.
2. The candidate is presented with a test item and four possible answers.
3. If the candidate answers the question correctly, a slightly more difficult item will follow, and the level of difficulty will increase with each item until the candidate misses an item.
4. If the candidate misses an item, a slightly less difficult item will follow, and the level of difficulty will decrease with each item until the candidate has answered an item correctly.
5. This process will continue until the candidate has achieved a definite "pass" or a definite "fail" score. There will be NO borderline "pass" or "fail" scores because the adaptive testing method will determine the candidate's level of performance before ending the exam.
6. The least number of items a candidate can take to complete the exam is 75, 15 of which will be "pilot items" and will not count toward the "pass" or "fail" score, and 60 of which will determine the candidate's score.
7. The number of the item the candidate is currently answering will appear in the upper right side of the screen.
8. When the candidate has answered enough items to determine a definite pass or fail score, a message will appear on the screen notifying the candidate that he/she has completed the exam.
9. The most number of items a candidate can take is 265, and the longest amount of time the candidate can take to complete the exam is 6 hours.
10. There will be a mandatory break after 2 hours and a voluntary break after an additional 1½ hours (breaks will not be calculated in the 6-hour time limit).
11. If a candidate has NOT obtained a pass/fail score at the end of the 6 hours and has NOT completed all 265 items in the 6-hour limit, but HAS answered ALL of the last 60 questions presented correctly, he/she will pass the exam.
12. If a candidate has NOT obtained a pass/fail score at the end of the 6 hours, has NOT completed all 265 items in the 6-hour limit, and has NOT answered ALL of the last 60 questions presented correctly, he/she will fail the exam.
13. A specific passing score is recommended by the National Council. All states require the same score to pass, so that if you pass in one state, you are eligible to practice nursing in any other state. However, states do differ in their requirements

regarding the number of times a candidate can take the NCLEX-RN®.

14. Although the Council has the ability to determine a candidate's score at the time of completion of the exam, it has been decided that it would be best for candidates to receive their scores from their Board of Nurse Examiners. The Council does not want the testing center to be in a position of having to deal with candidates' reactions to scores, nor does the Council want those waiting to take their exams to be influenced by such reactions.

15. Only two keys on the computer will be used: the space bar and the return key and both will have red tape on them so that they can easily be identified.

16. You must answer each question in order to proceed. You cannot omit a question or return to an item presented earlier. **THERE IS NO GOING BACK,** which works in your favor!

17. The examination is written at 10th grade reading level.

18. There is *no* penalty for guessing with four choices as you have a 25% chance of *guessing* the correct answer.

19. The NCSBN Candidate Bulletin is available at http://www.ncsbn.org. Select NLCLEX Candidate Bulletin.

> **HESI HINT:** One choice or more are likely to be VERY wrong. You will usually be able to rule out two of the four choices rather quickly. Reread the question and choices again, if necessary. Ask yourself which choice answers the question being asked. Even if you have absolutely NO idea what the correct answer is, you will have a 50/50 chance of GUESSING the right answer if you follow this process. Your first response will provide an "educated guess" and will usually be the correct answer. GO WITH YOUR GUT RESPONSE!

GENTLE REMINDERS OF GENERAL PRINCIPLES

Take care of yourself. Follow these "golden rules" for NCLEX-RN® SUCCESS!

1. **EAT WELL:** High-carbohydrate, high protien, and low-fat diet.
2. **SLEEP WELL:** Get a good night's sleep the night before the test. This is not the time to cram or to party. You have done your job, now enjoy the process.
3. **ELIMINATE ALCOHOL AND OTHER MIND-ALTERING DRUGS:** It goes without saying that such substances can inhibit your performance on the exam.
4. **SCHEDULE STUDY TIME:** Between now and the exam, review nursing content, focusing on areas that you identified as your "weak" points when taking the practice tests (review your computer scoring sheets). Use the HESI Study Schedule to block out the time needed for study, then be good to yourself, and use that blocked time for YOU; study.
5. **BE PREPARED:** Assemble all necessary materials the night before the exam (admission ticket, directions to the testing center, identification, money for lunch, glasses or contacts).
   A. **APPROVED ITEMS:** Candidates are only allowed to bring identification forms into the testing room. Watches, candy, chewing gum, food, drinks, purses, wallets, pens, pencils, beepers, cellular phones, post it notes, study materials or aids, and calculators are not allowed.
   B. **ALLOW PLENTY OF TIME:** Arrive early; it is better to be early than late. Allow for traffic jams, etc.
   C. **DRESS COMFORTABLY:** Dress in layers so that you can take off a sweater or jacket if you become too warm, or wear it if you become too cold.
6. **AVOID NEGATIVE PEOPLE:** From now until you have completed the exam, stay away from those who share their anxieties with you or project their insecurities onto you. Sometimes this is a fellow classmate or even your best friend. They will still be there when the exam is over. Right now you need to take care of yourself - avoid the negative, look for the positive.
7. **DO NOT DISCUSS THE EXAM:** Avoid talking about the exam during breaks and while waiting to take the exam.
8. **AVOID DISTRACTIONS:** Take earplugs with you and use them if you find that those around you distract you, e.g., those chewing gum, rattling paper, or getting up to leave the exam.
9. **THINK POSITIVELY:** Use the affirmation "I CAN BE SUCCESSFUL." Obtain the *HESI Relaxation and Affirmation* cassette tape and use it H.S. and PRN from now until you take the exam. Use the relaxation side at night (Not on the way to the exam or at breaks during the exam - you might fall asleep!) Use the affirmation side on the way to the exam or any time you feel the need to boost your confidence. Think: "I have the knowledge to successfully complete the NCLEX-RN®."

LEGAL ASPECTS OF NURSING
LAWS GOVERNING NURSING

Nurse Practice Acts provide the laws that control the practice of nursing in each state. Mandatory nurse practice acts mandate that, under the law, only licensed professionals can practice nursing. All states now have mandatory nurse practice acts.

Nurse Practice Acts govern the nurse's responsibility in making assignments.
1. Assignments should be commensurate with the nursing personnel's educational preparation, experience, and knowledge.
2. The nurse should supervise the care provided by nursing personnel for which he/she is administratively responsible.
3. Sterile or invasive procedures should be assigned to and/or supervised by a professional nurse.

TORTS:

DESCRIPTION: An act involving injury or damage to another (except breech of contract) resulting in civil liability, (i.e. the victim can sue) instead of criminal liability (see crime).

UNINTENTIONAL TORTS:
NEGLIGENCE AND MALPRACTICE

1. **Negligence**: Performing an act that a reasonable and prudent person would not do. Measure of negligence is "reasonableness" (i.e., would a reasonable and prudent nurse act in the same manner under the same circumstances?).
2. **Malpractice**: Negligence of professional personnel, e.g., professional misconduct, or unreasonable lack of skill in carrying out professional duties.

Four elements are necessary to prove negligence/malpractice; if any one element is missing, it cannot be proved.
1. Duty: Obligation to use due care (what a reasonable, prudent nurse would do). Failure to care for and/or to protect others against unreasonable risk. The nurse must ANTICIPATE foreseeable risks. Example: If a floor has water on it, the nurse is responsible for anticipating the risk to the client of falling.
2. Breach of Duty: Failure to perform according to the established standard of conduct in providing nursing care.
3. Injury/Damages: Failure to meet standard of care, which causes actual injury or damage to the client, either physical or mental.
4. Causation: A connection exists between conduct and the resulting injury referred to as "proximate cause" or "remoteness of damage."

Hospital policies provide a guide for nursing actions. They are NOT laws, but courts generally rule against nurses who have violated the employer's policies. Hospitals can be liable for poorly formulated or poorly implemented policies.

Incident reports alert administration to possible liability claims and the need for investigation; they do NOT protect against legal action being taken for negligence or malpractice.

Examples of negligence/malpractice:
1. Burning a client with a hot water bottle or heating pad.
2. Leaving sponges or instruments in a client in surgery.
3. Performing incompetent assessments.
4. Failing to heed warning signs of shock or impending MI.
5. Ignoring signs and symptoms of bleeding.
6. Forgetting to give a medication or giving the wrong medication.

INTENTIONAL TORTS:
ASSAULT AND BATTERY
1. **Assault**: Mental or physical threat, e.g., forcing (without touching) a client to take a medication or treatment.
2. **Battery**: Touching, with or without the intent to do harm, e.g., hitting or striking a client. If a mentally competent adult is forced to have a treatment he/she has refused, battery occurs.

INVASION OF PRIVACY: Encroachment or trespassing on another's body and/or personality.
1. **False imprisonment**: Confinement without authorization.
2. **Exposure of a person**: Exposure or discussion of the client's case. After death, the client has a right to be unobserved, excluded from unwarranted operations, and protected from unauthorized touching of the body.
3. **Defamation**: Divulgence of privileged information or communication, e.g., from charts, conversations, or observations.

FRAUD: Willful and purposeful misrepresentation that could cause, or has caused, loss or harm to a person or property.

EXAMPLES OF FRAUD:
1. Presenting false credentials for the purpose of entering nursing school, obtaining a license, or obtaining employment.
2. Describing a myth regarding a treatment, e.g., telling a client that a placebo has no side effects and will cure his disease, or telling a client that a treatment or diagnostic test will "not hurt," when indeed pain is involved in the procedure.

CRIME: Act contrary to a criminal statute. Crimes are wrongs punishable by the state, committed against the state, with intent usually present.

Commission of a crime requires:
1. Committing a deed contrary to criminal law.
2. Omitting an act when there is a legal obligation to perform such an act, e.g., refusing to assist with the birth of a child if such a refusal results in injury to the child.
3. Criminal conspiracy occurs when two or more persons agree to commit a crime.
4. Assisting or giving aid to a person in the commission of a crime makes that person equally guilty of the offense (awareness must be present that the crime is being committed).
5. Ignoring a law is **not** usually an adequate defense against committing a crime, e.g., a nurse who sees another nurse taking narcotics from the unit supply and ignores this observation is not adequately defended against committing a crime.
6. Assault is justified for self-defense. However, in order to be justified, only enough force can be used as to maintain self-protection.
7. Search warrants are required prior to searching a person's property.
8. It is a crime **not** to report suspected child abuse; i.e., **the nurse's legal responsibility is to report suspected child abuse.**

NURSING PRACTICE AND THE LAW

PSYCHIATRIC NURSING

Civil procedures: Methods used to protect the rights of psychiatric clients.

Voluntary admission: Client admits him/herself to an institution for treatment and retains civil rights.

Involuntary admission: Someone other than the client applies for admission to an institution.
1. Requires certification by healthcare provider that the person is a danger to self and/or others (depending on the state, one or two healthcare provider certifications are required.)
2. Individuals have the right to a legal hearing within a certain number of hours or days.
3. Most states limit commitment to 90 days.
4. Extended commitment is usually no longer than one year.

Emergency admission: Any adult may apply for emergency detention of another. However, medical or judicial approval is required to detain anyone beyond 24 hours.
1. Persons held against their will can file a habeas corpus to try and get the court to hear their case and release them.
2. The court determines the sanity and alleged unlawful restraint of a person.

Legal and civil rights of hospitalized clients:
1. Right to wear their own clothes, keep personal items, and a reasonable amount of cash for small purchases.
2. Right to have individual storage space for their own use.
3. Right to see visitors daily.
4. Right to have reasonable access to a telephone and the opportunity to have private conversations by telephone.
5. Right to receive and send mail (unopened).
6. Right to refuse shock treatments and/or lobotomy.

Competency hearing: Legal hearing that is held to determine a person's capability to make responsible decisions about self, dependents, or property.

Persons declared incompetent have the legal status of a minor, i.e., they cannot:
1. Vote.
2. Make contracts or wills.
3. Drive a car.
4. Sue or be sued.
5. Hold a professional license.

A guardian is appointed by the court for the incompetent person. Declaring a person incompetent can be initiated by the state or the family.

Insanity: A legal term meaning the accused is not criminally responsible for the unlawful act committed because he/she is mentally ill.

Inability to stand trial: The person accused of committing a crime is not mentally capable of standing trial. He/She:

1. Cannot understand the charge against him/her.
2. Must be sent to psychiatric unit until legally determined competent for trial.
3. Once the person is mentally fit, he/she must stand trial and serve any sentence, if convicted.

> **HESI HINT:** Often an NCLEX-RN® question asks who should explain the surgical procedure to the client. The answer is the PROVIDER. This is probably the only question where you refer to the healthcare provider. Remember, nurses are proud people - nurses wrote the test items, and they expect nurses to handle most client situations. Also remember it is the nurse's responsibility to be sure that the operative permit is signed and is on the chart. It is NOT the nurse's responsibility to explain the procedure to the client.

PATIENT IDENTIFICATION

The Joint Commission on Accreditation of Healthcare Organizations (JCAHO) has implemented new patient identification requirements to meet safety goals.

1. Use at least 2 patient identifiers whenever taking blood samples, administering medications, or administering blood products
2. The patient room number MAY NOT be used as a form of identification.

SURGICAL PERMIT

Consent to operate (surgical permit), must be obtained prior to any surgical procedure, however minor it might be.

Legally, the surgical permit must be:

1. Written.
2. Obtained voluntarily.
3. Explained to the client, i.e., "informed consent" must be obtained.

Informed consent means the operation has been fully explained to the client, including:

1. Possible complications and disfigurements.
2. Removal of any organs or parts of the body.

Surgery permits:

1. Must be witnessed by an authorized person such as the healthcare provider or a nurse.
2. Protect the client against unsanctioned surgery and protect the healthcare provider/surgeon, hospital, and hospital staff against possible claims of

unauthorized operations.

3. Adults and emancipated minors may sign their own operative permits if they are mentally competent.
4. Permission to operate on a minor child or an incompetent or unconscious adult must be obtained from a responsible family member or guardian.

CONSENT

The law does not *require* written consent to perform medical treatment.

1. Treatment can be performed if the client has been fully informed about the procedure.
2. Treatment can be performed if the client voluntarily consents to the procedure.
3. If informed consent cannot be obtained (e.g., client is unconscious) and immediate treatment is required to save "life or limb," the emergency laws can be applied. *(See Good Samaritan Act below)*

Verbal or written consent:

1. When verbal consent is obtained, a notation should be made which:
   A. Describes in detail how and why verbal consent was obtained.
   B. Is placed in the client's record or chart.
   C. Is witnessed and signed by TWO persons.
2. Written or verbal consent can be given by:
   A. Alert, coherent, or otherwise competent adults.
   B. Parent or legal guardian.
   C. Person "in loco parentis" (person standing in for a parent with a parent's rights, duties, and responsibilities) of minors or incompetent adults.

Consent of minors:

1. Minors 14 years of age and older must agree to treatment along with their parent or guardian.
2. Emancipated minors can consent for treatment themselves.

EMERGENCY CARE

Good Samaritan Act: Protects health practitioners against malpractice claims for care provided in emergency situations (e.g., the nurse gives aid at the scene to an automobile accident victim).

The nurse is required to perform in a "reasonable and prudent manner."

HEALTHCARE PROVIDERS/PHYSICIANS PRESCRIPTIONS

The nurse is required to obtain a healthcare provider/physician prescription (order) to carry out medical procedures.

Although verbal phone prescriptions should be avoided, the nurse should follow the agency's policy and procedures. Failure to follow such rules could be considered *negligence*. JCAHO requires that organizations implement a process for taking verbal or telephone orders that includes a "read-back" of critical values. The employee receiving the prescription should write the verbal order/critical value on the chart or record it in the computer and then read back the order/value to the healthcare provider.

If a nurse questions a healthcare providers/physicians prescription because he/she believes that it is *wrong* (e.g., the wrong dosage for a medication was prescribed), the nurse should do the following:
1. Inform the healthcare provider/physician.
2. Record that the healthcare provider/physician was informed and record the healthcare providers/physicians response to such information.
3. Inform the nursing supervisor.
4. Refuse to carry out the prescription.

If the nurse believes that a healthcare providers/physicians prescription was made with *poor judgment* (e.g., the nurse believes the client does not need as many tranquilizers as the healthcare provider/physician prescribeded) the nurse should:
1. Record that the healthcare provider/physician was notified and that the prescription was questioned.
2. Carry out the prescription because a nurse's nursing judgment cannot be substituted for a healthcare providers/physicians medical judgment.

If a nurse is asked to perform a task for which he/she has not been prepared educationally (e.g., obtain a urine specimen from a premature infant by needle aspiration of the bladder), or with the necessary experience (e.g., a nurse who has never worked in

labor and delivery is asked to perform a vaginal exam and determine cervical dilation), the nurse should do the following:
1. Inform the healthcare provider/physician that he/she does not have the education or experience necessary to carry out the prescription.
2. Refuse to carry out the prescription.

HESI HINT:
- If the nurse carries out a healthcare providers/physicians prescription for which he/she is not prepared and does not inform the Healthcare Provider/Physician of his/her lack of preparation, the nurse is solely liable for any damages.
- If the nurse INFORMS the healthcare provider/physician of his/her lack of preparation in carrying out a prescription and carries out the prescription anyway, the nurse AND the healthcare provider/physician are liable for any damages.

The nurse cannot, without a healthcare providers/physicians prescription, alter the amount of drug given to the client. For example, if a healthcare provider/physician has prescribeded pain medication in a certain amount and the client's pain is not, in the nurse's judgment, severe enough to warrant the dosage prescribed, the nurse *cannot* reduce the amount without first checking with the healthcare provider/physician. Remember, nursing judgment cannot be substituted for medical judgment.

HESI HINT: Assignments are often tested on the NCLEX-RN®. The Nurse Practice Acts of each state govern policies related to making assignments. Usually, when asked who should be assigned to do a sterile dressing change - it should be a licensed nurse - RN or LPN who has been "checked off" on this procedure.

RESTRAINTS
Clients may be restrained only under the following circumstances:
1. In an emergency.
2. For a limited time.
3. For the limited purpose of protecting the client from injury.

Nursing Responsibilities with regard to restraints:
1. The nurse must notify the Healthcare Provider/Physician immediately that the client has been restrained.
2. The nurse should document the facts regarding the

rationale for restraining the client.

When restraining a client, the nurse should do the following:
1. Use restraints after exhausting all reasonable alternatives.
2. Apply the restraints properly.
3. Check frequently to see that the restraints do not impair circulation, or cause pressure sores or other injuries. *(Record the monitoring of restraints.)*
4. Remove restraints as soon as possible.

HESI HINT:
- **Restraints of any kind may constitute false imprisonment.**
- **Freedom from unlawful restraint is a basic human right and is protected by law.**

HEALTH INSURANCE PORTABILITY AND ACCOUNTABILITY ACT OF 1996 (HIPAA)

Congress passed the Health Insurance Portability and Accountability Act of 1996 (HIPAA) to create a national patient record privacy standard.

WHO AND WHAT IS COVERED?

HIPAA privacy rules pertain to healthcare providers, health plans, and health clearinghouses and their business partners who engage in computer to computer transmissioin of healthcare claims, payment and remittance, benefit information, and/or health plan eligibility information, and who disclose personal health information that specifically identifies an individual and is transmitted electronically, in writing, or verbally. Patient privacy rights are of key importance. Patients must provide written approval for the disclosure of any of their health information for almost any purpose. Healthcare providers/ physicians must offer specific information to patients that explains how their personal health information will be used. Patients must have access to their medical records, and they can receive copies of these and request that changes be made if they identify inaccuracies. Healthcare providers/physicians who do not comply with HIPAA regulations, and/or make unauthorized disclosures, risk civil and criminal liability. According to the Department of Health and Human Services (DHHS), civil penalties can be assessed as high as $25,000 per year, and criminal penalties can be assessed at $50,000 with a year in prison to as much as $250,000 and ten years in prison.

For further information, use this link to the DHHS Web Site, Office of Civil Rights, which contains frequently asked questions about HIPAA, to access: Standards for Privacy of Individually Identifiable Health Information. (July, 2001). *http://aspe.hhs.gov/admnsimp/final/pvcguide1.htm*

REVIEW QUESTIONS LEGAL
1. What types of procedures should be assigned to professional nurses?
2. Negligence is measured by "reasonableness." What question might the nurse ask when determining such "reasonableness?"
3. List the four elements that are necessary to prove negligence.
4. Define an intentional tort, and give one example.
5. Differentiate between voluntary and involuntary admission.
6. List five activities a person who is declared incompetent cannot do.
7. Name three legal requirements of a surgical permit.
8. Who may give consent for medical treatment?
9. What law protects the nurse who provides care or gives aid in an emergency situation?
10. What actions should the nurse take if he/she questions a healthcare providers/physicians prescription, i.e., believes the prescription is wrong?
11. Describe the nurse's legal responsibility when asked to perform a task for which he/she is unprepared.
12. Describe nursing care of the restrained client.
13. Describe six patient rights guaranteed under HIPAA regulations that nurses must be aware of in the practice.

ANSWERS TO REVIEW QUESTIONS
1. Sterile or invasive procedures.
2. Would a reasonable and prudent nurse act in the same manner under the same circumstances?
3. Duty: Failure to protect client against unreasonable risk; Breach of Duty: Failure to perform according to established standards; Causation: Damage is done to client, physical or mental; Damages: A connection exists between conduct of the nurse and resulting injury.
4. Conduct causing damage to another person in a

willful or *intentional* way *without* just cause. Example: Hitting a client out of anger, not in a manner of self-protection.

5. Voluntary: Client admits self to an institution for treatment and retains his/her civil rights; he/she may leave at any time. Involuntary: Someone other than client applies for admission to an institution (relative, friend, or the state); requires certification by 1 to 2 healthcare providers/physicians that the person is a danger to self and/or others; person has a right to legal hearing (habeas corpus) to try and get released, the court determines justification for holding the person.

6. Vote, make contracts or wills, drive a car, sue or be sued, hold a professional license.

7. Voluntary, informed, written.

8. Alert, coherent, or otherwise competent adults; a parent or legal guardian; Person "in loco parentis" of minors or incompetent adults.

9. The Good Samaritan Act.

10. Inform the healthcare provider/physician, record the healthcare provider/physician was informed and the healthcare providers/ physicians response to such information; inform the nursing supervisor; refuse to carry out the prescription.

11. Inform the healthcare provider/physician or person asking the nurse to perform the task that he/she is unprepared to carry out the task; refuse to perform the task.

12. Apply restraints properly; check restraints frequently to see that they are not causing injury and *record* such monitoring; remove restraints as soon as possible; use restraints *only* as a last resort.

13. Patient must give written consent before healthcare providers can use or disclose personal health information; healthcare providers/physicians must give patients notice about provider responsibilities regarding patient confidentiality; patients must have access to their medical records; providers who restrict access must explain why, and must offer patients a description of the complaint process; patients have the right to request that changes be made in their medical records to correct inaccuracies; healthcare providers must follow specific tracking procedures for any disclosures made that ensure accountability for maintenance of patient confidentiality; patients have the right to request that healthcare providers/physicians restrict use and disclosure of their personal health information, though the provider may decline to do so.

LEADERSHIP MANAGEMENT

DESCRIPTION: Nurses act in both leadership and management roles.
1. A leader is an individual who influences people to accomplish goals.
2. A manager is an individual who works to accomplish the goals of the organization.
3. A nurse-manager acts to achieve the goals of safe, effective client care within the over-all goals of a Healthcare facility.

SKILLS AND CHARACTERISTICS OF THE NURSE-MANAGER	
SKILLS OF THE NURSE-MANAGER	CHARACTERISTICS OF THE NURSE-MANAGER
Communication	Authority
Organization	Accountability
Delegation	Responsibility
Supervision	Leadership
Critical thinking	Commitment to quality
HESI HINT: NCLEX-RN® questions often include examples of nursing interventions which DO or DO NOT demonstrate these skills and characteristics.	
CLASSIC LEADERSHIP STYLES	BEHAVIORS ASSOCIATED WITH LEADERSHIP STYLES
Democratic (participative)	Assertive
Authoritarian (autocratic)	Aggressive
Laissez-Faire (permissive)	Passive

Figure 1-6

HESI HINT: Effective leadership involves ASSERTIVE management skills. Look for responses that demonstrate the nurse using assertive communication skills.

COMMUNICATION SKILLS:
Assertive communication.
1. Clearly defined goals and expectations.
2. Verbal/Non-Verbal messages congruent.
3. Critical to directing phase of management..

HESI HINT: Assertive communication starts with "I need" rather than "You must."

HESI HINT: Motivation comes from within an individual. The nurse leader can provide an environment that will promote motivation through positive feedback, respect, and seeking input. Look for responses that DEMONSTRATE these behaviors.

ORGANIZATIONAL SKILLS:
Organizational skills encompass resource management of:
1. People.
2. Time.
3. Supplies.

DELEGATION SKILLS:

1. The authority, accountability, and responsibility of the RN are based on the State Nurse Practice Act, standards of professional practice, the policies of the healthcare organization, and ethical-legal models of behavior.
2. Definitions:

    A) DELEGATION is the process by which responsibility and authority are transferred to another individual.
    B) RESPONSIBILITY is the obligation to complete a task.
    C) AUTHORITY is the right to act or command the actions of others.
    D) ACCOUNTABILITY is the ability and willingness to assume responsibility for actions and related consequences.

3. The nurse transfers responsibility and authority for the completion of delegated tasks, BUT, the nurse retains accountability for the delegation process. This accountability involves ensuring that the five rights of delegation are achieved.

FIVE RIGHTS OF DELEGATION (DEFINED BY THE NATIONAL COUNCIL OF STATE BOARDS OF NURSING)

1. Right Task:
   Is this a task that can be delegated by a nurse?
2. Right Circumstance:
   Considering the setting and available resources, should delegation take place?
3. Right person:
   Is the task being delegated by the right person to the right person?
4. Right Direction/Communication:
   Is the nurse providing a clear, concise description of the task, including limits and expectations?
5. Right Supervision:
   Once the task is delegated, is appropriate supervision maintained?

SUPERVISION SKILLS

1. Direction/Guidance:
   A. Clear, concise directions.
   B. Expected outcome.
   C. Time frame.
   D. Limitations.
   E. Verification of assignment.
2. Evaluation/Monitoring
   A. Check in frequently.
   B. Communication lines.
   C. Achievement of outcome.
3. Follow-up:
   A. Communicate evaluation findings to the LPN or UAP and other appropriate personnel.
   B. Teaching/guidance needed.

CRITICAL THINKING SKILLS

Nurses are accustomed to using the Nursing Process as the model for problem-SOLVING in client care situations.
1. Use this model to think critically in leadership/management situations.
   A. Assessment:
      1) What are the needs/problems?
   B. Analysis:
      1) What has the highest priority?
   C. Planning:
      1) What outcomes and goals must be accomplished?
      2) What are the available resources?
         a) Nursing staff.
         b) Interdisciplinary team members.
         c) Time.
         d) Equipment.
         e) Space. (client rooms, home environment, etc.)
   D. Implementation:
      1) Communicating expectations.
      2) Is documentation complete?
   E. Evaluation:
      1) Were the desired outcomes achieved?
      2) Was safe, effective care provided?

HESI HINT: Delegating to the right person requires that the nurse be aware of the qualifications of the delegatee: appropriate education, training, skills, experience and demonstrated/documented competence.

HESI HINT: Remember Nursing Process: assessment, analysis, diagnosis, planning and evaluation (any activity requiring nursing judgment) MAY NOT be delegated to unlicensed assistive personnel. Delegated activities fall within the implementation phase of the nursing process.

HESI HINT: UAPs (Unlicensed Assistive Personnel) generally do NOT perform invasive or sterile procedures.

HESI HINT: The RN is accountable for adhering to the three basic aspects of supervision when delegating to other Healthcare personnel, such as LPNs, graduate nurses, inexperienced nurses, student nurses, and UAPs.

HESI HINT: Priorities often center on which client should be assessed FIRST by the nurse. Ask yourself: Which client is the most critically ill? Which client is most likely to experience a significant change in condition? Which client requires assessment by an RN?

HESI HINT: The nurse manager needs to analyze all the desired outcomes involved when assigning rooms for clients, or assigning client care responsibilities. A client with an infection should not be assigned to share a room with a surgical or immunocompromised client. A nurse's client care management should be based on the nurse's abilities, the individual client's needs, and the needs of the entire group of assigned clients. Safety and infection control are high priorities.

NURSE LEADERS/MANAGERS AS CHANGE AGENTS

LEWIN'S CHANGE THEORY:	NURSES OFTEN ACT AS CHANGE AGENTS, WHICH INVOLVES:
• Unfreezing	• Initiation of a change
• Moving	• Motivation toward a change
• Refreezing	• Implementation of a change

Figure 1-7

SKILLS NEEDED BY CHANGE AGENTS:
1. Problem-solving
2. Decision making
3. Interpersonal

NURSE LEADERS/MANAGERS AS COLLABORATORS
1. Collaborative healthcare teams require:
   A. Shared goals, commitment and accountability.
   B. Open and clear communication.
   C. Respect for the expertise of all team members.
2. Critical pathways:
   A. Interdisciplinary plan of care.
   B. For diagnoses and care that can be standardized.
   C. A guide to track client progress.
   D. Do NOT replace individualized care.
3. Case Management:
   A. Coordination of care provided by an interdisciplinary team.
   B. Manage resources effectively.
   C. Use critical pathways to organize care.
4. Quality assurance:
   A. CQI/TQM.
   B. An organized approach to the improvement of:
      1) Outcome achievement.
      2) Quality of care provided.

HESI HINT: Change causes anxiety. An effective nurse change agent uses problem-solving skills to recognize factors, such as anxiety, that contribute to resistance to change, and uses decision-making and interpersonal skills to overcome that resistance. Interventions that demonstrate these skills, include seeking input, showing respect, valuing opinions, and building trust.

REVIEW QUESTIONS
LEADERSHIP/MANAGEMENT
1. By what authority may RNs delegate nursing care to others?
2. An UAP may perform care that falls within which component of the nursing process?
3. Which types of communication skills are necessary to implement a democratic leadership style?
4. What are the five rights of delegation?
5. Which tasks can be delegated to an UAP?
   A. Inserting a Foley catheter.
   B. Measuring and recording output from a Foley catheter.
   C. Teaching a client how to care for a catheter when discharged.
   D. Assess for symptoms of a UTI.
6. What are the essential steps of effective supervision?
7. Which of the following is an example of assertive communication?
   A. "You need to improve the way you spend your time so that all of your care gets done."
   B. "I've noticed that many of your clients did not get their care today."

ANSWERS TO REVIEW QUESTIONS

1. State Nurse Practice Act.
2. Implementation.
3. Assertive communication skills.
4. Right task, right circumstance, right person, right direction or communication, and right supervision.
5. Which tasks:
   A. Is a sterile invasive procedure, which should not be delegated to an UAP.
   B. Falls within the implementation phase of the nursing process, and does not require nursing judgment. Evaluation of the I&O must be done by the nurse.
   C. Client teaching requires the abilities of the nurse, and should not be delegated. The UAP may be instructed to report anything unusual that is observed, or any symptoms reported by the client, but this does not replace assessment by the nurse.
   D. Assessment must be performed by the nurse, and should not be delegated. The UAP may be instructed to report anything unusual that is observed, or any symptoms reported by the client, but this does not replace assessment by the nurse.
6. Direction, Evaluation and Follow-up.
7. Example:
   A. This is an aggressive communication, which causes anger, hostility and a defensive attitude.
   B. Assertive communication begins with "I" rather than "You," and clearly states the problem.

Disaster Nursing

The role of the nurse takes place at all three levels of disaster management.
1. Disaster Preparedness
2. Disaster Response
3. Disaster Recovery

To achieve effective disaster management:
1. Organization is the key.
2. All personnel must be trained.
3. All personnel must know their role.

Levels of Prevention in Disaster Management
1. Primary Prevention
   A. Participate in development of disaster plan.
   B. Train rescue workers in triage/basic first aid.
   C. Educate personnel for shelter management.
   D. Educate the public on disaster plan and personal preparation for disaster.

2. Secondary Prevention
   A. Triage
   B. Treatment of injuries
   C. Treatment of other conditions, mental health
   D. Shelter supervision
3. Tertiary Prevention
   A. Follow-up care for injuries
   B. Follow-up care for psychological problems
   C. Recovery assistance
   D. Prevention of future disasters & their consequences

Triage
1. French word meaning to sort or categorize
2. Goal – maximize the number of survivors by sorting the injured according to treatable and untreatable victims *(see figure 1-8 color code system).*
3. Primary Criteria used
   A. Potential for survival
   B. Availability of resources

TRIAGE COLOR CODE SYSTEM				
	RED	**YELLOW**	**GREEN**	**BLACK**
URGENCY	Most Urgent – First priority	Urgent – Second priority	Third priority	Dying or dead
INJURY TYPE	Life threatening injuries	Injuries with systemic effects and complications	Minimal injuries with no systemic complications	Catastrophic injuries
MAY DELAY TREATMENT?	NO	30 to 60 minutes	Several Hours	No hope for survival – no treatment

Figure 1-8

NURSING INTERVENTIONS AND ROLES IN TRIAGE
1. Triage duties using a systemic approach such as the START method *(see figure 1-9)*
2. Treatment of injuries
   A. Render first aid for injuries
   B. Provide additional treatment as needed in definitive care areas
3. Treatment of other conditions, mental health
   A. Determine health needs other than injury
   B. Refer for medical treatment as required

   C. Provide treatment for other conditions based on medically approved protocols

SHELTER SUPERVISION
1. Coordinate activities of shelter workers
2. Oversee records of victims admitted & discharged from shelter
3. Promote effective interpersonal & group interactions of victims in shelter
4. Promote independence and involvement of victims housed in the shelter

SIMPLE TRIAGE AND RAPID TREATMENT (START METHOD FOR TRIAGE)

First: Separate the walking wounded - Move to a safe area – Evaluate later/GREEN Tag
Next: Three step evaluation of non-walking victims – ONE VICTIM AT A TIME

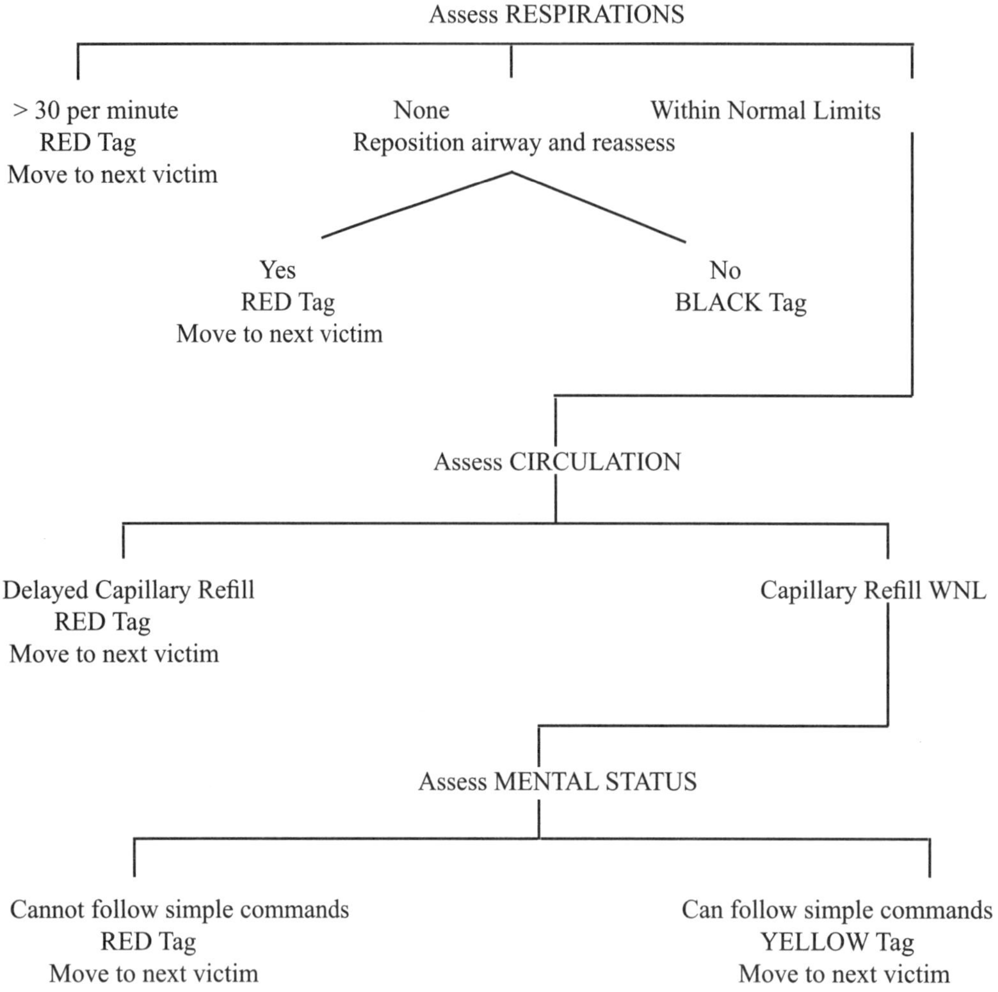

Assess RESPIRATIONS

> 30 per minute
RED Tag
Move to next victim

None
Reposition airway and reassess

Within Normal Limits

Yes
RED Tag
Move to next victim

No
BLACK Tag

Assess CIRCULATION

Delayed Capillary Refill
RED Tag
Move to next victim

Capillary Refill WNL

Assess MENTAL STATUS

Cannot follow simple commands
RED Tag
Move to next victim

Can follow simple commands
YELLOW Tag
Move to next victim

Figure 1-9

BIOTERRORISM

1. Learn symptoms of illnesses that are associated with exposure to likely biological and/or chemical agents.
2. Could appear days to weeks after exposure
3. Therefore nurses and other healthcare providers/physicians would be the "first responders"
   as victims seek medical evaluation after symptoms manifest. "First responders" are critical in identification of an outbreak, determination of cause of outbreak, identification of risk factors, implementation of measures to control and minimize the outbreak.

4. Possible agents *(see Figure 1-10 Biological and Chemical Agents and Radiation charts)*
   A. Biological agents
      - Anthrax
      - Pneumonic plague
      - Botulism
      - Smallpox
      - Inhalation tularemia
      - Viral hemorrhagic fever
   B. Chemical agents
      - Biotoxin agents
        - Ricin
      - Nerve agents
        - Sarin
   C. Radiation

BIOLOGICAL AGENTS			
	ANTHRAX	**PNEUMONIC PLAGUE**	**BOTULISM**
AGENT	• *Bacillus anthracis* • A bacterium that forms spores • 3 types: → Cutaneous → Inhalation → Digestive	• *Yersinia pestis* • A bacterium found in rodents and their fleas	• *Clostridium botulinum* • A toxin made by a bacterium
TRANSMISSION	• Inhalation of powder form • Inhalation of spores from infected animal products (such as wool) • Handling of infected animals • Eating undercooked meat from infected animals • Cannot be spread from person to person	• Aerosol release into the environment • Respiratory droplets from an infected person (six-foot range) • Untreated bubonic plague sequellae	• Foodborne botulism occurs when a person ingests pre-formed toxin • Wound botulism occurs when wounds are infected with *C. botulinum* that secretes the toxin • Cannot be spread person to person
INCUBATION PERIOD	• Within 7 days (all types) • Inhalation incubation period extends to 42 days	• 1 to 6 days	• Few hours to a few days • Foodborne: most commonly 12 to 36 hours, but range is 6 hours to 2 weeks

Figure 1-10

BIOLOGICAL AGENTS (CONTINUED)			
	ANTHRAX	**PNEUMONIC PLAGUE**	**BOTULISM**
SIGNS & SYMPTOMS	• Cutaneous: sores that develop into painless blisters, then ulcers with black centers • GI: nausea, anorexia, bloody diarrhea, fever, severe stomach pain • Inhalation: cold and flu symptoms including sore throat, mild fever, muscle aches, cough, chest discomfort, shortness of breath, tiredness, muscle aches	• Fever • Weakness • Rapidly developing pneumonia • Bloody or watery sputum • Nausea & vomiting • Abdominal pain • Without early treatment will see shock, respiratory failure, and rapid death	• Double and/or blurred vision • Drooping eyelids • Slurred speech • Difficulty swallowing • Descending muscle weakness
TREATMENT	• Prevention after exposure consists of the use of antibiotics such as ciprofloxacin, doxycycline, or penicillin and vaccination • Treatment after infection is usually a 60 day course of antibiotics • Success of treatment after infection depends on the type of anthrax and how soon the treatment begins	• If close contact with infected person and within 7 days of exposure will treat with antibiotics prophylactically • Recommended antibiotic treatment withing 24 hours of first symptom and treat for at least 7 days • Oral: tetracyclines, fluroquinolones • IV: Streptomycin or gentamycin	• Antitoxin to reduce severity of disease (most effective when administered early in course of disease) • Supportive care • May require mechanical ventilation
MISCELLANEOUS	• Vaccine available, but not to the general public • Given to those who may be exposed such as certain members of the U.S. armed forces, laboratory workers, and workers who enter or re-enter contaminated areas	• Easily destroyed by sunlight and drying • In air can survive up to one hour • No vaccine available	• No vaccine available

Figure 1-10 (continued)

BIOLOGICAL AGENTS (CONTINUED)			
	SMALLPOX	INHALATION TULAREMIA	VIRAL HEMORRHAGIC FEVER
AGENT	• *Variola virus* • An orthopoxvirus	• *Francisella tularensis* • A highly infectious bacterium	• Four families of viruses (examples: Ebola, Lassa, Dengue, Yellow, Marburg) • RNA viruses enveloped in a lipid coating
TRANSMISSION	• Aerosol release into the environment • Contact with infected person (direct and prolonged face-to-face • Bodily fluids • Contaminated objects • Air in enclosed settings (rare)	• Insect (usually tick and deerflies) bites • Handling sick or dead infected animals • Contaminated food or water • Inhalation of airborne bacterium • Cannot be spread from person to person	• From viral reservoirs such as rodents and arthropods or an animal host; some hosts remain unknown • May be transmitted person to person via close contact or bodily fluids • Objects contaminated with bodily fluids
INCUBATION PERIOD	• 7 to 17 days	• Most commonly 3 to 5 days, but may range from 1 to 14 days	• 2 to 21 days (varies by virus)
SIGNS & SYMPTOMS	• High fever • Head and body aches • Vomiting • Rash that progresses to raised bumps and pus-filled blisters that crust and scab then fall off in about 3 weeks leaving a pitted scar	• Skin ulcers • Swollen and painful lymph glands • Sore throat • Mouth sores • Diarrhea • Pneumonia • If inhaled: abrupt onset of fever and chills, headache, muscle aches, joint pain, dry cough, and progressive weakness • Those who develop pneumonia may exhibit chest pain, difficulty breathing, bloody sputum, and respiratory failure	• Varies by individual virus but common symptoms exist • Marked fever • Exhaustion • Muscle aches • Loss of strength • As disease worsens more severe symptoms emerge • Bleeding under skin, in internal organs, or from body orifices (mouth, eyes, ears) • Shock • CNS malfunction • Seizures • Coma • Renal failure

Figure 1-10 (continued)

BIOLOGICAL AGENTS (CONTINUED)			
	SMALL POX	INHALATION TULAREMIA	VIRAL HEMORRHAGIC FEVER
TREATMENT	• No proven treatment • Supportive therapy • Antibiotic treatment for secondary infections • Research being done with antivirals	• Antibiotics for 10 to 14 days • Oral: tetracyclines, fluoruquinolones IM or IV: Streptomycin, gentamycin	• Supportive therapy • Generally no established cure • May use Ribavirin with Lassa fever
MISCELLANEOUS	• A fragile virus – aerosolized die within 24 hours, even quicker if in sunlight • Vaccine available	• Can remain alive in water and soil for two weeks • No vaccine available	• Need a reservoir to survive: humans are not the natural reservoir but once infected by the host can transmit to one another • While these viruses were once geographically restricted to where the host lived, the increasing incidence of international travel brings outbreaks to places where the viruses have never been seen before • No vaccines available except for Argentine and Yellow fevers

Figure 1-10 (continued)

24

CHEMICAL AGENTS & RADIATION (CONTINUED)			
	RICIN	**SARIN**	**RADIATION**
AGENT	• Poison made from waste left over from processing castor beans • Forms include powder, mist, pellet • Dissolved in water or weak acid	• Human-made chemical • Similar to but far more potent than organophosphate pesticides • Clear, odorless, and tasteless liquid that can evaporate to a gas and spread into the environment	• A form of energy both man-made and natural
TRANSMISSION	• Deliberate act of poisoning by inhalation or injection [need miniscule amount (500 mcg) to kill] • Deliberate act of contamination of food and water supply (requires greater amount to kill) • Cannot be spread from person to person through casual contact	• Agent in air: exposed through skin, eyes, inhalation • Ingested in water or food • Clothing can release Sarin for approximately 30 minutes after contact	• External exposure comes from the sun or from man-made sources such as x-rays, nuclear bombs, or nuclear disasters (like Chernobyl) • Small quantities in air, water, food cause internal exposure
INCUBATION PERIOD	• Inhalation: within 8 hours • Ingestion: < 6 hours	• Vapor: a few seconds • Liquid: a few minutes to 18 hours	• Exposure is cumulative – low dose exposure effects may not be seen for several years • A high dose received in a matter of minutes results in Acute Radiation Syndrome (ARS)

Figure 1-10 (continued)

INTRODUCTION

CHEMICAL AGENTS & RADIATION (CONTINUED)

	RICIN	SARIN	RADIATION
SIGNS & SYMPTOMS	• Inhalation: respiratory distress, fever, nausea, tightness in chest, heavy sweating, pulmonary edema, decreased B/P, respiratory failure, death • Ingestion: vomiting and diarrhea that becomes bloody, severe dehydration, decreased B/P, hallucinations, seizures, hematuria, within several days liver, spleen, and kidney failure will occur • Skin and eyes: redness and pain	• Runny nose • Watery eyes • Pinpoint pupils • Eye pain and blurred vision • Drooling • Excessive sweating • Respiratory symptoms • Diarrhea • Altered LOC • Nausea and vomiting • Headache • Decreased or increased B/P • In large doses: loss of consciousness, convulsions, paralysis, respiratory failure, death	• ARS: nausea, vomiting, diarrhea, then bone marrow depletion, weight loss, loss of appetite, flu symptoms, infection, and bleeding • Mild effects include skin reddening • May lead to cancers (low dose or those surviving ARS)
TREATMENT	• Supportive care	• Remove from body as soon as possible • Supportive care • Antidote available: most effective if given as soon as possible after exposure	• Dependent on dose and type of radiation • Supportive care
MISCELLANEOUS	• Stable agent: not affected by very hot or very cold temperatures • Death usually occurs in about 36 to 72 hours • If survive for 3 to 5 days, victim will usually recover • No vaccine available	• A heavy vapor, this agent sinks to low lying areas • Mildly or moderately exposed people usually recover completely • Severely exposed people usually do not survive • May experience neurological problems lasting 1 to 2 weeks post exposure	• Survival dependent on dose • Full recovery may take a few weeks to a few years

Figure 1 - 10 (continued)

For further information see:
www.bt.cdc.gov/index.asp

26

> **HESI HINT:** It is important to remember that in disaster/bioterrorism management, the nurse must consider both the individual and the community.

NURSING ASSESSMENT
1. Community disaster risk assessment
2. Measures to mitigate distater effect
3. Exposure symptom identification

ANALYSIS (NURSING DIAGNOSIS)
1. Knowledge deficit related to . . .
2. Poisoning related to . . .
3. Trauma related to . . .
4. Suffocation related to . . .
5. Anxiety related to . . .
6. Fear related to . . .
7. Ineffective community coping related to . . .
8. Risk for post-trauma stress syndrome related to . . .

NURSING PLANS AND INTERVENTIONS
1. Participate in development of disaster plan
2. Educate the public on disaster plan & personal preparation for disaster
3. Train rescue workers in triage/basic first aid
4. Educate personnel for shelter management
5. Triage
6. Treatment of injuries and illness
7. Treatment of other conditions, mental health
8. Shelter supervision
9. Follow-up care for injuries
10. Follow-up care for psychological problems
11. Recovery assistance
12. Prevention of future disasters & their consequences

REVIEW QUESTIONS
DISASTER NURSING
1. **List the three levels of disaster management.**
2. **List examples of the three levels of prevention in disaster management.**
3. **Define Triage.**
4. **Identify 3 bioterrorism agents.**

ANSWERS TO REVIEW QUESTIONS
1. Disaster preparedness, disaster response, disaster recovery.
2. Primary: develop plan, train/educate personnel and public; Secondary: triage, treatment shelter supervision; Tertiary: follow-up, recovery assistance, prevention of future disasters.
3. To sort or categorize.
4. Anthrax, Pneumonic plague, botulism, smallpox, inhalation tularemia, viral hemorrhage fever, ricin, sarin, radiation.

RESPIRATORY FAILURE

ACUTE RESPIRATORY DISTRESS SYNDROME (ARDS)

DESCRIPTION: The exchange of oxygen for carbon dioxide in the lungs is inadequate for oxygen consumption and carbon dioxide production within the body's cells.

Acute respiratory distress syndrome is characterized by:
1. Hypoxemia: Po_2 below 50 mmHg.
2. Hypercapnia: Pco_2 above 45 mmHg.

> HESI HINT: ARDS is an unexpected, catastrophic pulmonary complication occurring in a person with no previous pulmonary problems. The mortality rate is high (50%).

During acute failure the arterial pH falls below 7.30, indicating acidosis.

> HESI HINT: In ARDS, a common laboratory finding is a lowered Po_2. However, these clients are not very responsive to high concentrations of oxygen.

> HESI HINT: Think about the physiology of the lungs by remembering PEEP: Positive end expiratory pressure is the instillation and maintenance of small amounts of air into the alveolar sacs to prevent them from collapsing each time the client exhales. The amount of pressure can be set with the ventilator and is usually around 5 to 10 cm of water.

Common causes of respiratory failure include:
1. COPD.
2. Pneumonia.
3. Tuberculosis.
4. Contusion.
5. Aspiration.
6. Inhaled toxins.
7. Emboli.
8. Drug overdose.
9. Fluid overload.
10. Disseminated intravascular coagulation (DIC).
11. Shock.

NURSING ASSESSMENT
1. Dyspnea, tachypnea.
2. Intercostal retractions.
3. Cyanosis.
4. Hypoxemia: $Po_2 < 50$ mmHg with $FiO_2 > 60\%$
5. Diffuse pulmonary infiltrates seen on chest x-ray as "white-out" appearance.
6. Verbalized anxiety; restlessness.

ANALYSIS (NURSING DIAGNOSES)
1. Impaired gas exchange related to…
2. Ineffective airway clearance related to…
3. Ineffective breathing pattern related to…
4. Decreased cardiac output related to…
5. Fluid volume excess related to…

NURSING PLANS AND INTERVENTIONS
1. Maintain client on a ventilator with the correct settings.
2. Provide care for either an oral airway or a tracheostomy.

> HESI HINT: Suction ONLY when secretions are present.

3. Monitor breath sounds for pneumothorax especially when positive end expiratory pressure (PEEP) is used to keep small airways open.
4. Provide emotional support to decrease anxiety and allow ventilator to "work" the lungs.
5. Monitor client hemodynamically with essential vital signs and cardiac monitor.
6. Monitor ABGs routinely.
7. Monitor vital organ status: central nervous system, level of consciousness, renal system output and myocardium (apical pulse, blood pressure).
8. Monitor fluid and electrolyte balance.
9. Monitor metabolic status through routine lab work. *(See figure 2-1, Blood Gases: Arterial/Venous)*

HESI HINT: Before drawing arterial blood gases from the radial artery, perform the Allen test to assess collateral circulation. Make the client's hand blanch by obliterating both the radial and ulnar pulses. Then release the pressure over the ulnar artery only. If flow through the ulnar artery is good, flushing will be seen immediately. The Allen test is then positive, and the radial artery can be used for puncture. If the Allen test is negative, repeat on the other arm. If this test is also negative, seek another site for arterial puncture. The Allen test ensures collateral circulation to the hand if thrombosis of the radial artery should follow the puncture.

BLOOD GASES: ARTERIAL/VENOUS

NORMAL VALUES	ARTERIAL	VENOUS
Ph	7.35 to 7.45	7.31 to 7.42
Po_2	80 to 100	35 to 45
Pco_2	35 to 45	39 to 52
HCO_3(mEq/L)	22 to 26	22 to 26
Anion gap (mEq/L)	10 to 18	8 to 16

Figure 2-1

HESI HINT: If the client does not have O_2 to his/her brain, the rest of the injuries do not matter because death will occur. However, they must be removed from any source of imminent danger, such as a fire.

RESPIRATORY FAILURE IN CHILDREN

DESCRIPTION: Common causes of respiratory failure in children include:
1. Congenital heart disease.
2. Respiratory distress syndrome.
3. Infection, sepsis.
4. Neuromuscular diseases.
5. Trauma and burns.
6. Aspiration.
7. Fluid overload or dehydration.
8. Anesthesia and narcotic overdose.

NURSING ASSESSMENT
1. "Bad" looking child.
2. Very slow or very rapid respiratory rate, apnea, gasping.
3. Tachycardia.
4. Cyanosis, pallor, or mottled color (connotes deterioration of systemic perfusion).
5. Irritability, and later, lethargy (connotes a deteriorating level of consciousness).
6. Retractions, nasal flaring, poor air movement.
7. Hypoxemia, hypercapnia, respiratory acidosis.
8. Laboratory data: values should be evaluated, keeping in mind the percent of oxygen the child is receiving.

HESI HINT:
- Pco_2 >45 or Po_2 <60 on 50% O_2 signifies respiratory failure.
- A child in severe distress should be on 100% O_2.

REVIEW QUESTIONS
RESPIRATORY FAILURE
1. What Po_2 value indicates hypoxemia?
2. What blood value indicates hypercapnia?
3. Identify the condition that exists when the Po_2 is less than 50 mmHg and FiO_2 is greater than 60%.
4. List three symptoms of respiratory failure in the adult.
5. List four common causes of respiratory failure in children.
6. What percentage of O_2 should a child in severe respiratory distress receive?

ANSWERS TO REVIEW QUESTIONS
1. Below 50 mmHg.
2. Pco_2 above 45 mmHg.
3. Hypoxemia.
4. Dyspnea/tachypnea, Intercostal retractions, Cyanosis.
5. Congenital heart disease, Infection or sepsis, Respiratory distress syndrome, Aspiration, Fluid overload or dehydration.
6. 100%.

Shock

Description: Widespread, serious reduction of tissue perfusion (lack of O_2 and nutrients), which, if prolonged, leads to generalized impairment of cellular functioning. *(See figure 2-2, Types of Shock; figure 2-3, Stages of Hypovolemic Shock; and figure 2-4, Medical Treatment for Shock)*

Arterial pressure is the driving force for blood flow through all the organs, and is dependent on:
1. Cardiac output to perfuse the body.
2. Peripheral vasomotor tone to return blood/fluid to the heart.
3. Amount of circulating blood.
4. Marked reduction in either cardiac output or peripheral vasomotor tone, without a compensatory elevation in the other, results in system HYPOTENSION.

5. Those at risk for development of shock include:
    A. The very young or the very old client.
    B. Post-MI clients.
    C. Clients with severe dysrhythmia.
    D. Clients with adrenocortical dysfunction.
    E. Persons with a history of recent hemorrhage or blood loss.
    F. Clients with burns.
    G. Clients with massive/overwhelming infection.

> **HESI HINT:** Early signs of shock are agitation and restlessness resulting from cerebral hypoxia.

TYPES OF SHOCK	
TYPE	**DESCRIPTION**
HYPOVOLEMIC	Related to external or internal blood/fluid loss (most common cause of shock).
CARDIOGENIC	Related to ischemia/impairment in tissue perfusion from myocardial infarction, serious arrhythmia, or congestive heart failure. All of this results in decreased cardiac output.
VASOGENIC	Related to allergens (anaphylaxis), spinal cord injury, or peripheral neuropathies, all resulting in venous pooling and decreased blood return to heart, which decreases cardiac output over time.
SEPTIC	Related to endotoxins released from bacteria, which cause vascular pooling, diminished venous return and reduced cardiac output.

Figure 2-2

> **HESI HINT:** If cardiogenic shock exists with the presence of pulmonary edema, i.e., from pump failure, position client to REDUCE venous return (HIGH-FOWLER'S with legs down) in order to decrease venous return further to the left ventricle.

STAGES OF HYPOVOLEMIC SHOCK		
STAGE	**SIGNS AND SYMPTOMS**	**CLINICAL DESCRIPTION**
STAGE I: INITIAL STAGE Blood loss of less than 10%. Compensatory mechanisms triggered.	• Apprehension and restlessness (first signs of shock) • Increased heart rate • Cool, pale skin • Fatigue	• Arteriolar constriction • Increased production of anti-diuretic hormone (ADH) • Arterial pressure is maintained • Cardiac output usually normal (for healthy individuals) • Selective reduction in blood flow to skin and muscle beds
STAGE II: COMPENSATORY STAGE Blood volume reduced by 15 to 25%. Decompensation begins.	• Flattened neck veins and delayed venous filling time • Increased pulse and respirations • Pallor, diaphoresis, and cool skin • Decreased urinary output • Sunken soft eyeballs • Confusion	• Marked reduction in cardiac output • Arterial pressure decline (despite compensatory arteriolar vasoconstriction) • Massive adrenergic compensatory response resulting in: tachycardia, tachypnea, cutaneous vasoconstriction, and oliguria • Decreased cerebral perfusion
STAGE III: PROGRESSIVE STAGE	• Edema • Increased blood viscosity • Excessively low BP • Dysrhythmia, ischemia, & myocardial infarction (MI) • Weak, thready, or absent peripheral pulses	• Rapid circulatory deterioration • Decreased cardiac output • Decreased tissue perfusion • Reduced blood volume

Figure 2-3

STAGES OF HYPOVOLEMIC SHOCK (CONTINUED)		
STAGE	SIGNS AND SYMPTOMS	CLINICAL DESCRIPTION
STAGE IV: IRREVERSIBLE STAGE	• Profound hypotension, unresponsive to vasopressor drugs • Severe hypoxemia, unresponsive to O_2 administration • Anuria, renal shut down • Heart rate slows, BP falls, with consequent cardiac and respiratory arrest	• Cell destruction so severe that death is inevitable • Multiple organ system failure • *It is the nurse's responsibility to recognize the signs and symptoms of shock. Every effort should be made to prevent the devastating clinical course that the progression of shock can take.*

Figure 2-3 (continued)

HESI HINT: Severe shock leads to widespread cellular injury and impairs the integrity of the capillary membranes. Fluid and osmotic proteins seep into the extra vascular spaces, further reducing cardiac output. A vicious cycle of decreased perfusion to ALL cellular level activities ensues. All organs are damaged, and if perfusion problems persist, the damage can be permanent.

MEDICAL TREATMENT FOR SHOCK

GOAL: Quick restoration of cardiac output and tissue perfusion.
• Rapid infusion of volume-expanding fluids:
  → Whole blood, Plasma, Plasma substitutes (colloid fluids). Note that while whole blood is an acceptable volume expander, it is rarely used due to a high risk of transfusion reactions.
  → Isotonic, electrolyte intravenous solutions such as Ringer's Lactate and Normal Saline.
• If shock is cardiogenic in nature, the infusion of volume-expanding fluids may result in pulmonary edema.
  → Restoration of cardiac function should take priority.
  → Administration of cardiotonic drugs (such as digitalis) may increase cardiac contractility.
  → Other drugs that enhance contractility include dopamine (Dopram).
  → Vasoconstricting agents such as dopamine (Dopram) and norepinephrine (Levophed) may be used as vasoconstrictors in cardiogenic shock.
• Central venous OR pulmonary artery catheters are inserted to monitor cardiogenic versus hypovolemic shock.
• Serial measurements of CVP, urine output, heart rate, and the clinical and mental state of the client are done every 5 to 15 minutes.
• Following immediate attention to improvement of perfusion, attention is directed toward treating the underlying cause of the condition.
• Administration of drugs is usually withheld until circulating volume has been restored.
• Administration of O_2.

Figure 2-4

NURSING ASSESSMENT
Vital Signs:
1. Tachycardia (pulse >100 BPM).
2. Tachypnea (respirations >24 min.).
3. Blood pressure decreased (systolic, <80 mmHg).
Mental status exam:
1. Early shock: restless, hyper-alert.
2. Late Shock: decreased alertness, lethargy, coma.
Skin changes:
1. Cool, clammy (warm skin in vasogenic and early septic shock).
2. Diaphoresis.
3. Pale.

Fluid status (acute renal tubular necrosis can happen quickly in shock):
1. Urine output decreases or an imbalance between intake and output occurs.
2. Abnormal CVP (<4 cm of H_2O).
3. Urine specific gravity > 1.020 (indicates hypovolemia).

ANALYSIS (NURSING DIAGNOSES)
1. Fluid volume deficit related to…
2. Decreased cardiac output related to…
3. Altered thought process related to…
4. Anxiety (family and individual) related to…

NURSING PLANS AND INTERVENTIONS

1. Monitor arterial pressure by understanding the concepts related to arterial pressure. *(See figure 2-5, Arterial Pressure)*
2. Monitor BP, pulse, respirations, and arrhythmias every 15 minutes or more often depending on stability of client.
3. Assess urine output every hour to maintain *at least* 30 ml/hour.
4. Notify healthcare provider if urine output drops below 30 cc/hr. (reflects decreased renal perfusion and may result in permanent renal damage).
5. Administer fluids as prescribed by provider: blood, colloids, or electrolyte solutions until designated CVP is reached. (In shock situations, the healthcare provider often orders fluids to elevate CVP 16 to 19 cm of H_2O as compensation for decreased cardiac output). *(See figure 2-6, Administration of Blood Products)*
6. Place client in modified Trendelenburg's position (feet up 45 degrees, head flat).
7. Administer medications IV (*not* IM or subq) until perfusion improves in muscles and subcutaneous tissue.
8. Keep client warm (increase heat in room or put warm blankets on client…not TOO hot).
9. Keep side rails up during all procedures. (Clients in shock experience mental confusion and may easily be injured by falls).
10. Obtain blood for lab work as prescribed: CBC, electrolytes, BUN, creatinine (renal damage), and blood gasses (oxygenation).

When administering vasopressors/adrenergic stimulants, such as epinephrine (Bronkaid), dopamine (Dopram), dobutamine (Dobutrex) norepinephrine (Levophed) or isoproterenol (Isuprel):
1. Administer through volume-controlled pump.
2. Monitor BP every 5 to 15 minutes.
3. Watch intravenous site carefully for extravasation and tissue damage.
4. Ask healthcare provider for target mean systolic blood pressure (usually 80 to 90 mmHg).

When administering vasodilators, such as hydralazine (Apresoline), nitroprusside (Nipride), or labetalol hydrochloride (Normodyne, Trandate) to counteract effects of vasopressors:

1. Wait for precipitous decrease or increase in BP, if prescribed together.
2. If drop in BP occurs, decrease vasodilator infusion rate first, then increase vasopressor.
3. If BP increases precipitously, decrease vasopressor rate first, then increase rate of vasodilator.
4. Obtain blood work as prescribed: CBC, electrolytes, BUN, creatinine (renal damage), and blood gases (oxygenation).

> **HESI HINT:** All vasopressor/vasodilator drugs are potent and dangerous and require weaning on and off. Do not change infusion rates simultaneously.

Provide family support:
1. Notify appropriate support persons for waiting family during crisis, i.e., call spiritual advisor, other family members, or anyone the family thinks will be supportive.
2. At intervals, notify family of actions/ progress or lack of progress in realistic terms.
3. Collaborate with healthcare provider before notifying family of medical interventions.

> **HESI HINT:** A client is brought into the hospital suffering shock symptoms as a result of a bee sting. What is the first priority? Maintaining an open airway (the allergic reaction damages the lining of the airways causing edema). Also, keep the client warm without constricting clothing; keep legs elevated (not Trendelenburg because the weight of the lower organs restricts breathing).
>
> Epinephrine: 1:1,000, 0.2 to 0.5 ml subq for mild
> or
> Epinephrine: 1:10,000, 5 ml IV for severe
>
> Volume-expanding fluids are usually given to clients in shock. However, if the shock is cardiogenic, pulmonary edema may result.
>
> Drugs of choice for shock:
> • Digitalis preparations: Increase the contractility of the heart muscle.
> • Vasoconstrictors (Levophed, Dopamine): Generalized vasoconstriction to provide more available blood to the heart to help maintain cardiac output.

ARTERIAL PRESSURE

CONCEPT	DEFINITION
MEAN ARTERIAL PRESSURE (MAP)	• Level of pressure in the central arterial bed measured indirectly by blood pressure measurement. • MAP = cardiac output x total peripheral resistance = systolic blood pressure + 2 (diastolic blood pressure) / 3. • In adults, usually approaches 100 mmHg. • Can be measured directly through arterial catheter insertion.
CARDIAC OUTPUT	• Volume of blood ejected by the left ventricle per unit of time. • Stroke volume (amount of blood ejected per beat) x heart rate. [Normal: 4-6 L/min]
PERIPHERAL RESISTANCE	• Resistance to blood flow offered by the vessels in the peripheral vascular bed.
CENTRAL VENOUS PRESSURE	• Pressure within the right atrium. Normal: 4 to 10 cm of H_2O.

Figure 2-5

HESI HINT: A common volume-expanding substance is plasma and possibly whole blood.

ADMINISTRATION OF BLOOD PRODUCTS

BLOOD PRODUCTS	REACTIONS/ COMPLICATIONS	ASSESSMENT	NURSING INTERVENTIONS
• Whole blood volume & RBC replacement (500ml bag with Saline) • Fresh frozen plasma volume	• Reactions: • Hemolytic reaction – caused by blood type or Rh incompatibility • Antigen – antibody reaction • Allergic reaction • Delayed hemolytic reaction • Non hemolytic febrile reaction	• Mild: fever and chills • Severe: DIC or circulatory collapse • Other symptoms include apprehension, headache, chest pain, sense of impending doom, flank pain, GI distress • Symptoms are usually immediate but may be delayed until other units are transfused. • Delayed reactions may occur 1 to 2 weeks after transfusion. Symptoms include unexplained fatigue, jaundice, and/or fever • Non-hemolytic febrile symptoms include fever, chills, malaise	• *STOP TRANSFUSION, CHANGE TUBING*, then continue saline IV • Notify MD immediately • Monitor vital signs • **For ABO incompatibilities:** • Treat shock • Send blood and urine specimens to lab • Send unit of blood to lab (complete) • **For allergic reactions**: • Treat anaphylaxis • **For Non-hemolytic febrile reactions:** • Assume hemolytic and treat as above until proven otherwise • Then treat with antipyretics • May treat prophylatically in future transfusions

NURSING SKILLS

- Use a 18-gauge or larger needle to administer.
- Use only blood administration tubing to infuse blood products.
- Run infusion slowly the first 15 minutes to detect early signs of transfusion reaction, thereafter may infuse more rapidly.
- Check vital signs frequently before, during, and immediately following infusion, and note any increase in temperature. Follow agency policy regarding specific timetable for blood infusion.
- Check and double check the product before infusing to see that it is:
  → Correct product, as prescribed; double check with a second licensed person.
  → Correct blood type and Rh factor, matched with the client's.

Figure 2-6

DISSEMINATED INTRAVASUCLAR CLOTTING (DIC)

DESCRIPTION: A coagulation disorder with paradoxical thrombosis and hemorrhage.

DIC is an acute complication of conditions such as hypotension and septicemia, suspected when there is bloody oozing from two or more unexpected sites.

The first phase involves abnormal clotting in the microcirculation, which uses up clotting factors, and results in an inability to form clots and hemorrhage occurs.

The diagnosis is based on laboratory findings:
1. Prothrombin time (PT): prolonged.
2. Partial thromboplastin time (PTT): prolonged.
3. Fibrinogen: decreased.
4. Platelet count decreased.
5. Fibrin degradation (split) products (FDP): increased

NURSING ASSESSMENT
1. Petechiae, purpura, hematomas.
2. Oozing from IV sites, drains, gums, and wounds.
3. GI and GU bleeding.
4. Hemoptysis.
5. Mental status change.
6. Hypotension, tachycardia.
7. Pain.

ANALYSIS (NURSING DIAGNOSES)
1. Potential for injury related to…
2. Alteration in tissue perfusion related to…

NURSING PLANS AND INTERVENTIONS:
1. Monitor client for bleeding.
2. Monitor vital signs.
3. Protect client from injury and bleeding.
   A. Provide gentle oral care with mouth swabs.
   B. Minimize needle sticks, use smallest gauge needle possible.
   C. Turn frequently to eliminate pressure points.
   D. Minimize number of BPs taken by cuff.
   E. Use gentle suction to prevent trauma to mucosa.
   F. Apply pressure to any oozing site.
4. Administer Heparin IV during the first phase to inhibit coagulation.
5. Provide emotional support to decrease anxiety.

HESI HINT: You are caring for a woman who was in a severe automobile accident several days ago. She has several fractures and internal injuries. The exploratory laparotomy was successful in controlling the bleeding. However, today you find that this client is bleeding from her incision, is short of breath, has a weak thready pulse, has cold and clammy skin, and hematuria.

What do you think is wrong with the client, and what would you expect to do about it?

These are typical signs and symptoms of DIC crisis. Expect to administer IV heparin to block the formation of thrombin (Coumadin does not do this). However, the client described is already past the coagulation phase and into hemorrhagic phase. Her management would be administration of clotting factors along with palliative treatment of the symptoms as they arise. (Her prognosis is poor.)

REVIEW QUESTIONS
SHOCK/DIC
1. Define shock.
2. What is the most common cause of shock?
3. What causes septic shock?
4. What is the goal of treatment for hypovolemic shock?
5. What intervention is used to restore cardiac output when hypovolemic shock exists?
6. It is important to differentiate between hypovolemic and cardiogenic shock. How might the nurse determine the existence of cardiogenic shock?
7. If a client is in cardiogenic shock, what might result from administration of volume expanding fluids, and what intervention can the nurse expect to perform in the event of such an occurrence?
8. List five assessment findings found in most shock victims.
9. What is the normal central venous pressure for an adult?
10. Once circulating volume is restored, vasopressors may be prescribed to increase venous return. List the main drugs that are used.
11. What is the established minimum renal output per hour?
12. List four measurable criteria that are the major expected outcomes of a shock crisis.

13. **Define DIC.**
14. **What is the effect of DIC on PT, PTT, platelets, FSPs (FDPs)?**
15. **What drug is used in the treatment of DIC?**
16. **Name four nursing interventions to prevent injury in clients with DIC.**

ANSWERS TO REVIEW QUESTIONS

1. Widespread, serious reduction of tissue perfusion, which leads to generalized impairment of cellular function.
2. Hypovolemia.
3. Release of endotoxins from bacteria which act on nerves in vascular space in periphery, causing vascular pooling, reduced venous return, and decreased cardiac output, resulting in poor systemic perfusion.
4. Quick restoration of cardiac output and tissue perfusion.
5. Rapid infusion of volume-expanding fluids.
6. History of MI with left ventricular failure or possible cardiomyopathy, with symptoms of pulmonary edema.
7. Pulmonary edema, administer cardiotonic drugs such as digitalis preparations.
8. Tachycardia; tachypnea; hypotension; cool clammy skin; decrease in urinary output.
9. 4 to 10 cm of H_2O.
10. Epinephrine (Bronkaid), dopamine (Dopram), dobutamine (Dobutrex), norepinephrine (Levophed), or isoproterenol (Isuprel)
11. 30 cc/hr.
12. BP mean of 80 to 90 mmHg; $Po_2 > 50$ mmHg; CVP above 6 cm of H_2O; urine output at least 30 cc/hr.
13. A coagulation disorder in which there is paradoxical thrombosis and hemorrhage.
14. Prothrombin time – Prolonged; Partial thromboplastin time – Prolonged; Platelets – Decreased; Fibrin split products – Increased.
15. Heparin
16. Gently provide oral care with mouth swabs. Minimize needle sticks and use the smallest gauge needle possible when injections are necessary. Eliminate pressure by turning the client frequently. Minimize the number of BPs taken by cuff. Use gentle suction to prevent trauma to mucosa. Apply pressure to any oozing site.

RESUSCITATION

CARDIOPULMONARY RESUSCITATION

Cardiopulmonary Arrest
Usually caused by myocardial infarction (MI): necrosis of the heart muscle caused by inadequate blood supply to heart.

MIs usually occur at rest or with moderate activity, contrary to the belief that they occur with strenuous activity.

Symptoms immediately preceding MI:
1. Chest pain/discomfort either at rest or with ordinary activity.
2. Change in previous stable anginal pain, i.e., an increase in frequency or severity or rest angina occurring for the first time.
3. Chest pain in a client with known coronary heart disease that is unrelieved by rest and/or nitroglycerin.

HESI HINT: NCLEX-RN® questions on CPR often deal with prioritization of actions. Question: What actions are required for each of the following situations?
- A 24-year-old motorcycle accident victim with a ruptured artery of the leg is pulseless and apneic.
- A 36-year-old first-time pregnant woman who arrests during labor.
- A 17-year-old with no pulse or respirations who is trapped in an overturned car, which is starting to catch fire.
- A 40-year-old businessman who arrests two days after a cervical laminectomy.

O_2 is necessary for survival; all other injuries are secondary – EXCEPT for removal of any source of imminent danger, such as a fire.

Chest pain of myocardial ischemia:
1. Is usually described as crushing, pressing, constricting, oppressive, or heavy.
2. Tends to increase in intensity over a few minutes.
3. May be substernal or more diffused.
4. May radiate to one or both shoulders and arms, or to neck, jaw or back.

Occasions for cardiopulmonary resuscitation are often *unwitnessed* cardiac arrests.

HESI HINT: WHEN TO SEEK EMERGENCY MEDICAL SERVICE (EMS)
- The symptoms of anterior myocardial infarction (AMI) characteristically last more than 15 minutes and are more intense than angina.
- THE AHA guidelines recommend that those at risk for acute coronary syndrome (ACS) should activate the EMS if chest discomfort worsens or is unimproved 5 minutes after taking one tablet or spray of nitroglycerin.

MANAGEMENT OF CARDIAC ARREST

OUT-OF-HOSPITAL (UNWITNESSED)

HESI HINT: It is important for the nurse to stay current with the American Heart Association's guidelines for Basic Life Support (BLS) by being certified every two years, as required.

- Position person supine, tap, and call out, "Are you all right?"
- If no response occurs, call for help or ask someone to call the local emergency number, usually 911. Get A.E.D.
- Establish an AIRWAY by extending neck with the head/tilt, chin/lift or jaw thrust maneuver. Clear airway of foreign body, if visible.
- Assess breathing by the look, listen, feel method:
  → Look for chest excursion.
  → Listen for breathing sounds through mouth/nose.
  → Feel for breath on rescuer's cheek/face.
  → Differentiate between Agonal breathing (ineffective gasps) and regular, effective breathing.
- If no breathing is noted:
  → Ventilate with 2 mouth-to-mouth, breaths over 1 second and make the chest rise.
  → Assess circulation by palpating carotid pulse for no more than 10 seconds.
  → If no pulse, initiate cardiac compressions by depressing lower half of the sternum at a rate of 100/min. "push hard, push fast"
  → Continue CPR until spontaneous respirations and pulse return.

HESI HINT: CPR is performed using a 30:2 ratio of compression to ventilations, at the compression rate of 100/min, continuously without pauses for ventilation. After 5 cycles, then reassess for breathing and pulse. The compressor role should be rotated about every 2 minute without interruption of the compression rate.

HESI HINT: At 20 weeks gestation and beyond, the gravid uterus should be shifted to the left by placing the woman in a 15°-30° angled left lateral position or using a wedge under her right side to tilt her to her left.

IN-HOSPITAL

HESI HINT: Initiate CPR with BLS guidelines immediately, then move on to Advanced Cardiac Life Support (ACLS) guidelines.

Determine responsiveness by tapping the client and shouting "Are you all right?"
- If no response occurs, call a "Code" or cardiac arrest in order to initiate response of cardiac arrest TEAM.
- Position client on cardiac board.
- Ventilate with 100% O_2 with oral airway and mouth-to-mask or use a bag-mask device.
- Initiate chest compressions.
Team leader arrives and assesses client, directs team members and obtains history and precipitating events to arrest.
- Without interrupting CPR, apply cardiac portable monitor "quick-look" paddles to determine if defibrillation is necessary or if asystole has occurred.
- Rapid defibrillation is indicated in ventricular fibrillation or pulseless ventriculator tachycardia.
- Resume CPR begining with compresions, immediately after defibrillations.

Figure 2-7

ADVANCED CLINICAL CONCEPTS

MANAGEMENT OF A FORGIEN BODY AIRWAY OBSTRUCTION (FBAO)

ADULTS AND CHILDREN ONE YEAR AND OLDER

- If unable to ventilate during CPR, suspect foreign body in airway.
- If conscious, stand behind person and grasp around waist with clenched fist (halfway between navel and xiphoid) and exert palmar thrust inward at epigastrium (Heimlich maneuver) in rapid sequence.
- Chest thrust should be used in obese or pregnant patients.
- Continue until object is expelled or person falls to ground unconscious, then activate EMS and begin CPR.
- Only use a fingersweep if the object is seen obstructing the airway.

Figure 2-8

RESUSCITATION

NEONATAL	CHILD AGE 1 TO 8
See Maternity Nursing • Ventilations are done over mouth and nose using a size 1 mask with a term neonate, size 0 for a preterm. • With neonates, initial ventilation with peak inflating pressures of 30-40 cm H2O at a rate of 40-60/ min is usually successful in unresponsive term infants. • If the heart rate is under 60, compressions are done with thumb side-by-side encircling the thorax and over the lower third of the sternum, to a depth of 1/3 the A/P chest diameter with a compression to ventilation ratio of 3:1 to achieve 120 events per min (90 compressions plus 30 breaths). • Compressions can also be accomplished with one hand under the back, and two fingers over the midsternum.	• Ventilations (mouth-mouth) should make the chest rise. Mouth and nose should be used for infants (under 1 year). • The chest is compressed with one palm at a rate of 100/min. "Push hard, push fast." • A ratio of 2 ventilations to 30 compressions, one rescuer (or 2: 15 for two rescuers) without pauses for ventilations (8-10/min) should be maintained. • The most common rhythm in pediatrics is asystole or bradycardia. • Epinephrine is the drug of choice given IV at 0.01 mg/ kg body weight using a 1:10,000 solution.

Figure 2-9

MANAGEMENT OF A FORGIEGN BODY AIRWAY OBSTRUCTION(FBAO): PEDIATRIC
INFANTS AND CHILDREN

• Open the conscious child's mouth and attempt to clear obstruction manually if the object can be seen. (NO blind sweeps – may push the foreign object further down throat).
• For a child, perform subdiaphragmatic abdominal thrusts (Heimlich maneuver) in rapid sequence until the obstruction is relieved.
• Only if the solid material is seen obstructing the airway should an attempt be made to remove it.
• If the infant is able to CRY, COUGH, OR BREATHE, do NOT interfere.
• If the infant is conscious and CANNOT cry, cough, or breathe:
  → Place infant face down, head lower than trunk, with legs straddling your arm and chest supported by upturned hand.
  → Give five firm blows to back with heel of hand (compresses rib cage between two hands).
  → Position face upward and give five chest thrusts as you would for cardiac massage.
  → Repeat until the object is expelled or the infant becomes unresponsive.
• If unresponsive, begin CPR:
  → Using tongue-jaw lift (use your thumbs to pull down the jaw, lowering the jaw in order to do a visual inspection), open the mouth. If the foreign object is seen, take it out.
  → Open airway (tilt the infant's head and lift the chin) and perform mouth to mouth/nose breathing – cover the infant's mouth and nose with your mouth and give the infant two breaths, and follow with chest compressions.

Figure 2 - 10

REVIEW QUESTIONS

RESUSCITATION

1. What is the first priority when a client with an unwitnessed cardiac arrest is found?
2. Define myocardial infarction.
3. What criteria should alert a client with known angina who takes nitroglycerin tablets sublingually to call the EMS?
4. After calling out for help and asking someone to dial for emergency services, what is the next action in CPR?
5. True or False: In feeling for presence of a carotid pulse, no more than 5 seconds should be used.
6. During one-rescuer CPR, what is the ratio of compressions to ventilations for an adult? During one-rescuer CPR, what is the ratio of compressions to ventilations for a child?
7. What is the FIRST drug most likely to be used for an in-hospital cardiac arrest?
8. A client in cardiac arrest is noted on bedside monitor to be in pulseless ventricular tachycardia. What is the first action that should be taken?
9. True or False: A precordial thump is routine activity for an in-hospital cardiac arrest.
10. How would the nurse assess the adequacy of compressions during CPR? How would the nurse assess for adequacy of ventilations during CPR?
11. If a person is choking, when should the rescuer intervene?
12. One should NEVER make blind sweeps into the mouth of a choking child or infant. Why?
13. Why do the ACLS guidelines recommend a decreased reliance on the use of bicarbonate during adult CPR?

ANSWERS TO REVIEW QUESTIONS

1. Begin CPR.
2. Necrosis of the heart muscle due to poor perfusion of the heart.
3. Unrelieved chest pain after nitroglycerin.
4. Call for help and begin CPR. For unresponsive infants & children, CPR should be performed for one minute before placing a 911 call for help.
5. FALSE: palpate for no more than 10 seconds, recognizing that arrhythmias or bradycardia could be occurring.
6. 30:2 X 5 cycles. 15:2 for a child and neonate with two rescuers.
7. Epinephrine.
8. Defibrillation.
9. FALSE: only indicated in pulseless VT or VF or when ventricular asystole on monitor responds to a thump with a QRS complex.

10. Check for a pulse. Watch for chest excursion and auscultate bilaterally for breath sounds.
11. When the person points to his/her throat and can no longer cough, talk, or make sounds.
12. Because the object might be pushed further down into the throat.
13. Because acidosis should be relieved with improved ventilation. Bicarbonate administration can actually contribute to increased CO_2.

FLUID AND ELECTROLYTE BALANCE

HOMEOSTASIS
DESCRIPTION: The process of maintaining a relative state of equilibrium.
1. Homeostasis occurs in relation to maintenance of the composition of fluids.
2. Fluid composition is maintained by: *(See figure 2-11, Fluid Volume Deficit/Excess)*

HESI HINT: Changes in osmolarity cause shifts in fluid. The osmolarity of the extracellular fluid (ECF) is almost entirely due to sodium. The osmolarity of intracellular fluid (ICF) is related to many particles, with potassium being the primary electrolyte. The pressures in the ECF and the ICF are almost identical. If either ECF or ICF change in concentration, fluid shifts from the area of lesser concentration to the area of greater concentration.

HESI HINT:
- **Dextrose 10% is a hypertonic solution and should be administered IV.**
- **Normal saline is an isotonic solution and is used for irrigations, such as bladder irrigations or IV flush lines with intermittent IV medication.**
- **Use only isotonic (neutral) solutions in irrigations, infusions, etc., unless the specific aim is to shift fluid to intracellular or extracellular spaces.**

Kidneys:
1. Selectively maintain and excrete body fluids.
2. Selectively retain needed substances and excrete unneeded substances, i.e., electrolytes.
3. Regulate pH by excreting or maintaining hydrogen ions and bicarbonate.
4. Excrete metabolic wastes and toxic substances.

Lungs:
1. Rid the body of approximately 300 ml of fluid per day and play a role in acid-base balance.
2. Regulate carbon dioxide concentration.

Heart: Pumps with sufficient force to perfuse the kidneys, necessary for their functioning.

Adrenal glands: Secrete aldosterone which causes sodium retention (which causes water retention) and potassium excretion.

Parathyroid glands: Regulate calcium and phosphorus balance.

Pituitary gland: Secretes antidiuretic hormone (ADH), which causes the body to retain water.

ELECTROLYTE IMBALANCE
NURSING ASSESSMENT
(See Figure 2-12, Electrolyte Imbalances)

PLANS AND INTERVENTIONS
(See Figure 2-12, Electrolyte Imbalances)

HESI HINT: Potassium imbalances are potentially life threatening; must be corrected immediately. A low magnesium often accompanies a low K+, especially with use of diuretics.

FLUID VOLUME		
VARIABLE	**DEFICIT**	**EXCESS**
DESCRIPTION	• Occurs when the body loses water and electrolytes isotonically, that is, in the same proportion as in the normal body fluid • Serum electrolyte levels remain normal • **Dehydration**: State in which the body loses water and serum sodium levels increase	• Occurs when the body retains water and electrolytes isotonically • **Water intoxication**: State in which the body retains water and serum sodium levels decrease.
CAUSES	• Vomiting • Diarrhea • GI suctioning • Sweating • Inadequate fluid intake • Massive edema, as with initial stage of major burns • Ascites • Elderly – forgetting to drink	• Congestive heart failure (CHF) • Renal failure • Cirrhosis, liver failure • Excessive ingestion of table salt • Over-hydration with sodium-containing fluid • Poorly controlled IV therapy, especially in young and old clients
SYMPTOMS	• Weight loss (one pint of fluid loss is equal to one pound of weight loss) • Decreased skin turgor • Oliguria, concentrated urine • Dry and sticky mucous membranes • Postural hypotension or weak, rapid pulse	• Peripheral edema • Increased bounding pulse • Elevated BP • Distended neck and hand veins • Dyspnea; moist crackles heard when lungs auscultated • Attention loss, confusion, aphasia • Altered level of consciousness
LAB FINDINGS	• Elevated BUN and creatinine • Increased serum osmolarity • Elevated Hgb and Hct	• Decreased BUN • Decreased Hgb and Hct • Decreased serum osmolality • Decreased urine osmolality and specific gravity
TREATMENT/ NURSING CARE	• Strict I & O • Replace fluids isotonically, preferably orally • ***WATER IS A HYPOTONIC FLUID*** • If intravenous hydration is needed, isotonic fluids are used	• Diuretics • Fluid restriction • Strict I & O • Sodium-restricted diet • Weigh daily • Monitor K+ serum

Figure 2-11

HESI HINT: Fluid Volume Deficit: Dehydration
• **Elevated BUN**: The BUN measures the amount of urea nitrogen in the blood. Urea is formed in the liver as the end product of protein metabolism. The BUN is directly related to the metabolic function of the liver and the excretory function of the kidneys.
• Creatinine, as with BUN, is excreted entirely by the kidneys and is therefore directly proportional to renal excretory function. However, unlike BUN, the creatinine level is affected very little by dehydration, malnutrition, or hepatic function. The daily production of creatinine depends on muscle mass, which fluctuates very little. Therefore, it is a better test of renal function than is the BUN. Creatinine is generally used in conjunction with the BUN test and they normally are in a 1:20 ratio.
• Serum osmolality measures the concentration of particles in a solution. It refers to the fact that the same amount of solute is present, but the amount of solvent (fluid) is decreased. Therefore, the blood can be considered "more concentrated."
• Urine osmolality and specific gravity increase.

ELECTROLYTE IMBALANCES

ABNORMALITIES & COMMON CAUSES	SIGNS/SYMPTOMS	TREATMENT
Hyponatremia (↓ Na) • Diuretics • GI fluid loss • Hypotonic tube feeding • D_5W or hypotonic IV fluids • Diaphoresis	• Anorexia, nausea & vomiting • Weakness • Lethargy • Confusion • Muscle cramps, twitching • Seizures • Na Below 135 mEq/L	• Restrict fluids (safer) • If IV saline solutions prescribed, administer very slowly. Use if fluid restriction not effective
Hypernatremia (↑Na) • Water deprivation • Hypertonic tube feeding • Diabetes insipidus • Heatstroke • Hyperventilation • Watery diarrhea • Renal failure • Cushing's syndrome	• Thirst • Hyperpyrexia • Sticky mucous membranes • Dry mouth • Hallucinations • Lethargy • Irritability • Seizures • Na above 145 mEq/L	• Restrict sodium in the diet • Beware of "hidden" sodium in foods and medications • Increase water intake
Hypokalemia (↓K) • Diuretics • Diarrhea • Vomiting • Gastric suction • Steroid administration • Hyperaldosteronism • Amphotericin B • Bulimia • Cushing's syndrome	• Fatigue • Anorexia • Nausea, vomiting • Muscle weakness • Decreased GI motility • Dysrhythmias • Paresthesia • Flat T waves on EKG • K less that 3.5 mEq/L	• Administer potassium supplements orally or IV • Oral forms of potassium are unpleasant tasting and are irritating to the GI tract (Do not give on empty stomach; dilute) • *Never* give IV bolus, MUST be well diluted • Assess renal status, i.e., urinary output prior to administering • Encourage foods high in potassium, e.g., banana, oranges, cantaloupe, avocado, spinach, potato
Hyperkalemia (↑K) • Hemolyzed serum sample produces pseudohyperkalemia • Oliguria • Acidosis • Renal failure • Addison's disease • Multiple blood transfusions	• Muscle weakness • Bradycardia • Dysrhythmias • Flaccid paralysis • Intestinal colic • Tall T waves on EKG • K above 5.0 mEq/L	• Eliminate parenteral potassium from IV infusions, medications • Administer 50% glucose with regular insulin • Administer cation exchange resin (Kayexalate) • Monitor EKG • Administer calcium gluconate to protect the heart • IV loop diuretics may be prescribed • Renal dialysis may be required
Hypocalcemia (↓ Ca) • Renal failure • Hypoparathyroidism • Malabsorption • Pancreatitis • Alkalosis	• Diarrhea • Numbness • Tingling of extremities • Convulsions • Positive Trousseau's sign • Chvostek's sign • Ca below 8.5 mEq/L • At risk for tetany	• Administer calcium supplements orally 30 minutes before meals • Administer calcium IV slowly; infiltration can cause tissue necrosis • Increase calcium intake, e.g., dairy products, greens

Figure 2-12

ELECTROLYTE IMBALANCES (CONTINUED)		
ABNORMALITIES & COMMON CAUSES	SIGNS/SYMPTOMS	TREATMENT
Hypercalcemia ($\uparrow$Ca) • Hyperparathyroidism • Malignant bone disease • Prolonged immobilization • Excess calcium supplementation	• Muscle weakness • Constipation • Anorexia • Nausea, vomiting • Polyuria • Polydipsia • Neurosis • Dysrhythmias • Ca above 10.5 mEq/L	• Eliminate parenteral calcium • Administer agents to reduce calcium such as Calcitonin • Avoid calcium-based antacids • Renal dialysis may be required
Hypomagnesemia ($\downarrow$Mg) • Alcoholism • Malabsorption • Diabetic ketoacidosis • Prolonged gastric suction • Diuretics	• Anorexia, distention • Neuromuscular irritability • Depression • Disorientation • Mg below 1.5 mEq/L	• Administer $MgSO_4$ IV • Encourage foods high in magnesium, e.g., meats, nuts, legumes, fish, and vegetables
Hypermagnesemia ($\uparrow$Mg) • Renal failure • Adrenal insufficiency • Excess replacement	• Flushing • Hypotension • Drowsiness, lethargy • Hypoactive reflexes • Depressed respirations • Bradycardia • Mg above 2.5 mEq/L	• Avoid magnesium-based antacids and laxatives • Restrict dietary intake of foods high in magnesium
Hypophosphatemia ($\downarrow$Ph) • Refeeding after starvation • Alcohol withdrawal • Diabetic ketoacidosis • Respiratory alkalosis	• Paresthesias • Muscle weakness • Muscle pain • Mental changes • Cardiomyopathy • Respiratory failure • Ph below 2.0 mEq/L	• Correct underlying cause • Administer oral replacement of phosphates with vitamin D
Hyperphosphatemia ($\uparrow$Ph) • Renal failure • Excess intake of phosphorus	• Short term: Tetany symptoms • Long term: Phosphorus precipitation in non-osseus sites • Ph above 4.5 mEq/L	• Administer aluminum hydroxide with meals to bind phosphorus • Dialysis may be required if renal failure is underlying cause

Figure 2-12 (continued)

INTRAVENOUS (IV) THERAPY

DESCRIPTION: IV solutions used to supply electrolytes, nutrients, and water.

ADMINISTRATION OF IV THERAPY

1. The purpose and duration of the IV therapy determines the type of equipment, such as IV tubing and size of needle that should be used, e.g., administration of blood requires a 19 gauge needle or larger (e.g., 18 or 16 gauge).

2. Gloves MUST be worn during venipuncture and when discontinuing an IV.

3. Assess the IV site frequently (minimum of every 2 hours). It is the nurse's legal responsibility to observe the client, to report any reactions, and to take measures necessary to prevent complications.

4. Intermittent IV therapy may be given through a saline lock; regular flushing maintains patency.

5. IV tubing and dressing should be changed according to hospital policy (usually every 72 hours).

6. When the IV is discontinued, apply pressure to the site for 1 to 3 minutes after the needle is removed.

TYPES OF IV SOLUTIONS

ISOTONIC	HYPOTONIC	HYPERTONIC

• Have an osmolality close to the ECF
• Do not cause red blood cells to swell or shrink
• Indicated for intravascular dehydration
• Isotonic solutions:
  → Normal saline (0.9%NS)
  → Lactated Ringer's (LR)
  → 5% Dextrose in water (D_5W)
    (D_5W is on the low end of isotonic - some sources classify as hypotonic)
• Used to treat intravascular dehydration (not enough fluid in vascular system)
• Common type of dehydration
• Examples: dehydration caused by running, labor, fever, etc.
	• Have an osmolarity lower than the ECF
	• Causes fluid to move from ECF to ICF
	• Indicated for cellular dehydration
	• Hypotonic solutions:
	  → 0.5% Normal saline (HNS or 0.45NS)
	  → 2.5% Dextrose in 0.45% saline ($D_{2.5}0.45\%NS$)
	• Used to treat intracellular dehydration (cells have too many osmoles, need to drive fluid into the cells)
	• Not a common occurance
	• Examples: dehydration caused by prolonged dehydration (may also see in clients who are on TPN for prolonged periods)
		• Have an osmolarity higher than the ECF
		• Indicated for intravascular dehydration with interstitial or cellular overhydration
		• Use with extreme caution
		• High concentrations of dextrose are given for caloric replacement such as intravenous hyperalimentation into a central vein for rapid dilution
		• Hypertonic saline solutions are available but used only when serum osmolality is dangerously low
		• Hypertonic solutions:
		  → 5% Dextrose in Lactated Ringer's (D_5LR)
		  → 5% Dextrose in 0.45% saline (D5 1/2 NS)
		  → 5% Dextrose in 0.9% saline (D_5NS)
		• Used to treat intravascular dehydration with cellular or interstitial overhydration.
		• Examples: dehydration resulting from surgery: blood loss causes intravascular dehydration but the tissue cuts inflame and pull fluid into the area causing interstitial overhydration
		• May also see with ascites and 3rd spacing

FLOW RATE CALCULATION

- Several formulas exist for calculating intravenous flow rates.
- Infusion pumps are used when measurement of exact flow is necessary.
- Using the following four steps for IV calculation will ensure proper calculation:

    1. ml/hr: $\dfrac{\text{Total ml fluid to be given}}{\text{Total hrs. to be administered}}$ = ml/hr. (Rate for IV infusions on a pump)

    2. gtts/min: $\dfrac{\text{Total ml fluid to be given}}{\text{Total mins. to be administered}}$ X gtts/ml = gtts/min (Rate for IV infusions by gravity)

Figure 2-13

HESI HINT: Check the IV tubing container to determine the drip factor because drip factors vary. The most common drip factors are 10, 12, 15, and 60 drops per milliliter. A microdrip is 60 drops per milliliter.

Hazards and Complications Associated with IV Administration

Infections such as septicemia and fungemia:
1. Use aseptic and antiseptic technique when starting an IV and when caring for IV site.
2. Inspect all fluids and containers before use to be sure they have not been opened or otherwise contaminated.
3. Change administration sets every 72 hours.
4. Do not leave primary solution hanging over 24°.
5. Do not irrigate blocked cannulas.

Pulmonary embolism: (Occurs when a substance or clot is propelled by venous circulation to the right side of the heart and subsequently into the pulmonary artery)
1. Use clot filters when infusing blood and blood products.
2. Avoid using veins in the lower extremities.
3. Do not irrigate plugged cannulas.

Air embolism: (Can be fatal if the pulmonary capillaries are blocked)
1. Prevent fluid containers from becoming empty.
2. Check valves, safety valves and micropore filters on vented Y-type infusions or piggyback infusions, which allow solutions to run simultaneously. Air may be introduced into the line if the containers become empty.

Circulatory overload: (Especially hazardous for clients with impaired renal and cardiac functioning)
1. Maintain infusion at prescribed rate (do not try to "catch up" if infusion is behind schedule).
2. Avoid administering fluids in excess of quantity prescribed for "keep-open" IVs.
3. Observe for signs of circulatory overload: weight gain, pitting edema, pulmonary edema (characterized by dyspnea, cough, sweating, and frothy or pinkish sputum), puffy eyelids, and ascites.

To reduce the risk of shock from a reaction to infusing substances:
1. Dilute drug, as recommended.
2. Inject drugs slowly, as recommended.
3. Use controlled volume chambers and micropore drip sets.

For phlebitis: (Can occur because of mechanical, chemical, and/or septic causes)
1. Avoid selecting a site over a joint.
2. Anchor cannulas well to prevent motion and reduce the risk of entry of microorganisms into the puncture wound.
3. Dilute medications adequately.
4. Use a cannula that is smaller than the vein.
5. Use aseptic and antiseptic technique.
6. Remove the cannula within 72 hours or immediately if one of the following occurs:
    A. Erythema.
    B. Induration.
    C. Tenderness when palpating the vein.

> **HESI HINT:** Flushing a saline lock requires approximately 1 1/2 times the amount of fluid that the tubing will hold in order to efficiently flush the tubing. REMEMBER to use sterile technique to prevent complications such as infiltration, emboli, and infection.

Acid-Base Balance

DESCRIPTION: An acid-base balance must be maintained in the body because alterations can result in alkalosis or acidosis.

Maintaining the acid-base balance is imperative and involves three systems:
1. A chemical buffer system.
2. The kidneys.
3. The lungs.

Acid-base balance is determined by the hydrogen ion concentration in body fluids.
1. Normal range is 7.35 to 7.45 expressed as the pH. *(See figure 2-14, Relationship of Sodium Bicarbonate to Carbonic Acid)*
2. pH below 7.35 indicates acidosis.
3. pH above 7.45 indicates alkalosis.
4. Measurement is by arterial blood gases (ABG). *(See figure 2-15, Arterial Blood Gas Comparisons)*

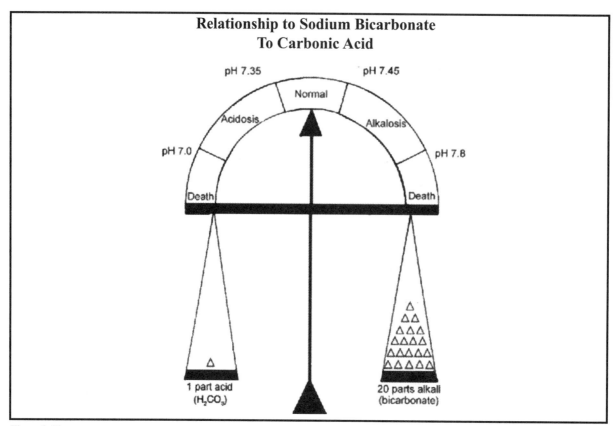

Relationship to Sodium Bicarbonate To Carbonic Acid

Figure 2-14

HESI HINT: A pH of less than 6.8 or more than 7.8 is NOT COMPATIBLE WITH LIFE.

CHEMICAL BUFFER SYSTEM

Chemical buffers act quickly to prevent major changes in body fluid pH by removing or releasing hydrogen ions.

The main chemical buffer is the bicarbonate-carbonic acid (HCO_3-H_2CO_3) system.
1. Normally there are 20 parts of bicarbonate to 1 part carbonic acid. If the 20:1 ratio is altered, the pH is changed (ratio is important, not absolute values).
2. Carbonic acid (H_2CO_3) is formed when carbon dioxide (CO_2) combines with water (H_2O).
3. Excess CO_2 in the body alters the ratio and creates an imbalance. Other buffer systems:
   A. Phosphate.
   B. Protein.
   C. Hemoglobin.

LUNGS
1. Control CO_2 content through respirations (carbonic acid content).
2. Control, to a small extent, water balance (CO_2 + H_2O = H_2CO_3).
3. Release excess CO_2 by increasing respiratory rate.
4. Retain CO_2 by decreasing respiratory rate.

KIDNEYS
1. Regulate bicarbonate levels by retaining and reabsorbing bicarbonate as needed.
2. Provide a very slow compensatory mechanism (can require hours or days).
3. Cannot help with compensation when metabolic acidosis is created by renal failure.

DETERMINING ACID-BASE DISORDERS
1. In uncompensated acid-base disturbances, it is easy to determine when a disorder exists. Draw arrows to indicate if the pH, pCO_2, or HCO_3 are increased ($\uparrow$), decreased ($\downarrow$), or within normal limits (WNL) ($\leftrightarrow$).
2. When pH is increased ($\uparrow$), alkalosis is present.
3. In respiratory disorders, the HCO_3 is normal and the arrows for pH and pCO_2 are in opposite directions.

4. In metabolic disorders, the pCO_2 is normal and the arrows for pH and HCO_3 are in the same direction or equal. *(See figure 2-16, Analysis of Arterial Blood Gases)*

5. The body will begin to compensate in acid-base disorders to bring the pH back within the normal range of 7.35 to 7.45.

EXAMPLE: For a client with a pH of 7.29 (↓), pCO_2 of 50 (↑), and a HCO_3 of 26 (↔):
1. Determine the pH: acidosis.
2. Determine the pCO_2: respiratory.
3. Determine HCO_3: not metabolic.
4. Respiratory acidosis is the disorder. *(See figure 2-17, Potential Etiologies of Acid-Base Conditions)*

> **HESI HINT:** The acronym ROME can help you remember: Respiratory, Opposite, Metabolic, Equal.

ARTERIAL BLOOD GAS COMPARISONS			
ACID-BASE CONDITIONS	**pH**	**pCO_2 (mmHg)**	**HCO_3 (mEq/L)**
Normal	7.35 to 7.45	35 to 45	22 to 26
Respiratory acidosis	↓	↑	Normal
Respiratory alkalosis	↑	↓	Normal
Metabolic acidosis	↓	Normal	↓
Metabolic alkalosis	↑	Normal	↑

Figure 2-15

ANALYSIS OF ARTERIAL BLOOD GASES		
COMPONENT	**DESCRIPTION**	**VALUES**
pH	• Measures hydrogen ion (H+) concentration	• 7.35 to 7.45
	• ↑ in ions (acidosis) reflects – in pH	• <7.35
	• ↓ in ions (alkalosis) reflects – in pH	• >7.45
pCO_2	• Partial pressure of CO_2 in arteries • Respiratory component of acid-base regulation	• 35 to 45 mmHg
	• Hypercapnia (Respiratory acidosis)	• >45 mmHg
	• Hyperventilation (Respiratory alkalosis)	• <35 mmHg
HCO_3	• Measures serum bicarbonate • May reflect primary metabolic disorder or compensatory mechanism to respiratory acidosis	• Normal 22 to 26 mEq/L
	• Metabolic acidosis	• <22 mEq/L
	• Metabolic alkalosis	• >26 mEq/L

Figure 2-16

POTENTIAL ETIOLOGIES OF ACID-BASE CONDITIONS		
CONDITION	PRIMARY ETIOLOGY	CONTRIBUTING ETIOLOGY
RESPIRATORY ACIDOSIS	• Hypoventilation	• COPD (primary etiology) • Pulmonary disease • Drugs • Obesity • Mechanical asphyxia • Sleep apnea
METABOLIC ACIDOSIS	• Addition of large amounts of fixed acids to body fluids	• Lactic acidosis (circulatory failure) • Ketoacidosis (diabetes, starvation) • Phosphates and sulfates (renal disease) • Acid ingestion (salicylates) • Secondary to respiratory alkalosis • Adrenal insufficiency
RESPIRATORY ALKALOSIS	• Hyperventilation	• Overventilation on a ventilator • Response to acidosis • Bacteremia • Thyrotoxicosis • Fever • Hepatic failure • Response to hypoxia • Hysteria
METABOLIC ALKALOSIS	• Retention of base or removal of acid from body fluids	• Excessive gastric drainage • Vomiting • Potassium depletion (diuretic therapy) • Burns • Excessive $NaHCO_3$ administration

Figure 2-17

REVIEW QUESTIONS

FLUID AND ELECTROLYTE BALANCE

1. **List four common causes of fluid volume deficit.**
2. **List four common causes of fluid volume overload.**
3. **Identify two examples of isotonic IV fluids.**
4. **List three systems which maintain acid-base balance.**
5. **Cite the ABG normals for the following:**
   A. **pH**
   B. **pCO_2**
   C. **HCO_3**
6. **Determine the following acid-base disorders:**
   A. **pH - 7.50, pCO_2 – 30, HCO_3 – 26:**
   B. **pH - 7.30, pCO_2 – 42, HCO_3 – 20:**
   C. **pH - 7.48, pCO_2 – 42, HCO_3 – 32:**
   D. **pH - 7.29, pCO_2 – 55, HCO_3 – 26:**

ANSWERS TO REVIEW QUESTIONS

1. GI causes: vomiting, diarrhea, GI suctioning. Decrease in fluid intake. Increase in fluid output such as sweating. Massive edema, ascites.
2. CHF, renal failure; cirrhosis; excess ingestion of table salt or over-hydration with sodium-containing fluids.
3. Ringer's lactate; normal saline.
4. Lungs; Kidneys; chemical buffers.
5. Normals:
   A. 7.35 to 7.45
   B. 35 to 45 mmHg
   C. 22 to 26 mEq/L
6. Disorders
   A. Respiratory Alkalosis
   B. Metabolic Acidosis
   C. Metabolic Alkalosis
   D. Respiratory Acidosis

ELECTROCARDIOGRAM
(ECG OR EKG)

DESCRIPTION: A visual representation of the electrical activity of the heart reflected by changes in the electrical potential at the skin surface.

> **HESI HINT:** Review the order of blood flow through the heart:
> Unoxygenated blood flows from the superior and inferior vena cava into the right atrium, then to the right ventricle. It flows out of the heart through the pulmonary artery, to the lungs for oxygenation. The pulmonary vein delivers oxygenated blood back to the left atrium, then to the left ventricle (largest, strongest chamber) and out the aorta.
>
> Review the three structures that control the one-way flow of blood through the heart:
> Valves
>   Atrioventricular valves
>   Tricuspid (right side)
>   Mitral (left side)
>   Semilunar valves
>   Pulmonic (in pulmonary artery)
>   Aortic (in aorta)
> Chordae tendinae
> Papillary muscles

1. The visual representation of an EKG can be recorded as a tracing on a strip of graph paper or seen on an oscilloscope.
2. The following conditions can interfere with normal heart functioning:
   A. Disturbances of rate or rhythm.
   B. Disorders of conductivity.
   C. Enlarged heart chambers.
   D. Presence of myocardial infarction.
   E. Fluid and electrolyte imbalances.
3. Each EKG should include identifying information:
   A. Client's name and identification number.
   B. Location, time, and date of recording.
   C. Client's age, sex, cardiac and noncardiac medications currently being taken.
   D. Height, weight, and BP.
   E. Clinical diagnosis and current clinical status.
   F. Any unusual position of the client during the recording.
   G. If present, thoracic deformities, respiratory distress, or muscle tremor.
4. The standard EKG is the 12 lead EKG.

5. Bedside monitoring through telemetry is more commonly seen in the clinical setting.
   A. Telemetry uses three or five leads transmitted to an oscilloscope.
   B. Graphic information is printed either upon request or at any time the set parameters are transcended.
6. A portable continuous monitor (Holter monitor) can be placed on the client to provide a magnetic tape recording. While wearing a Holter monitor, the client is instructed to keep a diary concerning:
   A. Activity.
   B. Medications.
   C. Chest pains.
7. The EKG graph paper consists of small and large squares. (*See figure 2-18, Composition of EKG paper*)
   A. The small squares represent 0.04 seconds each with five of these small squares combining to form one large square.
   B. Each large square represents 0.20 seconds (0.04 seconds x 5). Five large squares represent 1 second. Calculation of heart rate using the six-second rule: (*See figure 2-19, Calculation of Heart Rate*)
      1) The easiest means of calculating the heart rate.
      2) Cannot be used when the heart rate is irregular.
      3) 30 large squares equal one six-second time interval.
      4) Count the number of R-R intervals in the 30 large squares, and multiply by ten to determine the heart rate for one minute (the R is the high peak on the strip*). (See figure 2-20, Components of an EKG tracking)*

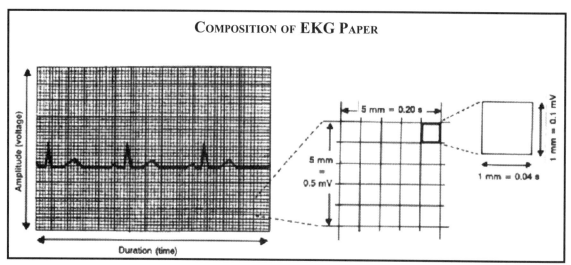

Figure 2-18

EKG waveforms are measured by amplitude (voltage) and duration (time).

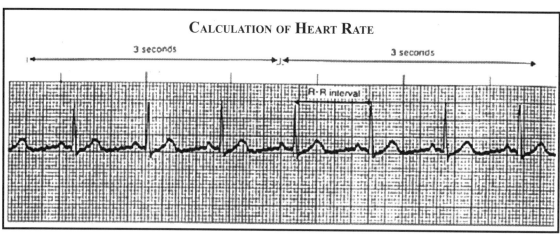

Figure 2-19

Determine the heart rate by doing the following:
1. Locate 30 large squares or 6 sections containing 5 large squares (sections noted above strip). This becomes the designated segment for counting heart rate.
2. Count the number of R-R intervals in the designated segment.
3. Multiply the number of R-R intervals counted in the designated segment by 10.
4. The heart rate for the above strip is 70.

COMPONENTS OF AN **EKG** TRACKING

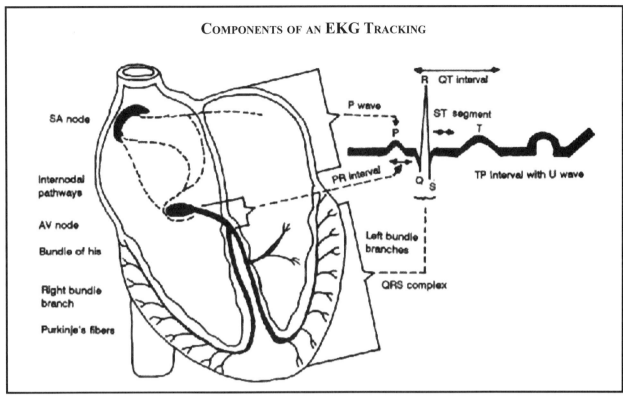

Figure 2-20

Composition of the EKG.
1. P wave: atrial systole.
   A. Represents depolarization of the atrial muscle.
   B. Should be rounded without peaking or notching.
2. QRS complex: ventricular systole.
   A. Represents depolarization of the ventricular muscle
   B. Normally follows the P wave.
   C. QRS interval measured from the beginning of the QRS to the end of the QRS (normal < .11 seconds)..
   D. T wave: ventricular diastole
      1) Represents repolarization of the ventricular muscle.
      2) Follows the QRS complex.
      3) Usually slightly rounded without peaking or notching.

> **HESI HINT:** Since the T wave represents repolarization of the ventricle, this is a critical time in the heartbeat. This action represents a resting and regrouping stage so that the next heartbeat can occur. If defibrillation occurs during this phase, the heart can be thrust into a life-threatening dysrhythmia.

3. ST segment:
   A. Represents early ventricular repolarization.
   B. Measured from the end of the S wave to the beginning of the T wave.
4. PR interval:
   A. Represents the time required for the impulse to travel through the atria (SA node), through the A-V node, to the Purkinje fibers in the ventricles.
   B. Measured from beginning of the P wave to the beginning of the QRS complex.
   C. Represents A-V nodal function (normal .12 to .20 seconds).
5. U wave:
   A. Not always present.
   B. Most prominent in the presence of hypokalemia.
6. QT interval:
   A. Represents the time required to completely depolarize and repolarize the ventricles.
   B. Measured from the beginning of the QRS complex to the end of the T wave.
7. R-R interval:
   A. Reflects the regularity of the heart rhythm.
   B. Measured from one QRS to the next QRS.

REVIEW QUESTIONS
ELECTROCARDIOGRAM, (ECG OR EKG)

1. Identify the waveforms found in a normal EKG.
2. In an EKG reading, which wave represents depolarization of the atrium?
3. In an EKG reading, what complex represents depolarization of the ventricle?
4. What does the PR interval represent?
5. If the U wave is most prominent, what condition might the nurse suspect?
6. Describe the calculation of the heart rate using an EKG rhythm strip.
7. What is the most important assessment data for the nurse to obtain on a client with an arrhythmia
8. Calculate the rate of this rhythm strip.

ANSWERS TO REVIEW QUESTIONS

1. P wave, QRS complex, T wave, ST segment, PR interval.
2. Represented by the P wave.
3. QRS complex.
4. The time required for the impulse to travel from the atria through the A-V node.
5. Hypokalemia.
6. Count the number of R-R intervals in the thirty large squares and multiply by 10 to determine the heart rate for one minute.
7. Ability of the client to tolerate the arrhythmia.
8. 90 to 100 depending on which set of 6 squares you use.

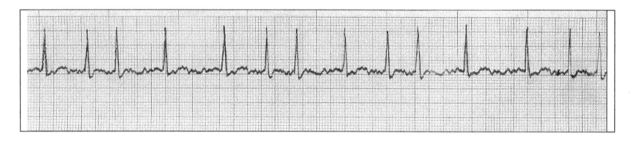

PERIOPERATIVE CARE

DESCRIPTION: The perioperative period includes client care before surgery (preoperative), during surgery (intraoperative), and after surgery (postoperative).

1. The nurse's role is to
   A. Demystify the experience.
   B. Reduce anxiety.
   C. Promote an uncomplicated perioperative period for the client and family.

2. Surgery is performed under aseptic conditions, in a hospital or alternate hospital setting (ambulatory surgical center or healthcare provider's office).

3. Many changes in perioperative care have occurred since 1983 as a result of Medicare mandates for outpatient care. Theses mandates tend to result in changes to all healthcare insurance coverage.

SURGICAL RISK FACTORS

- **AGE:** the very young and very old are greater surgical risks than children and adults.
- **NUTRITION:** obesity and malnutrition increase surgical risk.
- **FLUID AND ELECTROLYTE STATUS:** dehydration and hypovolemia increase surgical risk due to imbalances in calcium, magnesium, potassium and phosphorus.
- **GENERAL HEALTH:** any infection or pathology increases surgical risk.
  - → Cardiac conditions; angina, MIs, hypertension, congestive heart failure (well-controlled cardiac problems pose little risk).
  - → Blood coagulation disorders can lead to severe bleeding, hemorrhage, and shock.
  - → Upper respiratory tract infections (surgery is usually delayed when the client has an upper respiratory infection) and chronic obstructive pulmonary disease are exacerbated by general anesthesia and adversely affect pulmonary function.
  - → Renal disease, such as renal insufficiency, impairs fluid and electrolyte regulation.
  - → Diabetes mellitus predisposes clients to wound infection and delayed healing.
  - → Liver disease impairs the liver's ability to detoxify medications used during surgery to produce prothrombin or to metabolize nutrients for wound healing.
  - → Obesity.
- **CURRENT MEDICATIONS:** prescription and over-the-counter drugs. Medications which increase surgical risk include:
  - → Anticoagulants (increase blood coagulation time).
  - → Tranquilizers (may cause hypotension).
  - → Heroin (decreases central nervous system response).
  - → Antibiotics (may be incompatible with anesthetics).
  - → Diuretics (may precipitate electrolyte imbalance).
  - → Steroids.
  - → Over-the-counter herbal preparations.
  - → Vitamin E.

Figure 2-21

PREOPERATIVE CARE

Description: Care provided from the time the client/family makes the decision to have surgery until the client is taken to the operative suite.

DATA TO OBTAIN WHEN TAKING A PREOPERATIVE NURSING HISTORY

- Age
- Allergies to medications, foods, and topical antiseptics (especially iodine)
- Current medications: prescriptions, over-the-counter, and herbal preparations
- History of medical and surgical problems
- Previous surgical experiences
- Previous experience with anesthesia
- Tobacco, alcohol, and drug abuse
- Understanding of surgical procedure
- Coping resources

KEY COMPONENTS OF PREOPERATIVE TEACHING PLANS

- Regulations concerning valuables, jewelry, dentures
- Food and fluid restrictions such as NPO after midnight
- Invasive procedures such as urinary catheters, IVs, NG tubes, enemas, douches
- Preoperative medications
- Operating room, transportation, skin preparation, post anesthesia
- Postoperative procedures:
  - → Respiratory care such as ventilator, incentive spirometer, deep breather, splinting
  - → Activity such as ROM, leg exercises, early ambulation, turning
  - → Pain control such as IM medications, PCA (patient-controlled analgesia)
  - → Dietary restrictions
  - → Intensive care unit or post-anesthesia care unit orientation (recovery room)

PREOPERATIVE CHECKLIST INFORMATION

- "Informed consent," surgical consent, signed and witnessed consent for treatment within 24 hours; signature must be obtained prior to administration of any narcotics or other medications affecting client cognition.
- Accurate height and weight charted
- History and physical (by healthcare provider) in chart
- Chest x-ray, EKG, urinalysis
- Hgb, Hct, electrolytes, glucose, and type/crossmatch for blood
- Old chart
- Identification band on client, including allergies
- Addressograph information
- Contact lenses, glasses, dentures, partial plates, wigs, jewelry, artificial eye, prostheses, make-up, nail polish removed
- Voided or catheterized, time
- In hospital gown
- Vital signs: BP, temp, pulse, respirations
- Premedication given: type and time
- Skin preparation (if prescribed by Healthcare Provider/Physician):
  - → Wash with soap and water
  - → Shave using a razor that is new and sharp, as skin must NOT be broken
  - → Follow shave with scrub or shower with povidone/iodine or another antibacterial solution
- Signature of nurse certifying completion

Figure 2-22

HESI HINT: Marking the operative site is required for procedures involving right/left distinctions, multiple structures (fingers, toes), or levels (spinal procedures). Site marking should be done with the involvement of the client.

INTRAOPERATIVE CARE

Description: From the time the client is received in the operative suite until admission to the recovery room, an operating room nurse is in charge of care.

- **Maintain quiet during induction**
- **Maintain safety**:
  - → Conduct client identification - right client - right procedure - right site
  - → Ensure that sponge, needle, and instrument counts are accurate
  - → Position during procedure to prevent injury
  - → Apply grounding device to client if electrocautery is to be used
  - → Strictly adhere to asepsis during ALL intraoperative procedures
  - → Ensure adequate, functioning suction set-up(s)
  - → Responsible for correct labeling, handling and deposition of any and all specimens
- **Monitor physical status**:
  - → If excessive blood loss occurs, calculate effect on client
  - → Report changes in pulse, temperature, respirations, blood pressure to surgeon in conjunction with anesthesiologist/CRNA
- **Provide psychological support**:
  - → Provide emotional support to client/family immediately prior to, during, and after surgery
  - → Arrange with MD to provide information to the family if surgery is prolonged or complications or unexpected findings occur
  - → Communicate emotional state of client to other healthcare team members

Figure 2-23

POSTOPERATIVE CARE

Description: From admission to recovery room until client is recovered.

- Initially the client goes to the recovery room or post-anesthesia care unit
- Upon arrival, the client is assessed for vital signs (BP, pulse, respirations, temperature), level of consciousness, skin color and condition, dressing location and condition, intravenous fluids, drainage tubes, position, and oxygen saturation levels
- When stabilized and prescribed by the healthcare provider, the client is then transferred to the general nursing unit or the intensive care unit
- Immediate postoperative nursing care should include:
  - → Monitor for signs of shock and hemorrhage: Hypotension, narrow pulse pressure, rapid weak pulse, cold moist skin, increased capillary filling time (***See figure 2-25, Common Postoperative Complications)***
  - → Position on side (if not contraindicated) to prevent aspiration and allow client to cough out airway; side rails should be up at all times
  - → Provide warmth with heated blanket
  - → Manage nausea/vomiting with antiemetic drugs and NG suctioning
  - → Manage pain with intravenous analgesics
  - → Check with anesthesiologist about intraoperative medications before administering pain medications
  - → Determine intraoperative irrigations/instillations with drains to help evaluate amount of drainage on dressing and/or in drainage collection devices

Figure 2-24

COMMON POSTOPERATIVE COMPLICATIONS

POSTOPERATIVE COMPLICATION	OCCURRENCE	INTERVENTIONS FOR PREVENTIONS
URINARY RETENTIONS	8 to 12 hours postoperatively	• Monitor hydration status and encourage oral intake if allowed • Offer bedpan or assist to commode
PULMONARY PROBLEMS • Atelectasis • Pneumonia • Embolus	1 to 2 days postoperatively	• Assist client to turn, cough, deep breathe q2 hours • Keep client hydrated • Early ambulation • Early incentive spirometer
WOUND-HEALING PROBLEMS	5 to 6 days postoperatively	• Splint incision when client coughs • Monitor for signs of infection, malnutrition, dehydration • High-protein diet
HESI HINT: Wound dehiscence is separation of the wound edges and is more likely to occur with vertical incisions. It usually occurs after the early postoperative period, when the client's own granulation tissue is "taking over" the wound, after absorption of the sutures has begun. Evisceration of the wound is protrusion of intestinal contents (in an abdominal wound) and is more likely in clients who are older, diabetic, obese or malnourished and have prolonged paralytic ileus.		
URINARY TRACT INFECTIONS	5 to 8 days postoperatively	• Oral fluid intake • Emptying of bladder q4 to 6 hours • Monitor intake and output • Avoid catheterizations if possible
THROMBOPHLEBITIS	6 to 14 days postoperatively	• Leg exercises q8 hr. while in bed • Early ambulation • Apply antiembolus (TED) stockings or sequential hose as prescribed. Remove TEDS q8 hr. and reapply • Avoid pressure which may obstruct venous flow; don't raise knee gatch on bed, do not place pillows beneath knees, avoid crossing legs at knees • Low-dose heparin may be used prophylactically
DECREASED GASTROINTESTINAL PERISTALSIS • Constipation • Paralytic ileus	2 to 4 days postoperatively	• NG tubing to decompress GI tract • Client to limit use of narcotic analgesics which decrease peristalsis • Encourage early ambulation

Figure 2-25

HESI HINT: NCLEX-RN® items will focus on the nurse's role in terms of the entire perioperative process.
Sample: A 43-year-old mother of two teenage daughters enters the hospital to have her gallbladder removed in a same-day surgery using a scope instead of an incision. What nursing needs will dominate each phase of her short hospital stay?

Preparation phase: Education about postoperative care, NPO, assist with meeting family needs. **Operative phase:** Assessment, management of the operative suite. **Post-anesthesia phase:** Pain management, post-anesthesia precautions. **Postoperative phase:** Prevent and assess for complications, pain management, dietary restrictions, activity.

REVIEW QUESTIONS

PERIOPERATIVE CARE

1. List five variables that increase surgical risk.
2. Why is a client with liver disease at increased risk for operative complications?
3. Preoperative teaching should include demonstration and explanation of expected postoperative client activities. What activities should be included?
4. What items should the nurse assist the client in removing before surgery?
5. How and why is the client positioned in the immediate postoperative period?
6. List three nursing actions to prevent postoperative wound dehiscence/evisceration.
7. Identify three nursing interventions to prevent postoperative urinary tract infections.
8. Identify nursing/medical interventions to prevent postoperative paralytic ileus.
9. List four nursing interventions to prevent postoperative thrombophlebitis.
10. During the intraoperative period, what activities should the operating room nurse do to ensure safety during surgery?

ANSWERS TO REVIEW QUESTIONS

1. Age: very young and very old, obesity and malnutrition, preoperative dehydration/hypovolemia, preoperative infection, use of anticoagulants preoperative (aspirin).
2. Impairs ability to detoxify medications used during surgery. Impairs ability to produce prothrombin to reduce hemorrhage.
3. Respiratory activities: breathing, use of spirometer. Exercises: range of motion, leg exercises, turning. Pain management: medications, splinting. Dietary restrictions: NPO to progressive diet. Dressings and drains. Orientation to recovery room environment.
4. Contact lenses, glasses, dentures, partial plates, wigs, jewelry, prostheses, make-up and nail polish.
5. Usually on the side or with head to side in order to prevent aspiration of any emesis.
6. Splint incision when coughing, encourage coughing/deep breathing in EARLY postoperative period when sutures are STONG. Monitor for signs of infection, malnutrition, and dehydration. Encourage high-protein diet.
7. Avoid postoperative catheterization. Increase oral fluid intake. Empty bladder q4 to 6 hours, early ambulation.
8. Early ambulation. Limit use of narcotic analgesics. NG tube decompression.
9. Perform in-bed leg exercises. Early ambulation. Apply antiembolus stockings. Avoid positions/pressure which obstruct venous flow.
10. Ascertain correct sponge, needle, and instrument count. Position client to avoid injury. Apply ground during electrocautery use. Strict use of surgical asepsis.

HIV INFECTION

DESCRIPTION: Infection with Human Immunodeficiency Virus (HIV).

1. HIV was first documented in 1981. At that time, the constellation of symptoms was not known to be caused by a virus and the disease was named in a manner that describes what is now known to be the end stage of a very long, chronic infection from a virus. The name given to symptoms was Acquired Immunodeficiency Syndrome (AIDS).
2. It is now understood that the disease is caused by a retrovirus, which is attracted to CD4 T-cells lymphocytes, macrophages, and cells of the central nervous system.
3. The virus enters the cell and begins to replicate. Some event, such as co-factors (herpes simplex and CMV) can stimulate this replication.
4. The destruction of the CD4 T-cell causes depletion in the number of CD4 T-cells and a loss of the body's ability to fight infection. Individuals with fewer than 200 CD4 T-cells are at risk for opportunistic infections. (Normal CD4 T-cell count is 600 to 1200.)
5. Initially, the individual often suffers an acute infection, which is quite similar to mononucleosis. *(See figure 2-26, Stages of HIV)*
6. Initial symptoms usually occur within 3 weeks of initial exposure to HIV, after

which the person becomes asymptomatic. Persons infected with HIV can transmit the virus to others any time after infection has occurred, whether they are symptomatic or asymptomatic.

7. Current CDC definition of AIDS (end stage infection) includes persons with specific, serious, opportunistic infections such as pneumocystis carinii pneumonia (PCP), disseminated cytomegalovirus, or Kaposi's sarcoma.

8. Risk groups include the following:
    A. Homosexual or bisexual males.
    B. IV drug abusers or those who have had tattoos or acupuncture.
    C. Heterosexual partners of a risk group member.
    D. Recipients of blood products prior to blood product screening, e.g., those with hemophilia who were diagnosed and treated prior to 1985.
    E. Those taking medications such as steroids or other agents that cause immunosuppression.
    F. Infants born to infected mothers.

STAGES OF HIV	
STAGE	**DESCRIPTION/SYMPTOMS**
PRIMARY INFECTION (ACUTE HIV INFECTION OR ACUTE HIV SYNDROME) CD4 T-CELL COUNTS OF AT LEAST 800 CELLS/MM³	• Flu-like symptoms, fever, malaise • Mononucleosis like illness, lymphadenopathy, fever, malaise, rash • Symptoms usually occur within 3 weeks of initial exposure to HIV, after which the person becomes asymptomatic
HIV ASYMPTOMATIC (CDC CATEGORY A) CD4 T-CELL COUNTS MORE THAN 500 CELLS/MM³	• No clinical problems • Characterized by continuous viral replication • Can last for many years, 10 years or longer
HIV Symptomatic (CDC Category B) CD4 T-cell counts between 200 to 499 cells/mm³	• Persistent generalized lymphadenopathy • Persistent fever • Weight loss, diarrhea • Peripheral neuropathy • Herpes zoster • Candidiasis • Cervical dysplasia • Hairy leukoplakia, oral
AIDS (CDC CATEGORY C) CD4 T-CELL COUNTS LESS THAN 200 CELLS/MM³	• Occurs when a variety of bacteria, parasites or viruses overwhelm the body's immune system • Once classified as category C, the patient remains classified as category C. This has implications for entitlements (ie, health benefits, housing, food stamps, etc.)

Figure 2-26

NURSING ASSESSMENT

1. Laboratory testing:
    A. Positive ELISA (enzyme-linked immunosorbent assay) - can have false positive.
    B. Confirmation by the Western Blot test, which uses electrophoreses and evaluates virus specific bands.
    C. Polymerase chain reaction test (PCR) may be used to differentiate betwenn HIV infection in the neonate and antibodies neonates receive from the mother.
    D. Seroconversion to positive on these tests occurs usually within 6 weeks to 3 months, but may take as long as 12 months.
    E. Prior to seroconversion to antibody positive status, P24 antigen assay will be positive.

(This test detects the core antigen of the virus.)

2. Symptoms:
    A. Extreme fatigue.
    B. Loss of appetite and unexplained weight loss of more than ten pounds in two months.
    C. Swollen glands.
    D. Leg weakness or pain.
    E. Unexplained fever for more than a week.
    F. Night sweats.
    G. Unexplained diarrhea.
    H. Dry cough; may represent pneumocystis carinii pneumonia (PCP).
    I. White spots in the mouth and throat, may represent candidiasis.
    J. Painful blisters, may represent shingles..

K. Painless purple-blue lesions on the skin,

L. Confusion, disorientation.

M. In women, recurrent vaginal infections that

are resistant to treatment.

3. Opportunistic infections.

(See figure 2-27, Opportunistic Infections)

OPPORTUNISTIC INFECTIONS

PNEUMOCYSTIS CARINII PNEUMONIA	KAPOSI'S SARCOMA	CYPTOSPORIDIOSIS	CANDIDIASIS OF ORAL CAVITY AND ESOPHAGUS
• Fever • Dry cough • Dyspnea at rest • Chills	• Purple-blue lesions on skin, often arms and legs • Invasion of gastrointestinal tract, lymphatic system, lungs, and brain	• Severe, watery diarrhea (may be 30 to 40 stools per day) • Abdominal cramps • Nausea • Electrolyte imbalance • Malaise	• Thick white exudate in the mouth • Unusual taste to food • Retrosternal burning • Oral ulcers
CRYPTOCOCCAL MENINGITIS	CYTOMEGALOVIRUS (CMV) RETINITIS	CMV COLITIS	DISSEMINATED CMV
• Headache • Changes in level of consciousness • Nausea, vomiting • Stiff neck • Blurred vision	• Most common CMV infection in persons with AIDS • Impaired vision in one or both eyes • Can lead to blindness	• Diarrhea • Malabsorption of nutrients • Weight loss	• Malaise • Fever • Pancytopenia • Weight loss • Positive cultures from blood, urine or throat
PERIRECTAL MUCOCUTANEOUS HERPES SIMPLEX VIRAL INFECTIONS	LYMPHOMAS OF CENTRAL NERVOUS SYSTEM (CNS)	TUBERCULOSIS	HIV ENCEPHALOPATHY
• Severe pain • Bleeding, rectal discharge • Ulceration in the rectal area	• Change in mental status • Apathy • Psychomotor slowing • Seizures	• Pulmonary and extrapulmonary • Lymphatic and hematogenous TB are common **Negative skin testing does not rule out TB**	• Memory loss and impaired concentration • Apathy • Depression • Psychomotor slowing (most prominent symptom) • Incontinence • CAT scan findings: diffuse atrophy and ventricular enlargement

Figure 2-27

HESI HINT: HIV clients with tuberculosis require respiratory isolation. Tuberculosis is the only real risk to non-pregnant caregivers that is not related to a break in universal precautions (i.e., needle sticks, etc.).

ANALYSIS (NURSING DIAGNOSES)

1. Potential for infection related to…
2. Alteration in thought processes related to…
3. Alteration in nutrition: less than body requirements related to…
4. Alteration in elimination related to…
5. Alteration in breathing pattern related to…
6. Alteration in sexuality patterns related to…
7. Fatigue related to…
8. Anticipatory grieving related to…

NURSING PLANS AND INTERVENTIONS

1. Assess respiratory functioning frequently.
2. Avoid known sources of infection.
3. Use strict asepsis for all invasive procedures.
4. Obtain vital signs frequently.
5. Plan activities to allow rest periods.
6. Elevate head of bed.
7. Refer to nutritionist.
8. Offer small, frequent feedings.
9. Weigh daily.
10. Encourage client to avoid fatty foods.

11. Monitor for skin breakdown, offer good skin care.
12. Use safety precautions for clients with neurological symptoms or loss of vision.
13. Orient client who is confused.
14. Provide emotional support for grieving client who is losing all relationships and skills.
15. Provide emotional support for significant others: family, family of choice, lovers, friends.
16. Administer IV fluids for hydration, as prescribed.
17. Administer total parenteral nutrition (TPN) as prescribed.
18. Administer agents which treat specific, opportunistic infections and medications for HIV. *(See figure 2-28, HIV Drugs)*
19. Assist with pain management, administer prescribed narcotics or analgesics.

> **HESI HINT:** STANDARD PRECAUTIONS
> WASH HANDS, even if gloves have been worn to give care.
> WEAR GLOVES (latex) for touching blood or body fluids, or any non-intact body surface.
> WEAR GOWNS during any procedure that might generate splashes (changing clients with diarrhea).
> USE MASKS AND EYE PROTECTION during activity which might disperse droplets (suctioning).
> DO NOT RECAP NEEDLES, dispose of in puncture-resistant containers.
> USE MOUTH PIECE for resuscitation efforts.
> *REFRAIN FROM GIVING CARE* if you have open skin lesions.

> **HESI HINT:** Caregivers who are pregnant may choose not to care for a client with Cytomegalovirus (CMV).

HIV DRUGS
(CLIENT SHOULD HAVE REGULAR BLOOD COUNTS TO TRACK CD4 LEVELS AND VIRAL LOAD)

DRUGS	INDICATIONS	ADVERSE REACTIONS	NURSING IMPLICATIONS
NRT Inhibitors: • Didanosine (Videx) • Lamivudine (Epivir) • Abacavir (Ziagen) • Zalsitabine (Hivid)	HIV infection. Classifications used in various combinations to reduce viral load and slow development of resistance.	• Peripheral neuropathies • Pancreatitis • ↑Triglycerides • Fever, rash, N/V, abdominal cramps	• Monitor for neuropathies • Monitor amylase, lipase, triglycerides • Give on empty stomach
Protease Inhibitors • Indinavir (Crixivan) • Amprenivir (Agenerase) • Saguinavir (Invirase) • Ritonivir (Norvir, Kaletra) • Nelinavir (Viracept)		• Depression • Ketoacidosis • Seizures • Angioedema • Stevens-Johnson syndrome	• Many drug-drug interactions • Hi fat/hi protein foods reduce absorption • Give most of these WITH food • Reduces contraceptive effects • Do not confuse ritonivir (Norvir) with trade name zidovudine (Retrovir)
Non-NRT Inhibitors • Efavirenz (Sustiva) • Delaviridine (Rescriptor) • Nevirapine (Viramune)		• CNS changes • Nausea • Rash • ↑Triglycerides • Hepatotoxicity	• Many drug-drug interactions • Monitor liver function tests • Reduces contraceptive effects • Do not confuse Viramune with Viracept
Combination Products • Lamivudine + zidovudine (Combivir) • Avacavir+ lamivudine + zidovudine (Trizivir)		• Monitor for side effects associated with the individual drugs	• Note implications of the individual drugs in the combination product

Figure 2-28

HIV DRUGS (CONTINUED)

DRUGS	INDICATIONS	ADVERSE REACTIONS	NURSING IMPLICATIONS
Anti-infectives • Atovaquone (Mepron) • Trimethoprim/sullfamethoxazole (Bactrim)	Mepron used for PCP in those unable to tolerate trimethoprim/sulfamethoxazole prophylaxis	• CNX disturbances • Ageranulocytosis • Phlebitis if IV • Renal calculi with Bactrim	• Enhances effects of oral hypoglycemics • Increases thrombocytopenia risk if given with thiazide diuretics • Check for allergy to sulfonamide
Antivirals • Acyclovir sodium (Zovirax) • Gancyclovir (Cytovene)	Herpes simplex CMV retinitis	• Granulocytopenia • Thrombocytopenia	• Give with or without food • Many incompatibilities IV PO, IV, topical • Monitor liver function tests
Anti-fungals • Ampherotericin B (Fungizone)	IV: Cryptococcal meningitis PO: Oral candidiasis	• Nephrotoxicity • Hypotension • Hypokalemia • Febrile reaction • Muscle cramps • Circulatory problems	• Many drug-drug interactions • Vesicant-monitor IV site closely; premedicate with antipyretic; give slowly • Swish as long as possible before swallowing PO form
Anti-protozoals • Pentamidine isethionate (Pentam 300)	Prophylaxis for PCP Treatment of PCP	• Leukopenia • EKG abnormalities	• IV or aerosol-not oral • Use careful precautions against potential spread of TB

Figure 2-28 (continued)

PEDIATRIC HIV INFECTION

DESCRIPTION: Infection with HIV in infants and children.

1. Sources of infection for pediatric clients:
   A. Perinatal transmission. 30 to 50% children born to HIV positive mothers will be infected unless mother treated with zidovudine during pregnancy and neonate treated after birth, then rate decreases to 4 to 8%.
   B. HIV-infected blood products.
   C. Through breast milk.
   D. Sexual abuse.
2. Although maternal antibodies may be present at birth in some children, the antibody tests will convert to negative before 18 months of age.

NURSING ASSESSMENT

1. Risk groups:
   A. Infants born to mothers who are HIV positive.
   B. Hemophiliacs.
   C. Infants/children who have received blood transfusions.
2. Symptoms:
   A. Failure to thrive.
   B. Lymphadenopathy.
   C. Organomegaly.
   D. Neuropathy.
   E. Cardiomyopathy.
   F. Chronic recurrent infections, such as thrush.
   G. Unexplained fevers.

> **HESI HINT:** Pediatric HIV is often evidenced by lymphoid interstitial pneumonitis, pulmonary lymphoid hyperplasia, and opportunistic infections.

> **HESI HINT:** The focus of NCLEX-RN® questions is likely to be assessment of early signs of the disease and management of complications associated with HIV.

ANALYSIS (NURSING DIAGNOSES)

1. All diagnoses for adults may be experienced by children depending on the age of the child.
2. Alteration in family process related to …
3. Alteration in growth and development related to …

NURSING PLANS AND INTERVENTIONS

1. Avoid exposure to persons with infections, especially chickenpox.
2. Administer NO live virus vaccines.
3. Teach:
   A. Family to use gloves when diapering the

61

child, if child has diarrhea.

   B.   Family to clean any soiled surfaces (wearing gloves) with 10% bleach solution.

   C.   Family to identify signs of opportunistic infections.

4.   Monitor growth parameters.

5.   Administer gamma globulin as prescribed, usually each month.

6.   Support use of social services.

7.   Support child attending school as much as child is able.

8.   *See care plan for adult HIV client.*

9.   Assist in community and school education programs.

REVIEW QUESTIONS

HIV INFECTION

1.   Identify the way HIV is transmitted.

2.   Vertical transmission (from mother to fetus) occurs how often if mother is not treated during pregnancy?

3.   Describe universal precautions.

4.   What are the side effects of amphotericin B?

5.   What does the CD4 T cell count describe?

6.   Why does the CD4 T cell count drop in HIV infections?

7.   Describe the ways a pediatric client might acquire HIV infection.

ANSWERS TO REVIEW QUESTIONS

1.   Transmitted through blood and body fluids, e.g., unprotected sexual contact with an infected person, sharing needles among drug abusing persons, infected blood products (rare), maternal to fetus transmission through breast milk, or breaks in universal precautions (needle sticks or similar occurrences).

2.   Vertical transmission occurs 30 to 50% of the time.

3.   Protection from blood and body fluids is the goal of standard precautions. Standard precautions initiate barrier protection between caregiver and client through: Hand washing, use gloves, use gown and mask, eye protection as indicated, depending on activity of care and the likelihood of exposure. Prevent needle sticks by not capping needles.

4.   Side effects of amphotericin B (can be quite severe) include: Anorexia, Chills, Cramping, Muscle and joint pain, Circulatory problems.

5.   CD4 T cell count describes the number of infection-fighting lymphocytes the person has.

6.   CD4 T cell count drops because the virus destroys CD4 T cells as it invades them and replicates.

7.   Through infected blood products. Through sexual abuse. Through breast milk.

PAIN

DESCRIPTION: An individual's subjective experience.

Client's pain often goes unrecognized and untreated.

1.   Healthcare professionals are poorly educated about identifying, assessing, and managing pain.

2.   Healthcare professionals often cling to outdated beliefs and biases, including fear of addiction.

An individual's response to pain is influenced by several factors.

1.   Anxiety: reduction of anxiety can help control pain.

2.   Past experience with pain: the more pain experienced in childhood, the greater the perceptions of pain in adulthood.

3.   Culture and religion: cultural and religious practices from one's family play an important role in determining how a person experiences and expresses pain.

4.   Gender.

Pain is classified as either acute or chronic.

1.   Acute pain:

   A.   Temporary.

   B.   Occurs after an injury to the body.

   C.   Examples: postoperative pain, labor pain, renal calculi pain.

2.   Chronic pain:

   A.   Chronic non-malignant pain, e.g., low back pain or rheumatoid arthritis.

   B.   Chronic intermittent pain, e.g., migraine headaches.

   C.   Chronic malignant pain: associated with neoplastic diseases.

Theory of pain:

1.   Gate control theory: pain impulses travel from the periphery to the gray matter in the dorsal horn of the spinal cord along small nerve fibers.

   A.   A "gating" mechanism exists, called the substantia gelatinosa, which either opens or closes the transmission of pain impulses to the brain.

   B.   It is thought that stimulation of large, fast-conducting sensory fibers oppose the input from small pain fibers, thus blocking pain

transmission.
- C. Modalities used: stimulation of large fibers by massage, heat, cold, acupuncture, TENS.
2. Endorphin/enkephalin theory:
- A. Endorphins: naturally-occurring compounds that have morphine-like qualities which modulate pain by preventing the conduction of pain impulses in the CNS.
- B. Enkephalins: specific neurotransmitters that bind with opiate receptors in the dorsal horn of the spinal cord that modulate pain by closing the gate and stopping the pain impulse.
- C. Modalities used: stimulation of endogenous opiate release through acupuncture, placebos, TENS.

Nursing Assessment

1. Location: localized, radiating, or referred.
2. Intensity: ask client to rate pain before and after intervention such as medication (use scale such as 1 to 10 with 1 being no pain).
3. Comfort: often clients can describe what relieves pain better than the pain itself.
4. Quality: sharp, dull, aching, soreness, etc.
5. Chronology: ask client when pain started, what time of day if occurs, how often if appears, how long it lasts, is it constant or intermittent, has the intensity changed.
6. Subjective Experience: what decreases or aggravates pain, what other symptoms are associated with pain, what interventions provide relief, what limitations does the pain inflict.

Analysis (Nursing Diagnoses)

1. Pain related to…
2. Ineffective individual coping related to…
3. Sleep disturbance related to…
4. Activity intolerance related to…
5. Self-care deficit related to…

Nursing Plans and Interventions
Pain Management

Pharmacological interventions. *(See figure 2-29, Routes of Administration for Analgesics)*
1. Non-narcotics, Non-steroidal Anti-inflammatory Drugs (NSAIDs). *(See figure 3-35, NSAIDs)*
- A. Act by a peripheral mechanism at level of damaged tissue by inhibiting prostaglandin and other chemical mediator syntheses involved in pain.
- B. Antipyretic activity by action on the hypothalamic heat-regulating center to reduce fever.
- C. Examples: salicylates-aspirin (Bayer) nonsalicylates, acetaminophen (Tylenol), ibuprofen (Motrin).
2. Narcotic agonist/antagonist.
- A. Act as narcotics (agonists) that antagonize the "pure" agonists (counteract narcotic effects).
- B. Administration after client has been receiving narcotics may cause withdrawal symptoms.
- C. Side effects include drowsiness, occasional nausea and psychomimetic effects such as hallucinations and euphoria.
- D. Examples: butorphanol (Stadol), nalbuphine (Nubain).
3. Narcotics.
- A. Act as opioids, binding with specific opiate receptors throughout the CNS to reduce pain perception.
- B. Side effects include nausea and vomiting, constipation, respiratory depression, and CNS depression.
- C. Examples: meperidine (Demerol), morphine sulfate.

> **HESI HINT:** For narcotic-induced respiratory depression, administer Naloxone 0.1 mg to 0.4 mg IV every 2 to 3 minutes as needed, until 1.0 mg is achieved.

Adjuvant to analgesics:
1. Given in combination with an analgesic to potentiate or enhance the analgesic's effectiveness.
2. Helpful in controlling discomforts associated with pain such as nausea, anxiety, and depression, e.g., promethazine (Phenergan).

> **HESI HINT:** Use noninvasive methods for pain management when possible:
> - Relaxation exercises
> - Distraction
> - Imagery
> - Biofeedback
> - Interpersonal Skills
> - Physical care: altering positions, touch, hot and cold applications.

63

ROUTES OF ADMINISTRATION FOR ANALGESICS	
ROUTE	**ADMINISTRATION**
ORAL	• Preferred method of administration. • Drug levels usually peak at 1 to 2 hours.
INTRAMUSCULAR	• Acceptable method of managing acute, short-term pain. • Onset 30 minutes, peak effect 1 to 3 hours, duration of action 4 hours.
RECTAL	• Useful with clients who are nauseated and unable to take analgesics by mouth. • Useful for home care and with elderly clients as an alternative to po and IV administration. Reduced effectiveness with constipation.
IV BOLUS (IV PUSH)	• Provides the most rapid onset (5 minutes), but with the shortest duration (1 hour). • Useful with acute pain, such as a client in labor.
PATIENT-CONTROLLED ANALGESIA (PCA)	• Ideal method of pain control in that the client is able to prevent pain by administering to him/herself smaller doses of the narcotic (usually morphine) as soon as the first sign of discomfort arises. • Usually administered IV. • A predetermined dose and a set lockout interval (5 to 20 minutes) is prescribed by MD, and pump is calibrated to deliver the specified dose whenever client "hits the button." • Lock-out mechanism prevents overdosage. • Pump can record number of times the client uses the pump and the cumulative dose delivered.
CONTINUOUS SUBCUTANEOUS NARCOTIC INFUSION (CSI)	• Useful with clients who cannot take anything by mouth and who require prolonged administration of parenteral narcotics. • Provides a constant level of analgesia by continuous infusion of a narcotic. • Site should be inspected every 8 hours and changed at least every 7 days.
CONTINUOUS EPIDURAL ANALGESIA	• Catheter threaded into epidural space with continuous infusion of fentanyl citrate, morphine, or other narcotic analgesics. • Danger of respiratory depression.
TRANSDERMAL PATCHES	• Applied to skin (self-adhesive or with overlay to secure patch). • Also used to deliver hormonal therapy, nitroglycerin, and nicotine. • Sites for application and frequency of application are specific to each medication. • Document: removal of old patch, as well as site and application date/time of new patch.

Figure 2-29

NURSING ASSESSMENT
1. Pain. *(See figure 2-30, Pain Relief Techniques)*
2. Response to pharmacological intervention: tolerance to pharmacological interventions may occur, i.e., the client physiologically requires increasingly larger doses to provide the same effect.
   A. First sign of tolerance is a decreased duration of drug effectiveness.
   B. Increased dosages can be a result of increased pain rather than tolerance, e.g., clients with advanced cancer.

HESI HINT: Narcotic analgesics are preferred for pain relief because they bind to the various opiate receptor sites in the CNS. Morphine is often the preferred narcotic (REMEMBER, it causes respiratory depression).

Other agonists are meperidine and methadone. Narcotic antagonists block the attachment of narcotics to the receptors, such as Narcan (naloxone). Once Narcan has been given, additional narcotics cannot be given until the Narcan effects have passed.

PAIN RELIEF TECHNIQUES
NONINVASIVE: Cutaneous stimulation which is useful alone or in combination with other pain-management techniques.

- Heat and cold applications decrease pain and muscle spasm.
- Transcutaneous electrical nerve stimulation (TENS) provides continuous mild electrical current to the skin via electrodes.
- Massage provides a simple, inexpensive, and effective method of pain relief.
- Distraction diverts client's attention from the pain; useful during short periods of pain or during painful procedures such as IV venipunctures.
- Relaxation can be used as a distraction and to facilitate sedation or sleep; rarely decreases pain sensation.
- Biofeedback techniques: control of autonomic responses (tachycardia, muscle tension) to pain through electrical feedback.

INVASIVE: Any procedure used to relieve pain, which invades the body.

- Nerve blocks: injection of anesthetic into or near a nerve to decrease pain pathways, e.g., "deadening" area for dental work, regional anesthesia used in obstetrics.
- Neurosurgical procedures: surgical or chemical (alcohol) interruption of nerve pathways; commonly used in clients with cancer who have severe pain.
- Acupuncture: insertion of needles at various points into the body to relieve pain.

Figure 2-30

ONSET OF COMMONLY ADMINISTRATED NARCOTICS			
MEDICATION	**MODE**	**ONSET**	**COMMENTS**
codeine	PO	30 to 45 minutes	Do NOT administer discolored injection solutions; may also be prescribed as an antitussive or antidiarrheal.
	IM or SC	10 to 30 minutes	
hydromorphone (Dilaudid)	PO	30 minutes	Fast acting, potent narcotic, more likely to cause appetite loss than other narcotics.
	IM	15 minutes	
	IV	10 to 15 minutes	
meperidine HCL (Demerol)	PO	15 minutes	May be used by persons allergic to morphine. Use with extreme caution in clients with impaired renal function because its active metabolite accumulates in renal failure. Watch for signs of toxicity such as CNS hyperirritability. Less likely to cause smooth muscle spasm than any other narcotic, which is why it is commonly used for postoperative pain. Do not administer to children for longer than 48 hours..
	IM	10 to 15 minutes	
	IV	1 minute	
morphine sulfate	PO	60 to 90 minutes	Drug of choice in relieving pain associated with myocardial infarction. May cause transient decrease in blood pressure. Drug of choice for use with chronic cancer pain.
	IM	10 to 30 minutes	
	IV	10 minutes	
propoxyphene HCL	PO	15 to 60 minutes	May cause false decreases in urinary steroid secretion tests.
fentanyl citrate (Duragesic)	IM IV Intradermal Intrabuccal Intrathecal	7 to 15 minutes within 5 minutes within 12 hours 5 to 15 minutes immediate	Synthetic narcotic, MSO_4-like. Acts quicker; less duration

Figure 2-31

REVIEW QUESTIONS

PAIN

1. What modalities are associated with the Gate control pain theory?
2. How does past experiences with pain influence current pain experience?
3. What modalities are thought to increase the production of endogenous opiates?
4. What six factors should the nurse include when assessing the pain experience?
5. What mechanism is involved in the reduction of pain through the administration of nonsteroidal anti-inflammatory medications?
6. If narcotic agonist/antagonist drugs are administered to a client already taking narcotic drugs, what may be the result?
7. List four side effects of narcotic medications.
8. What is the antidote for narcotic-induced respiratory depression?
9. What is the first sign of tolerance to pain analgesics?
10. Which route of administration for pain medications has the quickest onset and the shortest duration?
11. List the six modalities that are considered non-invasive, non-pharmacologic pain relief measures.

ANSWERS TO REVIEW QUESTIONS

1. Massage, heat and cold, acupuncture, TENS.
2. The more pain experienced in childhood, the greater the perception of pain in adulthood or with current pain experience.
3. Acupuncture, administration of placebos, TENS.
4. Location, intensity, comfort measures, quality, chronology and subjective view of pain.
5. NSAIDs act by a peripheral mechanism at the level of damaged tissue by inhibiting prostaglandin synthesis and other chemical mediators involved in pain transmission.
6. Initiation of withdrawal symptoms.
7. Nausea/vomiting; constipation; CNS depression; respiratory depression.
8. Narcan (Naloxone)
9. Decreased duration of drug effectiveness.
10. Intravenous push or bolus.
11. Heat and cold applications; transcutaneous electrical nerve stimulation (TENS); massage; distraction, relaxation techniques; biofeedback techniques.

DEATH AND GRIEF

DESCRIPTION: Death is the last developmental task for an individual. It completes the life cycle. Grief is the process an individual goes through to deal with loss.

NURSING ASSESSMENT
Types of death:
1. Natural/expected.
2. Sudden/unexpected.
3. Suicide.

Stages of preparing for an expected death:
1. Denial.
   A. Coping style used to protect self/ego.
   B. May be noncompliant, refusing to seek treatment, ignoring symptoms.
   C. Client changes the subject when speaking about illness.
   D. Client might state, "Not me, it must be a mistake."
2. Anger.
   A. Often directed at family and/or healthcare team members.
   B. "Why me?" "It's not fair."
3. Bargaining.
   A. Usually makes a deal with God to prolong life.
   B. Usually does not share this with anyone, it is a very private experience.
4. Depression.
   A. Results from the losses experienced because of health status and hospitalization.
   B. Anticipation of the loss of life.
5. Acceptance.
   A. Accepts the inevitable.
   B. May begin to emotionally separate.

Stages of dealing with loss (grief).
1. Shock, disbelief, rejection or denial.
   A. Anger and crying.
   B. Conflicting emotions.
   C. Anger toward the deceased.
   D. Guilt.
   E. Preoccupation with loss.
2. Resolution.
   A. Process can take up to 1 year or more.
   B. Renewed interest in activities.

Complicated grief.
1. If grief unresolved, determine level of dysfunction.

2. Physical symptoms similar to the deceased.
3. Clinical depression.
4. Social isolation.
5. Failure to acknowledge loss.

ANALYSIS (NURSING DIAGNOSES)
1. Dysfunctional grief related to…
2. Powerlessness related to…

NURSING PLANS AND INTERVENTIONS
1. Encourage client to express anger in a supportive, non-threatening environment.
2. Discourage rumination.
3. Assist client in giving up idealized perception of deceased; point out misrepresentations.
4. Encourage interaction with others.
5. Assist client with identification of support systems.
6. Consult spiritual leader as indicated by client need and preference.
7. Assist client toward a comfortable, peaceful death.

> **HESI HINT:** Do not take away the coping style used in a crisis state… DENIAL. It is a very useful and needed tool at the initial stage for some. Support, do not challenge, unless it hinders/blocks treatment – endangering the patient.

REVIEW QUESTIONS
DEATH AND GRIEF
1. **Identify the five stages of death and dying.**
2. **A client has been told of a positive breast biopsy report. She asks no questions and leaves the healthcare provider's office. She is overheard telling her husband, "The doctor didn't find a thing." What coping style is operating at this stage of grief?**
3. **Your client, an incest survivor, is speaking of her deceased father, the perpetrator. "He was a wonderful man, so good and kind. Everyone thought so." What would be the most useful intervention at this time?**
4. **Your client feels responsible for his sister's death because he took her to the hospital where she died. "If I hadn't taken her there, they couldn't have**

killed her." It has been one month since her death. Is this response indicative of a normal or complicated grief reaction?
5. **Mrs. Green lost her husband three years ago. She has not disturbed any of his belongings and continues to set a place at the table for him nightly. Is this response indicative of a normal or complicated grief reaction?**

ANSWERS TO REVIEW QUESTIONS
1. Denial, Anger, Bargaining, Depression, Acceptance.
2. Denial.
3. Gently point out both the positive and negative aspects of her relationship with her father. Try to minimize the idealization of the deceased.
4. This is a normal expression of anger and guilt, which occurs. Try to minimize the rumination of these thoughts.
5. This is a dysfunctional grief reaction. Mrs. Green has never moved out of the denial stage of her grief work.

RESPIRATORY SYSTEM

PNEUMONIA

DESCRIPTION: Inflammation of the lower respiratory tract.

1. Pneumonia is commonly caused by infectious agents.
2. Pneumonia is generally classified according to causative agent:
   A. Bacterial (gram-positive and gram-negative).
   B. Viral.
   C. Fungal (rare).
3. Pneumonia may be community acquired or nosocomial (hospital/agency acquired).
4. High-risk groups include individuals who are:
   A. Debilitated with accumulated lung secretions.
   B. Cigarette smokers.
   C. Immobile.
   D. Immunosuppressed.
   E. Experiencing a depressed gag reflex.
   F. Sedated.
   G. Neuromuscular disorders.

NURSING ASSESSMENT

1. Tachypnea: shallow respirations, often with use of accessory muscles.
2. Abrupt onset of fever with shaking and chills (not reliable with elderly).
3. Productive cough with pleuritic pain.
4. Rapid, bounding pulse.
5. In the elderly, symptoms include:
   A. Confusion.
   B. Lethargy.
   C. Anorexia.
   D. Rapid respiratory rate.
6. Pain and dullness to percussion over the affected lung area.
7. Bronchial breath sounds; crackles.
8. Chest x-ray indication of infiltrates with consolidation or pleural effusion.
9. Elevated WBC.
10. ABGs indicate hypoxemia.

> **HESI HINT:** Fever can cause dehydration from excessive fluid loss in diaphoresis. Increased temperature also increases metabolism and the demand for oxygen.

> **HESI HINT:** High risk for pneumonia:
> - Any person, who has altered level of consciousness, has depressed or absent gag and cough reflexes, is susceptible to aspirating oropharyngeal secretions. (Alcoholics, anesthetized individuals, those with brain injury, drug overdose, or stroke victims.)
> - When feeding, raise the head of the bed and position the client on side - not on back.

ANALYSIS (NURSING DIAGNOSES)

1. Impaired gas exchange related to…
2. Ineffective airway clearance related to…
3. Activity intolerance related to…
4. Potential fluid volume deficit related to…

NURSING PLANS AND INTERVENTIONS

1. Assess sputum for volume, color, consistency, and clarity.
2. Assist client to cough productively by:
   A. Deep breathing every two hours (may use incentive spirometer).
   B. Using humidity to loosen secretions (may be oxygenated).
   C. Suctioning the airway, if necessary.
3. Provide fluids up to 3 liters/day unless contraindicated (helps liquefy lung secretions).
4. Assess lung sounds before and after coughing.
5. Assess rate, depth, and pattern of respirations regularly (normal adult rate is 16 to 20 breaths/min).
6. Monitor ABGs (pO_2> 80 mmHg; pCO_2 <45 mmHg).
7. Monitor O_2 saturation with pulse oximetry (ideally >95%).
8. Assess skin color.
9. Assess mental status, restlessness, irritability.
10. Administer O_2 as prescribed.
11. Monitor temperature regularly.
12. Provide adequate rest periods, including uninterrupted sleep.
13. Administer antibiotics as prescribed. *(See figure 3-1, Anti-Infectives)*
14. Teach high-risk client/family about risk factors and include preventive measures.
15. Encourage at-risk groups to get annual pneumonia and flu immunizations.

> **HESI HINT:** Bronchial breath sounds are heard over areas of density or consolidation. Sound waves are easily transmitted over consolidated tissue.

MEDICAL SURGICAL NURSING

ANTI-INFECTIVES			
DRUGS	**INDICATIONS**	**ADVERSE REACTIONS**	**NURSING IMPLICATIONS**
PENICILLINS • procaine penicillin G (Wycillin) • benzathine penicillin (BiCillin L-A) • penicillin V • (Pen.Vee.K)	• Anti-infectives • Used primarily for gram-positive infections	• Allergic reactions • Anaphylaxis • Phlebitis at IV site • Diarrhea • GI distress • Super infection • False positive for glucose using clinitest	• Use with caution in clients allergic to cephalosporins • Monitor for allergic reactions • Observe all clients for at least 30 minutes following parenteral administration • Oral penicillin G should be taken on an empty stomach • Probenecid decreases renal excretion, thereby resulting in an increased blood level of the drug • Alters contraceptive effectiveness
SEMI-SYNTHETIC • oxacillin sodium • naficillin sodium • cloxacillin sodium • dicloxacillin sodium	• Anti-infectives • Used primarily for gram-positive infections	• Allergic reactions • Anaphylaxis • Superinfection • *See Penicillins*	• Cannot be used in clients allergic to penicillin • Caution in clients allergic to cephalosporins • Monitor for superinfection (sore mouth, vaginal discharge, diarrhea, cough) • *See Penicillins*
ANTI-PSEUDOMONAL PENICILLINS & COMBINATIONS • ampicillin • ticarcillin + clavulanate (Timentin) • pipercillin + tazobactam (Zosyn) • ampicillin + sulbactam (Urasyn)	• Anti-infectives • Broad spectrums	• Similar to penicillin • Ampicillin rash	• Contraindicated in clients allergic to penicillin • *See Penicillins*

Figure 3-1

ANTI-INFECTIVES (CONTINUED)			
DRUGS	**INDICATIONS**	**ADVERSE REACTIONS**	**NURSING IMPLICATIONS**
TETRACYCLINES • tetracycline HCL • doxycycline hyclate (Vibramycin)	• Anti-infectives	• Hypersensitivity reactions • Photosensitivity	• Decrease the effectiveness of oral contraceptives • Avoid concurrent use of antacids, milk products • Inspect IV site frequently • Monitor for super infections • Avoid exposure to sunlight during use • Avoid use in pregnant clients and children under 8 years, can cause yellow-brown discoloration of teeth and growth retardation
AMINOGLYCOCIDES • gentamicin sulfate • tobramycin sulfate (Nebein) • amikacin sulfate **MISCELLANEOUS AGENT** • vancomycin hydrochloride • metronidazole (Flagyl)	• Anti-infectives • Used with gram-negative bacteria	• Neuromuscular blockade • Nephrotoxicity • Ototoxicity	• Monitor renal function, BUN, creatinine, and I&O • Monitor for ototoxicity; headache, dizziness, hearing loss, tinnitus • Monitor for super infection • Monitor for serum drug concentrations
CEPHALOSPORINS **First Generation**: • cefazolin (Kefzol) • cephalexin (Keflex) **Second Generation**: • cefaclor (Ceclor) • cefamandole (Mandol) • cefuroxime (Ceftin-po, Zinacef-IV) • cefoxitin (Mefoxin) **Third Generation**: • cefotaxime (Claforan) • ceftriaxone (Rocephin) • ceftazidime (Fortaz) • cefipime (Maxipime)	• Anti-infectives	• Allergic reactions • Thrombophlebitis • GI distress • Super infection	• Use with caution in clients allergic to penicillin and cephalosporins • *See Penicillins*
CARBAPENEMS • imipenem (Primaxin) • meropenem (Merrem) • ertapenem (Ivanz)			
MONOBACTAM • azactam	• Pseudomonas aeruginosa + many otherwise resistant organisms • Most effective against gram negatives	• Phlebitis • Pseudomembranous colitis • CNS changes • EEG changes • Headache/diplopia • Hypotension	• Monitor renal &hepatic function, especially in elderly • Carefully monitor for diarrhea • Assess motorsensory function and cardiac rhythm

Figure 3-1 (continued)

MEDICAL SURGICAL NURSING

ANTI-INFECTIVES (CONTINUED)			
DRUGS	**INDICATIONS**	**ADVERSE REACTIONS**	**NURSING IMPLICATIONS**
MACROLIDES • clarithromycin (Biaxin) • azithromycin (Zithromax) • erythromycin	• Biaxin (PO): URI, I including Strep; as adjunct treatment for *H. pylori* • Zithromax (IV)- gram negative & gram positive organism	• Pseudomembranous colitis • Phlebitis-a vesicant • Superinfections • Dizziness • Dyspnea	• Give Biaxin XL with food • Space MAO inhibitors 14 days before start & after end of Biaxin • Report diarrhea, abdominal cramping-all macrolides • Monitor liver, renal labs • PO Zithromax-give on empty stomach
FLUOROQUINOLONES • ciprofloxacin (Cipro) • levofloxacin (Levaquin) • gatifloxacin (Tequin)	• All 3 of the most difficult to treat respiratory infections, UTIs, skin, bone & joint infections • Has been used as conjunctive treatment for TB and AIDS	• Superinfections • CNS disturbances • Arrhyis & cataracts possible with Cipro • Cipro-a vesicant	• Prompt onset • Crosses placenta & in breast milk • Can lower seizure threshold • Monitor liver, renal & blood counts • Safety for children not known • Many drug-drug interactions
LINCOSAMIDES • clindamycin (Cleocin)	• PCP in AIDS • Severe infections resistant to penicillins & cephalosporins • Used in penicillin or erythromycin-sensitive clients	• Agranulocytosis • Pseudomembranous colitis • Superinfections	• Highly toxic drug; use only when absolutely necessary • Periodic liver, renal & blood counts • Report diarrhea immediately
STREPTOGRAMIN • Quinipristin/ dalfopristin (Synercid)	• Life-threatening VRE	• Arthralgia, myalgia • Severe versicant • Pseudomembranous colitis • N/V, diarrhea • Rash, pruritis	• Incompatible with any saline solutions or heparin • Functionally related to both macrolides & lincosamides • Monitor total bilirubin • Many drug-drug interactions
OXAZOLIDINONE • Zyvox	• Life-threatening VRE & MRSA	• GI disturbances • Headache • Pancytopenia • Pseudomembranous colitis • Superinfections	• Monitor renal & liver labs, + blood count • May exacerbate hypertension especially if ingests foods with tyramine • Report diarrhea immediately

Figure 3-1 (continued)

CHRONIC OBSTRUCTIVE PULMONARY (LUNG) DISEASE (COPD)

DESCRIPTION: A chronic, progressive condition characterized by obstruction of airflow entering or leaving the lungs.

1. Common to have exacerbations and remissions. During exacerbation, the client is acutely ill.
2. Illness types include:
    A. Emphysema.
    B. Chronic bronchitis.
    C. Asthma.
3. Alveoli beyond the chronic obstruction are over inflated, causing chronic hypoxemia, hypoxia, and hypercapnia (trapped CO_2).

> **HESI HINT:** Compensation occurs over time in clients with chronic lung disease, and arterial blood gasses (ABGs) are altered. It is imperative that baseline data are obtained on the client.

OBSTRUCTIVE LUNG DISORDERS

	CHRONIC BRONCHITIS	EMPHYSEMA	ASTHMA
PATHOPHYSIOLOGY	• Chronic sputum with cough production on a daily basis for a minimum of 3 months/ year • Chronic hypoxemia/ cor pulmonale • Increase in mucus, cilia production • Increase in bronchial wall thickness (obstructs air flow) • Reduced responsiveness of respiratory center to hypoxemic stimuli	• Reduced gas exchange surface area • Increased air trapping (increased A-P diameter) • Decreased capillary network • Increased work / increased O_2 consumption	• Narrowing or closure of the airway due to a variety of stimulants
PRECIPITATING FACTORS	• Higher incidence with smokers	• Cigarette smoking • Environment and/or occupational exposure • Genetic	• Mucosal edema • V/Q abnormalities • Increased work of breathing • Beta blockers • Respiratory infection • Allergic reaction • Emotional stress • Exercise • Environmental or occupational exposure • Reflux esophagitis
ASSESSMENT	• Generalized cyanosis • "Blue Bloaters" • Right-sided heart failure • Distended neck veins • Crackles • Expiratory wheezes	• "Pink puffers" • Barrel chest • Pursed lip breathers • Distant, quiet breath sounds • Wheezes • Pulmonary blebs on x-ray	• Dyspnea, wheezing, chest tightness • Assess precipitating factors • Medication history
NURSING PLANS AND INTERVENTIONS	• Lowest FiO_2 possible to prevent CO_2 retention • Monitor for s/s of fluid overload • Maintain PaO_2 between 55 to 60 • Baseline ABGs • Teach pursed lip breathing and diaphragmatic breathing • Teach tripod position	• Lowest FiO_2 possible to prevent CO_2 retention • Monitor for s/s of fluid overload • Maintain PaO_2 between 55 to 60 • Baseline ABG's • Teach pursed lip breathing and diaphragmatic breathing • Teach tripod position	• Administer bronchodialators • Administer fluids and humidification • Education (etiology, medication regime) • ABG's • Ventilatory patterns

Figure 3-2

MEDICAL SURGICAL NURSING

NURSING ASSESSMENT

1. Changes in breathing pattern (for example, an increase in rate with a decrease in depth).
2. Use of accessory breathing muscles (barrel chest).
3. Generalized cyanosis of lips, mucous membranes, face, nail beds ("blue bloater").
4. Cough (dry or productive).
5. Higher CO_2 than average.
6. Low O_2, as determined by pulse oximetry.
7. Decreased breath sounds.
8. Coarse crackles in lung fields which tend to disappear after coughing, wheezing.
9. Dyspnea, orthopnea.
10. Poor nutrition.
11. Activity intolerance.
12. Anxiety concerning breathing; manifested by:
    A. Anger.
    B. Fear of being alone.
    C. Fear of not being able to "catch breath."

> **HESI HINT:** Productive cough and comfort can be facilitated by semi-Fowler's or high Fowler's positions, which lessen pressure on the diaphragm from abdominal organs. Gastric distention becomes a priority in these clients because it elevates the diaphragm and inhibits full lung expansion.

> **HESI HINT:** NORMAL ABG VALUES
>
> | Bld. Gas | Adult | Child |
> |---|---|---|
> | pH | 7.35 to 7.45 | 7.36 to 7.44 |
> | Pco$_2$ | 35 to 45 mmHg | Same as adult |
> | Po$_2$ | 80 to 100 mmHg | Same as adult |
> | HCO$_3$ | 22 to 26 mEq/L | Same as adult |

> **HESI HINT:** Pink Puffer: Barrel chest is indicative of emphysema and is caused by use of accessory muscles to breathe, which causes the person to work harder to breathe, but the amount of O_2 taken in is adequate to oxygenate the tissues.
> Blue Bloater: Insufficient oxygenation occurs with chronic bronchitis and leads to generalized cyanosis and often right-sided heart failure.

ANALYSIS (NURSING DIAGNOSES)

1. Ineffective airway clearance related to…
2. Ineffective breathing pattern related to…
3. Impaired gas exchange related to…
4. Activity intolerance related to…

> **HESI HINT:** Cells of the body depend on oxygen to carry out their functions. Inadequate arterial oxygenation is manifested by cyanosis and slow capillary refill (<3 seconds). A chronic sign is clubbing of the fingernails, and a late sign is clubbing of the fingers.

NURSING PLANS AND INTERVENTIONS

1. Teach to sit upright and bend slightly forward to promote breathing.
    A. In bed - sitting with arms resting on overbed table (tripod position).
    B. In chair - leaning forward with elbows resting on knees (tripod position).
2. Teach diaphragmatic and pursed-lip breathing. Teach prolonged expiratory phase to clear trapped air.
3. Administer O_2 at 1 to 2 liters per nasal cannula. *(See figure 3-6, Nursing Skills: Respiratory Client)*

> **HESI HINT:** Caution must be used in administering O_2 to a COPD client. The stimulus to breathe is hypoxia (hypoxic drive) not the usual hypercapnia, the stimulus to breathe for healthy persons. Therefore, if too much oxygen is given, the client may stop breathing!

4. Pace activities to conserve energy.
5. Maintain adequate dietary intake.
    A. Small, frequent meals.
    B. Favorite foods.
    C. Dietary supplements.
6. Provide an adequate fluid intake (3 liters/day).
7. Instruct in relaxation techniques (teach when not in distress).
8. Teach prevention of secondary infections.
9. Teach about medication regime. *(See figure 3-3, Bronchodilators/Corticosteroids)*
10. Smoking cessation is imperative. Teach proper technique for inhalers.
11. Encourage health promotion activities.

BRONCHODILATORS/CORTICOSTEROIDS

DRUGS	INDICATIONS	ADVERSE REACTIONS	NURSING IMPLICATIONS
ADRENERGICS/ SYMPATHOMEMETICS • epinephrine • isoproterenol HCL (Isuprel) • albuterol (Proventil) • isoetharine (Bronuometer) • terbutaline (Brethine) • salmeterol (Serevent) metaproterenol (inhaled) (Alupint) • levalbuterol (Xopenex)	• Bronchodilator	• Anxiety • Increased heart rate • Nausea, vomiting • Urinary retention	• Check heart rate • Monitor for urinary retention especially in men over 40 • Instruct in proper use of inhaler • Use bronchodilator inhaler before steroid inhaler • May cause sleep disturbance
METHYLXANTHINE • aminophylline (IV) • theophylline (PO)	• Bronchodilator	• GI distress • Sleeplessness • Cardiac dysrhythmias • Hyperactivity	• Administer oral forms with food • Avoid foods containing caffeine • Check heart rate • Instruct in proper use of inhaler • Monitor therapeutic range 10 to 20 mg/ml • Crosses placenta
CORTICOSTEROIDS • prednisone (PO) • solu-medrol (IV) • beclomethasone dispropionate (inhaled) (Vanceril) • budesonide (inhaled) (Pulmicort) • fluticasone (inhaled) (Flovent) • triamcinolone (inhaled) (Azmacort) • flunisolide (inhaled) (Aerobid)	• Anti-inflammatory	• Cardiac dysrhythmias which occur with long-term steroid use	• *See Endocrine Disorders in Medical Surgical Nursing* • Instruct in proper use of inhaler
ANTICHOLINERGICS • ipratropium (Atrovent)	• Bronchodilator • Control rhinnorrhea	• Dry mouth • Blurred vision • Cough	• Do not exceed 12 doses in 24 hours

Figure 3-3

MEDICAL SURGICAL NURSING

BRONCHODILATORS/CORTICOSTEROIDS (CONTINUED)			
DRUGS	**INDICATIONS**	**ADVERSE REACTIONS**	**NURSING IMPLICATIONS**
COMBINATION PRODUCTS • fluticasone + salmetero (Advair) • ipratropium + albuterol (Combivent)	• See individual drugs	• See individual drugs	• See individual drugs

Figure 3-3 (continued)

HESI HINT: When asked to prioritize nursing actions, use the ABC rule:
• **Airway first**
• **Then breathing**
• **Then circulation**

HESI HINT: *Look and Listen!* If breath sounds are clear, but the client is cyanotic and lethargic, adequate oxygenation is not occurring.

HESI HINT: The key to respiratory status is assessment of breath sounds as well as visualization of the client. Breath sounds are better "described," not named, e.g., sounds should be described as "crackles," "wheeze," "high-pitched whistling-sound," rather than "rales," rhonchi," etc., which may not mean the same thing to each clinical professional.

HESI HINT: Watch for NCLEX-RN® questions that deal with oxygen delivery. In adults, O_2 must bubble through some type of water solution so it can be humidified if given at > 4 L/min or delivered directly to the trachea. If given at 1 to 4 L/min or by mask or nasal prongs, the oropharynx and nasal pharynx provide adequate humidification.

CANCER OF THE LARYNX

DESCRIPTION: Neoplasm occurring in the larynx, most commonly squamous cell in origin.
1. Prolonged use of alcohol and/or tobacco is directly related to development.
2. Other contributing factors include the following:
   A. Vocal straining.
   B. Chronic laryngitis.
   C. Family predisposition.
   D. Industrial exposure to carcinogens.
   E. Nutritional deficiencies.
3. Men are affected eight times more often than women.
4. Diagnosis usually occurs between ages 55 and 70.
5. Earliest sign is hoarseness or a change in vocal quality.
6. Medical management includes radiation therapy, often with adjuvant chemotherapy or surgical removal of the larynx (laryngectomy).

NURSING ASSESSMENT
1. MRI.
2. Direct laryngoscopy.
3. Hoarseness for greater than 2 weeks (early).
4. Color changes in mouth or tongue.

HESI HINT: With cancer of the larynx, the tongue and mouth often appear white, gray, dark brown, or black, and may appear patchy.

5. Later changes include: dysphagia, dyspnea, cough, hemoptysis, weight loss, neck pain radiating to the ear, enlarged cervical nodes, halitosis.
6. X-rays of head, neck, and chest.
7. CT scan of neck and biopsy.

ANALYSIS (NURSING DIAGNOSES)
Client undergoing a laryngectomy:
1. Anxiety related to…
2. Ineffective airway clearance related to…
3. Impaired verbal communication related to…

NURSING PLANS AND INTERVENTIONS
Provide preoperative teaching.
1. Allow client/family to observe and handle tracheostomy tubes and suctioning equipment.
2. Explain how and why suctioning will take place after surgery.
3. Plan for acceptable communication method after surgery. Consider literacy level.
4. Refer to speech pathologist.
5. Discuss the planned rehabilitation program.

Provide postoperative care.
1. Simplify communications.
2. Utilize planned alternate communication method.
3. Keep call bell/light within reach at all times.
4. Ask client yes/no questions whenever possible.

Promote respiratory functioning.
1. Assess respiratory rate and characteristics every 1 to 2 hours.
2. Keep bed in semi-Fowler's position at all times.
3. Keep laryngeal airway humidified at all times.
4. Auscultate lung sounds every 2 to 4 hours.
5. Provide tracheostomy care every 2 to 4 hours and PRN.

> **HESI HINT:** Tracheostomy care involves cleaning the inner cannula, suctioning, and applying a clean dressing.

6. Administer tube feedings as prescribed.
7. Encourage ambulation as early as possible.
8. Refer for speech rehabilitation with artificial larynx and/or to learn esophageal speech.

> **HESI HINT:** Air entering the lungs is humidified along the naso-bronchial tree. This natural humidifying pathway is gone for the client who has had a laryngectomy. If the air is not humidified before entering the lungs, secretions tend to thicken and become crusty.

> **HESI HINT:** A laryngectomy tube has a larger lumen and is shorter than the tracheostomy tube. Observe the client for any signs of bleeding or occlusion, which are the greatest immediate postoperative risks (first 24-hours).

> **HESI HINT:** Fear of choking is very real for laryngectomy clients. They cannot cough as before because the glottis is gone. Teach the "glottal stop" technique to remove secretions (take a deep breath, momentarily occlude the tracheostomy tube, cough, and simultaneously remove the finger from the tube).

TUBERCULOSIS
DESCRIPTION: Communicable lung disease caused by an infection with the *Mycobacterium tuberculosis* bacteria.

1. Airborne transmission.
2. After initial exposure, the bacteria encapsulates (forms Ghon's lesion).
3. Bacteria remain dormant until a later time when clinical symptoms appear.

NURSING ASSESSMENT
Often asymptomatic. Symptoms include:
1. Fever with night sweats.
2. Anorexia, weight loss.
3. Malaise, fatigue.
4. Cough, Hemoptysis.
5. Dyspnea, pleuritic chest pain with inspiration.
6. Cavitation or calcification as evidenced on chest x-ray.
7. Positive sputum culture.

> **HESI HINT:** TB SKIN TEST:
> A positive TB skin test is exhibited by an induration 10 mm or greater in diameter 48 hours after skin test. Anyone who has received a BCG vaccine will have a positive skin test and must be evaluated using a chest x-ray.

ANALYSIS (NURSING DIAGNOSES)
1. Knowledge deficit related to…
2. Potential for infection of others related to…
3. Altered nutrition: less than body requirements related to…

NURSING PLANS AND INTERVENTIONS
1. Provide client teaching.
   A. Cough into tissues and dispose of immediately into special bags.
   B. Take all prescribed medications daily for 9 to 12 months.
   C. **Wash hands** using proper handwashing technique.
   D. Report symptoms of deteriorating condition, especially hemorrhage.
2. Collect sputum cultures as needed; client may return to work after three (3) negative cultures.
3. Place client in respiratory isolation while hospitalized.
4. Administer antituberculosis medications as prescribed. *(See figure 3-4, Anti-tuberculosis Drugs)*
5. Refer client and high-risk persons to local or state health department for testing and prophylactic treatment.

ANTITUBERCULOSIS DRUGS

DRUGS	INDICATIONS	ADVERSE REACTIONS	NURSING INTERVENTION
ANTIMYCOBACTERIAL • **isoniazid** (INH) • **rifampin** (Rifabutin-Mycobutia) • **ethambutol** • **pyrazinamide** (Tebrazid)	Tuberculosis	• Hepatitis with INH and rifampin • Neuropathy with INH • Optic neuritis and skin rash with ethambutol • Hepatoxicity with pyrazinamide • Hyperuricemia	• Give pyridoxine (vitamin B6) with INH to counteract neuropathy • Antituberculosis agents are given together in treatment of TB • Monitor liver function tests • Use with caution in clients with renal disease
ANTIFUNGAL AGENTS • **amphotericin B** (Fungizone) • **nystatin** (Nilstat)	Systemic fungal infections	• Nausea, vomiting • Tinnitus • Nephrotoxicity • Febrile reactions	• Check IV site frequently for leakage – a vesicant • Observe for side effects which are common • Protect solutions from light • Monitor BUN, creatinine, and CBC • Monitor vital signs every 30 minutes for 4 hours during initial IV therapy

Figure 3-4

> **HESI HINT:** Teaching is very important with the TB client. Drug therapy is usually long term (9 months or longer). It is essential that the client take the medications as prescribed for the entire time. Skipping doses or prematurely terminating the drug therapy can result in a public health hazard.

> **HESI HINT:** TEACHING POINTS - Rifampin: Reduces effectiveness of oral contraceptives; should use other birth control methods during treatment; gives body fluids orange tinge; stains soft contacts. Isoniazid (INH): Increases Dilantin levels. Ethambutal: Vision check before starting therapy and monthly; may have to take 1 to 2 years longer.
>
> Teach rationale for combination drug therapy to increase compliance. Resistance develops more slowly if several anti-Tb drugs given, instead of just one drug at a time.

LUNG CANCER

DESCRIPTION: Neoplasm occurring in the lung.
1. Lung cancer is the number one cancer killer of men in the United States and is increasing rapidly among women.
2. Cigarette smoking is a common cause of lung cancer.
3. Exposure to occupational hazards such as asbestos and radioactive dust pose significant risk.
4. Lung cancer tends to appear years after exposure; it is most commonly seen in persons in the fifth or sixth decade of life.
5. Lung cancer has a poor prognosis; five-year survival rate is approximately 10%.

NURSING ASSESSMENT
1. Dry, hacking cough early with cough turning productive as disease progresses.
2. Hoarseness.
3. Dyspnea.
4. Hemoptysis; rust-colored or purulent sputum.
5. Pain in the chest area.
6. Diminished breath sounds, occasional wheezing.
7. Abnormal chest x-ray.
8. Positive sputum for cytology.

ANALYSIS (NURSING DIAGNOSES)
1. Pain related to…
2. Ineffective breathing pattern related to…
3. Impaired gas exchange related to…
4. Altered nutrition: less than body requirements related to…

Nursing interventions are similar to those implemented for the client with COPD:

1. Place client in semi-Fowler's position.
2. Teach pursed lip breathing to improve gas exchange.
3. Teach relaxation techniques; client often becomes anxious about breathing difficulty.
4. Administer oxygen, as indicated by pulse oximetry or arterial blood gases (ABGs).
5. Take measures to allay anxiety:
   A. Keep client/family informed of impending tests and procedures.
   B. Give client as much control as possible over personal care.
   C. Encourage client/family to verbalize concerns.
6. Decrease pain to manageable level by administering analgesics as needed (within safety range for respiratory difficulty).
7. Surgery – thoractomy for clients who have a resectable tumor.
   A. Pneumonectomy – removal of entire lung.
      1) Position on operative side or back.
      2) Chest tubes not usually used.
   B. Lobectomy and segmental resection.
      1) Position on back or non-operative side.
      2) Check that tubing is not kinked or obstructed.
      3) Chest tubes usually inserted. *(See figure 3-5, Chest Tubes)*

> **HESI HINT:** Some tumors are so large that they fill entire lobes of the lung. When removed, large spaces are left. Chest tubes are not usually used with these clients because it is helpful if the mediastinal cavity, where the lung used to be, fills up with fluid. This fluid helps prevent a shift of the remaining chest organs to fill the empty space

   C. Chest tubes:
      1) Encourage client to cough and deep breathe or to use incentive spirometry at least every two hours.
      2) Maintain a dry occlusive dressing to the chest tube site at all times.
      3) Check all connections in the drainage system every 4 to 8 hours. (Tape to prevent disconnections.)
      4) Monitor chest tube bottles if suctioning is used (bubbling in suction control chamber indicates proper suctioning).
      5) Monitor straw in water seal chamber for fluctuation with respirations.
      6) Measure chest tube drainage by marking on the exterior of the drainage unit.
      7) More than 100 cc/hour is considered a large amount for adults and must be reported to healthcare provider.

> **HESI HINT: CHEST TUBES**
> - If the chest tube becomes disconnected, do not clamp! Immediately place the end of the tube in a container of sterile saline or water until a new drainage system can be connected.
> - If the chest tube is accidentally removed from the client, the nurse should apply pressure immediately with an occlusive dressing and notify the healthcare provider.

8. Chemotherapy:
   A. Attend to immunosuppression factor. *(See Oncology)*
   B. Administer antiemetics prior to administration of chemotherapy.
   C. Take precautions for the administration of antineoplastics. *(See Oncology)*
9. Radiation therapy:
   A. Provide skin care according to healthcare provider's request.
   B. Instruct the client NOT to wash off the lines drawn by the radiologist.
   C. Instruct client to wear soft, cotton garments only.
   D. Avoid use of powders or creams to radiation site unless specified by radiologist.

CHEST TUBES

- Used to remove or drain blood or air from the intrapleural space, to expand the lung after surgery, or to restore sub-atmospheric pressure to the thoracic cavity.
- Many brands of commercial chest drainage systems are available; all are based upon the traditional three-bottle water seal system.

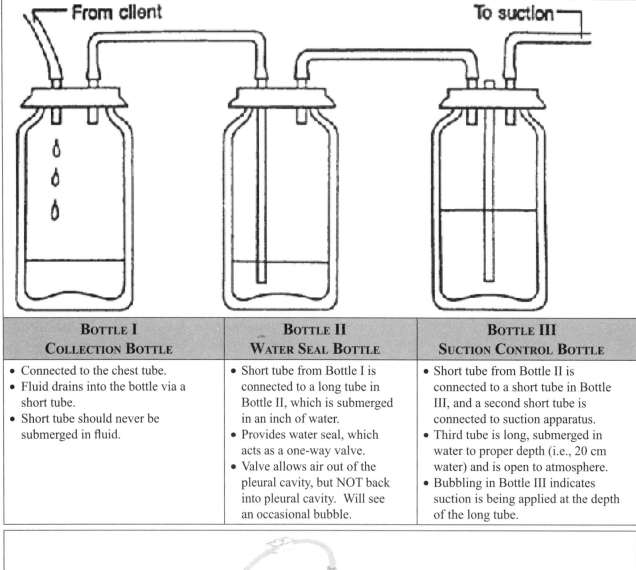

BOTTLE I COLLECTION BOTTLE	BOTTLE II WATER SEAL BOTTLE	BOTTLE III SUCTION CONTROL BOTTLE
• Connected to the chest tube. • Fluid drains into the bottle via a short tube. • Short tube should never be submerged in fluid.	• Short tube from Bottle I is connected to a long tube in Bottle II, which is submerged in an inch of water. • Provides water seal, which acts as a one-way valve. • Valve allows air out of the pleural cavity, but NOT back into pleural cavity. Will see an occasional bubble.	• Short tube from Bottle II is connected to a short tube in Bottle III, and a second short tube is connected to suction apparatus. • Third tube is long, submerged in water to proper depth (i.e., 20 cm water) and is open to atmosphere. • Bubbling in Bottle III indicates suction is being applied at the depth of the long tube.

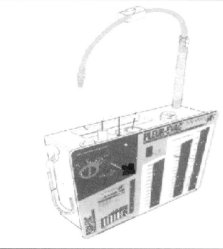

DISPOSABLE
CLOSED CHEST DRAINAGE SYSTEM

Figure 3-5

HESI HINT: Chest tube NCLEX-RN® content: Fluctuations (tidaling) in the fluid will occur if there is no external suction. These fluctuating movements are a good indicator that the system is intact and should move upward with each inspiration and downward with each expiration. If fluctuations cease, check for kinked tubing, accumulation of fluid in the tubing, occlusions, or change in the client's position, since expanding lung tissue may be occluding the tube opening. Remember, when external suction is applied the fluctuations cease. Most hospitals DO NOT MILK chest tubes as a means of clearing or preventing clots – it is too easy to remove chest tubes. Mediastinal tubes may have orders to be stripped because of location, compared to larger thoracic cavity tubes.

NURSING SKILLS: RESPIRATORY CLIENT

SUCTIONING (TRACHEAL)

- Suction when adventitious breath sounds are heard, when secretions are present at endotracheal tube, or when gurgling sounds are noted.
- Use aseptic/sterile technique throughout procedure.
- Wear mask and goggles.
- May liquefy secretions with 3 ml saline instilled prior to suctioning.
- Advance catheter until resistance is felt.
- Apply suction only when withdrawing catheter (gently rotate catheter when withdrawing).
- Never suction more than 10 to 15 seconds and only pass the catheter 3 times or less.
- Oxygenate with 100% O_2 for 1 to 2 minutes before suctioning and after to prevent hypoxia.

MAINTAIN VENTILATOR SETTING

- Verify that alarms are on.
- Maintain settings and check often to insure they are specifically set as prescribed by healthcare provider.
- Verify functioning of ventilator at least every four (4) hours.

OXYGEN ADMINISTRATION

- Nasal cannula: low oxygen flow for low oxygen concentrations (good for COPD).
- Simple face mask: low flow but effectively delivers high oxygen concentrations; cannot deliver <40% O_2.
- Non-rebreather mask: low flow but delivers high oxygen concentrations (60 to 90%).
- Partial rebreather mask: low flow oxygen reservoir bag attached; can deliver high oxygen concentrations.
- Venturi mask: high flow system; can deliver exact oxygen concentration.

PULSE OXIMETRY

- Easy measurement of oxygen saturation.
- Should be >90%, ideally above 95%.
- Noninvasive, fastens to finger, toe, or earlobe.

TRACHEOSTOMY CARE

- Aseptic technique (remove inner cannula only from stoma).
- Clean inner cannula with H_2O_2 – rinse with sterile saline.
- 4x4 gauze dressing is butterfly folded.

RESPIRATORY ISOLATION TECHNIQUE

- Mask required for anyone entering room.
- Private room required.
- Client must wear mask if leaving room.

PROPER USE OF AN INHALER

- Have client exhale completely.
- Only grip mouthpiece (in mouth) if client has a spacer, otherwise keep the mouth open to bring in volume of air with misted medication. While inhaling slowly, push down firmly on the inhaler to release the medication.
- Use bronchodilator inhaler before steroid inhaler.

Figure 3-6

HESI HINT: Various pathophysiological conditions can be related to the nursing diagnosis "Ineffective Breathing Patterns."

1. Inability of air sacs to fill and empty properly (emphysema, cystic fibrosis)
2. Obstruction of the air passages (carcinoma, asthma, chronic bronchitis)
3. Accumulation of fluid in the air sacs (pneumonia)
4. Respiratory muscle fatigue (COPD, pneumonia)

REVIEW QUESTIONS

RESPIRATORY SYSTEM

1. List four common symptoms of pneumonia the nurse might note on physical exam.
2. State four nursing interventions for assisting the client to cough productively.
3. What symptoms of pneumonia might the nurse expect to see in an older client?
4. What should the O_2 flow rate be for the client with COPD?
5. How does the nurse prevent hypoxia during suctioning?
6. During mechanical ventilation, what are three major nursing interventions?
7. When examining a client with emphysema, what physical findings is the nurse likely to see?
8. What is the most common risk factor associated with lung cancer?
9. Describe the preoperative nursing care for a client undergoing a laryngectomy.
10. List five nursing interventions after chest tube insertion.
11. What immediate action should the nurse take when a chest tube becomes disconnected from a bottle or suction apparatus? What should the nurse do if a chest tube is accidentally removed from the client?
12. What instructions should be given to a client following radiation therapy?
13. What precautions are required for clients with TB when placed on respiratory isolation?
14. List four components of teaching for the client with tuberculosis.

ANSWERS TO REVIEW QUESTIONS

1. Tachypnea, fever with chills, productive cough, bronchial breath sounds.
2. Deep breathing, fluid intake increased to 3 liters/day, use humidity to loosen secretions, suction airway to stimulate coughing.
3. Confusion, lethargy, anorexia, rapid respiratory rate.
4. 1 to 2 liters per nasal cannula, too much O_2 may eliminate the COPD client's stimulus to breathe. A COPD client has a hypoxic drive to breathe.
5. Deliver 100% oxygen (hyperinflating) before and after each endotracheal suctioning.
6. Monitor client's respiratory status and secure connections, establish a communication mechanism with the client, keep airway clear by coughing/suctioning.
7. Barrel chest, dry or productive cough, decreased breath sounds, dyspnea, crackles in lung fields.
8. Smoking.
9. Involve family/client in manipulation of tracheostomy equipment before surgery, plan acceptable communication method, refer to speech pathologist, discuss rehabilitation program.
10. Maintain a dry occlusive dressing to chest tube site at all times. Check all connections every 4 hours. Make sure Bottle III or end chamber is bubbling. Measure chest tube drainage by marking level on outside of drainage unit. Encourage use of incentive spirometry every 2 hours.
11. Place end in container of sterile water. Apply an occlusive dressing and notify healthcare provider STAT.
12. Do NOT wash off lines; wear soft cotton garments, avoid use of powders/creams on radiation site.
13. Mask for anyone entering room; private room; client MUST wear mask if leaving room.
14. Cough into tissues and dispose immediately into special bags. Long-term need for daily medication. Good handwashing technique. Report symptoms of deterioration, i.e., blood in secretions.

RENAL SYSTEM

ACUTE RENAL FAILURE (ARF)

DESCRIPTION: Abrupt deterioration of the renal system, a reversible syndrome.

> **HESI HINT:** Normally, kidneys excrete approximately 1 ml of urine per kg of body weight per hour, which is about 1 to 2 liters in a 24-hour period for adults.

1. Acute renal failure occurs when metabolites accumulate in the body and urinary output changes.
2. There are three major types of acute renal failure. *(See figure 3-7, Acute Renal Failure)*
3. There are three phases of acute renal failure.
   A. Oliguric phase.
   B. Diuretic phase.
   C. Recovery phase.

ACUTE RENAL FAILURE		
TYPES	**DESCRIPTION**	**ETIOLOGICAL FACTORS**
PRERENAL	Interference with renal perfusion	• Hemorrhage • Hypovolemia • Decreased cardiac output • Decreased renal perfusion
INTRARENAL	Damage to renal parenchyma	• Prolonged prerenal state • Nephrotoxins • Intratubular obstruction • Infections (glomerulonephritis) • Renal injury • Vascular lesions • Acute pyelonephritis
POSTRENAL	Obstruction in the urinary tract anywhere from the tubules to the urethral meatus	• Calculi • Prostatic hypertrophy • Tumors

NURSING ASSESSMENT
1. History of taking nephrotoxic drugs (salicylates, antibiotics, NSAIDS).
2. Alterations in urinary output.
3. Edema, weight gain (ask if waistbands have suddenly become too tight).
4. Change in mental status.

> **HESI HINT:** Electrolytes are profoundly affected by kidney problems (favorite NCLEX-RN® topic). There must be a balance between extracellular fluid and intracellular fluid to maintain homeostasis. A change in the number of ions or in the amount of fluid will cause a shift in one direction or the other. Sodium and chloride are the primary extracellular ions. Potassium and phosphate are the primary intracellular ions.

5. Diagnostic findings in the oliguric phase:
   A. Increased BUN and creatinine.
   B. Increased potassium (hyperkalemia).
   C. Decreased sodium (hyponatremia).
   D. Decreased pH (acidosis).
   E. Fluid overloaded (hypervolemic).
   F. High urine specific gravity >1.020.
6. Diagnostic findings in the diuretic phase:
   A. Decreased fluid volume (hypovolemia).
   B. Decreased potassium (hypokalemia).
   C. Further decrease in sodium (hyponatremia).
   D. Low urine specific gravity.
7. Diagnostic lab work returns to normal range in recovery phase.

> **HESI HINT:** In some cases, persons in ARF may not experience the oliguric phase but may progress directly to the diuretic phase during which the urine output may be as much as 10 liters per day.

ANALYSIS (NURSING DIAGNOSES)
1. Fluid volume overload related to…
2. Fluid volume deficit related to…
3. Anxiety related to…
4. Altered nutrition: Less than body requirements related to…

NURSING PLANS AND INTERVENTIONS

1. Monitor I&O accurately: give only enough fluids in oliguric phase to replace losses; usually 400 to 500 ml/24 hrs.
2. Document and report any change in fluid volume status.
3. Monitor lab values for both serum and urine to assess electrolyte status, especially hyperkalemia indicated by serum potassium levels over 7 mEq/L and ECG changes.
4. Assess level of consciousness for subtle changes.
5. Weigh daily: in oliguric phase gain up to 1 lb/day.
6. Prevent cross infection.
7. Kayexalate may be prescribed if K+ too high.

> **HESI HINT:** Body weight is a good indicator of fluid retention and renal status. Obtain accurate weights on all clients with renal failure – done on the same scale at the same time every day.

> **HESI HINT:** Fluid Volume Alterations
> **Fluid Excess symptoms:**
> - Dyspnea
> - Tachycardia
> - Jugular vein distension
> - Peripheral edema
> - Pulmonary edema
> **Fluid deficit symptoms:**
> - Decreased urine output
> - Reduction in body weight
> - Decreased skin turgor
> - Dry mucous membranes
> - Hypotension
> - Tachycardia

8. Provide low-protein, moderate-fat, high carbohydrate diet.

> **HESI HINT:** Watch for signs of hyperkalemia: dizziness, weakness, cardiac irregularities, muscle cramps, diarrhea, and nausea.

> **HESI HINT:** Potassium has a critical safe range (3.5 to 5.0 mEq/L) because it affects the heart, and any imbalance must be corrected by medications or dietary modification. *Limit high potassium foods* (bananas, avocados, spinach, fish) *and salt substitutes, which are high in potassium.*

> **HESI HINT:** Clients with renal failure retain sodium. With water retention, the sodium becomes diluted and serum levels may appear near normal. With excessive water retention, the sodium levels appear decreased (dilution). Limit fluid and sodium intake in ARF clients.

9. Monitor cardiac rate and rhythm (acute cardiac arrhythmias are usually related to hyperkalemia).
10. Monitor drug levels and interactions.

> **HESI HINT:** During oliguric phase, minimize protein breakdown and prevent rise in BUN by limiting protein intake. When the BUN and creatinine return to normal, ARF is determined to be resolved.

CHRONIC RENAL FAILURE END STAGE RENAL DISEASE (ESRD)

DESCRIPTION: Progressive, irreversible damage to the nephrons and glomeruli resulting in uremia.

1. Causes of chronic renal failure are multitudinous.
2. As renal function diminishes, dialysis becomes necessary.
3. Transplantation is an alternative to dialysis for some clients.

NURSING ASSESSMENT

1. History of high medication usage.
2. Family history of renal disease.
3. Increased BP.
4. Edema, pulmonary edema.
5. Neurologic impairment (weakness, drowsiness).
6. Decreasing urinary function:
   A. Hematuria.
   B. Proteinuria.
   C. Cloudy urine.
   D. Oliguric (100 to 400 ml/day).
   E. Anuric (less than 100 ml/day).

> **HESI HINT:** Accumulation of waste products from protein metabolism is the primary cause of uremia. Protein must be restricted in CRF clients. However, if protein intake is inadequate, a negative nitrogen balance occurs causing muscle wasting. The glomerular filtration rate (GFR) is most often used as an indicator of level of protein consumption.

7. Yellowish skin.
8. GI upsets.
9. Metallic taste in mouth.
10. Ammonia breath.
11. Dialysis. *(See figure 3-9, Renal Dialysis)*

HESI HINT:

DIALYSIS COVERED BY MEDICARE

- All persons in the United States are eligible for Medicare as of their first day of dialysis under special End Stage Renal Disease funding.
- Medicare card will indicate ESRD.
- Transplantation is covered by Medicare procedure; coverage terminates six months postoperative if dialysis is no longer required.

12. Previous kidney transplant.
13. Lab information:
    A. Azotemia.
    B. Increased creatinine and BUN.
    C. Decreased calcium.
    D. Elevated phosphorus and magnesium.

ANALYSIS (NURSING DIAGNOSES)

1. Fluid volume excess related to…
2. Altered nutrition: less than body requirements related to…
3. Decreased cardiac output related to…

NURSING PLANS AND INTERVENTIONS

1. Monitor serum electrolyte levels.
2. Weigh daily.
3. Strict I&O.
4. Check for jugular vein distension (JVD) and other signs of fluid overload.
5. Monitor edema, pulmonary edema.
6. Provide low-protein, low-sodium, low potassium, low phosphate diet.

HESI HINT: Protein intake is restricted until blood chemistry shows ability to handle protein catabolites: urea, creatinine. Ensure high calorie intake so protein is spared for its own work: give hard candy, jelly beans, flavored carbohydrate powders.

7. Administer aluminum hydroxide antacids to bind phosphates because client is unable to excrete phosphates (no magnesium-based antacids). Timing is important!
8. Encourage protein intake to be of high biologic value (eggs, milk, meat) because the client is on a low-protein diet.
9. Alternate periods of rest with periods of activity.
10. Encourage strict adherence to medication regime; teach client to obtain healthcare provider's permission before taking ANY over-the-counter medications.
11. Observe for complications:
    A. Anemia, administer antianemic drug. *(See figure 3-8, Antianemic)*
    B. Renal osteodystrophy (abnormal calcium metabolism causes bone pathology).
    C. Severe, resistant hypertension.
    D. Infection.
    E. Metabolic acidosis.
12. Living related or cadaver renal transplant.
    A. Monitor for rejection.
    B. Monitor for infection.
    C. Teach client to meticulously maintain immunosuppressive drug therapy.

ANTIANEMIC: BIOLOGIC RESPONSE MODIFIER (BRM)			
DRUGS	**INDICATIONS**	**ADVERSE REACTIONS**	**NURSING INTERVENTIONS**
erythropoietin (Epogen)	• Anemia due to decreased production of erythropoietin in end stage renal disease. • Stimulates RBC production, increases Hgb, reticulocyte count, and Hct	• Use with caution in the elderly because increased risk of thrombosis	• Monitor Hct weekly, report levels over 30 to 33% or increases of more than 4 points in less than 2 weeks. • Explain that pelvic and limb pain should dissipate after 12 hours. • Do not shake vial. Shaking may inactivate the glycoprotein. • Discard unused contents – does not contain preservatives.

Figure 3-8

HESI HINT: As kidneys fail, medications must often be adjusted. Of particular importance is digoxin toxicity since digitalis preparations are excreted by the kidneys. Signs of toxicity in adults include nausea, vomiting, anorexia, visual disturbances, restlessness, headache, cardiac arrhythmias, and pulse <60 beats per minute.

RENAL DIALYSIS

TYPES OF DIALYSIS	DESCRIPTION	NURSING IMPLICATIONS
HEMODIALYSIS	• Requires venous access (A-V shunt, fistula, or graft) • Treatment is 3 to 8 hours in length, 3 times per week • Correction of fluid and electrolyte imbalance is rapid • Potential blood loss • Does not result in protein loss	• Heparinization is required • Requires expensive equipment • Inconvenient for home use • Rapid shifts of fluid and electrolytes can lead to disequilibrium syndrome (an unpleasant sensation and potentially dangerous situation) • Potential hepatitis B and C • Do NOT take blood pressure or perform venipunctures on the arm with the A-V shunt, fistula or graft • Assess access site for thrill and bruit
CONTINUOUS HEMOFILTRATION	• Requires vascular access: usually femoral or subclavian catheters • Slow process • Correction of fluid and electrolyte imbalance is slow • Does not cause blood loss • Does not result in protein loss	• Requires heparinization of filter tubing • Filters are costly • Equipment is simple to use • Limited to special care units, NOT for home use • Filter may rupture causing blood loss

PERITONEAL	• Surgical placement of abdominal catheter is required (Tenckhoff, Gore-tex, column-disk)
	• Slow process
	• Correction of fluid and electrolyte imbalance is slow
	• Does not cause blood loss
	• Protein is lost in dialysate
		• Heparinization is NOT required
		• Fairly expensive
		• Simple to perform
		• Easy to use at home
		• Dialysate is similar to IV fluid and is prescribed for the individual client's electrolyte needs
		• Potential complications:
		  • Bowel or bladder perforation
		  • Exit-site and tunnel infection
		  • Peritonitis

Figure 3-9

HESI HINT: The major difference between dialysate for hemodialysis and peritoneal dialysis is the amount of glucose. Peritoneal dialysis dialysate is much higher in glucose. For this reason, if the dialysate is left in the peritoneal cavity too long, hyperglycemia may occur.

POSTOPERATIVE CARE: KIDNEY SURGERY		
ASSESSMENT	**NURSING INTERVENTIONS**	**RATIONALE**
RESPIRATORY STATUS	• Auscultate lung sounds to detect "wet" sounds indicating infection • Demonstrate method of splinting incision for comfort when coughing and deep breathing	• Flank incision causes pain with BOTH inspiration and expiration. Therefore, client avoids deep breathing and coughing which can lead to respiratory difficulties, including pneumonia
CIRCULATORY STATUS	• Check vital signs to detect early signs of bleeding, shock • Monitor skin color and temperature (pallor and cold skin are signs of shock) • Monitor urinary output (will decrease with circulatory collapse) • Monitor surgical site for frank bleeding	• The kidney is very vascular • Bleeding is a constant threat • Circulatory collapse will occur with hemorrhage and can occur very quickly
PAIN RELIEF STATUS	• Administer narcotic analgesics as needed to relieve pain	• Relief of pain will improve the client's cooperation with deep breathing exercises • Relief of pain will improve client's cooperation with early ambulation
URINARY STATUS	• Check urinary output and drainage from ALL tubes inserted during the surgery • Maintain accurate intake and output	• Mechanical drainage of bladder will be implemented after surgery

Figure 3-10

URINARY TRACT INFECTIONS

DESCRIPTION: Infection or inflammation at any site in the urinary tract.
(Kidney = pyelonephritis, urethra = urethritis, bladder = cystitis, prostate = prostatitis)
1. Normally, the entire urinary tract is sterile.
2. The most common infectious agent is *Escherichia coli.*
3. Persons at highest risk for acquiring UTI:
   A. Diabetics.
   B. Pregnant women.
   C. Men with prostatic hypertrophy.
   D. Immunosuppressed persons.
   E. Catheterized clients.
   F. Anyone with urinary retention, either short term or long term.
   G. Elderly women (bladder prolapse).
4. Diagnosis:
   A. Clean-catch midstream urine collection for culture to identify specific causative organism.
   B. Intravenous pyelogram (IVP) to determine kidney functioning.
   C. Cystogram to determine bladder functioning.
   D. Cystoscopy to determine bladder or urethral abnormalities.

NURSING ASSESSMENT
1. Signs of infection including fever and chills.
2. Urinary frequency or urgency, dysuria.
3. Hematuria.
4. Pain at the costovertebral angle.
5. Elevated serum WBC (greater than 10,000).

ANALYSIS (NURSING DIAGNOSES)
1. Pain related to…
2. Altered urinary elimination related to…
3. Knowledge deficit related to…

NURSING PLANS AND INTERVENTIONS
1. Administer antibiotics specific to infection agent.
2. Instruct client in the appropriate medication regimen.
3. Encourage fluid intake of 3,000 ml. fluid/day.
4. Maintain I&O.
5. Administer mild analgesics (acetaminophen or aspirin).
6. Encourage client to take warm tub baths or Sitz baths as a comfort measure (**no bubbles or oils**).
7. Encourage to void every 2 to 3 hours to prevent residual urine from stagnating in bladder.

MEDICAL SURGICAL NURSING

> **HESI HINT:** The key to resolving UTI with most antibiotics is to keep the blood level of the antibiotic constant. It is important to tell the client to take the antibiotics round-the-clock and not to skip doses so that a consistent blood level can be maintained for optimal effectiveness.

8. Develop and implement a teaching plan.
   A. Take entire prescription as directed.
   B. Force fluids to 3 liters/day (water, juices).
   C. Shower rather than bathe as a preventive measure. If bathing is necessary, never take a bubble or oil bath.
   D. Women/girls should cleanse from front to back after toileting.
    E. Avoid caffeine.
   F. Women should void immediately after intercourse.
   G. Void every 2 to 3 hours during the day.
   H. Wear cotton undergarments and loose clothing to help decrease perineal moisture.
   I. Practice good handwashing technique.
   J. Obtain follow-up care.

URINARY TRACT OBSTRUCTION (KIDNEY STONES)

DESCRIPTION: Partial or complete blockage of the flow of urine at any point in the urinary system.

1. Urinary tract obstruction is usually caused by calculi or stones.
2. When urinary tract obstruction occurs, urine is retained above the point of obstruction.
   A. Hydrostatic pressure builds, causing dilatation of the organs above the obstruction.
   B. If hydrostatic pressure continues to build, then hydronephrosis develops which can lead to renal failure.

NURSING ASSESSMENT

1. Pain, usually quite severe, acute.
2. Symptoms of obstruction:
   A. Fever, chills.
   B. Nausea, vomiting, diarrhea.
   C. Abdominal distention.

> **HESI HINT:** Location of the pain can help determine location of the stone.
> - Flank pain usually means the stone is in the kidney or upper ureter. If it radiates to the abdomen or scrotum, the stone is likely to be in the ureter or bladder.
> - Excruciating, spastic-type pain is called colic.
> - During kidney stone attacks, it is preferable to administer pain medications at regularly scheduled intervals rather than PRN to prevent spasm and optimize comfort.

3. Change in voiding pattern.
   A. Dysuria, hematuria.
   B. Urgency, frequency, hesitancy, nocturia, dribbling.
   C. Difficulty in starting a stream.
   D. Incontinence.
4. Those with the following conditions are at risk for developing calculi:
   A. Strictures.
   B. Prostatic hypertrophy.
   C. Neoplasms.
   D. Congenital malformations.
   E. History of calculi.
   F. Family history of calculi.

ANALYSIS (NURSING DIAGNOSES)

1. Pain related to…
2. Potential for infection related to…
3. Potential for injury related to…

NURSING PLANS AND INTERVENTIONS

1. Administer narcotic analgesics, IV best (usually Morphine or Meperidine).
2. Apply moist heat to the painful area unless prescribed otherwise.
3. Encourage high oral fluid intake to help dislodge the stone.
4. Administer intravenous antibiotics if infection is present.
5. STRAIN ALL URINE!
6. Send any stones found from straining to the laboratory for analysis.
7. Accurately document I&O.
8. Surgical management.
   A. Cystoscopy.
   B. Percutaneous nephrostomy (ultrasonic lithotripsy or perfusion chemolysis).
   C. Extracorporeal shock wave lithotripsy.
   D. Pyeolithotomy, ureterolithotomy.

HESI HINT: Percutaneous nephrostomy: A needle/catheter is inserted through the skin into the calyx of the kidney. The stone may be dissolved by percutaneous irrigation with a liquid which will dissolve the stone, or ultrasonic sound waves (lithotripsy) can be directed through the needle/catheter to break up the stone which then can be eliminated through the urinary tract.

9. Develop and implement a teaching plan to include:
   A. Encourage follow-up care, because stones tend to recur.
   B. Maintain a high fluid intake of 3 to 4 liters per day.
   C. Follow prescribed diet (based upon composition of stone).
   D. Avoid long periods of supine position.

BENIGN PROSTATIC HYPERPLASIA (BPH)

(Sometimes called hypertrophy of the prostate).
DESCRIPTION: Enlargement or hypertrophy of the prostate.
1. BPH tends to occur in men over 40 years of age.
2. Intervention is required when symptoms of obstruction occur.
3. The most common treatment is transurethral resection of the prostate gland (TURP). The prostate is removed by endoscopy (no surgical incision is made) allowing for a shorter hospital stay.

NURSING ASSESSMENT
1. Increased frequency with a decrease in amount of each voiding.
2. Nocturia.
3. Hesitancy.
4. Terminal dribbling.
5. Decrease in size and force of stream.
6. Acute urinary retention.
7. Bladder distention.

ANALYSIS (NURSING DIAGNOSES)
1. Pain related to…
2. Potential for injury: hemorrhage related to…
3. Potential for injury: infection related to…

NURSING PLANS AND INTERVENTIONS
1. Preoperative teaching to include information concerning pain from bladder spasms that occurs postoperative.
2. Maintain patent urinary drainage system to decrease the spasms.
3. Provide pain relief as prescribed: analgesics or antispasmotics such as Ditropan, Bentyl, or B&O suppositories.

HESI HINT: Bladder spasms frequently occur after TURP. Inform the client that the presence of the oversized balloon on the catheter (30 to 45 cc inflate) will cause a continuous feeling of needing to void. The client should not try to void around the catheter since this can precipitate bladder spasms. Medications to reduce or prevent spasms should be given.

4. Minimize catheter manipulation by taping catheter to abdomen or leg.
5. Maintain gentle traction on urinary catheter.
6. Check the urinary drainage system for clots.
7. Irrigate bladder as prescribed (may be continuous or intermittent). If continuous, keep Foley bag emptied to avoid retrograde pressure.

HESI HINT: Instillation of hypertonic or hypotonic solution into a body cavity will cause a shift in cellular fluid. *Use only sterile saline for bladder irrigation after TURP* since the irrigation must be isotonic to prevent fluid and electrolyte imbalance.

8. Observe the color and content of urinary output.
   A. Normal drainage after prostate surgery is reddish pink clearing to light pink within 24 hours after surgery.
   B. Monitor for bright red bleeding with large clots and increased viscosity.
9. Monitor vital signs frequently for indication of circulatory collapse.
10. Monitor Hgb and Hct for pattern of decreasing values that indicate bleeding.
11. After catheter is removed:
    A. Monitor amount and number of times client voids.
    B. Have the client use urine cups to provide a specimen with each voiding.
    C. Observe for hematuria after each voiding (urine should progress to clear yellow color by the fourth day).

D. Inform client that burning on urination and urinary frequency are usually experienced in the first postoperative week.

E. Generally the client is NOT impotent after surgery, but sterility may occur.

F. Instruct client to immediately report any frank bleeding to physician.

HESI HINT: Inform the client prior to discharge that some bleeding is expected after TURP. Large amounts of blood or frank bright bleeding should be reported. However, it is normal for the client to pass small amounts of blood during the healing process as well as small clots. He should rest quietly and continue drinking large amounts of fluid.

12. Instruct client to increase fluid intake to 3,000 ml/day.

13. Prepare client for discharge with instructions to:

A. Continue to drink 12 to 14 glasses of water a day.

B. Avoid constipation, straining.

C. Avoid strenuous activity, lifting, intercourse, or engaging in sports during the first 3 to 4 weeks after surgery.

D. Schedule a follow-up appointment.

REVIEW QUESTIONS
RENAL SYSTEM

1. **Differentiate between acute renal failure and chronic renal failure.**

2. **During the oliguric phase of renal failure, protein should be severely restricted. What is the rationale for this restriction?**

3. **Identify two nursing interventions for the client on hemodialysis.**

4. **What is the highest priority nursing diagnosis for clients in any type of renal failure?**

5. **A client in renal failure asks why he is being given antacids. How should the nurse reply?**

6. **List four essential elements of a teaching plan for clients with frequent urinary tract infections.**

7. **What are the most important nursing interventions for clients with possible renal calculi?**

8. **What discharge instructions should be given to a client who has had urinary calculi?**

9. **Following transurethral resection of the prostate gland (TURP), hematuria should subside by what postoperative day?**

10. **After the urinary catheter is removed in the TURP client, what are three priority nursing actions?**

11. **After kidney surgery, what are the primary assessments the nurse should make?**

ANSWERS TO REVIEW QUESTIONS

1. Acute renal failure: often reversible, abrupt deterioration of kidney function. Chronic renal failure: irreversible, slow deterioration of kidney function characterized by increasing BUN and creatinine. Eventually dialysis is required.

2. Toxic metabolites that accumulate in the blood (urea, creatinine) are derived mainly from protein catabolism.

3. Do NOT take BP or perform venipunctures on the arm with the A-V shunt, fistula, or graft. Assess access site for thrill and bruit.

4. Alteration in fluid and electrolyte balance.

5. Calcium and aluminum antacids bind phosphates and help to keep phosphates from being absorbed into blood stream thereby preventing rising phosphate levels, and must be taken with meals.

6. Fluid intake 3 liters/day; Good handwashing; Void every 2 to 3 hours during waking hours; Take all prescribed medications; Wear cotton undergarments.

7. Straining all urine is the MOST IMPORTANT intervention. Other interventions include accurate intake and output documentation and administering analgesics as needed.

8. Maintain high fluid intake of 3 to 4 liters per day. Follow-up care (stones tend to recur). Follow prescribed diet based on calculi content. Avoid supine position.

9. Fourth day.

10. Continued strict I&O. Continued observations for hematuria. Inform client burning and frequency may last for a week.

11. Respiratory status (breathing is guarded because of pain); circulatory status (the kidney is very vascular and excessive bleeding can occur); pain assessment; urinary assessment (most importantly, assessment of urinary output).

Cardiovascular System

> **HESI HINT:** What is the relationship of the kidneys to the cardiovascular system?
> - The kidneys filter about a liter of blood per minute.
> - If cardiac output is decreased, the amount of blood going through the kidneys is decreased; urinary output is decreased. Therefore, a decreased urinary output may be a sign of cardiac problems.
> - When the kidneys produce and excrete 0.5 ml of urine per kg of body weight or average 30 ml/hour output, the blood supply is considered to be minimally adequate to perfuse the vital organs.

Angina

Description: Chest discomfort or pain occurring when myocardial oxygen demands exceed supply.

Common causes:
1. Atherosclerotic heart disease.
2. Hypertension.
3. Coronary artery spasm.
4. Hypertrophic cardiomyopathy.

Nursing Assessment
1. Pain:
   A. Mild to severe intensity, described as: heavy, squeezing, pressing, burning, choking, aching, and feeling of apprehension.
   B. Substernal, radiating to left arm and/or shoulder, jaw, or right shoulder.
   C. Transient or prolonged with gradual or sudden onset; typically short duration.
   D. Often precipitated by: exercise, exposure to cold, heavy meal, mental tension, sexual intercourse.
   E. Relieved by rest or nitroglycerin.
2. Dyspnea, tachycardia, palpitations.
3. Nausea, vomiting.
4. Fatigue.
5. Diaphoresis, pallor, weakness.
6. Syncope.
7. Dysrhythmias.
8. Diagnostic information:
   A. EKG: generally at client baseline unless taken during anginal attack, when ST depression and T wave inversion may occur.
   B. Exercise stress test shows ST segment depression and hypotension.
   C. Stress echocardiogram: looks for changes in wall motion (indicated in women).
   D. Coronary angiogram: detects coronary artery spasms.
   E. Cardiac catheterization: detects arterial blockage.
9. Risk Factors:
   A. Nonmodifiable:
      1) Heredity.
      2) Gender, male > female until menopause, then equal risk.
      3) Ethnic background, American blacks.
      4) Age.
   B. Modifiable:
      1) Hyperlipidemia.
      2) Serum cholesterol above 300 mg/dl has four times greater risk of developing coronary artery disease (CAD) than those with levels less than 200 mg/dl (desirable level).
      3) Low density lipoprotein (LDL) **"Bad Cholesterol."** A molecule of LDL is approximately 50% cholesterol by weight (< 100 mg/dl optimal, <130 mg/dl desirable).
      4) High-density lipoprotein (HDL) **"Good Cholesterol."** HDL is inversely related to the risk of developing CAD (>60 mg/dl is desirable). In fact, HDL may serve to remove cholesterol from tissues.
      5) Hypertension.
      6) Cigarette smoking.
      7) Obesity.
      8) Physical inactivity.
      9) Diabetes mellitus.
      10) Stress.

Analysis (Nursing Diagnoses)
1. Pain related to…
2. Anxiety related to…

Nursing Plans and Interventions
1. Monitor medications and instruct client in proper administration.
2. Determine factors precipitating pain, and assist client/family in adjusting lifestyle to decrease these factors.
3. Teach risk factors, and identify client's own risk factors.
4. During an attack:
   A. Provide immediate rest.
   B. Take vital signs.
   C. Record an EKG.
   D. Administer no more than three nitroglycerin tablets, 5 minutes apart. *(See figure 3-12, Antianginals)*

E. Seek emergency treatment if no relief has occurred after taking nitroglycerin.

5. Physical activity.
   A. Avoid isometric activity.
   B. Implement an exercise program.
   C. Sexual activity may be resumed after exercise is tolerated, usually when able to climb two flights of stairs without exertion. Nitroglycerin can be taken prophylactically before intercourse.

6. Provide nutritional information modifying fats (saturated) and sodium. Antilipemic medications may be prescribed to lower cholesterol levels. *(See figure 3-11, Antilipemic; and Appendix B, Foods High in Sodium)*

7. Medical interventions include:
   A. Percutaneous Transluminal Coronary Angioplasty (PTCA): a balloon catheter is repeatedly inflated to split or fracture plaque and the arterial wall is stretched, enlarging the diameter of the vessel. A rotoblade is used to pulverize plaque.
   B. Arthrectomy: a catheter with a collection chamber is used to remove plaque which is trapped in the chamber.
   C. Coronary Artery Bypass Graft (CABG).
   D. Coronary Laser Therapy.
   E. Coronary artery stent.

ANTILIPEMIC			
DRUGS	**INDICATIONS**	**ADVERSE REACTIONS**	**NURSING IMPLICATIONS**
BILE SEQUESTRANTS: • **colestipol HCL** (Colestid) • **colesevelam** (Welchol) • **cholestyramine** (Questran)	• Treat type IIA hyper-lipidemia (hyper-cholesterolemia) when dietary changes fail	• Abdominal pain, N/V, distention, flatulence, belching, constipation • Reduced absorption of lipid-soluble vitamins: A, D, E, & K • Alters absorption of other oral medications	• Teach client to mix with powder forms with liquid or fruits high in moisture content such as applesauce to prevent accidental inhalation or esophageal distress • Monitor prothrombin times • Assess for visual changes & rickets • Administer other oral medications 1 hour before or 6 hours after giving bile sequestrants
HNG-CoA REDUCTASE INHIBITORS: (statins) • **atorvastatin** (Lipitor) • **fluvastatin** (Lescol) • **pravastatin** (Pravachol) • **simvastatin** (Zocor) • **lovostatin** (Mevacor)		• S.E. similar to bile sequestrants • May elevate liver enzymes • Hepatitis &/or pancreatitis • Rhabdomyolysis	• Obtain liver enzymes baseline & monitor every 6 months • Monitor CPK levels • Review specific drug/food interactions; avoid grapefruit juice • Timing with or without food varies with drug • Instruct client to report any muscle tenderness

Figure 3-11

ANTILIPEMIC (CONTINUED)			
DRUGS	**INDICATIONS**	**ADVERSE REACTIONS**	**NURSING IMPLICATIONS**
FIBRIC ACID DERIVATIVES: • **gemfibrate** (Lopid) • **fenofibrate** (Tricor) • **clofibrate** (Claripex)	Used with diet changes to lower both elevated cholesterol and triglycerides	• Abdominal/epigastric pain, diarrhea-most common • Flatulence, N/V • Heartburn • Dyspepsia • Gallstones • Tricor: weakness, fatigue, H/A • Myopathy	• Obtain baseline labs: liver function, CBC and electrolytes and monitor every 3 to 6 months Administer: • Lopid: 30 minutes before breakfast and dinner • Tricor: with meals
WATER-SOLUBLE VITAMIN: • **niacin** (Niaspan) • **nicotinic acid** (Nicobid)	Large doses decrease lipoprotein and triglyceride synthesis and increase HDL	• Flushing of face/neck • Pruritis • H/A • Orthostatic hypotension • (ER form): Hepatotoxicity • Hyperglycemia • Hyperuricemia • Upper GI distress	• Give with milk or food to avoid GI irritation • Client to change positions slowly • Instruct clients taking ER form to report darkened urine, light-colored stools, anorexia, yellowing of eyes or skin, severe stomach pain

Figure 3-11 (continued)

> **HESI HINT:** Angina is caused by myocardial ischemia. Which cardiac medications would be appropriate for acute angina?
>
> **Digoxin** - *Not appropriate* – Increases the strength and contractility of the heart muscle; the problem in angina is that the muscle is not receiving enough oxygen. Digoxin will not help.
>
> **Nitroglycerin** – *Appropriate* – Causes dilation of the coronary arteries, allowing more oxygen to get to the heart muscle.
>
> **Atropine** – *Not appropriate* - Increases heart rate by blocking vagal stimulation, which suppresses the heart rate. Does not address the lack of O_2 to the heart muscle.
>
> **Propanolol (Inderal)** – *Not appropriate* – for acute angina attack; however, is appropriate for long-term management of stable angina because it acts as a beta-blocker to control vasoconstriction.

ANTIANGINALS			
DRUGS	**INDICATIONS/ ACTIONS**	**ADVERSE REACTIONS**	**NURSING IMPLICATIONS**
NITRATES • nitroglycerin (NTG) • isosorbide dinitrate (Isordil) • isosorbide mononitrate (Imdur)	• Anginal prophylaxis • Acute attack • Reduces vascular resistance	• Headache • Flushing • Dizziness • Weakness • Hypotension • Nausea	• Monitor relief • Have client rest • Monitor vital signs • Store in original container • Replace NTG tablets every 3 to 5 months
BETA BLOCKERS • propranolol HCL (Inderal) • atenolol (Tenormin) • nadolol Corgard)	• Anginal prophylaxis • Reduce oxygen demand	• Fatigue • Lethargy • Hallucinations • Impotence • Bradycardia • Hypotension • CHF • Wheezing	• Monitor apical heart rate • Assess for decreased BP • Do not stop abruptly • Clients with CHF, bronchitis, asthma, COPD, renal or hepatic insufficiency have increased likelihood of incurring adverse reactions
CALCIUM CHANNEL BLOCKERS • Verapamil (Calan) • nifedipine HCL (Procardia) • diltiazem HCL (Cardizem, Norvasc)	• Anginal prophylaxis • Inhibits influx of calcium ions	• Dizziness • Hypotension • Fatigue • Headache • Syncope • Peripheral edema • Hypokalemia • Dysrhythmia • CHF	• Clients with CHF and the elderly have an increased likelihood of incurring adverse reactions • Assess for decreased BP • Monitor serum potassium • Swallow pills whole • Store at room temperature • Do not stop abruptly • Take 1 hour before meals or 2 hours after meals

Figure 3-12

Myocardial Infarction (MI)

Description: Disruption or deficiency of coronary artery blood supply resulting in necrosis of myocardial tissue.

Etiology of MI:
1. Thrombus or clotting.
2. Shock or hemorrhage.

Nursing Assessment

1. Sudden onset of pain in the lower sternal region (substernal).
   A. Severity increases until it becomes nearly unbearable.
   B. Heavy and vise-like pain often radiating to the shoulders and down arms.
   C. Differs from angina pain in its sudden onset.
   D. Pain *not* relieved by rest.
   E. Pain *not* relieved by nitroglycerin.
   F. May persist for hours or days.
   G. May *not* have pain (silent MI) especially in those with diabetic neuropathy.
2. Rapid, irregular, and feeble pulse.
3. Decreased level of consciousness indicating decreased cerebral perfusion.
4. Left heart shift sometimes occurs post-MI.
5. Cardiac dysrhythmias occur in about 90% of MI clients.
6. Cardiogenic shock or fluid retention.
7. Narrowed pulse pressure, e.g., 90/80.
8. Bowel sounds absent or high-pitched indicating possibility of mesenteric artery thrombosis which acts as an intestinal obstruction. *(See Gastrointestinal System)*
9. CHF indicated by wet lung sounds.
10. EKG changes; occur as early as 2 hours post MI or as late as 72 hours post-MI. *(See figure 3-13, Post-MI Cardiac Enzyme Elevations)*

Analysis (Nursing Diagnoses)
1. Alteration in tissue perfusion related to…
2. Decreased cardiac output related to…
3. Activity intolerance related to…
4. Alteration in comfort: pain related to …

POST-MI CARDIAC ENZYME ELEVATIONS			
Enzyme/Marker	**Onset**	**Peak**	**Return To Normal**
CK-2 (non-cardiac specific)	3 to 6 hours	12 to 24 hours	3 to 5 days
CK-MB (Recognized indicator of MI by most clinicians)	2 to 4 hours	12 to 20 hours	48 to 72 hours
Myoglobin	1 to 4 hours (elevate prior to CK-MB)	4 to 8 hours	24 hours
Cardiac Troponins	As early as 1 hour post injury	10 to 24 hours	5 to 14 days
LDH Total	24 hours	3 to 6 days	10 to 14 days
LDH$_1$ (A higher LDH$_1$ than LDH$_2$ indicates MI)	12 to 24 hours	48 hours	10 days
LDH$_2$	12 to 24 hours	48 hours	10 days

Figure 3-13

Nursing Plans and Interventions
1. Administer medications as prescribed.
   A. For pain and to increase O$_2$ perfusion, intravenous morphine sulfate (acts as a peripheral vasodilator and decreases venous return).
   B. Other medications often prescribed include: *(See figure 3-12, Antianginals)*
      1) Nitrates, e.g., nitroglycerin.
      2) Beta-blockers.
      3) Calcium channel blockers.
      4) Aspirin.
      5) Antiplatelet aggregates.
2. Obtain vital signs including EKG rhythm strip regularly per agency policy.
3. Administer oxygen at 2 to 6 liters per nasal cannula.
4. Obtain cardiac enzymes as prescribed.
5. Provide a quiet, restful environment.

6. Assess breath sounds for rales (indicating pulmonary edema).
7. Maintain patent IV line for administration of emergency medications.
8. Monitor fluid balance.
9. Keep in semi-Fowler's position to assist with breathing.
10. Maintain bedrest for 24 hours.
11. Encourage client to gradually resume activity.
12. Encourage verbalization of fears.
13. Provide information about the disease process and cardiac rehabilitation.
14. Medical interventions. *(See Angina)*
    A. Thrombolytic agents, within 1 to 4 hours of MI. *(See figure 3-14, Thrombolytic Agents)*
    B. Intra-aortic balloon pump (IABP) to improve myocardial perfusion.

THROMBOLYTIC AGENTS			
DRUGS	**INDICATIONS**	**ADVERSE REACTIONS**	**NURSING IMPLICATIONS**
streptokinase (Streptase) (Kabikinase)	• Deep vein thrombosis • Pulmonary embolism • Arterial thrombosis and embolism • Coronary thrombosis • Dissolving clots in arterio-venus cannula	• Anaphylactic response ranging from breathing difficulties to bronchospasm, periobital swelling, or angioneurotic edema • Increased risk of bleeding • Hemorrhagic infarction at site of myocardial damage • Reperfusion dysrhythmias	• Assess for bleeding at puncture site; apply pressure to control bleeding • Assess for allergic reactions and dysrhythmias during intracoronary perfusion • Immobilize client's leg for 24 hours after femoral coronary cannulation and perfusion; assess pedal pulses for adequate circulation • Monitor client's thrombin time after therapy. Do NOT administer heparin or oral anticoagulants until thrombin time is less than twice that of control • Do NOT shake vial when reconstituting; roll and tilt vial gently to mix
tenecteplase (TNKase) **reteplase** (Retavase)	• Acute management of coronary thrombosis	• Do not give is history of uncontrolled hypertension • Can cause hypotension	• Obtain baseline studies prior to administration: PT, PTT, CBC, fibrinogen level, renal studies, cardiac enzymes • Check for abnormal pulse, neuro signs, and presence of skin lesions which may indicate coagulation defects • Avoid needle punctures because of the possibility of bleeding – apply pressure for 10 minutes to venous puncture sites and 30 minutes to arterial puncture sites; follow with pressure dressing • Be prepared to treat reperfusion arrhythmias
urokinase (Abbokinase)	• Pulmonary embolism • Coronary thrombosis • IV catheter clearance	• Is nonantigenic and does not cause allergic reactions; otherwise has the same adverse reactions as those cited for streptokinase	• Infuse heparin and an oral anticoagulant following urokinase therapy to prevent rethrombosis • Much more expensive than streptokinase, but does not cause allergic reactions found with streptokinase therapy • Reconstitute immediately before use

Figure 3-14

96

THROMBOLYTIC AGENTS (CONTINUED)			
DRUGS	**INDICATIONS**	**ADVERSE REACTIONS**	**NURSING IMPLICATIONS**
tissue-type plasminogen activator (t-PA), Activase	• Deep vein thrombosis • Pulmonary embolism • Coronary thrombosis	• Interacts with heparin, oral anticoagulants, and antiplatelet drugs to increase the risk of bleeding	• Alters coagulation ONLY at the thrombus, ***not*** systemically (bleeding complications associated with streptokinase and urokinase are reduced with t-PA therapy) • Because t-PA is a human protein, allergic response is unlikely to occur • Half-life 3 to 7 minutes. Use immediately

Figure 3-14 (continued)

HYPERTENSION

DESCRIPTION: Persistent blood pressure levels greater than 140/90.
1. Essential (primary) hypertension has no known etiology.
2. Secondary hypertension develops in response to an identifiable mechanism.

> **HESI HINT:** Blood pressure is created by the difference in the pressure of the blood as it leaves the heart and the resistance it meets flowing out to the tissues. Therefore, any factor that alters cardiac output or peripheral vascular resistance will alter blood pressure. Diet and exercise, smoking cessation, weight control, and stress management can control many factors that influence the resistance blood meets as it flows from the heart.

NURSING ASSESSMENT
1. BP greater than 140/90 or diastolic BP greater than or equal to 90 on three separate occasions:
   A. Obtain BP lying, sitting, and standing.
   B. Compare readings taken lying, sitting, and standing. A difference of more than 10 mmHg of either systolic or diastolic indicates postural hypotension. **TAKE IN BOTH ARMS.**
2. Genetic risk factors (non-modifiable):
   A. Positive family history for hypertension.
   B. Gender (men have greater risk of being hypertensive at an earlier age than women).
   C. Age (increasing risk with increasing age).
   D. Ethnicity (African Americans at greater risk than Whites).
3. Life style and habits which increase risk of becoming hypertensive (modifiable):
   A. Use of alcohol, tobacco, and caffeine.
   B. Sedentary lifestyle, obesity.
   C. Socioeconomic level (incidence is greater in lower socioeconomic groups).
   D. Nutrition history of high salt and fat intake.
   E. Use of oral contraceptives or estrogens.
   F. Stress.

> **HESI HINT:** Remember the risk factors for hypertension: heredity, race, age, alcohol abuse, increased salt intake, obesity, and use of oral contraceptives.

4. Associated physical problems:
   A. Renal failure.
   B. Respiratory problems, especially COPD.
   C. Cardiac problems, especially valvular disorders.
5. Pharmacological history:
   A. Steroids (increase BP).
   B. Estrogens (increase BP).
6. Assess for headache, edema, nocturia, nosebleeds, vision changes (may be asymptomatic).
7. Assess level of stress and source of stress (job-related, economic, family).
8. Assess personality type, i.e., determine if client exhibits "Type A" behavior.

ANALYSIS (NURSING DIAGNOSES)
1. Knowledge deficit related to…
2. Potential noncompliance related to…
3. Altered tissue perfusion related to…

NURSING PLANS AND INTERVENTIONS
   Develop a teaching plan to include:
1. Information about disease process.
   A. Risk factors.
   B. Causes.
   C. Long-term complications.
   D. Life style modifications.
   E. Relationship of treatment to prevention of complications.
2. Information about treatment plan.

A. How to take own blood pressure.

B. Reasons for each medication. *(See figure 3-15, Diuretics; and figure 3-16, Antihypertensives)*

C. How and when to take each medication.

D. Necessity of consistency with medication regime.

E. Need for ongoing assessment while taking antihypertensives.

> **HESI HINT:** The number one cause of CVA with hypertensive clients is non-compliance with medication regime. Hypertension is often symptomless, and antihypertensive medications are expensive and have side effects. Studies have shown that the more clients know about their antihypertensive medications, the more likely they are to take them – teaching is important!

F. Monitor serum electrolytes every 90 to 120 days for duration of treatment.

G. Monitor renal functioning (BUN and creatinine) every 90 to 120 days for duration of treatment.

H. Monitor BP and pulse rate, usually weekly.

3. Encourage client to implement non-pharmacological measures to assist with BP control such as:

A. Stress reduction.

B. Weight loss.

C. Tobacco cessation.

D. Exercise.

4. Determine medication side effects experienced by client.

A. Impotence.

B. Insomnia.

5. Provide nutritional guidance including a sample meal plan and how to eat out (low-salt, low-fat/low cholesterol diet).

DIURETICS			
DRUGS	**INDICATIONS**	**ADVERSE REACTIONS**	**NURSING IMPLICATIONS**
THIAZIDES • **chlorthalidone** (Hygroton) • **hydrochlorothiazide** (Esidrex, Microzide) • **indapamide** (Lozol) • **metolazone** (Zaroxolyn)	• To decrease fluid volume • Inexpensive • Effective • Useful in severe hypertension • Effective orally • Enhances other antihypertensives	• Hypokalemia symptoms include: → Dry mouth → Thirst → Weakness → Drowsiness → Lethargy → Muscle aches → Tachycardia • Hyperuricemia • Glucose intolerance • Hypercholesterolemia • Sexual dysfunction	• Observe for postural hypotension, can be potentiated by: → Alcohol → Barbiturates → Narcotics • Caution with: → Renal failure → Gout → Client taking lithium • Hypokalemia increases risk of digitalis toxicity • Administer potassium supplements
LOOP • **furosemide** (Lasix) • **forsemide** (Demadex) • **bumetanide** (Bumex)	• Rapid action • Potent for use when thiazides fail • Cause volume depletion	• Hypokalemia • Hyperuricemia • Glucose intolerance • Hypercholesterolemia • Hypertriglyceridemia • Sexual dysfunction • Weakness	• Volume depletion and electrolyte depletion are rapid • All nursing implications cited for Thiazides
POTASSIUM SPARING • **spironolactone** (Aldactone) • **amiloride** (Midamor)	• Volume depletion without significant potassium loss	• Hyperkalemia • Gynecomastia • Sexual dysfunction	• Watch for hyperkalemia or renal failure in those treated with ACE inhibitors or NSAIDs • Watch for increase in serum lithium levels • Give after meals to decrease GI distress

Figure 3-15

DIURETICS (CONTINUED)

DRUGS	INDICATIONS	ADVERSE REACTIONS	NURSING IMPLICATIONS
COMBINATION LOOPS & POTASSIUM-SPARING • **HCTZ and triamterene** (Maxide) • **HCTZ + amiloride** (Moduretic) • **HCTZ + spironolactone** (Aldactizide)	• Decrease fluid volume while minimizes K+ loss	• S.E.s of individual drugs offset or minimized by its partner	• Caution client previously on a loop or thiazide alone, not to overdo K+ foods now because of K+ sparing component in new drug • Follow scheduling dosage to avoid sleep disruption

Figure 3-15 (continued)

ANTIHYPERTENSIVES

DRUGS	INDICATIONS	ADVERSE REACTIONS	NURSING IMPLICATIONS
ALPHA-ADRENERGIC BLOCKERS • **prazosin HCL** (Minipress) • **terazosin** (Hytrin) • **pentolamine meysalate** (Regitine) • **doxazosin** (Cardura)	• Used as peripheral vasodilator which acts directly on the blood vessels • Used in extreme hypertension of pheochromocytoma	• Orthostatic hypotension • Weakness • Palpitations	• Use cautiously in elderly clients • Occasional vomiting and diarrhea • Warn clients of possible: → Drowsiness → Lack of energy → Weakness
COMBINED ALPHA BETA BLOCKERS • **labetalol** (Normodyne) • **carvedilol** (Coreg)	• Produces decrease in BP without reflex tachycardia or bradycardia	• CHF • Ventricular dysrhythmias • Blood dyscrasias • Bronchospasm • Orthostatic hypotension	• Contraindicated with: → CHF → Heart block → COPD
BETA BLOCKERS • **metoprolol tartrate** (Lopressor) • **nadolol** (Corgard) • **propranolol HCL** (Inderal) • **timolol maleate** (Blocadren) • **atenolol** (Tenormin) • **bisoprolol** (Zebeta) • **metropolol** (Lopressor, Toprol)	• Blocks the sympathetic nervous system especially to the heart • Produces a slower heart rate • Lowers blood pressure • Reduces O$_2$ consumption during myocardial contraction	• Bradycardia • Fatigue • Insomnia • Bizarre dreams • Sexual dysfunction • Hypertriglyceridemia • Decreased HDL • Depression	• Check apical or radial pulse daily • Monitor for GI distress • Do not discontinue abruptly • Watch for shortness of breath, give cautiously with bronchospasm • Do not vary how taken (with or without food) • Do not vary time taken • May mask symptoms of hypoglycemia or may prolong a hypoglycemic reaction
CENTRAL-ACTING INHIBITORS • clonidine (Catapres) • guanabenz acetate (Wytensin) • methyldopa (Aldomet)	• Decrease BP by stimulating central alpha receptors resulting in decreased sympathetic outflow from the brain	• Drowsiness • Dry mouth • Fatigue • Sexual dysfunction	• Watch for rebound hypertension if abruptly discontinued • Caution to make position changes slowly, avoid standing still, or taking hot baths and showers

Figure 3-16

 MEDICAL SURGICAL NURSING

99

ANTIHYPERTENSIVES (CONTINUED)			
DRUGS	**INDICATIONS**	**ADVERSE REACTIONS**	**NURSING IMPLICATIONS**
VASODILATORS • **hydralazine HCL** (Apresoline) • **minoxidil** (Loniten)	• Decreases BP by decreasing peripheral resistance	• Headache • Tachycardia • Fluid retention (CHF, pulmonary edema) • Postural hypotension	• Monitor BP, pulse routinely • Observe for peripheral edema • Monitor I&O • Weigh daily
ANGIOTENSIN II RECEPTOR ANTAGONISTS • **losartan** (Cozaar) • **valsartan** (Diovan) • **irbesartan** (Avapro)	• Blocks the vasoconstrictor and aldesterone – producing effects of angiotensin II at various sites (vascular smooth muscle and adrenal glands)	• Hypotension • Fatigue • Hepatitis • Renal failure • Hyperkalemia (rare)	• Monitor liver enzymes, electrolytes • Monitor for angioedema in those with history of it when on ACE inhibitors previously
ANGIOTENSIN-CONVERTING ENZYME (ACE) INHIBITORS • **captopril** (Capoten) • **enalapril maleate** (Vasotec) • **lisinopril** (Zestril) • **ramipril** (Altace) • **benazepril** (Lotensin) • **quinapril** (Accupril)	• Decreases BP by suppressing renin – angiotensin aldosterone system and inhibiting conversion of angiotensin I to angiotensin II • Useful with diabetics	• Proteinuria • Neutropenia • Skin rash • Cough	• Observe for acute renal failure (reversible) • Routine renal function tests • Remain in bed 3 hours after first dose
CALCIUM CHANNEL BLOCKERS • **diltiazem** (Cardizem) • **nifedipine** (Procardia, Adalat) • **verapamil** HCL (Calan, Isoptin) • **nisoldipine** (Sular)	• Inhibits calcium ion influx during cardiac depolarization • Decreases SA/AV node conduction	• Headache • Hypotension • Dizziness • Edema • Nausea • Constipation • Tachycardia • CHF • Dry cough	• Check BP and pulse routinely • Limit caffeine consumption • Take medications before meals • Avoid grapefruit juice with these drugs as it will increase serum levels causing hypotension • High fat meals elevate serum levels

Figure 3-16 (continued)

PERIPHERAL VASCULAR DISEASE (PVD)

DESCRIPTION: PVD involves circulatory problems that can be due to either arterial or venous pathology.

1. The signs, symptoms, and treatment of PVD can be opposite, depending on the source of pathology. Therefore, careful assessment is very important.

2. *See figure 3-17, Assessment of Arterial and Venous Insufficiency; and figure 3-18, Treatment of Arterial and Venous Insufficiency.*

ANALYSIS (NURSING DIAGNOSES)

1. Altered peripheral tissue perfusion related to…
2. Activity intolerance related to…
3. Impaired skin integrity related to…
4. Potential for infection related to…
5. Pain related to…

ASSESSMENT OF ARTERIAL AND VENOUS INSUFFICIENCY

AREA	ARTERIAL	VENOUS
PREDISPOSING FACTORS	• Arteriosclerosis. 95% of all cases are caused by atherosclerosis • Advanced age	• History of deep vein thrombosis (DVT) • Valvular incompetence
ASSOCIATED DISEASES	• Raynaud's Disease (non-atherosclerotic, triggered by extreme heat or cold) • Buerger's Disease (occlusive inflammatory disease, strongly associated with smoking) • Diabetes • Acute occlusion (emboli/thrombi)	• Varicose veins • Thrombophlebitis • Venous stasis ulcers
SKIN	• Smooth • Shiny • Loss of hair • Thick nails	• Brown pigment around ankles
COLOR	• Pallor on elevation • Rubor when dependent	• Cyanotic when dependent
TEMPERATURE	• Cool	• Warm
PULSES	• Decreased or absent	• Normal
PAIN	• Sharp • Increase with walking and elevation • Intermittent claudication: CLASSIC presenting symptom, occurs in skeletal muscles during exercise; relieved by rest • Rest pain: occurs when the extremities are horizontal; may be relieved by dependent position; often appears when collateral circulation fails to develop	• Persistent, aching, full feeling, dull sensation • Pain relieved when horizontal • Elevate and use elastic stockings
ULCERS	• Very painful • Occur on lateral lower leg, toes, heel • Demarcated edges • Necrotic • Not edematous	• Slightly painful • Occur on medial leg, ankle • Uneven edges • Superficial • Marked edema

Figure 3-17

NURSING PLANS AND INTERVENTIONS

1. Monitor extremities at designated intervals.
   A. Color.
   B. Temperature.
   C. Sensation and pulse quality in extremities.
2. Schedule activities within client's tolerance level.
3. Encourage rest at the first sign of pain.
4. Encourage to keep extremities elevated (if venous) when sitting and change position often.
5. Avoid crossing legs and wear nonrestrictive clothing.
6. Keep the extremities warm by wearing extra clothing such as socks and slippers. Do ***not*** use external heat sources such as electric heating pads.
7. Teach methods to prevent further injury.
   A. Change position frequently.
   B. Wear nonrestrictive clothing.
   C. Avoid crossing legs or keeping legs in a dependent position.
   D. Wear shoes when ambulating.
   E. Obtain proper foot and nail care.

> **HESI HINT:** Decreased blood flow results in diminished sensation in the lower extremities. Any heat source can cause severe burns before the client actually realizes the damage is being done.

8. Discourage cigarette smoking (causes vasoconstriction and spasm of arteries).
9. Provide preoperative and postoperative care if surgery is required.
   A. Preoperative: Maintain affected extremity at a level position, if venous, or slightly dependent

position, if arterial, (15 degrees), at room temperature, and protected from trauma.

B. Postoperative: Assess surgical site frequently for hemorrhage.

C. Anticoagulants may be continued after surgery to prevent thrombosis of affected artery and to diminish development of thrombi at the initiating site.

TREATMENT OF ARTERIAL AND VENOUS INSUFFICIENCY		
AREA	**ARTERIAL**	**VENOUS**
NON-INVASIVE TREATMENT	• Elimination of smoking • Topical antibiotic • Saline dressing • Bed rest/immobilization • Thrombolytic agents: if clots are the problem-not used for Raynaud's or Buerger's *Disease (See figure 3-14, Thrombolytic Agents)*	• Systemic antibiotics • Compression dressing (snug) • Limb elevation • For thrombosis, thrombolytic agents are *administered (See figure 3-14, Thrombolytic Agents)* and anticoagulants *(See figure 3-19, Anticoagulants)*
SURGERY	• Embolectomy: removal of clot • Endarterectomy: removal of clot and stripping of plaque • Arterial Bypass: Teflon/Dacron graft or autograft • Percutaneous transluminal angioplasty (PTA): compression of plaque • Amputation: removal of extremity	• Vein ligation • Thrombectomy • Debridement

Figure 3-18

ABDOMINAL AORTIC ANEURYSM (AAA)

DESCRIPTION: Dilation of the abdominal aorta caused by an alteration in the integrity of its wall.

1. Most common cause of AAA is atherosclerosis. Late manifestation of syphilis.
2. Without treatment, rupture and death will occur.
3. AAA is often asymptomatic.
4. Most common symptom is abdominal pain or low back pain with the complaint that the client can feel "heart beating."
5. Those taking antihypertensive drugs are at risk of developing AAA.

> **HESI HINT:** A client is admitted with severe chest pain and states that he feels a terrible, tearing sensation in his chest. He is diagnosed with a dissecting aortic aneurysm. What assessment should the nurse obtain in the first few hours?
> • **Vital signs q1 hour**
> • **Neurological vital signs**
> • **Respiratory status**
> • **Urinary output**
> • **Peripheral pulses**

NURSING ASSESSMENT

1. Bruit (swooshing sound heard over a constricted artery when auscultated) heard over abdominal aorta, pulsation in upper abdomen.
2. Abdominal or lower back pain.
3. Abdominal x-ray will confirm diagnosis if aneurysm is calcified (aortagram, angiogram, abdominal ultrasound).
4. Symptoms of rupture: hypovolemic or cardiogenic shock with sudden, severe abdominal pain.

ANALYSIS (NURSING DIAGNOSES)

1. Activity intolerance related to...
2. Impaired skin integrity related to...
3. Anxiety related to...

NURSING PLANS AND INTERVENTIONS

1. Assess all peripheral pulses and vital signs regularly.
   A. Radial.
   B. Femoral.
   C. Popliteal.
   D. Posterior tibial.
   E. Dorsalis pedis.
2. Observe for signs of occlusion after graft.
   A. Change in pulses.
   B. Severe pain.
   C. Cool to cold extremities below graft.

D. White or blue extremities.
3. Observe renal functioning for signs of kidney damage (artery clamped during surgery may result in kidney damage).
    A. Output of less than 30 ml/hour.
    B. Amber urine.
    C. Elevated BUN and creatinine (early signs of renal failure).

> **HESI HINT:** During aortic aneurysm repair, the large arteries are clamped for a period of time and kidney damage can result. Monitor daily BUN and creatinine levels. Normal BUN is 10 to 20 mg/dl and normal creatinine is 0.6 to 1.2 mg/dl. The ratio of BUN to creatinine is 20:1. When this ratio increases or decreases, suspect renal problems.

4. Observe for postoperative ileus.
    A. NG tube 1 to 2 days postoperative (may help prevent ileus).
    B. Check bowel sounds every shift.

THROMBOPHLEBITIS

DESCRIPTION: Inflammation of the venous walls with the formation of a clot. Also known as venous thrombosis, phlebothrombosis, deep vein thrombosis (DVT).

NURSING ASSESSMENT
1. Calf or groin pain. Positive Homan's sign (Note: only about 50% with phlebitis will manifest this sign).

> **HESI HINT:** A positive Homan's sign is considered an early indication of thrombophlebitis. However, it may also indicate muscle inflammation. If a deep vein thrombosis has been confirmed, a Homan's sign should *not* be elicited because of the increased risk of embolization.

2. Functional impairment of extremity.
3. Edema and warmth in extremity.
4. Asymmetry.
    A. Inspect legs from groin to feet.
    B. Measure diameter of calf.
5. Tender areas noted on affected extremity with very gentle palpation.
6. Occlusion noted with diagnostic testing.
    A. Venogram.
    B. Doppler ultrasound.
    C. Fibrinogen scanning.
7. Risk factors:
    A. Prolonged strict bed rest.

B. General surgery.
C. Leg trauma.
D. Previous venous insufficiency.
E. Obesity.
F. Oral contraceptives.
G. Pregnancy.
H. Malignancy.

ANALYSIS (NURSING DIAGNOSES)
1. Pain related to…
2. Altered tissue perfusion related to…

> **HESI HINT:** Heparin prevents conversion of fibrinogen to fibrin and prothrombin to thrombin, thereby inhibiting clot formation. Since the clotting mechanism is prolonged, do not cause tissue trauma which may lead to bleeding when giving heparin subcutaneously. Do *not* massage area or aspirate; give in the abdomen between the pelvic bones; 2 inches from umbilicus; rotate sites.

NURSING PLANS AND INTERVENTIONS
1. Administer anticoagulant therapy as prescribed. *(See figure 3-19, Anticoagulants)*

> **HESI HINT:** ANTICOAGULANTS
> HEPARIN
> ANTAGONIST: PROTAMINE SULFATE
> LAB: PTT or APTT determines efficacy
> Keep 1.5 to 2.5 times normal control
> COUMADIN
> ANTAGONIST: Vitamin K
> LAB: PT determines efficacy
> Keep 1.5 to 2.5 times normal control
>
> INR (International Normalized Ratio)
> Desirable therapeutic level usually 2 to 3 seconds (reflects how long it takes a blood sample to clot)

A. Observe for side effects, especially bleeding.
B. Teach client side effects of medications included in treatment regime.
C. Monitor laboratory data to determine the efficacy of medications included in treatment regime.
D. Include information on all lab requests that client is receiving anticoagulants.
E. Partial Thromboplastin Time (PTT) determines efficacy of heparin.
F. Prothrombin Time (PT) determines efficacy of Coumadin.

G. Maintain pressure on venipuncture sites to minimize hematoma formation.

H. Notify physician of any unusual bleeding.
   1) Abnormal vaginal bleeding.
   2) Nosebleeds.
   3) Melena.
   4) Hematuria.
   5) Gums.
   6) Hemoptysis.

I. Use soft toothbrush, floss with waxed floss.

J. Wear medical alert symbol.

K. Avoid alcoholic beverages.

L. Avoid safety razor if taking Coumadin.

M. No ASA.

2. Use anti-embolic stockings. Elevate extremity and/or shock blocks for foot of bed.

3. Bedrest; strict, if prescribed, means no bathroom privileges! Prevent straining.

4. Monitor for decreasing symptomatology.
   A. Pain.
   B. Edema.

5. Monitor for pulmonary embolus (chest pain, shortness of breath).

6. Teach client that there is increased risk for DVT formation in the future.

ANTICOAGULANTS			
DRUGS	**INDICATIONS**	**ADVERSE REACTIONS**	**NURSING IMPLICATIONS**
heparin sodium (Hepalean, Hep-lock)	• Administered parenterally (SQ or IV) as an antagonist to thrombin and prevent the conversion of fibrinogen to fibrin	• Hemorrhage • Agranulocytosis • Leukopenia • Hepatitis	• Assess PTT, Hgb, Hct, platelets • Assess stools for occult blood • Avoid IM injection • Notify anyone performing diagnostic testing of medication **ANTAGONIST: Protamine Sulfate**
warfarin sodium (Coumadin, Coufarin, Panwarfin)	• Blocks the formation of prothrombin from vitamin K	• Hemorrhage • Agranulocytosis • Leukopenia • Hepatitis	• See heparin • Given orally • Assess PT • Avoid sudden change in intake of foods high in vitamin K **ANTAGONIST: Vitamin K**
antiplatelet agent ticlopidine (Ticlid) **diperidimole** (Persantine) **clopidrogrel** (Plavix)	• Short term use after cardiac interventions • Reduce risk of thrombolytic stroke for those intolerant to aspirin • Prevention of thrombolytic disorders	• Neutropenia • Thrombocytopenia • Agranulocytosis • Leukopenia • Hemorrhage • GI irritation, bleeding • Pancytopenia	• Give p.c. or with food to decrease gastric irritation (Ticlid) • Advise not to take antacids within 2 hours of taking ticlopidine • Monitor CBC q2 weeks for three months, and thereafter if signs of infection develop • Monitor for signs of bleeding • Give 1 hour a.c. (Persantine); (Plavix) no regard for meals
low molecular weight heparin enoxaparin (Lovenox)	• Prevention of thrombolytic formation (deep vein)	• Hemorrhage • GI irritation, bleeding • Thrombocytopenia	• Monitor for signs of bleeding • Given subcutaneously • Monitor CBC • Use soft toothbrush, avoid cuts

Figure 3-19

DYSRHYTHMIAS

DESCRIPTION: Disturbance in heart rate and/or heart rhythm.

1. Dysrhythmias are caused by a disturbance in the electrical conduction of the heart, NOT by abnormal heart structure.
2. Client is often asymptomatic until cardiac output is altered.
3. Common causes of dysrhythmias:
   A. Drugs, e.g., digoxin, quinidine, caffeine, nicotine, alcohol.
   B. Acid-base and electrolyte imbalances (potassium, calcium, and magnesium).
   C. Marked thermal changes.
   D. Disease and trauma.
   E. Stress.

NURSING ASSESSMENT
1. Change in pulse rate and/or rhythm.

   A. Tachycardia: fast rates (>100 BPM).
   B. Bradycardia: slow rates (<60 BPM).
   C. Irregular rhythm.
   D. Pulselessness.
2. EKG changes.
3. Complaints of:
   A. Palpitations.
   B. Syncope.
   C. Pain.
   D. Dyspnea.
4. Diaphoresis.
5. Hypotension.
6. Electrolyte imbalance.

ANALYSIS (NURSING DIAGNOSES)
1. Alteration in tissue perfusion related to…
2. Activity intolerance related to…

SELECTED DYSRHYTHMIAS				
	ATRIAL FIBRILLATION	**ATRIAL FLUTTER**	**VENTRICULAR TACHYCARDIA**	**VENTRICULAR FIBRILLATION**
DESCRIPTION	• Chaotic activity in the AV node • No true P waves visible • Irregular ventricular rhythm	• Saw toothed wave form • Fluttering in chest • Ventricular rhythm states regular	• Wide bizarre QRS	• Cardiac emergency • No cardiac output
ASSESSMENT AND TREATMENT	• Anticoagulent therapy is needed due to risk for CVA • Administer antiarrhythmic drugs	• May use cardioversion to treat either atrial dysrhythmia • Administer antiarrhythmic drugs	• Assess whether client has a pulse • Is cardiac output impaired • Prepare for synchronized cardioversion • Administer antiarrhythmic drugs	• Start CPR • Defibrillate as quickly as possible • Administer antiarrhythmic drugs

Figure 3-20

NURSING PLANS AND INTERVENTIONS
1. Determine medications client is currently taking.
2. Determine serum drug levels, especially digitalis.
3. Determine serum electrolyte levels, especially K+ and Mg++.
4. Obtain EKG reading upon admission and monitor continuously.

> **HESI HINT:** A Holter monitor offers continuous observation of the client's heart rate. To make assessment of the rhythm strips most meaningful, teach the client to keep a record of:
> • **Medication times and doses**
> • **Chest pain episodes -- type and duration**
> • **Valsalva maneuver (straining at stool, sneezing, coughing)**
> • **Sexual activity**
> • **Exercise**

5. Approach client in a calm, reassuring manner.
6. Monitor client's activity, and observe for any symptoms occurring during activity.
7. Ensure proper administration of medications, and monitor for side effects. *(See figure 3-21, Antiarrhythmics)*
8. Be prepared for emergency measures such as cardioversion or defibrillation.

> **HESI HINT:** Cardioversion is the delivery of synchronized electrical shock to the myocardium.

9. Be prepared for pacemaker insertion.
    A. Temporary pacemaker – used temporarily in emergency situations. Pacing wire is threaded into the right ventricle via the superior vena cava, or an epicardial wire is put in place (through the client's chest incision) during cardiac surgery.
    B. Permanent internal pacemaker with pulse generator implanted in the abdomen or shoulder. May be single or dual chambered. Programmable pacemakers can be reprogrammed by placing a magnetic device over the generator.
    C. Instruct the client to:

1) Report pulse rate lower than the set rate of the pacemaker.
2) Avoid leaning over an automobile with the engine running.
3) Stand 4 to 5 feet away from electromagnetic sources, such as operating microwave ovens or radar detectors that are operating.
4) Avoid MRI diagnostic testing.

> **HESI HINT:** Difference in synchronous and asynchronous pacemakers:
> - Synchronous or demand pacemaker fires only when the client's heart rate falls below a rate set on the generator.
> - Asynchronous or fixed pacemaker fires at a constant rate.

10. Recognize and treat PVCs as prescribed (tend to be precursors of ventricular tachycardia and ventricular fibrillation).
    A. Occur more often than once in 10 beats.
    B. Occur in groups of 2 and/or 3.
    C. Occur near the T wave.
    D. Take on multiple configurations.

ANTIARRHYTHMICS			
DRUGS	**INDICATIONS**	**ADVERSE REACTIONS**	**NURSING IMPLICATIONS**
CLASS I (I: A,B,C) • **quinidine** • **disopyramide phosphate** (Norpace) • **moricizine** (Ethmozine) • **lidocaine HCL** (Xylocaine) • **mexiletine** (Mexitil) • **tocainide HCL** (Tonocard) • **phenytoin sodium** (Dilantin) • **propafenone** (Rythmol) • **flecainide acetate** (Tambocor)	• Premature beats • Atrial flutter, fibrillation Contraindicated in heart block • Ventricular dysrhythmias • Unlabelled Use: Digitalis – induced arrhythmias • Ventricular dysrhythmias	• Diarrhea • Hypotension • EKG changes • Cinchonism • Interacts with many common drugs • Hypotension • CNS effects • Seizures • GI distress • Bradycardia • Dizziness • Slurred speech • Ventricular dysrhythmias	• Instruct client to monitor pulse rate and rhythm • Monitor EKG • Monitor for tinnitus and visual disturbances • Lidocaine administered IV bolus and by infusion • Monitor for confusion, drowsiness, slurred speech, seizures with lidocaine • Administer oral drugs with food • Monitor EKG • Monitor EKG • May cause digoxin toxicity
CLASS II • **propranolol HCL** (Inderal)	• Supraventricular and ventricular tachydysrythmias	• Hypotension • Bradycardia • Bronchospasm	• Monitor vital signs • Contraindicated in asthma, COPD

Figure 3-21

ANTIARRHYTHMICS (CONTINUED)			
DRUGS	**INDICATIONS**	**ADVERSE REACTIONS**	**NURSING IMPLICATIONS**
CLASS III (Intropics) • **bretylium tosylate (Bretylol)** • **amiodarone HCL** (Cordarone) • **milrinone** (Primacor) • **inamrinone** (Inocor) • **sotalol** (Betapace)	• Ventricular dysrhythmias	• Dysrhythmias • Hypertension or hypotension • Muscle weakness, tremors • Photophobia	• Amiodarone is now one of the first choice drugs • Monitor vital signs, EKG • Instruct client taking amiodarone to wear sunglasses and sunscreens when outside
CLASS IV • **verapamil HCL** (Isoptin, Calan)	• Supraventricular dysrhythmias	• Hypotension • Bradycardia • Constipation	• Monitor BP and pulse • Instruct client to change positions slowly
MISCELLANEOUS AGENTS			
• **atropine sulfate** (Atropisol)	• Bradycardia	• Chest pain • Urinary retention • Dry mouth	• Monitor heart rate and rhythm • Assess for chest pain • Assess for urinary retention • Avoid use in glaucoma
• **digoxin** (Lanoxin) • **digitoxin** (Crystodigin)	• Supraventricular dysrhythmias • Atrial fibrillation	• Bradycardia • Dysrhythmias • Anorexia, nausea, vomiting, diarrhea, visual disturbances	• Monitor pulse rate and rhythm • Instruct client to report signs of toxicity • Hypokalemia increases the risk of toxicity • Causes hypercalcemia
• **epinephrine** (Adrenaline)	• Cardiac arrest	• Tachycardia • Hypertension	• Impaired renal function can cause toxicity – monitor BUN and creatinine • Monitor pulse return in asystole • Monitor vital signs

Figure 3-21 (continued)

MEDICAL SURGICAL NURSING

ANTIARRHYTHMICS (CONTINUED)			
ADDITIONAL DRUGS THAT PROMOTE CARDIOVASCULAR PERFUSION IN THE FAILING HEART			
VASOPRESSORS • **levarterenol** (Levophed)	• Dilated coronary arteries & causes peripheral vasoconstriction for emergency hypotensive states not caused by blood loss, vascular thrombosis, or anesthesia using cyclopropane or halothane	• Can cause SEVERE tissue necrosis, sloughing & gangrene if infiltrates (blanching along vein pathway = preliminary sign of extravasation)	• Rapidly inactivated by various body enzymes; need to ensure IV patency • Use cautiously in previously hypertensive clients • Check BP q 2 to 5 minutes • Use large veins to avoid complications of prolonged vasoconstriction • Pressor effects poentiated by many drugs; check drug-drug interactions • Have pentolamine (Regitine) diluted per protocol for local injection if infiltrates
CARDIOTONIC/ **VASODILATOR (human** **B-type naturidic** **peptide: HBNP)** • **nesuritide** (Natecor)	• Treatment of acutely decompensated CHF in clients who have dyspnea at rest or with minimal activity • Reduces PCWP & reduces dyspnea	• Hypotension is primary side effect & can be dose limiting • Arrhythmias • H/A, dizziness, insomnia, tremors, paresthesias • Abdominal pain, N/V	• Many drug-drug interactions • Monitor BP & telemetry • As diuresis occurs, monitor electrolytes, especially K+ • Watch for over-response to treatment in elderly
GROUP IIA-IIIB **INHIBITOR (platelet** **antiaggregate)** • **eptifibatide** (Integrilin)	• Acute coronary syndrome (unstable angina or non-Q waver MI) • Used in combination with heparin, aspirin & in selected situations, Ticlid & Plavix.	• Bleeding, most frequent • Hypotension • Thrombocytopenia • Acute toxicity: decreased muscle tone, dyspnea, loss of righting reflex	• Check drug-drug interactions before giving other meds • Obtain baseline PT/aPTT, H&H, platelet count & monitor • Dose adjusted by weight for elderly • Same client teaching as with heparin re. activities to avoid • Watch for bleeding • Quickly reversible, so emergency procedures may still be performed shortly after discontinuing infusion

Figure 3-21 (continued)

CONGESTIVE HEART FAILURE (CHF)

DESCRIPTION: Inability of the heart to pump enough blood to meet the tissue's oxygen demands.
Primary underlying conditions causing CHF are:
1. Ischemic heart disease.
2. MI.
3. Cardiomyopathy.
4. Valvular heart disease.
5. Hypertension.

NURSING ASSESSMENT
1. Observe for symptoms associated with left-sided or right-sided failure. *(See figure 3-22, Left-Sided/Right-Sided Heart Failure)*
2. Enlargement of ventricles as indicated by chest x-ray.

ANALYSIS (NURSING DIAGNOSES)
1. Decreased cardiac output related to…
2. Altered patterns of urinary output related to…
3. Activity intolerance related to…
4. Anxiety related to…
5. Tissue perfusion decrease related to…

NURSING PLANS AND INTERVENTIONS
1. Monitor vital signs at least q 4 hours for changes.
2. Monitor apical heart rate with vital signs to detect dysrhythmias, S_3 or S_4.
3. Assess for hypoxia.
   A. Restlessness.
   B. Tachycardia.
   C. Angina.
4. Auscultate lungs for indication of pulmonary edema (wet sounds/crackles).
5. Administer oxygen as needed.
6. Elevate head of bed to assist with breathing.
7. Observe for signs of edema.
   A. Weigh daily.
   B. Monitor I&O.
   C. Measure abdominal girth; observe ankles and fingers.
8. Limit sodium intake.
9. Elevate lower extremities while sitting.
10. Check apical heart rate prior to administration of digitalis, withhold medication and call physician if rate is below 60 BPM. *(See figure 3-23, Digitalis Preparations)*
11. Administer diuretics in morning if possible. *(See figure 3-15, Diuretics)*
12. Provide periods of rest after periods of activity.

LEFT-SIDED HEART FAILURE		RIGHT-SIDED HEART FAILURE	
PULMONARY EDEMA (LEFT VENTRICULAR FAILURE)		PERIPHERAL EDEMA (RIGHT VENTRICULAR FAILURE)	
DESCRIPTION	**SYMPTOMS**	**DESCRIPTION**	**SYMPTOMS**
Results in pulmonary congestion due to the inability of the left ventricle to pump blood to the periphery.	• Dyspnea • Orthopnea • "Wet" lung sounds • Cough • Fatigue • Tachycardia • Anxiety • Restlessness • Confusion	Results in peripheral congestion due to the inability of the right ventricle to pump blood out to the lungs. Often results from left-sided failure or pulmonary disease.	• Peripheral edema • Weight gain • Distended neck veins • Anorexia, nausea • Nocturia • Weakness

Figure 3-22

HESI HINT: Restricting sodium reduces salt and water retention, thereby reducing vascular volume and preload.

HESI HINT: Digitalis
- Side effects of digitalis are increased when the client is hypokalemic.
- Has a negative chronotropic effect, i.e., it slows the heart rate. Hold the digitalis if the pulse rate is <60, >120, or has markedly changed rhythm.
- Bradycardia, tachycardia, or dysrhythmias may be signs of digitalis toxicity: these signs include nausea, vomiting, and headache in adults.
- If withheld, consult with physician.

DIGITALIS PREPARATIONS

DRUGS	INDICATIONS	ADVERSE REACTIONS	NURSING IMPLICATIONS
• digitoxin (Crystodigin, Purodigin) • digoxin (Lanoxin, Lanoxicaps)	• CHF • Increases the contractility of cardiac muscle • Slow heart rate and conduction	• Severe: A-V block • Headache • Dysrhythmias • Nausea • Vomiting • Blurred vision • Yellow-green halos • Hypotension • Fatigue	• Monitor serum electrolytes; hypokalemia increases risk of digoxin toxicity • Monitor serum digitalis levels if any side effects are present • Check apical pulse prior to administration; call healthcare provider if rate is below 60 BPM • Teach client to take radial pulse prior to administration and call healthcare provider if below 60 BPM in adults • Therapeutic range: 0.5 to 2 mg
• digoxin-immune FAB (Digibind)	• Antidote for digitalis toxicity • Binds with digitoxin or digoxin to prevent binding at their site of action	• Decreased cardiac output • Atrial tachyarrhythmias • Use with caution in children and elderly	• Use with 0.22 micron filter • Place client on continuous cardiac monitor • Have resuscitation equipment at bed side before giving first dose

Figure 3-23

INFLAMMATORY AND INFECTIOUS HEART DISEASE

DESCRIPTION: Inflammatory and infectious process involving the endocardium and pericardium.
1. Endocarditis is an inflammatory disease involving the inner surface of the heart including the valves. Organisms travel through the blood to the heart where vegetations, which can become emboli, form.
2. Causes of endocarditis:
    A. Rheumatic heart disease.
    B. Congenital heart disease.
    C. IV drug abuse.
    D. Cardiac surgery.
    E. Immunosuppression.
    F. Dental procedures.
    G. Invasive procedures.
3. Pericarditis is an inflammation of the outer lining of the heart.

4. Causes of pericarditis:
    A. Post MI.
    B. Trauma.
    C. Neoplasm.
    D. Connective tissue disease.
    E. After heart surgery.
    F. Idiopathic.
    G. Infections.

NURSING ASSESSMENT
1. Endocarditis:
    A. Fever.
    B. Chills, malaise, night sweats, fatigue.
    C. Murmurs.
    D. Symptoms of heart failure.
    E. Atrial embolization.
2. Pericarditis:
    A. Pain: sudden, sharp, severe.
        1) Substernal, radiating to the back or arm.
        2) Aggravated by coughing, inhalation,

deep breathing.
   3) Relieved by leaning forward.
   B. Pericardial friction rub.
   C. Fever.

> **HESI HINT: Infective Endocarditis**
> damage to heart valves occurs with the growth
> of vegetative lesions on valve leaflets. These
> lesions pose a risk of embolization; erosion/
> perforation of the valve leaflets; or abcesses
> within adjacent myocardial tissue. Valvular
> stenosis or regurgitation (insufficiency), most
> commonly of the mitral valve, can occur
> depending upon the type of damage inflicted
> by the lesions, leading to symptoms of left- or
> right-sided heart failure. *(See Valvular Heart
> Disease & Congestive Heart Failure)*

> **HESI HINT: Acute & Subacute Infective
> Endocarditis**
> There are 2 types of infective endocarditis:
> <u>acute</u>, which often affects individuals with pre-
> viously normal hearts and healthy valves, and
> carries a high mortality rate; and <u>subacute</u>,
> which typically affects individuals with pre-
> existing conditions, such as rheumatic heart
> disease, mitral valve prolapse, or immunosu-
> pression. Intravenous drug abusers are at risk
> for both acute and subacute bacterial endocar-
> ditis. When this population develops Subacute
> Infective Endocarditis, the valves on the right
> side of the heart (tricuspid and pulmonic)
> are typically affected due to the introduction
> of common pathogens which colonize on the
> skin (*S. epidermis or Candida*) into the venous
> system.

> **HESI HINT: Pericarditis**
> Presence of a friction rub is an indication of
> pericarditis (inflammation of the lining of the
> heart). ST segment elevation and T wave inver-
> sion are also signs of pericarditis.

ANALYSIS (NURSING DIAGNOSES)
1. Decreased cardiac output related to…
2. Potential for injury: emboli related to…

NURSING PLANS AND INTERVENTIONS

ENDOCARDITIS
1. Monitor hemodynamic status (vital signs, level of consciousness, urinary output).
2. Administer antibiotics IV for 4 to 6

weeks. The American Heart Association recommends administration of erythromycin before dental or genitourinary procedures. Clients may be instructed in IV therapy for home healthcare.
3. Teach clients about anticoagulant therapy if prescribed.
4. Encourage client to maintain good hygiene.
5. Instruct client to inform dentist or other healthcare providers of history.

PERICARDITIS
1. Provide rest and maintain position of comfort.
2. Administer analgesics and anti-inflammatory drugs.

Valvular Heart Disease
Description: Heart valves are unable to fully open (stenosis) or fully close (insufficiency or regurgitation).
1. Valve dysfunction most commonly occurs on the left side of the heart with the mitral valve most frequently involved, followed by the aortic valve.

> **HESI HINT:** With mitral valve stenosis,
> blood is regurgitated back into the left atrium
> from the left ventricle. In early period, there
> may be no symptoms; but, as the disease pro-
> gresses, the client will exhibit excessive fatigue,
> dyspnea on exertion, orthopnea, dry cough,
> hemoptysis, or pulmonary edema. There will
> be a rumbling apical diastolic murmur, and
> atrial fibrillation is common.

2. Common causes of valvular disease:
   A. Rheumatic fever.
   B. Congenital heart diseases.
   C. Syphilis.
   D. Endocarditis.
   E. Hypertension.
3. Prevention of rheumatic heart disease would reduce the incidence of valvular heart disease.

NURSING ASSESSMENT
1. Fatigue.
2. Dyspnea, orthopnea.
3. Hemoptysis and pulmonary edema.
4. Murmurs.
5. Irregular cardiac rhythm.
6. Angina.

ANALYSIS (NURSING DIAGNOSES)
1. Decreased cardiac output related to...
2. Impaired gas exchange related to...
3. Activity intolerance related to...

NURSING PLANS AND INTERVENTIONS
1. *See Congestive Heart Failure*.
2. Monitor client for atrial fibrillation with thrombus formation.
3. Teach the necessity for prophylactic antibiotic therapy before any invasive procedure, e.g., dental procedures.
4. Prepare the client for surgical repair or replacement of heart valves.
5. Instruct clients receiving valve replacement of the need for lifelong anticoagulant therapy to prevent thrombus formation.

REVIEW QUESTIONS
CARDIOVASCULAR SYSTEM
1. **How do clients experiencing angina describe that pain?**
2. **Develop a teaching plan for the client taking nitroglycerin.**
3. **List the parameters of blood pressure for diagnosing hypertension.**
4. **Differentiate between essential and secondary hypertension.**
5. **Develop a teaching plan for the client taking antihypertensive medications.**
6. **Describe intermittent claudication.**
7. **Describe the nurse's discharge instructions to a client with venous peripheral vascular disease.**
8. **What is often the underlying cause of abdominal aortic aneurysm?**
9. **What lab values should be monitored daily for the client with thrombophlebitis who is undergoing anticoagulant therapy?**
10. **When do PVCs (premature ventricular contractions) present a grave danger?**
11. **Differentiate between the symptoms of left-sided cardiac failure and right-sided cardiac failure.**
12. **List three symptoms of digitalis toxicity.**
13. **What condition increases the likelihood of digitalis toxicity occurring?**
14. **What life style changes can the client who is at risk for hypertension initiate to reduce the likelihood of becoming hypertensive?**
15. **What immediate actions should the nurse implement when a client is having a myocardial infarction?**
16. **What symptoms should the nurse expect to find in the client with hypokalemia?**
17. **Bradycardia is defined as a heart rate below _____ BPM. Tachycardia is defined as a heart rate above _____ BPM.**
18. **What precautions should clients with valve disease take prior to invasive procedures or dental work?**

ANSWERS TO REVIEW QUESTIONS
1. Described as squeezing, heavy, burning, radiates to left arm or shoulder, transient or prolonged.
2. Take at first sign of anginal pain. Take no more than 3, five minutes apart. Call for emergency attention if no relief in 10 minutes.
3. >140/90.
4. Essential has no known cause while secondary hypertension develops in response to an identifiable mechanism.
5. Explain how and when to take med, reason for med, necessity of compliance, need for follow-up visits while on med, need for certain lab tests, vital sign parameters while initiating therapy.
6. Pain related to peripheral vascular disease occurring with exercise and disappearing with rest.
7. Keep extremities elevated when sitting, rest at first sign of pain, keep extremities warm (but do NOT use heating pad), change position often, avoid crossing legs, wear unrestrictive clothing.
8. Atherosclerosis.
9. PTT, PT, Hgb, and Hct, platelets.
10. When they begin to occur more often than once in 10 beats, occur in 2s or 3s, land near the T wave, or take on multiple configurations.
11. Left-sided failure results in pulmonary congestion due to back-up of circulation in the left ventricle. Right-sided failure results in peripheral congestion due to back-up of circulation in the right ventricle.
12. Dysrhythmias, headache, nausea, and vomiting.
13. When the client is hypokalemic (which is more common when diuretics and digitalis preparations are given together.)
14. Cease cigarette smoking if applicable, control weight, exercise regularly, and

maintain a low-fat/low-cholesterol diet.

15. Place the client on immediate strict bedrest to lower oxygen demands of heart, administer oxygen by nasal cannula at 2 to 5 l/min., take measures to alleviate pain and anxiety (administer prn pain medications and anti-anxiety medications.)
16. Dry mouth and thirst, drowsiness and lethargy, muscle weakness and aches, and tachycardia.
17. 60 BPM. 100 BPM.
18. Take prophylactic antibiotics.

GASTROINTESTINAL SYSTEM

HIATAL HERNIA

DESCRIPTION: Herniation of the stomach and other abdominal viscera through an enlarged esophageal opening in the diaphragm.
1. The etiology of hiatal hernia is unknown.
2. Contributing factors include congenital defects and trauma.

NURSING ASSESSMENT
1. Heartburn after eating.
2. Feeling of fullness and discomfort after eating.
3. Positive diagnosis determined by fluoroscopy or barium swallow.

ANALYSIS (NURSING DIAGNOSES)
1. Pain related to…
2. Knowledge deficit related to…
3. Anxiety related to…

NURSING PLANS AND INTERVENTIONS
1. Determine eating pattern which alleviates symptoms.
    A. Encourage small, frequent meals.
    B. Eliminate foods that are determined to aggravate symptoms (these foods are client specific).
    C. Sit up while eating and remain in upright position for at least one hour after eating.
    D. Stop eating 3 hours before bedtime.
    E. Teach about frequently prescribed medications (H_2 antagonists, antacids).

> **HESI HINT:** A Fowler's or semi-Fowler's position is beneficial in reducing the amount of regurgitation as well as preventing the encroachment of the stomach tissue upward through the opening in the diaphragm.

2. Teaching plan for client/family should include the following:
    A. Differentiate between the symptoms of hiatal hernia and MI.
    B. Be alert to the possibility of aspiration.

PEPTIC ULCER DISEASE (PUD)

DESCRIPTION: Ulceration which penetrates the mucosal wall of the GI tract.
1. Gastric ulcers tend to occur in the lesser curvature of the stomach.
2. Duodenal ulcers occur in the duodenum.
3. Esophageal ulcers occur in the esophagus.
4. The etiology of some peptic ulcer disease is unknown. A significant number of gastric ulcers are caused by a bacteria, helicobactor pylori (*H. pylori*) and can be successfully treated with drug therapy. Risk factors for development of peptic ulcers include:
    A. Drugs (NSAIDs, corticosteroids).
    B. Alcohol.
    C. Cigarette smoking.
    D. Acute medical crisis or trauma.
5. Symptoms common to all types of ulcers include the following:
    A. Belching.
    B. Bloating.
    C. Epigastric pain radiating to the back (not associated with the type of food eaten) and relieved by antacids.

NURSING ASSESSMENT
1. Determine how food intake affects pain.
2. History of antacid or histamine antagonist use.
3. Melena.
4. Presence and/or location of peptic ulcers as determined by:
    A. Barium swallow.
    B. Upper endoscopy.
    C. Gastric analysis indicating increased levels of stomach acid.
5. Potential complications:
    A. Hemorrhage.
    B. Perforation (always demands surgery).
    C. Obstruction.

ANALYSIS (NURSING DIAGNOSES)

1. Pain related to…
2. Altered nutrition related to…
3. Knowledge deficit related to…
4. Potential for injury related to…

NURSING PLANS AND INTERVENTIONS

1. Determine symptom onset and how symptoms are relieved.
2. Monitor color, quantity, consistency of stools and emesis, and test for occult blood.
3. Administer medications as prescribed, usually 1 to 2 hours after meals and at bedtime. *(See figure 3-24, Anti-ulcer Drugs)*

ANTI-ULCER DRUGS			
DRUGS	**INDICATIONS**	**ADVERSE REACTIONS**	**NURSING IMPLICATIONS**
ANTACIDS • **aluminum hydroxide/ magnesium hydroxide** (Maalox) (Mylanta) (Riopan) (Gelusil II)	• Treatment of peptic ulcers • Work by neutralizing or reducing acidity of stomach contents • Differences in absorption rate	• Constipation • Diarrhea • Drug interactions	• Need to take several times a day • Administer after meals • Assess for history of renal diseases when client is taking magnesium products; electrolyte readjustment occurs and can result in renal insufficiency and calcinosis
HISTAMINE₂ ANTAGONISTS • **ranitidine HCL** (Zantac) • **cimetidine** (Tagament) • **famotidine** (Pepcid) • **nizatidine** (Axid)	• Treatment of peptic ulcers • Prophylactic treatment for clients at risk for developing ulcers (those on steroids, or highly stressed)	• Multiple drug interactions	• Cigarette smoking interferes with drug action • Expensive

MUCOSAL HEALING AGENTS
• **sucralfate** (Carafate)
	• Treatment of peptic ulcers	• Constipation
		• Drug interaction with:
		  • tetracycline
		  • phenytoin sodium
		  • digoxin
		  • cimetidine
			• Medication to be taken at least one hour before meals
			• Antacids interfere with absorption

PROTON PUMP INHIBITORS • **lansoprazole** (Prevacid) (PO only) • **pantoprazole** (Protonix) (available PO & IV) • **esomeprazole** (Nexium) (PO only)	• Treatment of erosive esophagitis associated with gastroesophageal reflux disease (GERD)	• Constipation • Heartburn • Anxiety • Diarrhea • Abdominal pain, hepatocellular damage, pancreatitis, gastroenteritis • Tinnitis, vertigo, confusion, H/A • Blurred vision, hypokinesia • Chest pain, dyspnea	• Taken before meals • Do not crush or chew **Pantoprazole IV:** • Resume oral therapy as soon as feasible • Long-lasting effects of drug may inhibit absorption of other drugs • Not removed by hemodialysis • Monitor for indications of adverse reactions

Figure 3-24

4. Administer mucosal healing agents at least one hour before meals, as prescribed. *(See figure 3-24, Anti-Ulcer Drugs)*
5. Encourage small, frequent meals with no bedtime snack. Avoid beverages containing caffeine.
6. Prepare for surgery if uncontrolled bleeding, obstruction, or perforation occurs.
   A. Gastric resection.
   B. Vagotomy.
   C. Pyloroplasty.
7. Dumping syndrome may occur postoperatively.
   A. Secondary to rapid entry of hypertonic food into jejunum (pulls water out of bloodstream).
   B. Occurs 5 to 30 minutes after eating.
   C. Characterized by vertigo, syncope, sweating, pallor, tachycardia.
   D. Provide small, frequent meals: high-protein, high-fat, low-carbohydrate diet.
   E. Avoid liquids with meals and encourage client to lie down after eating.
   F. This syndrome can also be observed in clients on hypertonic tube feeding.
8. Teach client to avoid medications that increase the risk for developing peptic ulcers.
   A. Salicylates.
   B. Nonsteroidal anti-inflammatory drugs such as ibuprofen.
   C. Corticosteroids in high doses.
   D. Reserpine (antihypertensive).
   E. Anticoagulants.
9. Teach client the importance of informing all healthcare personnel of ulcer history.
10. Teach client symptoms of GI bleeding.
    A. Dark, tarry stools.
    B. Coffee-ground emesis.
    C. Bright red, rectal bleeding.
    D. Fatigue.
    E. Pallor.
    F. Severe abdominal pain should be reported immediately (could denote perforation).
11. Teach client importance of smoking cessation and stress management.

> **HESI HINT:** Stress can cause or exacerbate ulcers. Teach stress reduction methods and encourage those with a family history of ulcers to obtain medical surveillance for ulcer formation.

> **HESI HINT: CLINICAL MANIFESTATIONS OF GI BLEEDING:**
> - **Pallor: conjunctival, mucous membranes, nail beds.**
> - **Dark, tarry stools.**
> - **Bright red or coffee-ground emesis.**
> - **Abdominal mass or bruit.**
> - **Decreased BP, rapid pulse, cool extremities (shock).**

INFLAMMATORY BOWEL DISEASES
DESCRIPTION: Consists of Crohn's disease and ulcerative colitis.

CROHN'S DISEASE (REGIONAL ENTERITIS)
DESCRIPTION: Subacute, chronic inflammation extending throughout the entire intestinal mucosa (most frequently found in terminal ileum).

NURSING ASSESSMENT
1. Abdominal pain (unrelieved by defecation).
2. Diarrhea and weight loss, with client becoming emaciated.
3. Constant fluid loss.
4. Perforation of the intestine may occur due to severe inflammation and constitutes a medical emergency.

> **HESI HINT:** The GI tract usually accounts for only 100 to 200 ml fluid loss per day, although it filters up to 8 liters per day. *Large fluid losses can occur if vomiting and/or diarrhea exists.*

ULCERATIVE COLITIS
DESCRIPTION: Disease which affects the superficial mucosa of the colon, causing the bowel to eventually narrow, shorten, and thicken due to muscular hypertrophy. Occurs in the large bowel and rectum.

NURSING ASSESSMENT
1. Diarrhea.
2. Abdominal pain and cramping.
3. Intermittent tenesmus (anal contractions) and rectal bleeding.
4. Liquid stools containing blood, mucous and pus (may pass 10 to 20 liquid stools per day).
5. Weakness and fatigue.
6. Anemia.

ANALYSIS (NURSING DIAGNOSES)
1. Fluid volume deficit related to…
2. Pain related to…
3. Altered nutritional status: less than body requirements related to…

NURSING PLANS AND INTERVENTIONS
1. Determine bowel elimination pattern and control diarrhea with diet and medication as indicated.
2. Provide a nutritious, well-balanced, low-residue, low-fat, high-protein, high-calorie diet. *No dairy products*.
3. Administer vitamin supplements and iron.
4. Avoid foods which are known to cause diarrhea, such as milk products and spicy food.
5. Avoid smoking, caffeinated beverages, pepper, and alcohol.
6. Provide complete bowel rest with intravenous hyperalimentation if necessary.
7. Administer medications as prescribed, often steroids, antidiarrheals, sulfasalazine (Azulfidine).
8. Monitor I&O and serum electrolytes.
9. Weigh at least twice a week.
10. Provide emotional support and encourage use of support groups such as local Ileitis and Colitis Foundation.
11. Encourage client to talk with the enterostomal therapists BEFORE surgery.
12. If ileostomy performed, teach stoma care. *(See figure 3-25 Stoma Care)*

> **HESI HINT:** Opiate drugs tend to depress gastric motility. However, they should be given with care, and those receiving them should be closely monitored because a distended intestinal wall accompanied by decreased muscle tone may lead to intestinal perforation.

DIVERTICULAR DISEASES
DESCRIPTION: Manifested in two clinical forms, diverticulosis and diverticulitis.
1. Diverticulosis: bulging pouches in the GI wall (diverticula) push the mucosa lining through the surrounding muscle.
2. Diverticulitis: inflamed diverticula, (may cause obstruction, infection, and/or hemorrhage.)

> **HESI HINT:** Diverticulosis is the presence of pouches in the wall of the intestine. There is usually no discomfort, and the problem goes unnoticed unless seen on radiological examination (usually prompted by some other condition). Diverticulitis is an inflammation of the diverticula (pouches), which can lead to perforation of the bowel.

NURSING ASSESSMENT
1. Left lower quadrant pain.
2. Increased flatus.
3. Rectal bleeding.
4. Signs of intestinal obstruction.
    A. Constipation alternating with diarrhea.
    B. Abdominal distention.
    C. Anorexia.
    D. Low-grade fever.
5. Barium enema positive for diverticular disease. Obstruction, ileus, or perforation confirmed with abdominal x-ray. Barium not done during acute phase of illness.

ANALYSIS (NURSING DIAGNOSES)
1. Altered tissue perfusion related to…
2. Pain related to…
3. Altered nutrition less than body requirements related to…

NURSING PLANS AND INTERVENTIONS
1. Provide a well-balanced, high-fiber diet unless inflammation is present, at which time client is NPO followed by low-residue, bland foods.

> **HESI HINT:** A client admitted with complaints of severe lower abdominal pain, cramping, and diarrhea is diagnosed with diverticulitis. What are the nutritional needs of this client throughout recovery?
> - Acute phase – NPO graduating to liquids.
> - Recovery phase – no fiber or foods that irritate the bowel.
> - Maintenance phase – high-fiber diet, with bulk-forming laxatives to prevent pooling of foods in the pouches where they can become inflamed. Avoid small, poorly digested foods such as popcorn, nuts, seeds, etc.

2. Include bulk-forming laxatives such as Metamucil in daily regimen.
3. Increase fluid intake to 3 liters/day.

4. Monitor I&O, bowel elimination, avoid constipation.
5. Observe for complications.
    A. Obstruction.
    B. Peritonitis.
    C. Hemorrhage (with ruptured diverticuli, a temporary colostomy is performed and maintained for approximately 3 months to allow the bowel to rest).
    D. Infection.

INTESTINAL OBSTRUCTION

DESCRIPTION: Partial or complete blockage of intestinal flow (fluids, feces, gas).
1. Mechanical causes of intestinal obstruction include:
    A. Adhesions (most common cause).
    B. Hernia (strangulates the gut).
    C. Volvulus (twisting of the gut).
    D. Intussusception (telescoping of the gut within itself).
    E. Tumors, develop slowly; usually mass of feces becomes lodged against the tumor.
2. Neurogenic causes of intestinal obstruction:
    A. Paralytic ileus (usually occurs in postoperativeclients).
    B. Spinal cord lesion.
3. Vascular cause: mesenteric artery occlusion (leads to gut infarct).

> **HESI HINT: Bowel Obstructions:**
> - **Mechanical** – due to disorders outside the bowel (hernia, adhesions), due to disorders within the bowel (tumors, diverticulitis), or due to blockage of the lumen in the intestine (intussusception, gall stone).
> - **Non-Mechanical** – paralytic ileus, which does not involve any actual physical obstruction, but results from inability of the bowel itself to function.

NURSING ASSESSMENT
1. Sudden onset of abdominal pain, tenderness or guarding.
2. History of abdominal surgeries.
3. History of obstruction.
4. Distention.
5. Increased peristalsis when obstruction first occurs, then peristalsis become absent when paralytic ileus occurs.
6. Bowel sounds are high-pitched with early mechanical obstruction and diminished to absent with neurogenic, or late mechanical

obstruction.

ANALYSIS (NURSING DIAGNOSES)
1. Altered (GI) tissue perfusion related to…
2. Fluid volume deficit related to…
3. Pain related to…

> **HESI HINT:** Blood gas analysis will show an alkalotic state if the bowel obstruction is high in the small intestine where gastric acid is secreted. If the obstruction is in the lower bowel where base solutions are secreted, the blood will be acidic.

NURSING PLANS AND INTERVENTIONS
1. NPO, IV fluids, and electrolyte therapy.
2. I&O, Foley catheter to maintain strict output.
3. Nasogastric intubation:
    A. Attach to low suction (intermittent 80 mmHg).
    B. Document output every 8 hours.
    C. Irrigate with normal saline if policy dictates.
4. Cantor, Miller-Abbott, Harris tubes are passed through the nose and into the stomach, usually by the healthcare provider.
    A. Advance tube every 1 to 2 hours.
    B. Do *not* secure to nose until tube reaches specified position.
    C. Reposition client every 2 hours to assist with placement of the tube.
    D. Connect to suction.
    E. Irrigate with air only.
    F. Note amount, color, consistency, and any unusual odor of drainage.
5. Document pain; medicate as prescribed.
6. Assess abdomen regularly for distention, rigidity, change in status of bowel sounds.
7. If conservative medical interventions fail, surgery will be required to remove obstruction.
    (See Perioperative Care)

> **HESI HINT:** A client admitted with complaints of constipation, thready stools, and rectal bleeding over the past few months is diagnosed with a rectal mass. What are the nursing priorities for this client?
> - **NPO**
> - **NG tube (possibly an intestinal tube such as a Miller-Abbott)**
> - **IV fluids**
> - **Surgical preparations of bowel (if obstruction is complete)**
> - **Teaching (preoperative, nutrition, etc.)**

CANCER OF THE COLON

DESCRIPTION: Tumors occurring in the colon.

1. Cancer of the colon is the second most common cancer in the U.S.
2. The estimated cure rate for cancer of the colon is 50%.
3. Forty-five percent of cancerous tumors of the colon occur in the rectal or sigmoid area, 25% in the cecum & ascending colon, and 30% in the remainder of colon.
4. Highest incidence is in persons over 60 years of age.
5. A diet of high-fiber, low-fat foods including cruciferous vegetables may be a factor in prevention of colon cancer.

HESI HINT: Diet recommended by the American Cancer Society to prevent bowel cancer:
- Eat more cruciferous vegetables (from the cabbage family such as broccoli, cauliflower, Brussels sprouts, cabbage, and kale).
- Increase fiber intake.
- Maintain average body weight.
- Eat less animal fat.

---

6. Early detection is important.

HESI HINT: AMERICAN CANCER SOCIETY RECOMMENDATIONS
For Early Detection of Colon Cancer:
- A digital rectal examination every year after 40.
- A stool blood test every year after 50.
- A sigmoidoscopy examination every 3 to 5 years after the age of 50, based on the advice of a physician.

---

7. Usual treatment is surgical removal of the tumor with adjuvant radiation or antineoplastic chemotherapy.
8. Diagnosis is made by digital examination, flexible fiber optic sigmoidoscopy with biopsy, colonoscopy, and barium enema.
9. Carcinoembryonic antigen (CEA) serum level is used to evaluate effectiveness of chemotherapy.

NURSING ASSESSMENT

1. Rectal bleeding.
2. Change in bowel habits.
3. Sense of incomplete evacuation.
4. Abdominal pain, nausea, vomiting.
5. Weight loss, cachexia.
6. Abdominal distention or ascites.
7. Family history of cancer, particularly cancer of the colon.
8. History of polyps.

ANALYSIS (NURSING DIAGNOSES)

1. Knowledge deficit related to…
2. Potential for ineffective coping related to…
3. Altered body image related to…

NURSING PLANS AND INTERVENTIONS

1. Prepare client for surgery. *(See Perioperative Care)*
2. Bowel preparation may include laxatives and gut lavage with polyethylene glycol (Golytely).
3. If colostomy performed, teach stoma care. *(See figure 3-25, Stoma Care)*
4. Provide high-calorie, high-protein diet.
5. Promote prevention of constipation with high-fiber diet.
6. Encourage early detection by screening with hemoccult (guiac) tests.

HESI HINT: Cancer of the colon is the most common cancer in the U.S. when considering men and women together. An early sign is rectal bleeding. Encourage patients 50 years of age or older, or those with increased risk factors, to be screened yearly with fecal occult blood testing. Routine colonoscopy at 50 is also recommended.

STOMA CARE

GENERAL INFORMATION

The more distal the stoma is, the greater the chance for continence.

- An ileostomy drains liquid material; peristomal skin is prone to breakdown from enzymes.
- As the stoma's location descends the GI tract, the effluence (stoma drainage) becomes more solid or formed.
- The greatest chance for continence is with a stoma created from the descending colon on the left side of the abdomen.
- Consultation with an enterostomal therapist is essential.

PREOPERATIVE CARE

Inform client/family what to expect postoperatively.

- Proposed location of the stoma.
- Approximate size.
- What it will look like, provide a picture if indicated.
- Include the family in teaching but emphasize that the client is ultimately responsible for his/her own care.

POUCH CARE

Ostimates will often wear pouches.

- The adhesive-backed opening, designed to cover the stoma, should provide about 1/8 inch clearance from the stoma.
- Use rubber band or clip to secure the bottom of the pouch and prevent leakage.
- Use simple squirt bottle to remove effluence from the sides of the bag. Change pouch system every 3 to 7 days.
- Clients should maintain an extra supply of pouches so that they never run out, and change the pouch even when bowel is inactive.
- Empty pouch when 1/3 to 1/2 full.

IRRIGATION

Those with descending colon colostomies can irrigate to provide control over effluence.

- Irrigate at approximately the same time daily.
- Use warm water (cold or hot water will cause cramping).
- Wash around stoma with lukewarm water and a mild soap.
- Commercial skin barriers may be purchased for home use.
- Odor control.
- Commercial preparations are available.
- Eliminate foods in diet which cause offensive odors.

DIET

Ileostomy

- Instruct client to chew food thoroughly.
- High-fiber foods can cause severe diarrhea and may need to be eliminated (popcorn, peanuts, unpeeled vegetables).

Colostomy

- Instruct client to resume the regular diet gradually. Foods that were a problem preoperative should be tried cautiously.

Figure 3-25

CIRRHOSIS

DESCRIPTION: Degeneration of liver tissue causing enlargement, fibrosis, and scarring.

1. Etiology of cirrhosis includes the following:
   A. Chronic alcohol ingestion (Laennec's cirrhosis).
   B. Viral hepatitis.
   C. Exposure to hepatotoxins (including medications).
   D. Infections.
   E. Congenital abnormalities.
   F. Chronic biliary tree obstruction.
   G. Chronic severe right congestive heart failure (CHF).
   H. Idiopathy.
2. Initially, hepatomegaly occurs; later, the liver becomes hard and nodular.

NURSING ASSESSMENT

1. History of alcohol and street drug intake.
2. Work history of exposure to toxic chemicals (pesticides, fumes, etc.).
3. Medication history of long-term use of hepatotoxic drugs.
4. Family health history of liver abnormalities.
5. Physical findings include the following:
   A. Weakness, malaise.
   B. Anorexia, weight loss.
   C. Palpable liver (early), abdominal girth increases as liver enlarges.
   D. Jaundice.
   E. Fetor hepaticus (fruity or musty breath).

> **HESI HINT: CLINICAL MANIFESTATIONS JAUNDICE**
> - Yellow skin, sclera, and/or mucous membranes (bilirubin in skin).
> - Dark-colored urine (bilirubin in urine).
> - Chalky or clay-colored stools (absence of bilirubin in stools).

> **HESI HINT:** Fetor hepaticus is a distinctive breath odor of chronic liver disease. It is characterized by a fruity or musty odor which results from the damaged liver's inability to metabolize and detoxify mercaptan which is produced by the bacterial degradation of methionine, a sulfurous amino acid.

   F. Asterixis (hand-flapping tremor that often accompanies metabolic disorders).

   G. Mental and behavioral changes.
   H. Bruising, erythema.
   I. Dry skin, spider angiomas.
   J. Gynecomastia (breast development), testicular atrophy.
   K. Ascites, peripheral neuropathy.
   L. Hematemesis.
   M. Palmar erythema (redness in palms of the hands).

> **HESI HINT:** For treatment of ascites, paracentesis and peritoneovenous shunts (LaVeen and Denver shunts) may be indicated.

> **HESI HINT:** Esophageal varices may rupture and cause hemorrhage. Immediate management includes insertion of an esophagogastric balloon tamponade – a Blakemore-Sengstaken or Minnesota tube. Other therapies include vasopressors, vitamin K, coagulation factors, and blood transfusions.

6. Clotting defects noted in laboratory findings include:
   A. Elevated bilirubin, AST, ALT, alkaline phosphatase, PT, and ammonia.
   B. Decreased Hgb, Hct, electrolytes, and albumin.

> **HESI HINT:** Ammonia is not broken down as usual in the damaged liver; therefore, the serum ammonia level rises.

7. Complications include:
   A. Ascites, edema.
   B. Portal hypertension.
   C. Esophageal varices.
   D. Encephalopathy.
   E. Respiratory distress.
   F. Coagulation defects.

ANALYSIS (NURSING DIAGNOSES)

1. Fluid volume excess related to…
2. Potential for injury (bleeding) related to…
3. Pain related to…
4. Ineffective breathing pattern related to…
5. Altered nutrition, less than body requirement related to…
6. Potential for infection related to…

NURSING PLANS AND INTERVENTIONS

1. Eliminate causative agent (alcohol, hepatotoxin).
2. Administer vitamin supplements (A, B

complex, C, K) and teach client/family the need for continuing these supplements.

3. Observe mental status frequently (at least every two hours); note any subtle changes.
4. Avoid initiating bleeding and observe for bleeding tendencies.
   A. Avoid injections whenever possible.
   B. Use small bore needles for IV insertion.
   C. Maintain pressure to venipuncture sites for at least 5 minutes.
   D. Use electric razor.
   E. Provide a soft-bristle toothbrush and encourage careful mouth care.
   F. Check stools and emesis for frank or occult blood.
   G. Prevent straining at stool.
      1) Administer stool softeners as prescribed.
      2) Provide high-fiber diet.
5. Provide special skin care.
   A. Avoid soap, rubbing alcohol, and perfumed products (are drying to the skin).
   B. Apply moisturizing lotion or baby oil frequently.
   C. Observe skin for any lesions including scratch marks.

D. Turn frequently and provide lotion to exposed skin.
6. Monitor fluid and electrolyte status daily.
   A. I&O (accurate output may require Foley catheter).
   B. Observe for edema, pulmonary edema.
   C. Measure abdominal girth (determines increase or decrease of ascites).
   D. Weigh daily (determines increase or decrease of edema and ascites).
   E. Restrict fluids to 1500 ml/day (may help to reduce edema and ascites).
7. Monitor dietary intake carefully, especially protein intake. Restrict protein if client has hepatic coma, otherwise encourage foods with high biologic protein.
8. Explain dietary restrictions: low-sodium, low potassium, low-fat, high-carbohydrate.
9. If encephalopathy is present, lactulose is used. *(See figure 3-26, Ammonia Detoxicant/ Stimulant Laxative)*
10. If esophageal varices are present, esophagogastric balloon tamponade (Blakemore tube), sclerotherapy, and/or portal systemic shunts may be used for treatment.

AMMONIA DETOXICANT/STIMULANT LAXATIVE			
DRUG	**INDICATIONS**	**ADVERSE REACTIONS**	**NURSING IMPLICATIONS**
lactulose (Cephulac)	• Encephalopathy • Used to decrease ammonia levels and bowel pH	• Diarrhea	• Instruct client regarding need for medication • Observe for diarrhea • Monitor ammonia levels

Figure 3-26

HEPATITIS

DESCRIPTION: Widespread inflammation of liver cells usually caused by a virus. *(See figure 3-27, Comparison of Three Types of Hepatitis)*

NURSING ASSESSMENT
1. Known exposure to hepatitis.
2. Recent transfusions or hemodialysis.
3. Individuals at risk for contracting hepatitis:
   A. Homosexual males.
   B. IV drug users (disease transmitted by dirty needles).
   C. Those who have recently had ears pierced or had tattoos drawn (disease transmitted by dirty needles).
   D. Those living in crowded conditions.

   E. Healthcare workers employed in high-risk areas:
      1) Labs.
      2) Emergency rooms.
      3) Critical care units.
      4) Hemodialysis units.
      5) Oncology.
      6) Centers for care of the mentally challenged.
4. Fatigue, malaise, weakness.
5. Anorexia, nausea and vomiting.
6. Jaundice, dark urine, clay-colored stools.
7. Myalgia (muscle aches), joint pain.
8. Dull headaches, irritability, depression.
9. Abdominal tenderness in right upper quadrant.

10. Fever with hepatitis A.
11. Elevations of liver enzymes (ALT, AST, alkaline phosphatase), bilirubin.

ANALYSIS (NURSING DIAGNOSES)

1. Activity intolerance related to…
2. Altered nutrition: less than body requirements related to…
3. Potential for infection related to…

NURSING PLANS AND INTERVENTIONS

1. Assess client's response to activity and plan periods of rest after periods of activity.
2. Assist client with care as needed, encourage client to get help with daily activities at home (caring for children, preparing meals, etc.).
3. Provide high-calorie, high-carbohydrate diet with moderate fats and proteins.
   A. Serve small, frequent meals.
   B. Provide vitamin supplements.
   C. Provide foods the client prefers.
4. Administer antiemetics as needed.

5. Teach client importance of adhering to personal hygiene, using individual drinking and eating utensils, toothbrushes, and razors. Prevention of spread to others must be emphasized.
6. Teach client to avoid hepatotoxic substances such as alcohol, aspirin, acetaminophen, and sedatives.

> **HESI HINT:** Liver tissue is destroyed by hepatitis. Rest and adequate nutrition are necessary for regeneration of liver tissue being destroyed by the disease. Since many drugs are metabolized in the liver, drug therapy must be scrutinized carefully. Caution the client that recovery takes many months, and previously taken medications should not be resumed without the healthcare provider's directions.

> **HESI HINT: PROVIDE AN ENVIRONMENT CONDUCIVE TO EATING**
> For clients who are anorexic and/or nauseated:
> - Remove strong odors immediately; they can be offensive and increase nausea.
> - Encourage client to sit up for meals; this can decrease the propensity to vomit.
> - Serve small, frequent meals.

COMPARISON OF THREE TYPES OF HEPATITIS			
CHARACTERISTIC	**HEPATITIS A (INFECTIOUS HEPATITIS)**	**HEPATITIS B (SERUM HEPATITIS)**	**HEPATITIS C**
SOURCE OF INFECTION	• Contaminated food • Contaminated water	• Contaminated blood products • Contaminated needles or surgical instruments	• Contaminated blood products • Contaminated needles; IV drug use • Dialysis
ROUTE OF INFECTION	• Oral • Fecal • Parenteral	• Parenteral • Oral • Fecal • Direct contact • Breast milk • Sexual contact	• Parenteral • Sexual contact
INCUBATION PERIOD	• 2 to 6 weeks	• 6 to 20 weeks	• Ave: 6 to 7 weeks
ONSET	• Abrupt	• Insidious	• Insidious
SEASONAL VARIATION	• Autumn • Winter	• All year	• All year
AGE GROUP AFFECTED	• Children • Young adults	• Any age	• Any age
VACCINE	• Yes	• Yes	• No
INOCULATION	• Yes	• Yes	• Yes
POTENTIAL FOR CHRONIC LIVER DISEASE	• No	• Yes	• Yes
IMMUNITY	• Yes	• Yes	• No

Figure 3-27

PANCREATITIS

DESCRIPTION: Nonbacterial inflammation of the pancreas.
1. Acute pancreatitis occurs when there is digestion of the pancreas by its own enzymes, primarily trypsin.
2. Alcohol ingestion and biliary tract disease are major causes of acute pancreatitis.
3. Chronic pancreatitis is a progressive, destructive disease with permanent dysfunction.
4. Long-term alcohol use is the major factor in chronic pancreatitis.
5. Alcohol consumption should be stopped when acute pancreatitis is suspected and consumption completely avoided in chronic pancreatitis.

NURSING ASSESSMENT
ACUTE PANCREATITIS
1. Severe mid-epigastric pain radiating to back. Usually related to excess alcohol ingestion or a fatty meal.
2. Abdominal guarding; rigid, board-like abdomen.
3. Nausea and vomiting.
4. Elevated temperature, tachycardia, decreased BP.
5. Bluish discoloration of flanks (Grey Turner's sign) or periumbilical area (Cullen's sign).
6. Elevated amylase, lipase, and glucose levels.

CHRONIC PANCREATITIS
1. Continuous burning or gnawing abdominal pain.
2. Ascites.
3. Steatorrhea, diarrhea.
4. Weight loss.
5. Jaundice, dark urine.
6. Signs and symptoms of diabetes mellitus.

123

..

ANALYSIS (NURSING DIAGNOSES)

1. Acute or chronic pain related to…
2. Altered nutrition: less than required related to…
3. Fluid volume deficit related to…

NURSING PLANS AND INTERVENTIONS
ACUTE PANCREATITIS

1. NPO.
2. Maintain NG tube to suction; TPN given.
3. Administer meperidine (Demerol) or morphine as needed.
4. Administer antacids, histamine-2, receptor-blocking drugs, anticholinergics, proton pump inhibitors.
5. Assist client to assume position of comfort on side with legs drawn up to chest.
6. Teach to avoid alcohol, caffeine, fatty and spicy foods.
7. If severe, blood sugar monitoring and regular insulin coverage may be needed, temporarily.

> **HESI HINT:** Acute pancreatitic pain is located retroperitoneally. Any enlargement of the pancreas causes the peritoneum to stretch tightly. Therefore, sitting up or leaning forward will reduce the pain.

CHRONIC PANCREATITIS

1. Administer analgesics such as meperidine or morphine (narcotic dependency may be a problem).
2. Administer pancreatic enzymes such as pancreatin (Creon) or pancrelipase (Viokase) with meals or snacks. Powdered forms should be mixed with fruit juice or applesauce (mixing with proteins should be avoided).
3. Monitor client's stools for number and consistency to determine effectiveness of enzyme replacement.
4. Teach client about bland, low-fat diet and to avoid rich foods, alcohol, and caffeine.
5. Monitor for signs and symptoms of diabetes mellitus.

CHOLECYSTITIS AND CHOLELITHIASIS

DESCRIPTION: Cholecystitis: An acute inflammation of the gallbladder. Cholelithiasis: The formation or presence of stones in the gallbladder.

1. Incidence of these diseases is greater in females who are multiparous and overweight.
2. Treatment for cholecystitis consists of IV hydration, administration of antibiotics, and pain control with meperidine or morphine.
3. Treatment for cholelithiasis consists of non-surgical removal of stones.
   A. Dissolution therapy (administration of bile salts, used rarely).
   B. Endoscopic retrograde cholangiopancreatography (ERCP).
   C. Lithotripsy (not covered by many insurance carriers, thereby limiting its use).
4. Cholecystectomy is performed if stones are not removed non-surgically and inflammation is *absent*. May be done through laproscope.

> **HESI HINT:** Following an endoscopic retrograde cholangiopancreatography (ERCP), the client may feel sick. The scope is placed in the gallbladder and the stones are crushed and left to pass on their own. These clients may be prone to pancreatitis.

NURSING ASSESSMENT

1. Pain, anorexia, vomiting, and/or flatulence precipitated by ingestion of fried, spicy, or fatty foods.
2. Fever, elevated WBC, and other signs of infection (cholecystitis).
3. Abdominal tenderness.
4. Jaundice and clay-colored stools (blockage).
5. Elevated liver enzymes, bilirubin, and WBC.

ANALYSIS (NURSING DIAGNOSES)

1. Pain related to…
2. Knowledge deficit related to…

NURSING PLANS AND INTERVENTIONS

1. Administer analgesic for pain as needed.
2. NPO.
3. Maintain NG tube to suction if indicated.
4. Administer IV antibiotics for cholecystitis, and administer antibiotics prophylactically for cholelithiasis.
5. I&O.
6. Monitor electrolyte status regularly.
7. Teach client to avoid fried, spicy, or fatty foods, and to reduce intake of calories if indicated.

MEDICAL SURGICAL NURSING

> **HESI HINT:** Non-surgical management of the client with cholecystitis includes:
> - Low-fat diet
> - Medications for pain and clotting if required
> - Decompression of the stomach via NG tube

8. Provide preoperative and postoperative care if surgery is indicated.
   (See Perioperative Care)
9. Monitor T-tube drainage.

REVIEW QUESTIONS
GASTROINTESTINAL SYSTEM

1. List four nursing interventions for the client with a hiatal hernia.
2. List three categories of medications used in the treatment of peptic ulcer disease.
3. List the symptoms of upper and lower gastrointestinal bleeding.
4. What bowel sound disruptions occur with an intestinal obstruction?
5. List four nursing interventions for postoperative care of the client with a colostomy.
6. List the common clinical manifestations of jaundice.
7. What are the common food intolerances for clients with cholelithiasis?
8. List five symptoms indicative of colon cancer.
9. In a client with cirrhosis, it is imperative to prevent further bleeding and observe for bleeding tendencies. List six relevant nursing interventions.
10. What is the main side effect of lactulose, which is used to reduce ammonia levels in clients with cirrhosis?
11. List four groups who have a high risk of contracting hepatitis.
12. How should the nurse administer pancreatic enzymes?

ANSWERS TO REVIEW QUESTIONS

1. Sit up while eating and one hour after eating. Eat small, frequent meals. Eliminate foods that are problematic.
2. Antacids, Histamine-2, receptor-blockers, mucosal healing agents, proton pump inhibitors.
3. Upper GI: Melena, hematemesis, tarry stools. Lower GI: Bloody stools, tarry stools. Similar: Tarry stools.

4. Early mechanical obstruction: high-pitched sounds; late mechanical obstruction: diminished or absent bowel sounds.
5. Irrigate daily at same time; Use warm water for irrigations; Wash around stoma with mild soap/water after each ostomy bag change; Pouch opening should extend at least 1/8 inch around the stoma.
6. Sclera-icteric (yellow sclera), dark urine, chalky or clay-colored stools.
7. Fried, spicy, and/or fatty foods.
8. Rectal bleeding, change in bowel habits, sense of incomplete evacuation, abdominal pain with nausea, weight loss.
9. Avoid injections, use small bore needles for IV insertion, maintain pressure for 5 minutes on all venipuncture sites, use electric razor, use soft-bristle toothbrush for mouth care, check stools and emesis for occult blood.
10. Diarrhea.
11. Homosexual males, IV drug users, recent ear piercing or tattooing, and healthcare workers.
12. Give with meals or snacks. Powder forms should be mixed with fruit juices.

ENDOCRINE SYSTEM

HYPERTHYROIDISM
(GRAVES' DISEASE, GOITER)

DESCRIPTION: Excessive activity of thyroid gland resulting in an elevated level of circulating thyroid hormones.

1. Hyperthyroidism can result from a primary disease state; as a result of replacement hormone therapy; or from excess thyroid stimulating hormone (TSH) from anterior pituitary tumor.
2. Graves' disease is thought to be an autoimmune process.
3. Diagnosis is made with serum hormone levels.
4. Common treatment for hyperthyroidism.
   A. Thyroid ablation with medication.
   B. Radiation.
   C. Thyroidectomy.
   D. Adnectomy of portion of anterior pituitary where TSH-producing tumor located.
5. *All* treatments leave the client hypothyroid, requiring hormone replacement.

NURSING ASSESSMENT
1. Enlarged thyroid gland.
2. Acceleration of body processes:
    A. Weight loss.
    B. Increased appetite.
    C. Diarrhea.
    D. Heat intolerance.
    E. Tachycardia, palpitations, increased BP.
    F. Diaphoresis, wet moist skin.
    G. Nervousness, insomnia.
3. Exophthalmos.
4. T_3 elevated above 220.
5. T_4 elevated above 12.
6. Thyroid stimulating hormone (TSH) level decreased if primary disease; elevated T_4 level suppresses TRH (thyroid-releasing hormone), which suppresses TSH secretion. If source is anterior pituitary, both will be elevated.
7. Radioactive iodine uptake (I_{131}) indicates presence of goiter.
8. Thyroid scan indicates presence of goiter.

ANALYSIS (NURSING DIAGNOSES)
1. Potential altered cardiac output related to…
2. Knowledge deficit related to…
3. Altered nutrition: less than body requirements related to…
4. Potential for injury related to…

NURSING PLANS AND INTERVENTIONS
1. Provide a calm, restful atmosphere.
2. Observe for signs of thyroid storm (life-threatening, sudden over secretion of thyroid hormone).

> **HESI HINT:** Thyroid storm is a life-threatening event that occurs with uncontrolled hyperthyroidism due to Graves' disease. Symptoms include fever, tachycardia, agitation, anxiety, and hypertension. Primary nursing interventions include maintaining an airway and adequate aeration.
> Propylthiouracil (PTU) or methimazole (Tapazole) are antithyroid drugs used to treat thyroid storm. Propanolol (Inderal) may be given to decrease excessive sympathetic stimulation.

3. Teach the following:
    A. After treatment, resulting hypothyroidism will require daily hormone replacement.
    B. Client should wear medic alert jewelry in case of emergency.
    C. Signs of hormone replacement overdosage are the signs for hyperthyroidism. *(See Nursing Assessment, Hyperthyroidism)*
    D. Signs of hormone replacement under-dosage are the signs for hypothyroidism. *(See Nursing Assessment, Hypothyroidism)*
4. Explain to client the recommended diet: high-calorie, high-protein, low-caffeine, low-fiber diet if diarrhea is present.
5. Perform eye care for exophthalmos:
    A. Artificial tears to maintain moisture.
    B. Sunglasses when in bright light.
    C. Annual eye exams.
6. Prepare client for treatment of hyperthyroidism.
    A. Thyroid ablation:
        1) Propylthiouracil (PTU) or methimazole (Tapazole) acts by blocking synthesis of T_3 and T_4.
        2) Dosage is calculated based on body weight and given over several months.
        3) Client should take medication exactly as prescribed so that the desired effect can be achieved.
        4) The expected effect is to make the client euthyroid; often given to prepare the client for thyroidectomy.
    B. Radiation:
        1) Iodine$_{131}$ is given to destroy thyroid cells. Beta rays remain radioactive for a few days.
        2) Iodine$_{131}$ is very irritating to the GI tract.
        3) Clients often vomit (vomitus is radioactive).
        4) Place client on radiation precautions. Use time, distance, and shielding as means of protection against radiation. *(See Reproductive System)*
    C. Thyroidectomy:

> **HESI HINT:** Postoperative thyroidectomy: Be prepared for the possibility of laryngeal edema. Put a tracheostomy set at bedside along with oxygen and a suction machine; Ca++ gluconate easily accessible.

1) Check frequently for bleeding.
2) Support the neck when moving client (do not hyperextend).
3) Check for laryngeal edema damage by watching for hoarseness or inability to speak clearly.
4) Determine number of parathyroid glands that have been removed.
5) Keep drainage devices compressed/ empty.

D. Adenectomy: TSH-secreting pituitary tumors resected using transnasal approach (trans-sphenoidal hypophysectomy).

> **HESI HINT:** Normal serum calcium is 9.0 to 10.5 mEq/L. The best indicator of parathyroid problems is a decrease in the client's calcium compared to the preoperative value.

> **HESI HINT:** If two or more parathyroid glands have been removed, the chance of tetany increases dramatically:
> - Monitor serum calcium levels (9.0 to 10.5 mg/dl is normal range)
> - Check for tingling of toes, fingers, and around the mouth
> - Check Chvostek's sign (tap over the parotid gland and watch for twitching of lip = positive)
> - Check Trousseau's sign (carpopedal spasm after inflating BP cuff above systolic pressure = positive)

HYPOTHYROIDISM
(HASHIMOTO'S DISEASE, MYXEDEMA)
DESCRIPTION: Hypofunction of the thyroid gland with resulting insufficiency of thyroid hormone.
1. Early symptoms of hypothyroidism are nonspecific but gradually intensify.
2. Treated with hormone replacement.
3. Endemic goiters occur in individuals living in areas where there is a deficit of iodine. Iodized salt has helped to prevent this problem.

> **HESI HINT:** Myxedema coma can be precipitated by acute illness, withdrawal of thyroid medication, anesthesia, use of sedatives, or hypoventilation (with the potential for respiratory acidosis and carbondioxide narcosis). *The airway must be kept patent,* and ventilator support used as indicated.

NURSING ASSESSMENT
1. Fatigue.
2. Thin, dry hair; dry skin.
3. Thick, brittle nails.
4. Constipation.
5. Bradycardia, hypotension.
6. Goiter.
7. Periorbital edema, facial puffiness.
8. Cold intolerance.
9. Weight gain.
10. Dull emotions and mental processes.
11. Diagnosed by:
    A. Low T_3 (below 70).
    B. Low T_4 (below 5).
    C. T_4 antibody present, indicating that T_4 is being destroyed by the body.

ANALYSIS (NURSING DIAGNOSES)
1. Knowledge deficit related to…
2. Potential non-compliance related to…
3. Activity intolerance related to…

NURSING PLANS AND INTERVENTIONS
1. Teach the following:
    A. Medication regime: daily dosage of prescribed hormone replacement.
    B. Medication effects and side effects. *(See figure 3-28, Thyroid Preparations)*
    C. Ongoing follow-up with serum hormone levels.
    D. Signs and symptoms of myxedema coma (hypotension, hypothermia, hyponatremia, hypoglycemia, respiratory failure).
2. Develop a bowel elimination plan to prevent constipation:
    A. Increase fluid intake to 3 liters a day.
    B. High-fiber diet including fresh fruits and vegetables.
    C. Increase activity.
    D. Discourage use of enemas and laxatives.
3. Avoid sedation, which can lead to respiratory difficulties.

THYROID PREPARATIONS			
DRUGS	**INDICATIONS**	**ADVERSE REACTIONS**	**NURSING IMPLICATIONS**
• **levothyroxine** (Synthroid) • **liothyronine** sodium (Cytomel) • **desiccated thyroid** (Armour Thyroid)	• Action is to increase metabolic rates • Synthetic T$_4$	• Anxiety • Insomnia • Tremors • Tachycardia • Palpitations • Angina • Dysrhythmias	• Check serum hormone levels routinely • Check BP and pulse regularly • Weigh daily • Report side effects to Healthcare provider • Avoid foods and products containing iodine • Initiate cautiously in clients with cardiovascular disease

Figure 3-28

ADDISON'S DISEASE
(PRIMARY ADRENOCORTICAL DEFICIENCY)

DESCRIPTION: Autoimmune process often found in conjunction with other endocrine diseases of an autoimmune nature. A primary disorder.

1. Sudden withdrawal from corticosteroids may precipitate symptoms of Addison's disease. *(See figure 3-29, Corticosteroids)*
2. Addison's disease is characterized by lack of cortisol, aldosterone, and androgens.
3. Definitive diagnosis is made using an ACTH stimulation test.
4. If ACTH production failure by anterior pituitary, then is considered secondary Addison's.

HESI HINT: Many people take steroids for a variety of conditions. NCLEX-RN® questions often focus on the need to teach clients the importance of precisely following the prescribed regimen. They should be cautioned against suddenly stopping the medications and be informed that it is necessary to taper off taking steroids.

NURSING ASSESSMENT
1. Fatigue, weakness.
2. Weight loss, anorexia, nausea, vomiting.
3. Postural hypotension.
4. Hypoglycemia.
5. Hyponatremia.
6. Hyperkalemia.
7. Hyperpigmentation (only if primary Addison's; not seen in secondary Addison's).
8. Signs of shock when in Addison's crises. *(See Advanced Clinical Concepts)*
9. Loss of body hair.
10. Hypovolemia, signs include:
    A. Hypotension.
    B. Tachycardia.
    C. Fever.

ANALYSIS (NURSING DIAGNOSES)
1. Fluid volume deficit related to…
2. Knowledge deficit related to…

NURSING PLANS AND INTERVENTIONS
1. Take vital signs frequently (every 15 minutes if in crisis).
2. Monitor I&O and weigh daily.
3. Instruct client to rise slowly because of the possibility of postural hypotension.
4. During Addison's crises administer intravenous glucose with parenteral glucocorticoids and requires large fluid volume replacement.
5. Monitor serum electrolyte levels.
6. Teaching should include:
    A. Need for lifelong hormone replacement.
    B. Need for close medical supervision.
    C. Need for medical alert jewelry.
    D. Signs and symptoms of over and under dosage of medication.
    E. Diet: high-sodium, low-potassium, and high-carbohydrate (complex carbohydrates).
    F. Encourage fluid intake of at least 3 liters of fluid per day.
7. Provide ulcer prophylaxis.

HESI HINT: Addison's Crisis Is A Medical Emergency: Brought on by sudden withdrawal of steroids or a stressful event (trauma, severe infection).

- Vascular Collapse: Hypotension and tachycardia occur; administer IV fluids at rapid rate until stabilized.
- Hypoglycemia: Administer IV glucose.
- *Administer Parenteral Hydrocortisone: Essential to reversing the crisis.*
- Aldosterone Replacement: Administer fludrocortisone acetate (Florinef) PO (only available as oral preparation) with simultaneous administration of salt (sodium chloride) if client has a sodium deficit.

CORTICOSTEROIDS

DRUGS	INDICATIONS	ADVERSE REACTIONS	NURSING IMPLICATIONS
STEROIDS • hydrocortisone • prednisone • dexamethasone	• Hormone replacement • Severe rheumatoid arthritis • Autoimmune disorders	• Emotional lability • Impaired wound healing • Skin fragility • Abnormal fat deposition • Hyperglycemia • Hirsutism • Moon face • Osteoporosis • *All symptoms of Cushing's syndrome if overdosage occurs*	• Wean slowly (administer a high dose then taper off) – careful monitoring required during withdrawal • Monitor serum potassium, glucose (can become diabetic), and sodium • Weigh daily; report weight gain of more than 5 pounds per week • Administer with anti-ulcer drugs or food • Use care to prevent injuries • Teach symptoms of Cushing's syndrome • Monitor BP and pulse closely

Figure 3-29

CUSHING'S SYNDROME

DESCRIPTION: Excess adrenalcorticoid activity.
1. Etiology is usually chronic administration of corticosteroids.
2. Cushing's syndrome can also be caused by adrenal, pituitary, or hypothalamus tumors.

NURSING ASSESSMENT
1. Physical symptoms include:
   A. Moon face.
   B. Truncal obesity.
   C. Buffalo hump.
   D. Abdominal striae.
   E. Muscle atrophy.
   F. Thinning of the skin.
   G. Hirsutism in females.
   H. Hyperpigmentation.
   I. Amenorrhea.
   J. Edema, poor wound healing, easy bruising.
2. Hypertension.
3. Susceptible to multiple infections.
4. Osteoporosis.
5. Peptic ulcer formation.
6. Many false positives and false negatives in laboratory testing.

7. Lab data often include the following findings:
   A. Hyperglycemia.
   B. Hypernatremia.
   C. Hypokalemia.
   D. Decreased eosinophils and lymphocytes.
   E. Increased plasma cortisol.
   F. Increased urinary 17-hydroxycorticoids.

ANALYSIS (NURSING DIAGNOSES)
1. Potential fluid volume excess related to…
2. Potential for infection related to…
3. Altered body image related to…

NURSING PLANS AND INTERVENTIONS
1. Protect from exposure to infection.
2. **WASH HANDS**; use good handwashing technique.
3. Monitor for signs of infection:
   A. Fever.
   B. Oral candida.
   C. Vaginal yeast infections.
   D. Adventitious lungs.
   E. Skin lesions.
   F. Elevated WBCs.
4. Teach safety measures.

A. Position bed close to floor with call light within easy reach.
B. Encourage use of side rails.
C. Be sure walkways are unobstructed.
D. Encourage wearing shoes when ambulating.
5. Provide low-sodium diet; encourage foods with vitamin D and calcium.
6. Provide good skin care.
7. Discuss possibility of weaning from steroids. (If weaning is done too quickly, Addison's symptoms will occur).
8. Encourage selection of clothing that minimizes visible aberrations; encourage maintenance of normal physical appearance.
9. Monitor I&O and weigh daily.
10. Provide ulcer prophylaxis.

> **HESI HINT:** Teach clients to take steroids with meals to prevent gastric irritation. They should never skip doses. If they have nausea or vomiting for more than 12 to 24 hours, they should contact the physician.

DIABETES MELLITUS

DESCRIPTION: Metabolic disorder in which there is an absence or insufficient production of insulin.

Diabetes mellitus is characterized by hyperglycemia.
1. Diabetes mellitus affects protein, carbohydrate, and fat metabolism.
2. Most recent diagnostic parameter is fasting glucose, either serum or capillary, of greater than 140 mg/dl.
3. Two major classifications of diabetes are Type I, insulin-dependent diabetes mellitus (IDDM) and Type II, non-insulin-dependent diabetes mellitus (NIDDM). *(See figure 3-30, Variables Related to Diabetes Mellitus)*
4. Many Type II diabetics use insulin but retain some degree of pancreatic function. *(See figure 3-31, Clinical Characteristics and Treatment of Diabetes Mellitus)*
5. Obesity is a major factor in NIDDM.
6. All diabetics develop diabetes-associated complications to some degree. The degree of pathologic changes is related to control of blood glucose levels.

NURSING ASSESSMENT
1. Integument:

A. Breaks in skin, infections on skin.
B. Diabetic dermapathy (skin spots).
C. Unhealed injection sites.

> **HESI HINT:** Why do diabetics have trouble with wound healing? High blood glucose contributes to damage of the smallest vessels, the capillaries. This damage causes permanent capillary scarring, which inhibits the normal activity of the capillary. This phenomenon causes disruption of capillary elasticity and promotes problems such as diabetic retinopathy, poor healing of breaks in the skin, cardiovascular abnormalities, etc.

2. Oral cavity:
    A. Caries.
    B. Periodontal disease.
    C. Candidiasis (raised, white patchy areas on mucous membranes).
3. Eyes:
    A. Cataracts.
    B. Retinal problems often exist.
4. Cardiopulmonary:
    A. Angina.
    B. Dyspnea.
5. Periphery:
    A. Hair loss on extremities indicating poor perfusion.
    B. Other signs of poor peripheral circulation:
        1) Coolness.
        2) Skin shininess and thinness.
        3) Peripheral pulses weak or absent.
        4) Ulcerations on extremity.
        5) Pallor.
        6) Thick nails with ridges.
6. Kidneys:
    A. Edema of face, hands, feet.
    B. Symptoms of urinary tract infection (UTI): fatigue, pallor, and weakness.
    C. Urinary retention.
7. Neuromusculature:
    A. Atrophy of hands and feet.
    B. Neuropathies with symptoms of numbness, tingling, pain, burning.
8. Gastrointestinal disturbances:
    A. Nighttime diarrhea.
    B. Emesis falling into a pattern, i.e., client vomits every night one hour after dinner.
    C. Gastroporesis = faulty absorption

9. Reproductive:
   A. Male impotence.
   B. Vaginal dryness, frequent vaginal infections.
   C. Menstrual irregularities.
10. Glycosylated hemoglobin confirms existence of hyperglycemia in previous 4 months.

VARIABLES RELATED TO DIABETES MELLITUS		
VARIABLE	TYPE I (IDDM)	TYPE II (NIDDM)
AGE AT ONSET	• Usually under 30 years of age	• School age to older adult
INSULIN PRODUCTION	• Absent	• Present, but inadequate
ONSET	• Rapid	• Insidious
SYMPTOMS	• Polydipsia • Polyphagia • Polyuria • Weight loss • Weakness	• Often unnoticed • Same symptoms as Type I, plus blurred vision
WEIGHT	• Usually thin	• Usually obese, sometimes normal
KETOSIS	• Common	• Rare
GENETICS	• No overwhelming predisposition	• Strong predisposition
PATHOGENESIS	• Viral, autoimmune	• Obesity, nutrition – major factor
CONTROL	• Difficult, with wide glycemic swings	• Often only dietary restrictions and exercise required
MEAL PLANNING	• Imperative	• Imperative
EXERCISE	• Imperative	• Imperative
MEDICATION	• Insulin required by all	• Maybe none, oral hypoglycemics, or insulin
LONG-TERM COMPLICATIONS	• Frequent	• Frequent

Figure 3-30

CLINICAL CHARACTERISTICS AND TREATMENT OF DIABETES MELLITUS		
CHARACTERISTICS	TYPE I (IDDM)	TYPE II (NIDDM)
DESCRIPTION	• Can become hyperglycemic relatively easily (they are "brittle diabetics") • Can go into ketoacidosis	• Rarely develop ketoacidosis • With extreme hyperglycemia, non-ketotic hyperosmolar hyperglycemia occurs
CLINICAL CHARACTERISTIC	• Serum glucose of 350 and above • Ketonuria in large amounts • Venous pH of 6.8 to 7.2 • Serum bicarbonate below 15 mEq/dl	• Hyperglycemia • Plasma hyperosmolality • Dehydration • Changed mental status
TREATMENT	• Usual treatment is with isotonic intravenous fluids • Slow intravenous infusion by IV pump of regular insulin with IM or SC bolus as needed • Careful replacement of potassium based upon lab data	• Usual treatment is with isotonic intravenous fluid replacement and careful monitoring of potassium and glucose levels • Intravenous insulin is not always necessary

Figure 3-31

HESI HINT: Glycosylated Hgb (Hgb A1C)
- **Indicates glucose control over previous 120 days (life of RBC).**
- **Valuable measurement of diabetes control.**

ANALYSIS (NURSING DIAGNOSES)
1. Knowledge deficit related to…
2. Ineffective individual coping related to…
3. Potential for injury related to…

NURSING PLANS AND INTERVENTIONS
1. Determine baseline lab data.
   A. Serum glucose.
   B. Electrolytes.
   C. Creatinine.
   D. BUN.
   E. ABGs as indicated.
2. Teach injection technique; lift skin, use 90°
   A. Identify the prescribed dose and type of insulin. *(See figure 3-33, Oral Hypoglycemics and figure 3-34, Types/ Actions of Insulin)*
   B. Store unopened insulin in refrigerator. If opened, may be kept at room temperature 3 months.
   C. May re-use syringes for same person: recap needle and store in refrigerator.
   D. Rotate injection sites (abdomen preferred for type I).
   E. Draw regular insulin into syringe FIRST when mixing insulins.
3. Diet:
   A. Work with dietitian to reinforce specific meal plan.
   B. Encourage use of exchange list; can be used when eating out.
   C. Meals should be timed according to medication peak times.
   D. Diet:

1) 55 to 60% carbohydrates.
2) 12 to 15% protein.
3) 30% or less fat.
4) Encourage foods high in complex carbohydrates, high in fiber, and low in fat whenever possible.
5) Alcoholic beverages can be included with proper exchanges made.
6) Bedtime snack can prevent insulin reactions due to long-acting insulin peak

E. Manage sick days (illness *raises* blood glucose).
   1) Teach client to keep taking insulin.
   2) Monitor glucose more frequently.
   3) Watch for signs of hyperglycemia.

HESI HINT: The body's response to illness/ stress is to produce glucose. Therefore, any illness results in hyperglycemia.

4. Exercise regimen:
   A. Regular non-strenuous exercise.
   B. Exercise should be done after mealtime; either exercise with someone or let someone know where exercise will take place to ensure safety.
   C. May need snack before or during exercise.
   D. Monitor blood glucose before, during, and after exercise when beginning a new regimen.
5. Teach signs and symptoms of hyperglycemia and hypoglycemia. *(See figure 3-32, Hyperglycemia/ Hypoglycemia Signs and Symptoms)*

HESI HINT: If in doubt whether a client is hyperglycemic or hypoglycemic, treat for hypoglycemia.

HYPERGLYCEMIA		HYPOGLYCEMIA	
SIGNS & SYMPTOMS	NURSING ACTION	SIGNS & SYMPTOMS	NURSING ACTION
• Polydipsia • Polyuria • Polyphagia • Blurred vision • Weakness • Weight loss • Syncope	• Encourage water intake • Check blood glucose frequently • Assess for ketoacidosis: → Urine ketones → Urine glucose → Administer insulin as directed	• Headache • Nausea • Sweating • Tremors • Lethargy • Hunger • Confusion • Slurred speech • Tingling around mouth • Anxiety, nightmares	• Usually occurs rapidly and is potentially life-threatening; treat immediately with complex CHO: example: graham cracker and peanut butter twice and, if no response, seek medical attention • Check blood glucose (may seize if < 40).

Figure 3-32

6. Foot care:
    A. Check feet daily for changes; report signs of injury, breaks in skin to Healthcare provider.
    B. Wash daily with mild soap and warm water. Do not soak. Dry well, especially between toes.
    C. Moisturize with a lanolin product, but not between the toes.
    D. Wear well-fitting shoes; never go barefoot or wear sandals.
    E. Wear clean socks daily.
    F. Never wear garters tight elastic-topped

7. Enc
    A. Re
    B. Refer t
8. Immediate atten
    or infection occurs.
9. Refer to the American D
    information and emotional s

ORAL HYPOGLYCEMICS

DRUGS	INDICATIONS	ADVERSE REACTIONS	NURSING IMPLICAT
SULFONYLUREAS ***First Generation*** • **tolbutamide** (Oranase) • **chlorpropamide** (Diabinese) ***Second Generation*** • **glyburide** (Micronase, DiaBeta) • **glipizide** (Glucotrol) • **glimepride** (Amaryl)	• Lowers blood sugar by stimulating the release of insulin by the beta cells of the pancreas + causes tissues to take up and store glucose more easily. • First generation are low potency and short acting • Second generation are high potency & longer acting	***First Generation*** • Hypoglycemia • Nausea, heartburn, constipation, anorexia • Agranulocytosis • Allergic skin reactions ***Second Generation*** • Weight gain • Hypoglycemia, particularly in the elderly	***First Generation*** • Responsiveness may decline over time • Given once daily with first meal • Monitor blood sugar • Hard to detect hypoglycemia if elderly or also on beta blockers ***Second Generation*** • Less likely to interact with other medications
BIGUINIDES • **metformin** (Glucophage)	• Lower serum glucose levels by inhibiting hepatic glucose production and increasing sensitivity of peripheral tissue to insulin	• Hypoglycemia • Abdominal discomfort • Diarrhea	• Many drug-drug interactions • Extended-release tablets should be taken with the evening meal • Use cautiously with pre-existing renal or liver disease, or CHF • Wait 48 hours to restart dosage after diagnostic studies requiring IV iodine contrast media
ALPHA-GLULCOSIDASE INHIBITORS • **acarbose** (Precose) • **miglitol** (Glyset)	• Lowers blood glucose by blunting sugar levels after meals	• Hypoglycemia	• Optimally, must be taken with the FIRST bite of each meal • May be taken with other classes of oral hypoglycemics • Monitor blood sugar

Figure 3-33

ED)

	S	NURSING IMPLICATIONS
	gain	• Many drug-drug interactions • Skip dose if meal skipped • No known drug interactions • Monitor liver function • Caution with use in CAD – may precipitate CHF
	pain ack pain sia, or diarrhea	• May be used with metformin • Give before meals; if a meal is skipped, skip the dose • Monitor blood sugar
	sible adverse of BOTH ycemia (severe)	• Note implications of both classes of drugs

(rotated text, partially visible, top-left):
socks.
G. Never try to remove corns or calluses (should
H. be done by professional).
Cut or file nails straight across.
Wear warm socks if feet are cold.
rage regular healthcare follow-up:
er to ophthalmologist.
podiatrist.
on should be sought if any sign
iabetes Association for
port.

MEDICAL SU NURS

OF INSULIN

TYPE			PEAK ACTION	NURSING IMPLICATIONS
RAPID-ACTING	• prompt zinc suspens. insulin (Semilente) • human insulin lispro (Humalog) • insulin aspart (Novolog)	 0.5 to 1 hr. 5 to 15 min.	2 to 3 hrs. 2 to 4 hrs 0.75 to 1.5 hr	• Lispro may be given intravenously • Give within 15 min. of a meal (lispro and aspart)
SHORT ACTING	• regular insulin (human)	30 to 60 min.	2 to 3 hrs.	• Regular insulin may be given IV
INTERMEDIATE ACTING	• isophane insulin (NPH) (Iletin) • insulin zinc suspension (Humulin L)	1 to 2 hrs.	6 to 12 hrs.	• Not to be given IV • Mixtures combine rapid-acting regular insulin with intermediate- acting NPH insulin in a 30% regular with 70% NPH proportion or at 50/50 combination
LONG-ACTING	• protamine zinc (PZI) Iletin) • extended zinc suspension (Ultralente) • insulin glargine (Lantus)	4 to 8 hrs. 1.1 hrs.	14 to 20 hrs. 5 hrs. (some sources say there is no peak)	• Not to be given IV • Recommended give once daily, se, at bedtime. In some cases, given bid. Acts as basalinsulin. Caution: CLEAR solution but bottle is distinctly different shape from regular insulin. *DO NOT CONFUSE INSULINS.* Do not shake solution Do not mix other insulins with Lantus Use cautiously if patient is NPO.

Figure 3-34

TYPES/ACTION OF INSULIN (CONTINUED)				
TYPE	NAME	ONSET	PEAK ACTION	NURSING IMPLICATIONS
PREMIX				**For all premixes:** Offer when food readily available
	• **Humalog 75/25**			25% lispro 75% humulin N (NPH)
	• **Human 70/30**			30% regular 70% NPH
	• **Novolog 70/30**			30% aspart 70% NPH

Figure 3-34 (continued)

HESI HINT: SELF-MONITORING BLOOD GLUCOSE (SMBG)
- Provides tight glucose control thereby decreasing the potential for long-term complications.
- Technique is specific to each meter if meter is used.
- Monitor before meals, at bedtime, and any time symptoms occur.
- Record results and report to healthcare provider at time of visit.

REVIEW QUESTIONS

ENDOCRINE SYSTEM

1. What diagnostic test is used to determine thyroid activity?
2. What condition results from all treatments for hyperthyroidism?
3. State three symptoms of hyperthyroidism and three symptoms of hypothyroidism.
4. List five important teaching aspects for clients who are beginning corticosteroid therapy.
5. Describe the physical appearance of clients who are Cushinoid.
6. Which type of diabetic always requires insulin replacement?
7. What type of diabetic sometimes requires no medication?
8. List five symptoms of hyperglycemia.
9. List five symptoms of hypoglycemia.
10. Name the necessary elements to include in teaching the new diabetic.
11. In less than ten steps, describe the method for drawing up a mixed dose of insulin (regular with NPH).
12. Identify the peak action time of the following types of insulin: rapid-acting regular insulin, intermediate-acting, long-acting.
13. When preparing the diabetic for discharge, the nurse teaches the client the relationship between stress, exercise, bedtime snacking, and glucose balance. State the relationship between each of these.
14. When making rounds at night, the nurse notes that an insulin-dependent client is complaining of a headache, slight nausea, and minimal trembling. The client's hand is cool and moist. What is the client most likely experiencing?
15. Identify five foot-care interventions that should be taught to the diabetic client.

ANSWERS TO REVIEW QUESTIONS

1. T_3, T_4.
2. Hypothyroidism, requiring thyroid replacement.
3. Hyperthyroidism: weight loss, heat intolerance, diarrhea. Hypothyroidism: fatigue, cold intolerance, weight gain.
4. Continue medication until weaning plan is begun by physician, monitor serum potassium, glucose, and sodium frequently; weigh daily, and report gain of >5 lbs./wk; monitor BP and pulse closely; teach symptoms of Cushing's syndrome.
5. Moon face, obesity in trunk, buffalo hump in back, muscle atrophy, and thin skin.
6. Type I, Insulin-dependent diabetes mellitus (IDDM).
7. Type II, Non-insulin-dependent diabetes mellitus (NIDDM).

MEDICAL SURGICAL NURSING

135

8. Polydipsia, polyuria, polyphagia, weakness, weight loss.

9. Hunger, lethargy, confusion, tremors or shakes, sweating.

10. Teach the underlying pathophysiology of the disease, its management/treatment regime, meal planning, exercise program, insulin administration, sick-day management, symptoms of hyperglycemia (not enough insulin), symptoms of hypoglycemia (too much insulin, too much exercise; not enough food).

11. Identify the prescribed dose/type of insulin per physician order; Store unopened insulin in refrigerator. If opened, may be kept at room temperature for up to 3 months. Draw up regular insulin FIRST; Rotate injection sites; May re-use syringe by recapping and storing in refrigerator.

12. Rapid-acting regular insulin: 2 to 4 hrs. Immediate-acting: 6 to 12 hrs. Long-acting: 14 to 20 hrs.

13. Stress and stress hormones usually increase glucose production and increase insulin need; exercise can increase the chance for an insulin reaction, therefore, the client should always have a sugar snack available when exercising (to treat hypoglycemia); bedtime snacking can prevent insulin reactions while waiting for long-acting insulin to peak.

14. Hypoglycemia/insulin reaction.

15. Check feet daily and report any breaks, sores or blisters to Healthcare provider, wear well-fitting shoes; never go barefoot or wear sandals; never personally remove corns or calluses; cut or file nails straight across; wash daily with mild soap and warm water.

MUSCULOSKELETAL SYSTEM

RHEUMATOID ARTHRITIS
DESCRIPTION: Chronic, systematic, progressive deterioration of the connective tissue (synovium) of the joints characterized by inflammation.

1. The exact cause unknown, but it is classified as an immune complex disorder.

2. Joint involvement is bilateral and symmetrical.

3. Severe cases may require joint replacement. *(See Joint Replacement)*

HESI HINT: A client comes to the clinic complaining of morning stiffness, weight loss, and swelling of both hands and wrists. Rheumatoid arthritis is suspected. Which methods of assessment might the nurse use and which methods would the nurse *not* use? Use inspection, palpation, and strength testing. Do not use range of motion (this activity promotes pain because ROM is limited).

NURSING ASSESSMENT
1. Fatigue.
2. Generalized weakness.
3. Weight loss.
4. Anorexia.
5. Morning stiffness.
6. Bilateral inflammation of joints with the following symptoms:
   A. Decreased range of motion.
   B. Joint pain.
   C. Warmth.
   D. Edema.
   E. Erythema.
7. Joint deformity.

HESI HINT: In the joint, the normal cartilage becomes soft, fissures and pitting occur, and the cartilage thins. Spurs form and inflammation sets in. The result is deformity marked by immobility, pain, and muscle spasm. The prescribed treatment regimen is corticosteroids for the inflammation; splinting, immobilization, and rest for the joint deformity; and NSAIDs for the pain.

8. Diagnosis confirmed by the following:
   A. Elevated erythrocyte sedimentation rate (ESR).
   B. Positive rheumatoid factor (RF).
   C. Presence of antinuclear antibody (ANA).
   D. Joint space narrowing indicated by arthroscopic exam (provides joint visualization).
   E. Abnormal synovial fluid (fluid in joint) indicated by arthrocentesis.

HESI HINT: Synovial tissues line the bones of the joints. Inflammation of this lining causes destruction of tissue and bone. Early detection of rheumatoid arthritis can decrease the amount of bone and joint destruction. Often the disease will go into remission. Decreasing the amount of bone and joint destruction will reduce the amount of disability.

ANALYSIS (NURSING DIAGNOSES)

1. Chronic pain related to…
2. Impaired physical mobility related to…
3. Self-care deficit related to…
4. Impaired individual coping related to…

NURSING PLANS AND INTERVENTIONS

1. Implement pain relief measures.
    A. Utilize moist heat.
        1) Warm, moist compresses.
        2) Whirlpool baths.
        3) Hot shower in the morning.
    B. Utilize diversionary activities.
        1) Imaging.
        2) Distraction.
        3) Self-hypnosis.
        4) Biofeedback.
    C. Administer medications and teach client about medications. *(See figure 3-35, NSAIDs; and figure 3-29, Corticosteroids)*
2. Provide periods of rest after periods of activity.
    A. Encourage self-care to maximal level.
    B. Allow adequate time for the client to perform activities.
    C. Perform activities during time of day when client feels most energetic.

3. Do not overexert. Encourage the client to maintain proper posture and joint position.

> **HESI HINT:** What activity recommendations should the nurse provide a client with rheumatoid arthritis?
> - **Do not exercise painful, swollen joints.**
> - **Do not exercise any joint to the point of pain.**
> - **Perform exercises slowly and smoothly; avoid jerky movements.**

4. Encourage use of assistive devices.
    A. Elevated toilet seat.
    B. Shower chair.
    C. Cane, walker, and/or wheelchair.
    D. Reachers.
    E. Adaptive clothing with Velcro closures.
    F. Straight-backed chairs with elevated seat.
5. Develop a teaching plan to include the following:
    A. Medication regime.
    B. Need for routine follow-up for evaluation of possible side effects.
    C. Range of motion and stretching exercises tailored to specific client needs.
    D. Safety tips/precautions on equipment use and environment.

NSAIDS (NONSTEROIDAL ANTI-INFLAMMATORY DRUGS)

DRUGS	INDICATIONS	ADVERSE REACTIONS	NURSING IMPLICATIONS
• **aspirin** (Anacin) • **ibuprofen** (Motrin, Nuprin, Advil) • **indomethacin** (Indocin) • **ketorolac tromethamine** (Toradol) • **celecoxib** (Celebrex) • **etodolac** (Lodine) • **diclofenac** (Voltaren) • **naproxen** (anaprox, Naprocin)	• Used as anti-inflammatory • Antipyretic • Analgesic • Can be used with other agents	• GI irritation, bleeding • Nausea, vomiting, constipation • Elevated liver enzymes • Prolonged coagulation time • Tinnitus • Thrombocytopenia • Fluid retention • Nephrotoxicity • Blood dyscrasias	• Teach to take with food or milk to reduce GI symptoms • Therapeutic serum salicylates level 20 to 25 mg%. • Teach to watch for signs of bleeding • Teach to avoid alcohol • Teach to observe for tinnitus • Administer corticosteroids for severe rheumatoid arthritis *(See figure 3-29)* • NSAIDs reduce the effect of ACE inhibitors in hypertensive clients • Note name similarity of Celebrex with other drugs having one letter difference in spelling • Encourage routine appointments to check liver/renal labs & CBC

Figure 3-35

LUPUS ERYTHEMATOSUS

DESCRIPTION: A systemic, inflammatory connective tissue disorder.

1. There are two classifications of lupus erythematosus:
    A. Discoid lupus erythematosus (DLE) affects skin only.
    B. Systemic lupus erythematosus (SLE).
2. SLE is more prevalent than DLE.
3. Lupus is an autoimmune disorder.
4. Kidney involvement is the leading cause of death in clients with lupus, followed by cardiac involvement.

HESI HINT: NCLEX-RN® questions often focus on the fact that avoiding sunlight is key in management of lupus erythematosus – this is what differentiates it from other connective tissue diseases.

5. Factors that trigger lupus:
    A. Sunlight.
    B. Stress.
    C. Pregnancy.
    D. Drugs.

NURSING ASSESSMENT
1. DLE: Dry, scaly rash on face or upper body (butterfly rash).
2. SLE:
    A. Joint pain and decreased mobility.
    B. Fever.
    C. Nephritis.
    D. Pleural effusion.
    E. Pericarditis.
    F. Abdominal pain.
    G. Photosensitivity.

ANALYSIS (NURSING DIAGNOSES)
1. Impaired skin integrity related to…
2. Pain related to…
3. Body image disturbance related to…

NURSING PLANS AND INTERVENTIONS
1. Instruct client to avoid prolonged exposure to sunlight.
2. Instruct client to clean the skin with mild soap.
3. Monitor and instruct client in administration of steroids.

DEGENERATIVE JOINT DISEASE (DJD)

DESCRIPTION: Non-inflammatory arthritis.

1. DJD is characterized by a degeneration of cartilage, a "wear and tear" process.
2. Usually affects one or two joints.
3. Occurs asymmetrically.
4. Obesity and over-use are a predisposing factor.

HESI HINT: Degenerative joint disease (DJD) and osteoarthritis are often described as the same disease, and indeed they both result in hypertrophic changes in the joints. However, they differ in that osteoarthritis is an inflammatory disease and DJD is characterized by non-inflammatory degeneration of the joints.

NURSING ASSESSMENT
1. Joint pain, which increases with activity and improves with rest.
2. Morning stiffness.
3. Asymmetry of affected joints.
4. Crepitus (grating sound in the joint).
5. Limited movement.
6. Visible joint abnormalities indicated in x-rays.
7. Joint enlargement and bony nodules.

ANALYSIS (NURSING DIAGNOSES)
1. Pain (chronic) related to…
2. Impaired physical mobility related to…
3. Self-care deficit related to…
4. Knowledge deficit related to…

NURSING PLANS AND INTERVENTIONS
See Rheumatoid Arthritis
1. Instruct in weight-reduction diet.
2. Remind client that excessive use of the involved joint aggravates pain and may accelerate degeneration.
3. Teach the client:
    A. Correct posture and body mechanics.
    B. Sleep with rolled terry cloth towel under cervical spine if neck pain a problem.
    C. To relieve pain in fingers and hands, wear stretch gloves at night.
    D. Keep joints in functional position.

OSTEOPOROSIS

DESCRIPTION: Metabolic disease in which bone demineralization results in decreased density and subsequent fractures.

1. Many fractures in the elderly occur as result of osteoporosis and often occur prior to the client's falling, rather than the client sustaining a fracture due to a fall.
2. The etiology of osteoporosis is unknown.
3. Postmenopausal women are at highest risk.

NURSING ASSESSMENT

1. Classic Dowager's hump or kyphosis of the dorsal spine.
2. Loss of height, often 2 to 3 inches.
3. Back pain, often radiating around the trunk.
4. Pathologic fractures, often occurring in the distal end of the radius and the upper third of the femur.
5. Compression fracture of spine can occur: assess ability to void and defecate.

> **HESI HINT:** Postmenopausal, thin, Caucasian women are at highest risk for development of osteoporosis. Encourage exercise, a diet high in calcium, and supplemental calcium. While TUMS is an excellent source of calcium, it is also high in sodium and hypertensive or edematous individuals should seek another source for supplemental calcium.

ANALYSIS (NURSING DIAGNOSES)

1. Potential for injury related to…
2. Impaired physical mobility related to…
3. Knowledge deficit related to…

NURSING PLANS AND INTERVENTIONS

1. Create a hazard-free environment.
2. Keep bed in low position.
3. Encourage client to wear shoes or slippers when out of bed.
4. Encourage environmental safety.
   A. Provide adequate lighting.
   B. Keep floor clear.
   C. Discourage use of throw rugs.
   D. Clean spills promptly.
   E. Keep side rails up at all times.

> **HESI HINT:** The main cause of fractures in the elderly, especially women, is osteoporosis. The main fracture sites seem to be hip, vertebral bodies, and Colles' fracture of forearm.

5. Provide assistance with ambulation.
   A. May need walker or cane.
   B. May need standby assistance when initially getting out of bed or chair.
6. Teach regular exercise program.
   A. Range of motion several times a day.
   B. Ambulate several times a day.
   C. Use of proper body mechanics.
7. Provide diet that is high in protein, calcium, and vitamin D; discourage use of alcohol and caffeine.
8. Encourage preventive measures for females.
   A. Estrogen replacement therapy after menopause.
   B. High calcium and vitamin D intake beginning in early adulthood.
   C. Calcium supplementation after menopause (TUMS is excellent source of calcium).
   D. Weight-bearing exercise.
9. Bone density study as a baseline after menopause, with frequence as recommended by healthcare provider.

FRACTURE

DESCRIPTION: Any break in the continuity of the bone.

> **HESI HINT:** NCLEX-RN® questions focus on safety precautions. Improper use of assistive devices can be very risky. When using a non-wheeled walker, the client should lift and move the walker forward, then take a step into it. The client should avoid scooting the walker or shuffling forward into it which takes more energy and is less stable than a single movement.

1. Fractures are described by type and extent of the break.
2. Fractures are caused by a direct blow, crushing force, sudden twisting motion, or disease such as cancer or osteoporosis.
   A. Complete fracture: Break across the entire cross-section of the bone.
   B. Incomplete fracture: Break occurs across only part of the bone.
   C. Closed fracture: Doesn't produce a break in the skin.
   D. Open fracture: Extends through skin or mucous membranes (much more prone to infection).
3. Five types of fractures are:
   A. Greenstick: One side of a bone is broken, the other side is bent.

B. Transverse: Across the bone.
C. Oblique: At an angle across the bone.
D. Spiral: Twisting around the bone.
E. Comminuted: Having more than three fragments.

> **HESI HINT:** What type of fracture is more difficult to heal, an extra capsular fracture (below the neck of the femur) or an intracapsular fracture (in the neck of the femur)?
> The blood supply enters the femur below the neck of the femur. Therefore, an intra-capsular fracture is much harder to heal and has a greater likelihood of necrosis since it is cut off from the blood supply.

NURSING ASSESSMENT
1. Signs and symptoms of fracture include:
   A. Pain, swelling, tenderness.
   B. Deformity, loss of functional ability.
   C. Discoloration, bleeding at the site through an open wound.
   D. Crepitus: crackling sound between two broken bones.

2. Fracture evident on x-ray.
3. Therapeutic management is based on:
   A. Reduction of the fracture.
   B. Maintenance of realignment by immobilization.
   C. Restoration of function.
4. Observe client's use of assistive devices.
   A. Crutches:
      1) There should be two to three finger widths between axilla and the top of the crutch.
      2) Three-point gait is most common. The client advances both crutches and the impaired leg at the same time. The client then swings uninvolved leg to the crutches.
   B. Cane:
      1) Placed on the unaffected side.
      2) Top of cane should be parallel to the greater trochanter.
   C. Walker:
      1) Upper extremity and unaffected leg strength assessed and improved with exercises, if necessary, so that upper body is strong enough to use walker.
      2) Client lifts and advances the walker and steps forward.

5. See Pediatric Nursing for cast care and care of the client in traction.

> **HESI HINT:** The risk of a fat embolism, a syndrome in which fat globules migrate into the bloodstream and combine with platelets to forme emboli, is greatest in the first 36 hours after a fracture. It is more common in clients with multiple fractures, fractures of long bones, and fractures of the pelvis. *The initial symptom of a fat embolism is confusion* due to hypoxemia (check blood gases for PO_2). Assess for respiratory distress, restlessness, irritability, fever, and petechiae. If an embolus is suspected, notify physician STAT, draw blood gases, administer oxygen, and assist with endotracheal intubation.

> **HESI HINT:** In clients with hip fractures, thromboembolism is the most common complication. Prevention includes passive range of motion exercises, elastic stocking use, elevation of the foot of the bed 25 degrees to increase venous return, and low-dose heparin therapy.

> **HESI HINT:** Clients with fractures, casts, or edema to the extremities need frequent neurovascular assessment distal to the injury. Skin color, temperature, sensation, capillary refill, mobility, pain and pulses should be assessed.

> **HESI HINT:** Assess the "5 Ps" of neurovascular functioning: pain, paresthesia, pulse, pallor, and paralysis.

JOINT REPLACEMENT
DESCRIPTION: A surgical procedure in which a mechanical device, designed to act as a joint, is used to replace a diseased joint.
1. Most commonly replaced joints include:
   A. Hip.
   B. Knee.
   C. Shoulder.
   D. Finger.
2. Prostheses may be ingrown or cemented.
3. Accurate fitting is essential.
4. Must have healthy bone stock for adequate healing.
5. Joint replacement provides excellent pain relief in 85 to 90% of the clients who have the surgery.

6. Infection is primary concern postoperatively.

Nursing Assessment
1. Joint pathology.
   A. Arthritis.
   B. Fracture.
2. Pain not relieved with medication.
3. Poor range of motion in the affected joint.

Analysis (Nursing Diagnoses)
1. Potential for infection related to…
2. Pain related to…
3. Potential for injury to affected limb related to…

Nursing Plans and Interventions
1. Provide postoperative care for wound and joint.
   A. Monitor incision site.
      1) Assess for bleeding and drainage.

> **HESI HINT:** Orthopedic wounds have a tendency to ooze more than other wounds. A suction drainage device usually accompanies the client to the postoperative floor. Check drainage often.

      2) Assess suture line for erythema and/or edema.
      3) Assess suction drainage apparatus for proper functioning.
      4) Assess for signs of infection.

> **HESI HINT:** NCLEX-RN® questions about joint replacement focus on complications. A big problem after joint replacement is *infection*.

   B. Monitor functioning of extremity.
      1) Check circulation, sensation, and movement of extremity distal to replacement.
      2) Provide proper alignment of affected extremity (client will return from the operating room with alignment for initial postoperative period).
      3) Provide abductor appliance (hip replacement) or continuous passive motion (CPM) device if indicated.
2. Monitor I&O every shift, including suction drainage.

> **HESI HINT:** Fractures of bone predispose the client to anemia, especially if long bones are involved. Check hematocrit every 3 to 4 days to monitor erythropoiesis.

3. Encourage fluid intake of 3 liters/day.
4. Encourage client to perform self-care activities at maximal level.
5. Coordinate rehabilitation: work closely with healthcare team to gradually increase client's mobility.
   A. Get client out of bed as soon as possible.
   B. Keep client out of bed as much as possible.
   C. Keep abductor pillow in place while client is in bed (hip replacement).
   D. Use elevated toilet seat and chairs with high seats for those who have had hip or knee replacement (prevents dislocation).
   E. Do not flex hip more than 90 degrees (hip replacement).

> **HESI HINT:** Instruct the client not to lift the leg upward from a lying position or to elevate the knee when sitting. This upward motion can pop the prosthesis out of the socket.

6. Provide discharge planning to include rehabilitation on an outpatient basis as prescribed.

> **HESI HINT:** Immobile clients are prone to complications: skin integrity problems, formation of urinary calculi (may limit milk intake), and venous thrombosis (may be on prophylactic anticoagulants).

Amputation
Description: Surgical removal of a diseased part or organ.
1. Causes for amputation include the following:
   A. Peripheral vascular disease, 80% (75% of these are diabetics).
   B. Trauma.
   C. Congenital deformities.
   D. Malignant tumors.
   E. Infection.
2. Amputation necessitates major life style and body image adjustments.

NURSING ASSESSMENT

1. Prior to amputation, symptoms of peripheral vascular disease include:
   A. Cool extremity.
   B. Absent peripheral pulses.
   C. Hair loss on affected extremity.
   D. Necrotic tissue and/or wounds.
      1) Blue or blue-gray turning black.
      2) Drainage possible, with or without odor.
   E. Leathery skin on affected extremity.
   F. Decrease of pain sensation in affected extremity.
2. Inadequate circulation determined by the following:
   A. Arteriogram.
   B. Doppler flow studies.

ANALYSIS (NURSING DIAGNOSES)

1. Pain related to…
2. Impaired physical mobility related to…
3. Self-care deficit related to…
4. Impaired body image related to…

NURSING PLANS AND INTERVENTIONS

1. Provide wound care.
   A. Monitor surgical dressing for drainage.
      1) Mark dressing for bleeding and check marking at least every 8 hours.
      2) Measure suction drainage every shift.
   B. Change dressing as needed (physician usually performs initial dressing change).
      1) **Maintain aseptic technique**.
      2) Observe wound color and warmth.
      3) Observe for wound healing.
      4) Monitor for signs of infection.
         a) Fever.
         b) Tachycardia.
         c) Redness of incision area.
2. Maintain proper body alignment in and out of bed.
3. Position client to relieve edema and spasms at residual limb (stump) site.
   A. Elevate residual limb (stump) the first 24 hours postoperatively.

> **HESI HINT:** The residual limb (stump) should be elevated on one pillow. If the residual limb (stump) is elevated too high, the elevation can cause a contracture.

   B. Do not elevate residual limb (stump) after 48 hours postoperatively.
   C. Keep residual limb (stump) in extended position and turn prone three times a day to prevent hip flexion contracture.
4. Be aware that phantom pain is REAL, will eventually disappear, and responds to pain medication.
5. Handle affected body part gently and with smooth movements.
6. Provide passive range of motion until client is able to perform active range of motion.
7. Collaborate with rehabilitation team members for mobility improvement.
8. Encourage independence in self-care, allowing sufficient time for client to complete care and to have input into care.

REVIEW QUESTIONS
MUSCULOSKELETAL SYSTEM

1. **Differentiate between rheumatoid arthritis and degenerative joint disease in terms of joint involvement.**
2. **Identify the categories of drugs commonly used to treat arthritis.**
3. **Identify pain relief interventions for clients with arthritis.**
4. **What measures should the nurse encourage female clients to take to prevent osteoporosis?**
5. **What are the common side effects of salicylates?**
6. **What is the priority nursing intervention used with clients taking NSAIDs?**
7. **List three of the most common joints that are replaced?**
8. **Describe postoperative residual limb (stump) care (after amputation) for the first 48 hours.**
9. **Describe nursing care for the client who is experiencing phantom pain after amputation.**
10. **A nurse discovers that a client who is in traction for a long bone fracture has a slight fever, is short of breath, and is restless. What does the client most likely have?**
11. **What are the immediate nursing actions**

if fat embolization is suspected in a fracture/ orthopedic client?

12. **List three problems associated with immobility.**
13. **List three nursing interventions for the prevention of thromboembolism in immobilized clients with musculoskeletal problems.**

1. Rheumatoid arthritis occurs bilaterally. Degenerative joint disease occurs asymmetrically.
2. NSAIDs (nonsteroidal anti-inflammatory drugs) of which salicylates are the cornerstone of treatment, and corticosteroids (used when arthritic symptoms are severe).
3. Warm, moist heat (compresses, baths, showers), diversionary activities (imaging, distraction, self-hypnosis, biofeedback), and medications.
4. Estrogen replacement after menopause, high-calcium and vitamin D intake beginning in early adulthood, calcium supplements after menopause, and weight-bearing exercise.
5. GI irritation, tinnitus, Thrombocytopenia, mild liver enzyme elevation.
6. Administer or teach client to take drugs with food or milk.
7. Hip, knee, finger.
8. Elevate residual limb (stump) first 24 hours. Do not elevate residual limb (stump) after 48 hours. Keep residual limb (stump) in extended position and turn prone three times a day to prevent flexion contracture.
9. Be aware that phantom pain is real and will eventually disappear. Administer pain medication; phantom pain responds to medication.
10. Fat embolism, which is characterized by hypoxemia, respiratory distress, irritability, restlessness, fever, and petechiae.
11. Notify physician STAT, draw blood gases, administer oxygen according to blood gas results, assist with endotracheal intubation and treatment of respiratory failure.
12. Venous thrombosis, urinary calculi, skin integrity problems.
13. Passive range of motion exercises, elastic stockings, and elevation of foot of bed 25 degrees to increase venous return.

NEUROSENSORY SYSTEM

GLAUCOMA
Chronic open-angle is also known as simple adult primary, and primary open-angle glaucoma.
DESCRIPTION: Condition characterized by increased intraocular pressure (IOP)

1. Gradual, painless vision loss.
2. Glaucoma may lead to blindness if untreated.
3. Glaucoma is the second leading cause of blindness in the U.S.
4. There is an increased incidence in the elderly population.
5. Glaucoma usually occurs bilaterally in those who have a family history of the condition.
6. Aqueous fluid is inadequately drained from the eye.
7. Generally asymptomatic, especially in early stages.
8. Tends to be diagnosed during routine visual exams.
9. Cannot be cured, but can be treated with success pharmacologically and surgically.

NURSING ASSESSMENT
1. Early signs include:
   A. Increase in intraocular pressure, >22 mmHg.
   B. Decreased accommodation or ability to focus.

HESI HINT: Glaucoma is often painless and symptom-free. It is usually picked up as part of a regular eye exam.

2. Late signs include:
   A. Loss of peripheral vision.
   B. Halos around lights.
   C. Decreased visual acuity, not correctable with glasses.
   D. Headache or eye pain which may be so severe as to cause nausea and vomiting (acute closed-angle glaucoma).
3. Diagnostic tests include the following:
   A. Tonometer used to measure intraocular pressure.
   B. Electronic tonometer used to detect drainage of aqueous humor.
   C. Gonioscopy used to obtain a direct visualization of the lens.
4. Risk factors include the following:
   A. Family history of glaucoma.

B. Family history of diabetes.
C. History of previous ocular problems.
D. Medication use.
1) Glaucoma is a side effect of many medications (e.g., antihistamines, anticholinergics).
2) Glaucoma can result from the interaction of medications.

ANALYSIS (NURSING DIAGNOSES)
1. Anxiety related to…
2. Sensory/perceptual alterations: visual related to…
3. Impaired health maintenance related to…

NURSING PLANS AND INTERVENTIONS
1. Administer eye drops as prescribed. *(See figure 3-36, Treatment of Glaucoma)*

HESI HINT: Eye drops are used to cause pupil constriction since movement of the muscles to constrict the pupil also allows aqueous humor to flow out, thereby decreasing the pressure in the eye. Pilocarpine is often used. Caution client that vision may be blurred 1 to 2 hours after administration of pilocarpine and adaptation to dark environments is difficult because of pupillary constriction (desired effect of the drug).

2. Orient client to surroundings.
3. Avoid nonverbal communication which requires visual acuity (e.g., facial expressions).
4. Develop a teaching plan to include the following:
A. Careful adherence to eye drop regime can prevent blindness.
B. Vision already lost cannot be restored.
C. Eye drops are needed the rest of life.
D. Proper eye drop instillation technique. OBTAIN A RETURN DEMONSTRATION. *(See figure 3-37, Eye Drop Administration)*
E. Safety measures to prevent injuries.
1) Remove throw rugs.
2) Adjust lighting to meet client's needs.
F. Avoid activities that may increase intraocular pressure.
1) Emotional upsets.
2) Exertion: pushing, heavy lifting, shoveling.
3) Coughing severely or excessive sneezing; get medical attention before upper respiratory infection (URI) worsens.
4) Constrictive clothing: tight collar or tie; belt or girdle too tight.
5) Straining at stool or constipation.

NURSING PLANS AND INTERVENTIONS
THE NON-SEEING (BLIND) CLIENT
1. Upon entering room, announce clearly your presence and identify yourself, address client by name.
2. Do *not* ever touch client unless he/she knows you are there.
3. Upon admission, orient client thoroughly to surroundings:
A. Demonstrate use of the call bell.
B. Walk client around the room and acquaint him/her with all objects: chairs, bed, TV, phone, etc.
4. Guide client when walking
A. Walk ahead of client and place his/her hand in the bend of your elbow.
B. Describe where you are walking. Note if passageway is narrowing or you are approaching stairs, curb, or an incline.
5. Always raise side rails for the "newly" sightless person, e.g., postoperative eye patch clients.
6. Assist with meal enjoyment by describing food and its placement in terms of face of a clock, e.g., "meat at 6 o'clock."
7. When administering medications, inform client of number of pills, give only ½ glass of water (to avoid spill).

TREATMENT OF GLAUCOMA

DRUGS	INDICATIONS	ADVERSE REACTIONS	NURSING IMPLICATIONS
PARA-SYMPATHOMIMETICS • **pilocarpine HCL** (multiple brands available) 0.5 to 0.6% is the drug of choice	• Enhance papillary constriction (Available in drops, gel and time-release wafer)	• Bronchospasm • Nausea, vomiting, diarrhea • Blurred vision, twitching eye lids, eye pain with focusing	• Use cautiously with: → Pregnancy → Asthma → Hypertension • Teach proper drop instillation technique • Need for ongoing use of the drug at prescribed intervals • Blurred vision tends to decrease with regular use of this drug
BETA-ADRENERGIC RECEPTOR-BLOCKING AGENTS • **timolol maleate optic** (Timoptic Solution) • **carteolol** (Ocupress)	• Inhibit formation of aqueous humor	• Side effects are insignificant • Hypotension	• Use cautiously with: → Hypersensitive → Asthmatic → 2nd or 3rd degree heart block → CHF → Congenital glaucoma → Pregnancy • Teach proper drop instillation technique • Need for ongoing use of the drug at prescribed intervals • Blurred vision tends to decrease with regular use of this drug
CARBONIC ANHYDRASE INHIBITORS • **acetazolamide** (Diamox) • **brinzolamide** (Azopt) • **dorzolamide** (Trusopt)	• Reduce aqueous humor production	• Numbness, tingling hands and feet • Nausea • Malaise	• Administer orally or IV • Produces diuresis • Assess for metabolic acidosis
PROSTAGLANDIN AGONISTS **latanoprost** (Xalatan) **travoprost** (Travatan) **bimateorost** (Lumigan)	• Lowers intraocular pressure of glaucoma by increasing outflow of aqueons humor	• Local irritation • Foreign body sensation • Increased brown pigmentation of iris • Increased eyelash growth	

HESI HINT: There is an increased incidence of glaucoma in the elderly population. Older clients are prone to problems associated with constipation. Therefore, the nurse should assess these clients for constipation and postoperative complications associated with constipation, and implement a plan of care directed at prevention, and, if necessary, treatment for constipation.

EYE DROP ADMINISTRATION
• Wash hands and external eye. • Tilt head back slightly. • Instill drop into lower lid, without touching the lid with the tip of the dropper. • Release the lid and sponge excess fluid from lid and cheek. • Close eye gently and leave closed 3 to 5 minutes. • Apply gentle pressure on inner canthus to decrease systematic absorption.

Figure 3-37

CATARACT

DESCRIPTION: Condition characterized by opacity of the lens.
1. Aging accounts for 95% of cataracts (senile).
2. Remaining 5% are from trauma, toxic substances, systemic diseases, or are congenital.
3. Safety precautions may reduce incidence of traumatic cataracts.
4. Surgical removal is done when vision impairment interferes with daily activities. Intraocular lens implants may be used.
5. Most surgeries are done under local anesthesia as an outpatient.

HESI HINT: The lens of the eye is responsible for projecting light, which enters onto the retina so that images can be discerned. Without the lens, which becomes opaque with cataracts, light cannot be filtered and vision is blurred.

NURSING ASSESSMENT
1. Early signs include:
   A. Blurred vision.
   B. Decreased color perception.
2. Late signs include:
   A. Diplopia.
   B. Reduced visual acuity progressing to blindness.
   C. Clouded pupil, progressing to a milky-white appearance.
3. Diagnostic tests include the following:
   A. Ophthalmoscope.
   B. Slit lamp biomicroscope.

ANALYSIS (NURSING DIAGNOSES)
1. Sensory/perceptual alterations: visual related to…
2. Anxiety related to…

NURSING PLANS AND INTERVENTIONS
1. Preoperative: demonstrate and request a return demonstration of eye medication instillation from client and/or family member.
2. Develop a postoperative teaching plan to include:
   A. Warning not to rub or put pressure on eye.
   B. Glasses or shaded lens should be worn during waking hours. Eye shield should be worn during sleeping hours.
   C. Avoid lifting objects over 15 pounds, bending, straining, coughing, or any activity that can increase intraocular pressure.
   D. Use stool softener to prevent straining at stool.
   E. Avoid lying on operative side.
   F. Need to keep water from getting into eye while showering or washing hair.
   G. Observe and report signs of increased intraocular pressure and infection (e.g., pain, changes in vital signs).

HESI HINT: When the cataract is removed, the lens is gone, making prevention of falls important. If the lens is replaced with an implant, vision is better than if a contact lens is used (some visual distortion) or if glasses are used (greater visual distortion – everything has a curved shape).

EYE TRAUMA

DESCRIPTION: Injury to the eye sustained from sharp or blunt trauma, chemicals, or heat.
1. Permanent visual impairment can occur.
2. Every eye injury should be considered an

MEDICAL SURGICAL NURSING

146

emergency.

3. Protective eye-shields in hazardous work environments and during athletic sports may prevent injuries.

NURSING ASSESSMENT
1. Determine type of injury and symptoms.
2. Diagnostic tests include the following:
   A. Slit lamp examination.
   B. Fluorescein to detect corneal injury.
   C. Visual acuity for medical documentation and legal protection.

ANALYSIS (NURSING DIAGNOSES)
1) Sensory/perceptual alterations: visual related to…
2) Pain related to…

NURSING PLANS AND INTERVENTIONS
1. Position the client relative to the type of injury; sitting position will decrease intraocular pressure.
2. Remove conjunctival foreign bodies unless embedded.
3. Never attempt to remove a penetrating or embedded object. Do NOT apply pressure.
4. Apply cold compresses to eye contusion.
5. Irrigate the eye following chemical injuries with copious amounts of water.
6. Administer eye medications as prescribed.
7. Explain that an eye patch may be applied to rest the eye. Reading and watching TV may be restricted for 3 to 5 days.
8. Explain that sudden increase in eye pain should be reported.

DETACHED RETINA

DESCRIPTION: A hole, tear, separation of the sensory retina from the pigmented epithelium.
1. Can be result of blunt trauma astigmatism.
2. Resealing is done by surgery:
   A. Cryotherapy – freezing
   B. Photocoagulation – laser
   C. Deathermy – heat
   D. Scleral Buckling – most often used

NURSING PLANS AND INTERVENTIONS
1. Activity (allow retina to "lie back")
2. Eye patch over affected eye
3. Eye Rx to inhibit accommodation and constriction. Cycloplegics to dilate (mydriatic): homatropine – an anticholinergic
4. Postoperative for pain – Tylenol, Demerol,

oxycodone
5. If gas bubble used (inserted in vitreous), position so bubble can "rise" against area to be reattached.

HEARING LOSS

CONDUCTIVE HEARING LOSS
DESCRIPTION: Hearing loss in which sound does not travel well to the sound organs of the inner ear. The volume of sound is less, but the sound remains clear. If volume is raised, hearing is normal.
1. Hearing loss is the most common disability in the U.S.
2. Usually results from cerumen (wax) impaction or middle ear disorders.

> **HESI HINT:** The ear consists of three parts: the external ear, the middle ear, and the inner ear. Inner ear disorders, or disorders of the sensory fibers going to the CNS, often are neurogenic in nature and may not be helped with a hearing aid. External and middle ear problems (conductive) may result from infection, trauma or wax buildup. These types of disorders are treated more successfully with hearing aids.

SENSORINEURAL HEARING LOSS
DESCRIPTION: A form of hearing loss in which sound passes properly through the outer and middle ear but is distorted by a defect in the inner ear.
1. Perceptive loss, usually progressive and bilateral.
2. Involves damage to the eighth cranial nerve.
3. Detected easily by use of a tuning fork.
4. Common causes include:
   A. Infections.
   B. Ototoxic drugs.
   C. Trauma.
   D. Neuromas.
   E. Noise.
   F. Aging process.

NURSING ASSESSMENT
1. Inability to hear a whisper from 1 to 2 feet away.
2. Inability to respond if nurse covers mouth when talking, indicating that client is lip

reading.

3. Inability to hear a watch tick 5 inches from ear.
4. Shouting in conversation.
5. Straining to hear.
6. Turning head to favor one ear.
7. Answering questions incorrectly or inappropriately.
8. Raising volume of radio/TV.

ANALYSIS (NURSING DIAGNOSES)

1. Sensory/perceptual alterations (auditory) related to…
2. Impaired communication related to…

NURSING PLANS AND INTERVENTIONS

1. The nurse should do the following to enhance therapeutic communication with the hearing impaired:
   A. Prior to starting conversation, reduce distraction as much as possible.
   B. Turn the television or radio down or off, close the door, or move to a quieter location.
   C. Devote full attention to the conversation; don't try to do two things at once.
   D. Look and listen during the conversation.
   E. Begin with casual topics and progress to more critical issues slowly.
   F. Do not switch topics abruptly.
   G. If you do not understand, let the client know.
   H. If the client is a lip reader, face them directly.
   I. Speak slowly and distinctly; determine whether you were understood.
   J. Allow adequate time for the conversation to take place; try to avoid hurried conversations.
   K. Use active listening techniques.

> **HESI HINT:** NCLEX-RN® questions often focus on communicating with older adults who are hearing impaired.
> - Speak in a low-pitched voice, slowly, and distinctly.
> - Stand in front of the person with the light source behind the client.
> - Use visual aids if available.

2. Be sure to inform the healthcare staff of the client's hearing loss.
3. Helpful aids may include a telephone amplifier, earphone attachments for the radio and TV, and lights or buzzers that ring for the doorbell in the most used rooms of the house.

NEUROLOGICAL SYSTEM
ALTERED STATE OF CONSCIOUSNESS

NURSING ASSESSMENT

1. Use agency neuro vital sign assessment tool. It will sometimes contain a scale for scoring, such as the Glasgow Coma Scale, which objectively documents the client's level of consciousness. *(See figure 3-38, Glasgow Coma Scale)*
   A. Maximum total is 15, minimum is 3.
   B. A score of 7 or less indicates COMA.
   C. Clients with low scores, i.e., 3 to 4, have a high mortality and poor prognosis.
   D. Clients with scores greater than 8 have a good prognosis for recovery.

> **HESI HINT:** Use of the Glasgow Coma Scale eliminates ambiguous terms to describe neurologic status such as lethargic, stuporous, or obtunded.

2. Neuro vital sign sheet will also address pupil size (with sizing scale), limb movement (with scale), and vital signs (blood pressure, temperature, pulse, respirations).
3. Assess skin integrity and corneal integrity.
4. Check bladder for fullness, auscultate lungs, and monitor cardiac status.
5. Family members and significant others should be assessed for knowledge of client status, coping skills, need for extra support, and the ability to assist or provide care on an ongoing basis.

HESI HINT: Almost every diagnosis in the NANDA format is applicable, as severely neurologically impaired persons require total care.

1. Ineffective breathing pattern related to…
2. Ineffective airway clearance related to…
3. Impaired gas exchange related to…
4. Decreased cardiac output related to…
5. Altered body temperature (especially if hypothalamus is involved) related to…
6. Potential for injury related to…
7. Impaired physical mobility related to…
8. Potential impaired skin integrity related to…
9. Anxiety related to…
10. Self-care deficit: eating, toileting, dressing, grooming related to…
11. Altered nutrition: less than body requirements related to…
12. Altered patterns of urinary elimination: incontinence related to…
13. Altered bowel elimination: constipation related to…

HESI HINT: Clients with an altered state of consciousness are fed by enteral routes since the likelihood of aspiration with oral feedings is great. Residual feeding is the amount of previous feeding still in the stomach. The presence of 100 ml residual in adults usually indicates poor gastric emptying and the feeding should be held.

HESI HINT: Paralytic ileus is common in comatose clients. Gastric tube aids in gastric decompression.

HESI HINT: Any client on bedrest/immobilized must have range of motion exercises often and very frequent position changes. Do not leave the client in any one position for longer than 2 hours. Any position that decreases venous return is dangerous, i.e., sitting with dependent extremities for long periods.

MEDICAL SURGICAL NURSING

GLASGOW COMA SCALE

VARIABLE	RESPONSE	SCORE
EYE OPENING	Spontaneously	4
	To verbal command	3
	To pain	2
	No response	1
MOTOR RESPONSE	To verbal command	6
	To painful stimuli • Localizes pain	5
	• Flexes/withdraws	4
	• Flexor posturing (decorticate)	3
	• Extensor posturing (decerebrate)	2
	• No response	1
VERBAL RESPONSE	Oriented and converses	5
	Disoriented, converses	4
	Uses inappropriate words	3
	Incomprehensible sounds	2
	No response	1

Figure 3-38

ALTERED STATES OF CONSCIOUSNESS
NURSING PLANS AND INTERVENTIONS

1. Maintain adequate respirations, airway, oxygenation:
   A. Document and report breathing pattern changes.
   B. Position for maximum ventilation: ¾ prone or semi-prone to prevent tongue from obstructing airway and slightly to one side with arms away from chest wall.
   C. Insert airway if tongue is obstructing or if client is paralyzed.
   D. Prepare for insertion of cuffed endotracheal tube.
   E. Keep airway free of secretions with suctioning. *(See figure 3-6, Nursing Skills: Respiratory Client)*
   F. Monitor arterial pO_2 and pCO_2.
   G. Prepare for tracheostomy if prolonged ventilator support is needed.
   H. Provide chest physiotherapy as prescribed by physician.
   I. Hyperventilate with 100% O_2 before and after suctioning.

2. Provide nutritional and fluid and electrolyte support.
   A. Keep client NPO until responsive and provide mouth care q4 hours.
   B. Maintain calorie count.
   C. Administer feedings as prescribed. *(See figure 3-39, Unconscious Client)*
   D. Monitor I&O.
   E. Record client's weight (weigh same time each day).

3. Prevent complications of immobility:
   A. Impairment in skin integrity:
      1) Turn q2 hours and assess bony prominences.
      2) Utilize egg crate, alternating pressure mattress, or waterbed.
      3) Use minimal amount of linens and underpads.
   B. Potential for thrombus formation:
      1) Assess Homan's sign every 8 hours if client is alert.
      2) Perform passive ROM exercises to lower extremities every 4 hours.
      3) Use elastic hose; remove and reapply q 8 hours.
      4) Avoid positions that decrease venous return.
      5) Avoid pillows under knees or gatched bed.
   C. Urinary calculi:

   1) Increase fluid intake PO or gastric tube.
   2) Assess urine for high specific gravity (dehydration) and balance between intake and output.
   D. Contractures/joint immobility:
      1) Passive ROM q4 hours.
      2) Sit client up in bed or chair if possible, or use neuro chair if necessary.
      3) Reposition q2 hours maintaining proper body alignment.
      4) Apply splints or other assistive devices to prevent foot drop, wrist drop, or other improper alignment.

4. Monitor and evaluate the vital sign changes indicating changes in condition:
   A. Pulse: a pulse rate change to <60 or >100 BPM can indicate increased ICP. Fast rate (>100 BPM) can indicate infection, thrombus formation, or dehydration.
   B. Blood pressure: rising BP or widening pulse pressure can indicate increased ICP.
   C. Temperature: report any abnormalities (temperature elevation can indicate worsening condition, damage to temperature regulating area of brain, and/or infection).
   D. Level of consciousness changes: active to somnolent.
   E. Pupillary changes: prompt to sluggish, increase in size.

HESI HINT: If temperature elevates, take quick measures to decrease it since fever increases cerebral metabolism and can increase cerebral edema.

HESI HINT: Safety Features for Immobilized Clients:
- **Prevent skin breakdown with frequent turning.**
- **Maintain adequate nutrition.**
- **Prevent aspiration with slow, small feedings or NG feedings.**
- **Monitor neurological signs to detect the first signs that intracranial pressure may be increasing.**
- **Provide range of motion exercises to prevent deformities.**
- **Prevent respiratory complications – frequent turning and positioning for optimal drainage.**

---

5. Prevent injury/promote safety:

A. Place bed in low position and keep side rails up at all times.
B. Pad side rails if client is agitated or if there is a history of seizure activity.
C. Restrain if client is trying to remove tubes or attempting to get out of bed.
D. Touch gently and talk softly and calmly to the client, remembering that hearing is often intact.

HESI HINT: Restlessness may indicate a return to consciousness but can also indicate anoxia, distended bladder, covert bleeding, or increasing cerebral anoxia. Do *not* over-sedate, and report any symptoms of restlessness.

E. Avoid over-sedating the client as sedatives/narcotics depress responsiveness and affect papillary reaction (an important assessment in neuro vital signs).
F. During all activities, tell the client what you are doing no matter what the level of consciousness.
6. Maintain hygiene/cleanliness:

A. Provide bathing, grooming and dressing.
B. Provide oral hygiene.
C. Wash hair weekly.
D. Provide nail care within agency guidelines.
7. Observe for bladder elimination problems:
A. Insert indwelling catheter if prescribed.
B. Remove indwelling catheter as soon as possible; use diaper or condom catheter.
8. Document and record bowel movements and report abnormal patterns of constipation or diarrhea.
A. Rapid infusion of tube feedings may cause diarrhea, while lack of fiber/inadequate fluids may cause constipation.
B. Initiate bowel program. *(See figure 3-39, Unconscious Client)*
9. Prevent corneal injury/drying:
A. Remove contact lenses if present.
B. Irrigate eyes with sterile prescribed solution and instill ophthalmic ointment in each eye every 8 hours to prevent corneal ulceration.
10. See Seizure Disorders in Pediatric section.

MEDICAL SURGICAL NURSING

UNCONSCIOUS CLIENT
GASTRIC GAVAGE
• Begin feeding when GI peristalsis returns.   • Place client in high Fowler's position.   • Place towel over chest.   • Connect gastrostomy tube to funnel or large syringe.   • Check gastric residual to assess absorption and client tolerance; return residual.   • Pour feeding into tilted funnel and unclamp tubing to allow feeding to flow by GRAVITY.   • Regulate flow by raising or lowering container. Feeding too fast causes diarrhea, gastric distension, pain. Feeding too slow causes possible obstruction of flow.   • After feeding, irrigate tube with water (tepid) and clamp tube.   • Apply small dressing over tube opening, coil tube and attach to dressing. May cover with an abdominal binder.
BOWEL MANAGEMENT PROGRAM

• Get bowel history from reliable source.
 • Establish specific time for evacuation. Regularity is essential.
     → In an unconscious client, can evacuate the bowel after the last tube feeding of day, because the gastro colic and duodenocolic reflexes are active after "meal."
     → Stimulate anorectal reflex with insertion of glycerin suppository 15 to 30 minutes before scheduled evacuation time. May need stronger suppository, such as bisacodyl (Dulcolax).
     → Ensure adequate fiber in tube feedings and adequate fluid intake of 2 to 4 liters/day.
     → May apply a rectal pouch to contain fecal material (ostomy bag with seal over anal opening).

Figure 3-39

Head Injury

Description: Any traumatic damage to the head.

1. Open head injury occurs when there is a fracture of the skull or penetration of the skull by an object.
2. Closed head injury (CHI) is the result of blunt trauma (more serious due to chance of increased intracranial pressure in "closed" vault).
3. Increased ICP is the main concern in head injury related to edema, hemorrhage, impaired cerebral auto-regulation and hydrocephalus.

> **HESI HINT:** The forces of impact influence the type of head injury. They include acceleration injury, which is caused by the head in motion, and deceleration injury, which occurs when the head stops suddenly. Helmets are a GREAT preventive measure for motorcyclists and bicyclists.

Nursing Assessment

1. Unconsciousness or disturbances in consciousness.
2. Vertigo.
3. Confusion, delirium and/or disorientation.
4. Symptoms of increased intracranial pressure (ICP).
   A. Change in level of responsiveness is the most important indicator of increased ICP.

> **HESI HINT:** Even subtle behavior changes, such as restlessness, irritability, or confusion, may indicate increased ICP.

   B. Changes in vital signs:
      1) Slowing of respirations or respiratory irregularities.
      2) Increase or decrease in pulse.
      3) Rising BP or widening pulse pressure.
      4) Temperature rise.
   C. Headache.
   D. Vomiting (projectile).
   E. Pupillary changes reflecting pressure on optic/oculomotor nerves.
      1) Pupils decrease or increase in size or become unequal.
      2) Lack of conjugate eye movement.
      3) Papilledema.
5. Seizures.
6. Ataxia.
7. Abnormal posturing (decerebrate or decorticate).

8. Cerebral spinal fluid (CSF) leakage through nose (rhinorrhea) or through ear (otorrhea).

> **HESI HINT:** CSF leakage carries the risk of meningitis and indicates a deteriorating condition. Because of CSF leakage, the usual signs of increased ICP may not occur.

9. Computerized axial tomography (CAT) scan or magnetic resonance imaging (MRI) will show lesion such as epidural or subdural hematomas requiring surgery.
10. EEG determines presence of seizure activity.

Analysis (Nursing Diagnoses)

1. Altered cerebral tissue perfusion related to…
2. Sensory/perceptual alterations related to…
3. Potential for injury related to…
4. Ineffective family coping related to…

Nursing Plans and Interventions

1. Maintain adequate ventilation/airway.
   A. Monitor pO_2 and pCO_2 for the development of hypoxia and hypercapnia.
   B. Position client semi-prone or lateral recumbent to prevent aspiration.
   C. Turn from side-to-side to prevent lung secretion stasis.
2. Keep head of bed elevated 30 to 45 degrees to aid venous return from the neck and decrease cerebral volume.
3. Obtain neurologic vital signs as prescribed (at least q1 to 2 hours) and maintain a continuous record of observations and Glasgow Coma Scale ratings.
4. Notify physician at **FIRST** sign of deterioration or improvement in condition.
5. Avoid activities that increase intracranial pressure such as:
   A. Change in bed position for caregiving, extreme hip flexion.
   B. Endotracheal suctioning.
   C. Compression of jugular veins (keep head straight and not to one side).
   D. Coughing, vomiting, or straining of any type (no Valsalva: increased intrathoracic pressure increases ICP).
6. If temperature increases, take immediate measures to reduce it (aspirin, acetaminophen, cooling blanket) since increased temperature increases cerebral blood flow drastically; avoid shivering.
7. Use intracranial monitoring system when available:
   A. Catheter inserted into lateral ventricle, sensor placed on the dura, or a screw into the subarachnoid space attached to pressure transducer.

B. Elevations of intracranial pressure over 20 mmHg should be reported **STAT**.
8. Administer medications prescribed by physician to reduce intracranial pressure:
   A. Hyperosmotic agents/diuretics: to dehydrate brain and reduce cerebral edema.
      1) Mannitol. *(See figure 3-40 Osmotic Diuretic)*
      2) Urea.
   B. Steroids: Dexamethasone (Decadron), methylprednesilone sodium/succinate (Solumedrol) to reduce brain edema.
   C. Barbiturates: to reduce brain metabolism and systemic blood pressure.
9. Insert indwelling Foley catheter to prevent restlessness caused by distended bladder and to monitor balance between restricted fluid intake and output, especially if placed on osmotic diuretics.

> **HESI HINT:** TRY NOT to use restraints; they only increase restlessness. AVOID narcotics since they mask level of responsiveness.

10. Physician may order passive hyperventilation on ventilator: leads to respiratory alkalosis, which causes cerebral vasoconstriction, decreased cerebral blood flow and therefore decreased ICP.
11. Continue seizure precautions. Healthcare provider may order prophylactic phenytoin (Dilantin).
12. Prevent complications of immobility. *(See Nursing Plans and Interventions for the Unconscious/Immobilized Client)*
13. Inform at discharge of possible aftereffects of head injury:
    A. Post-traumatic syndrome: headache, vertigo, emotional instability, inability to concentrate, impaired memory.
    B. Post-traumatic epilepsy.
    C. Post-traumatic neuroses/psychoses.

OSMOTIC DIURETIC			
DRUG	**INDICATIONS**	**ADVERSE REACTIONS**	**NURSING IMPLICATIONS**
mannitol (Osmitrol)	• Acts on renal tubules by osmosis to prevent water reabsorption • In bloodstream, draws fluid from the extra vascular spaces into the plasma	• Disorientation, confusion, and headache • Nausea and vomiting • Convulsions and anaphylactic reactions	• Use for short-term therapy ONLY • Never give to clients with cerebral hemorrhage • IV infusion is usually adjusted to urine output – filter and watch for crystals • Never give to clients with no urine output (Anuria); if output is <30 cc/hr, accumulation can cause pulmonary edema and water intoxication

Figure 3-40

SPINAL CORD INJURY

DESCRIPTION: Disruption in nervous system function, which may result in complete or incomplete loss of motor and sensory function. Changes occur in the function of all physiological systems.
1. Injuries are described by location in the spinal cord. Most common sites are: Fifth, sixth, and seventh cervical (C-5, C-6, C-7), the twelfth thoracic (T-12), and the first lumbar (L-1).
2. Damage can range from contusion to complete transection.
3. Permanent impairment cannot be determined until spinal cord edema has subsided, usually by one week.

NURSING ASSESSMENT
1. Assess breathing pattern, auscultate lungs.

> **HESI HINT:** Physical assessment should concentrate on respiratory status, especially in clients with injury at C-3 to C-5, as cervical plexus innervates diaphragm.

153

2. Check neuro/vital signs frequently, especially sensory and motor functions. Assess cardiovascular status.
3. Assess abdomen: Girth, bowel sounds, lower abdomen for bladder distention.
4. Assess temperature remembering hyperthermia often occurs.
5. Assess psychosocial status.
6. Hypotension and bradycardia occur with any injury above T-6 because sympathetic outflow is affected.

ANALYSIS (NURSING DIAGNOSES)
1. Ineffective breathing pattern related to…
2. Altered tissue perfusion related to…
3. Impaired skin integrity related to…
4. Self-care deficit related to…
5. Urinary retention related to…
6. Ineffective individual coping related to…

NURSING PLANS AND INTERVENTIONS
IN ACUTE PHASE OF SPINAL CORD INJURY:
1. ***See Nursing Plans and Interventions for the Unconscious/Immobilized Client.***
2. Maintain client in an extended position with cervical collar on during any transfer.
3. Stabilize the client from the accident scene to the emergency room. The client will be realigned and stabilized in the emergency room.
4. Maintain a patent airway – most important.
5. In cervical injuries, skeletal traction is maintained by use of skull tongs or halo ring (Crutchfield tongs or Gardner-Wells fixation device).
6. High-dose corticosteroids are often given to help control edema first 8 to 24 hours.
7. Use a kinetic therapy treatment table (Rotorest bed), which provides continuous side-to-side motion.
8. Use Stryker frame or **VERY FIRM** mattress with board underneath.
9. Assess for respiratory failure especially in clients with high cervical injuries.
10. Further loss of sensory/motor function below injury can indicate additional damage to cord from edema and should be reported **immediately**.
11. Evaluate for presence of spinal shock (a complete loss of all reflex, motor, sensory, and autonomic activity below the lesion). This is a **MEDICAL EMERGENCY,** which occurs immediately after the injury.
    A. Hypotension, bradycardia.
    B. Complete paralysis and lack of sensation below lesion.
    C. Bladder and bowel distension.

> **HESI HINT: It is imperative to reverse spinal shock as quickly as possible. Permanent paralysis can occur if a spinal cord is compressed for 12 to 24 hours.**

12. Evaluate for **autonomic dysreflexia** (exaggerated autonomic responses to stimuli), which occurs in clients with lesions at or above T-6. This is a **MEDICAL EMERGENCY** that usually occurs after the period of spinal shock is completed, usually triggered by a noxious stimulus, such as bowel or bladder distension. It may also be triggered by vaginal examination.
    A. Elevated BP.
    B. Pounding headache, sweating, nasal congestion, goose bumps, bradycardia.
    C. Bladder and bowel distension.
13. Watch for acute paralytic ileus, lack of gastric activity.
    A. Assess bowel sounds frequently.
    B. Initiate gastric suction to reduce distension, prevent vomiting/aspiration.
    C. May use rectal tube to relieve gaseous distension.
14. Suction with caution to prevent vagus nerve stimulation, which can cause cardiac arrest.
15. Administer high-dose corticosteroids to decrease edema and reduce cord damage.

IN REHABILITATIVE PHASE:
1. Encourage deep-breathing exercises.
2. Chest physiotherapy.
3. Kinetic bed to promote blood flow to extremities.
4. Antiembolic stockings.
5. Range of motion exercises.
6. Mobilize to chair as soon as possible.
7. Turn frequently.
8. Keep client clean and dry.
9. Observe for impending skin breakdown.
10. Teach client importance of impeccable skin care.
11. Intermittent catheterization every four hours.
    A. Begin teaching client catheterization technique.
    B. Teach family member if client is unable.

13. Teach bladder emptying techniques depending on level of injury and bladder muscle respose.
    A. UMN (spastic) bladder
    B. LMN (flaccid) bladder
14. Instruct client in I&O.
15. Acidify urine with vitamin C.

> **HESI HINT:** A common cause of death after spinal cord injury is urinary tract infection. Bacteria grow best in alkaline media, so keeping urine dilute and acidic is prophylactic against infection. Also, keeping the bladder emptied assists in avoiding bacterial growth in urine, which is stagnated in the bladder.

16. Begin bowel-training program.
17. Talk with client and family about permanence of disability.
18. Encourage rehabilitation facility staff to visit client.
19. Encourage client and family to visit rehabilitation facility.
20. Assist family to find support group and refer to community resources after dismissal from rehabilitation facility.

BRAIN TUMOR

DESCRIPTION: Neoplasm occurring in the brain.
1. Primary tumors arise in any tissue of the brain.
2. Secondary tumors are a result of metastasis from other areas (most often from the lungs, followed by breast metastasis).
3. Without treatment, benign as well as malignant tumors lead to death.

> **HESI HINT:** Benign tumors continue to grow and take up space in the confined area of the cranium causing neural and vascular compromise for the brain, increased intracranial pressure, and necrosis of brain tissue – even benign tumors must be treated as they may have malignant effects.

NURSING ASSESSMENT
1. Headache that is more severe upon awakening.
2. Vomiting not associated with nausea.
3. Papilledema with visual changes.
4. Behavioral and personality changes.
5. Seizures.
6. Aphasia, hemiplegia, ataxia.
7. Cranial nerve dysfunction.

8. Abnormal CAT scan.

ANALYSIS (NURSING DIAGNOSES)
1. Altered cerebral tissue perfusion related to…
2. Pain related to…
3. Potential for injury related to…
4. Anxiety and fear related to…

NURSING PLANS AND INTERVENTIONS
Nursing plans and interventions are similar to those implemented for the head injury client with increased ICP.
1. Elevate the head of the bed 30 to 40 degrees, maintain head in neutral position.
2. Radiation therapy:
    A. Provide skin care with non-oil-based soap and water. Avoid alcohol, powder, or oils on the skin.
    B. Explain that alopecia is temporary.
    C. Instruct client NOT to wash off the lines drawn by the radiologist.
3. Chemotherapy: medications may be injected intraventricularly or intravenously.
4. Surgical removal (craniotomy).
    A. Preoperative: shave head.
    B. Postoperative:
        1) Frequent neurologic and vital sign assessment.
        2) Position client with head of bed elevated for supratentorial lesions and flat for infratentorial lesions. Position client off the operative site.
        3) Monitor dressings for signs of drainage (excess amount of CSF).
        4) Monitor respiratory status to prevent hypoventilation.
        5) Avoid activities that cause increased ICP.
        6) Monitor for seizure activity.
        7) Administer medications. *(See Head Injuries)*

> **HESI HINT:** Craniotomy preoperative medications:
> - **Corticosteroids to reduce swelling**
> - **Agents and osmotic diuretics to reduce secretions (atropine, robinul)**
> - **Agents to reduce seizures (phenytoin)**
> - **Prophylactic antibiotics**

MULTIPLE SCLEROSIS

DESCRIPTION: Demyelinating disease resulting in the destruction of CNS myelin and consequent disruption in the transmission of nerve impulses.

1. Onset is insidious with 50% of clients still ambulatory 25 years after diagnosis.
2. Diagnosis determined by combination of data.
   A. Presenting symptoms.
   B. Increased white matter density seen on CT scan.
   C. MRI shows presence of plaques.
   D. CSF electrophoresis showing presence of oligoclonal (IgG) bands.
3. Current thinking is that multiple sclerosis is autoimmune in origin.

> **HESI HINT:** Symptoms involving motor function usually begin in the upper extremities with weakness progressing to spastic paralysis. Bowel and bladder dysfunction occurs in 90% of the cases. MS is more common in women. Progression is not "orderly."

NURSING ASSESSMENT

1. Nursing history of client to include:
   A. History of symptoms.
   B. Progression of illness.
   C. Types of treatment received and the response.
   D. Additional health problems.
   E. Current medications.
   F. Client/family's perception of illness.
   G. Community resources used by the client.
2. Physical assessment to include:
   A. Optic neuritis (loss of vision or blind spots).
   B. Visual or swallowing difficulties.
   C. Gait disturbances; intention tremors.
   D. Unusual fatigue, weakness and clumsiness.
   E. Numbness, particularly on one side of face.
   F. Impaired bladder and bowel control.
   G. Speech disturbances.
   H. Scotomas (white spots in visual field, diplopia).

ANALYSIS (NURSING DIAGNOSES)

1. Impaired physical mobility related to…
2. Sensory/perceptual alterations related to…
3. Fatigue related to…
4. Altered urinary elimination pattern related to…
5. Impaired home management related to…

NURSING PLANS AND INTERVENTIONS

1. Allow hospitalized client to keep own routine.
2. Orient client to environment and teach strategies to maximize vision.
3. Encourage self-care and frequent rest periods.
4. With exercise programs, encourage client to work up to the point just short of fatigue.
5. For muscle spasticity, stretch-hold-relax exercises are helpful as are riding a stationary bicycle and swimming; fall precautions.
6. Initially, work with client on a voiding schedule.
7. As incontinence worsens, the female may need to learn clean self-catheterization; the male may need a condom catheter.
8. Encourage adequate fluid intake, high-fiber foods, and a bowel regime for constipation problems.
9. Encourage the client and the family to verbalize their concerns with ongoing care issues.
10. Encourage client to maintain contact with a support group.
11. Refer client for home healthcare services.
12. Contact the local MS Society for emotional and direct service support.
13. Steroid therapy and chemotherapeutic drugs are administered in acute exacerbations to shorten length of attack.

> **HESI HINT:** Drug therapy for MS clients: ACTH, cortisone, Cytoxan, and other immunosuppressive drugs. Nursing implications for administration of these drugs should focus on prevention of infection.

14. Biologic response modifiers such as Interferon-B products have shown recent success in relapsing MS.

MYASTHENIA GRAVIS

DESCRIPTION: Disorder affecting the neuromuscular transmission of impulses in the voluntary muscles of the body.

1. Considered an autoimmune disease characterized by presence of acetylcholine

receptor antibodies (AChR) which interfere with neuronal transmission.

2. Usually affects females between ages 10 and 40 and males between ages 50 and 70.

NURSING ASSESSMENT

1. Diplopia (double vision), ptosis (eyelid drooping).
2. Mask-like affect: sleepy appearance due to facial muscle involvement.
3. Weakness of laryngeal and pharyngeal muscles: dysphagia, choking, food aspiration, difficulty speaking.
4. Muscle weakness improved by rest, worsened by activity.
5. Advanced cases respiratory failure, bladder and bowel incontinence.
6. Myasthenic crisis (attributed to disease worsening) symptoms associated with under-medication.
7. Cholinergic crisis (attributed to anticholinesterase over dosage): diaphoresis, diarrhea, fasciculations, cramps, marked worsening of symptoms from over-medication.

> **HESI HINT:** In clients with Myasthenia Gravis, be alert for changes in respiratory status – the most severe involvement may result in respiratory failure.

ANALYSIS (NURSING DIAGNOSES)

1. Ineffective airway clearance and breathing pattern related to…
2. Potential for injury related to…
3. Impaired physical mobility related to…
4. Nutrition: potential for less than body requirements related to…

NURSING PLANS AND INTERVENTIONS

1. If hospitalized, have tracheostomy kit available at bedside for possible myasthenic crisis.
2. Teach client the importance of wearing a medic alert bracelet.
3. Administer cholinergic drugs as prescribed. *(See figure 3-41, Treatment of Myasthenia Gravis)*
4. Schedule nursing activities to conserve energy, i.e., complete daily hygiene activities, administration of medications, and treatments **all at once** and allow rest periods. Plan activities during high-energy times, often in the early morning.
5. Instruct client to avoid situations that produce fatigue or physical/emotional stress (any type of stress can exacerbate symptoms).

> **HESI HINT:** Bedrest often relieves symptoms. Bladder and respiratory infections are often a recurring problem. Need for health promotion teaching.

6. Encourage coughing and deep breathing q4 to 6 hours. (Muscle weakness limits ability to cough up secretions, promotes URI).
7. If symptoms worsen, identify type of crisis: myasthenic or cholinergic crisis.

> **HESI HINT:** Myasthenic crisis is associated with a positive edrophonium (Tensilon) test, while a cholinergic crisis is associated with a negative test.

TREATMENT OF MYASTHENIA GRAVIS			
DRUG	**INDICATIONS**	**ADVERSE REACTIONS**	**NURSING IMPLICATIONS**

pyridostigmine bromide (Mestinon)	• Inhibits the action of cholinesterase at the cholinergic nerve endings
	• To promote accumulation of acetylcholine at cholinergic receptor sites
		• Cholinergic crisis can occur with overdose	• Atropine is antidote for drug-induced bradycardia
			• Take drug with milk/food to decrease GI side effects
			• Dosage regulation required; record keeping, re: side effects, drug response
			• Observe for symptoms of cholinergic crisis
			  → Fasciculations
			  → Abdominal cramps, diarrhea, incontinence of stool or urine
			  → Hypotension, bradycardia, respiratory depression
			  → Lacrimation, blurred vision
			• Drug therapy is lifelong and requires family teaching and support

Figure 3-41

PARKINSON'S DISEASE

DESCRIPTION: Disorder affecting movement involving the basal ganglia and substantia nigra.

NURSING ASSESSMENT
1. Rigidity of extremities.
2. Mask-like facial expressions with associated difficulty in chewing, swallowing, and speaking.
3. Drooling.
4. Stooped posture and slow, shuffling gait.
5. Tremors at rest, "pill rolling" movement.
6. Emotional lability.

> **HESI HINT:** NCLEX-RN® questions often focus on the features of Parkinson's disease – tremors (a coarse tremor of fingers and thumb on one hand which disappears during sleep and purposeful activity – also called "pill-rolling"), rigidity, hypertonicity, and stooped posture. Focus: SAFETY!

ANALYSIS (NURSING DIAGNOSES)
1. Self-care deficit related to…
2. Impaired physical mobility related to…
3. Nutrition: potential for less than body requirements related to…
4. Impaired verbal communication related to…
5. Body image disturbances related to…

NURSING PLANS AND INTERVENTIONS
1. Schedule activities later in the day to allow sufficient time for client to perform self-care activities without rushing.
2. Encourage activities and exercise. A cane or walker may be needed.
3. Eliminate environmental noise and encourage the client to speak slowly and clearly, pausing at intervals.
4. Serve soft diet, which is easy to swallow.
5. Administer antiparkinsonian drugs as prescribed. *(See figure 3-42, Antiparkinsonian Drugs)*

> **HESI HINT:** An important aspect of Parkinson's treatment is drug therapy. Since the pathophysiology involves an imbalance between acetylcholines and dopamine, symptoms can be controlled by administering dopamine precursor (Levodopa).

ANTIPARKINSONIAN DRUGS			
DRUGS	**INDICATIONS**	**ADVERSE REACTIONS**	**NURSING IMPLICATIONS**
ANTICHOLINERGICS (parasympatholytics) • **atropine sulfate** (Atropisol) • **benztropine mesylate** (Cogentin)	• Reduce cholinergic activity	• Increased heart rate • Postural hypotension • Dry mouth • Constipation • Urinary retention	• Review client's history for glaucoma, urinary obstruction • Warn to avoid rapid position changes • Avoid extreme heat • Provide gum, hard candy, and frequent mouth care
DOPAMINE AGONISTS • **levodopa** (Dopar) • **levodopa-carbidopa** (Sinemet) **DOPAMINE-RELEASING AGENTS** • **amantadine HCL** (Symmetrel) **DOPAMINE-RECEPTOR AGENTS** • **bromocriptine mesylate** (Parlodel) • **pramipexole** (Mirapol) • **pergolide** (Permax)	• Stimulates dopamine production or increases sensitivity of dopamine receptors • Newer drugs require less dosage	• Involuntary movements • Nausea • Vomiting	• Explain drugs may take months to achieve desired effects • Warn to avoid sudden position changes • Avoid foods high in Vitamin B_6 (meats, liver, i.e., high protein foods) • If insomnia occurs, suggest taking last dose earlier in day • May initially cause drowsiness; teach to avoid driving until response is determined
MONOAMINE OXIDASE TYPE B INHIBITOR • **selegiline** (Eldepryl)	• Used with dopamine agonist when client symptoms do not respond	• Confusion, dizziness • Nausea, dry mouth • Insomnia	• Review drug-drug interaction carefully • Not an option if client on antidepressants (SSRIs or trycyclics)

Figure 3-42

GUILLAIN-BARRÉ SYNDROME

DESCRIPTION: Clinical syndrome of unknown origin involving peripheral and cranial nerves.

1. Usually preceded by a respiratory or gastrointestinal infection 1 to 4 weeks prior to the onset of neurologic deficits.
2. Constant monitoring of these clients is required to prevent the life-threatening problem of acute respiratory failure.
3. Full recovery usually occurs within several months to a year after onset of symptoms.
4. About 10% of those diagnosed with Guillain-Barré Syndrome are left with a residual disability.

NURSING ASSESSMENT

1. Paresthesia (tingling and numbness).
2. Muscle weakness of legs progressing to the upper extremities, trunk, and face.
3. Paralysis of the ocular, facial, and oropharyngeal muscles causing marked difficulty in talking, chewing, and swallowing. Assess for the following:
   A. Breathlessness while talking.
   B. Shallow and irregular breathing.
   C. Use of accessory muscles while breathing.
   D. Any change in respiratory pattern.
   E. Paradoxical inward movement of the upper abdominal wall, while in a supine position, indicating weakness and impending paralysis of the diaphragm.
4. Increasing pulse rate and disturbances in rhythm.
5. Transient hypertension, orthostatic hypotension.
6. Possible pain in the back and in calves of legs.
7. Weakness or paralysis of the intercostal and diaphragm muscles may develop quickly.

ANALYSIS (NURSING DIAGNOSES)

1. Ineffective breathing pattern related to…
2. Altered nutrition less than body requirements related to…
3. Impaired verbal communication related to…

NURSING PLANS AND INTERVENTIONS

1. Monitor for respiratory distress and initiate mechanical ventilation if necessary.
2. See *(Nursing Plans and Interventions for the Unconscious/Immobilized Client.)*

STROKE: CEREBRAL VASCULAR ACCIDENT (CVA)

DESCRIPTION: Sudden loss of brain function resulting from a disruption of the blood supply to a part of the brain. Classified as thrombotic or hemorrhagic.

> **HESI HINT:** CNS involvement related to cause of CVA:
> - **Hemorrhagic** – caused by a slow or fast hemorrhage into the brain tissue – often related to hypertension.
> - **Embolytic** – caused by a clot, which has broken away from some vessel and has lodged in one of the arteries of the brain, blocking the blood supply. It is often related to atherosclerosis (may happen again).

1. Risk factors include the following:
   A. Hypertension.
   B. Previous Transient Ischemic Attacks (TIAs).
   C. Cardiac disease: atherosclerosis, valve disease, history of arrhythmias (particularly atrial flutter/fibrillation).
   D. Advanced age.
   E. Diabetes.
   F. Oral contraceptives.
   G. Smoking

> **HESI HINT:** Atrial flutter/fibrillation has a high incidence of thrombus formation following arrhythmia due to turbulence of blood flow through all valves/heart chambers.

2. Diagnosis is made by observation of clinical signs and confirmed by:
   A. Cranial computed tomography (CT scan).
   B. Magnetic resonance imaging (MRI).
   C. Doppler flow studies.
   D. Ultrasound imaging.
3. Presenting symptoms will relate to the specific area of the brain that has been damaged. *(See figure 3-43, Location of Disruption)*
4. Generally there is:
   A. Motor loss, usually exhibited as hemiparesis or hemiplegia.
   B. Communication loss exhibited as dysarthria, dysphasia, aphasia, or apraxia.
   C. Perceptual disturbance that can be visual, spatial, and/or sensory.
   D. Impaired mental acuity or psychological changes such as decreased attention span, memory loss, depression, lability, and hostility.
5. Bladder dysfunction, which may be either incontinence or retention.

6. Rehabilitation is begun as soon as the client is stable.

NURSING ASSESSMENT

1. Change in level of consciousness.
2. Paresthesia, paralysis.
3. Aphasia, agraphia.
4. Memory loss.
5. Vision impairment.
6. Bladder and bowel dysfunction.
7. Behavioral changes.
8. Assess client's functional abilities including:
    A. Mobility.
    B. Activities of daily living (ADL).
    C. Elimination.
    D. Communication.
9. Assess ability to swallow, eat, and drink without aspiration.

ANALYSIS (NURSING DIAGNOSES)

1. Impaired mobility related to…
2. Self-care deficit related to…
3. Altered pattern of urinary elimination related to…
4. Impaired communication related to…
5. Ineffective family/individual coping related to…
6. Body image disturbances related to…

LOCATION OF DISRUPTION		
FEATURE	**LEFT HEMISPHERE**	**RIGHT HEMISPHERE**
LANGUAGE	• Aphasia • Agraphia	• May be alert and oriented
MEMORY	• No deficit	• Disoriented • Cannot recognize faces
VISION	• Unable to discriminate words and letters • Reading problems • Deficits in right visual field	• Visual/spatial deficits • Neglect of left visual fields • Loss of depth perception
BEHAVIOR	• Slow • Cautious • Anxious when attempting a new task • Depression or catastrophic response to illness • Sense of guilt • Feeling of worthlessness • Worries over future • Quick anger and frustration	• Impulsive • Unaware of neurologic deficits • Confabulates • Euphoric • Constantly smiles • Denies illness • Poor judgment • Overestimates abilities • Impaired sense of humor
HEARING	• No deficit	• Loses ability to hear tonal variations

Figure 3-43

1. Control hypertension to help prevent future CVA.
2. Maintain proper body alignment while in bed. Use splints or other assistive devices (including bed rolls and pillows) to maintain functional position.
3. Position client to minimize edema, prevent contractures and maintain skin integrity.
4. Perform full ROM qid. Follow up with program initiated by other team members.
5. Encourage client to participate in or manage own personal care.
6. Set realistic goals; add new tasks daily.
7. Appropriate self-care activities for the hemiparetic person include:
   A. Bathing.
   B. Brushing teeth.
   C. Shaving with electric razor.
   D. Eating.
   E. Combing hair.
8. Encourage client to assist with dressing activities and modify them as necessary (client will wear street clothes during waking hours).
9. Analyze bladder elimination pattern.
   A. Offer bedpan or urinal according to client's particular pattern of elimination.
   B. Reassure client that bladder control tends to be regained quickly.
10. Follow up speech program initiated by the speech/language therapist.
    A. Ensure consistency with this program.
    B. Reassure the client that regaining speech is a very slow process.
11. Do not sensory overload client, i.e., give only one set of instructions at a time.
12. Encourage total family involvement in rehabilitation.
13. Encourage client/family to join a support group.
14. Encourage family members to allow the client to perform self-care activities as outlined by the rehabilitation team.
15. Refer for outpatient follow-up or for home healthcare.
16. Swallowing modifications may include: pureed/soft diet, thickened liquids, and head positioning.

> **HESI HINT:** Steroids are administered after a stroke to decrease cerebral edema and retard permanent disability. H_2 inhibitors are administered to prevent peptic ulcers.

REVIEW QUESTIONS
NEUROSENSORY/NEUROLOGICAL SYSTEMS

1. What are the classifications of the commonly prescribed eye drops for glaucoma?
2. Identify two types of hearing loss.
3. Write four nursing interventions for the care of the blind person and four nursing interventions for the care of the deaf person.
4. In your own words describe the Glasgow Coma Scale.
5. List four nursing diagnoses for the comatose client in order of priority. (Remember Maslow's Hierarchy of Needs to help you determine priority).
6. State four independent nursing interventions to maintain adequate respirations, airway, and oxygenation in the unconscious client.
7. Who is at risk for cerebral vascular accidents?
8. Complications of immobility include the potential for thrombus development. State three nursing interventions to prevent thrombi.
9. List four rationales for the appearance of restlessness in the unconscious client.
10. What nursing interventions prevent corneal drying in a comatose client?
11. When can a comatose client on IV hyperalimentation begin to receive tube feedings instead?
12. What is the most important principle in a bowel management program for a neurologic client?
13. Define cerebral vascular accident.
14. A client with a diagnosis of CVA presents with symptoms of aphasia, right hemiparesis, but no memory or hearing deficit. In what hemisphere has the client suffered a lesion?
15. What are the symptoms of spinal shock?
16. What are the symptoms of autonomic dysreflexia?
17. What is the most important indicator of increased ICP?
18. What vital sign changes are indicative of increased ICP?
19. A neighbor calls the neighborhood nurse stating that he was knocked hard to the floor by his very hyperactive dog. He is wondering what symptoms would indicate the need to visit an emergency room. What should the nurse tell him to do?
20. What activities and situations should be avoided that increase ICP?
21. How do Hyperosmotic agents (osmotic diuretics) used to treat intracranial pressure act?

MEDICAL SURGICAL NURSING

22. **Why should narcotics be avoided in clients with neurologic impairment?**
23. **Headache and vomiting are symptoms of many disorders. What characteristics of these symptoms would alert the nurse to refer a client to a neurologist?**
24. **How should the head of the bed be positioned for post-craniotomy clients with infratentorial lesions?**
25. **Is multiple sclerosis thought to occur because of an autoimmune process?**
26. **Is paralysis always a consequence of spinal cord injury?**
27. **What types of drugs are used in the treatment of myasthenia gravis?**

ANSWERS TO REVIEW QUESTIONS

1. Parasympathominetics for pupillary constriction, Beta-adrenergic receptor-blocking agents to inhibit formation of aqueous humor, carbonic anhydrase inhibitors to reduce aqueous humor production, and prostaglandin agonists to increase aqueous humor outflow.
2. Conductive (transmission of sound to inner ear is blocked) and sensorineural (damage to eighth cranial nerve).
3. **Care of blind**: announce presence clearly, call by name, orient carefully to surroundings, guide by walking in front of client with his/her hand in your elbow. **Care of deaf**: reduce distraction before beginning conversation, look and listen to client, give client full attention if they are a lip reader, face client directly.
4. An objective assessment of the level of consciousness based on a score of 3 to 15, with scores of 7 or less indicative of coma.
5. Ineffective breathing pattern, ineffective airway clearance, impaired gas exchange, and decreased cardiac output.
6. Position for maximum ventilation (prone or semi-prone and slightly to one side), insert airway if tongue obstructing; suction airway efficiently, monitor arterial pO_2 and pCO_2 and hyperventilate with 100% oxygen before suctioning.
7. Persons with history of hypertension, previous TIAs, cardiac disease (atrial flutter/fibrillation), diabetes, oral contraceptive use, and the elderly.
8. Frequent range of motion exercises, frequent (q2 hours) position changes, and avoidance of positions which decrease venous return.
9. Anoxia, distended bladder, covert bleeding, or a return to consciousness.
10. Irrigation of eyes PRN with sterile prescribed solution, application of ophthalmic ointment q8 hours, close assessment for corneal ulceration/drying.
11. When peristalsis resumes as evidenced by active bowel sounds, passage of flatus or bowel movement.
12. Establishment of REGULARITY.
13. A disruption of blood supply to a part of the brain, which results in sudden loss of brain function.
14. Left.
15. Hypotension, bladder and bowel distension, total paralysis, lack of sensation below lesion.
16. Hypertension, bladder and bowel distention, exaggerated autonomic responses, headache, sweating, goose bumps, and bradycardia.
17. A change in the level of responsiveness.
18. Increased BP, widening pulse pressure, increased or decreased pulse, respiratory irregularities and temperature increase.
19. Call his physician now and inform him/her of the fall. Symptoms needing medical attention would include vertigo, confusion or any subtle behavioral change, headache, vomiting, ataxia (imbalance), or seizure.
20. Change in bed position, extreme hip flexion, endotracheal suctioning, compression of jugular veins, coughing, vomiting, or straining of any kind.
21. Dehydrate the brain and reduce cerebral edema by holding water in the renal tubules to prevent reabsorption, and by drawing fluid from the extravascular spaces into the plasma.
22. Narcotics mask the level of responsiveness as well as pupillary response.
23. Headache which is more severe upon awakening and vomiting not associated with nausea are symptoms of a brain tumor.
24. Supratentorial – elevated; Infratentorial - flat.
25. Yes.
26. No.
27. Anticholinesterase drugs, which inhibit the action of cholinesterase at the nerve endings to promote the accumulation of acetylcholine at receptor sites, which should improve neuronal transmission to muscles.

MEDICAL SURGICAL NURSING

HEMATOLOGY/ONCOLOGY

ANEMIA

DESCRIPTION: Deficiency of erythrocytes (RBCs) reflected as decreased hematocrit (Hct), hemoglobin (Hgb), and RBCs.

NURSING ASSESSMENT

1. Pallor, especially of the ears and nail beds; palmar crease; conjunctiva.
2. Fatigue, exercise intolerance, lethargy, orthostatic hypotension.
3. Tachycardia, heart murmurs, heart failure.
4. Signs of bleeding such as hematuria, melena, menorrhagia.
5. Dyspnea.
6. Irritability, difficulty concentrating.
7. Cool skin, cold intolerance.
8. Risk factors:
   A. Diet lacking in iron, folate, and/or vitamin B_{12}.
   B. Family history of genetic diseases such as sickle cell or congenital hemolytic anemia.
   C. Medication history of anemia-producing drugs such as salicylates, and thiazide diuretics.
   D. Exposure to toxic agents such as lead or insecticides.
9. Diagnostic tests indicate abnormally low results.
   A. Hgb below 10 g/dl.
   B. Hct below 36 percent.
   C. RBCs below $4.0 \times 10^{12.}$
   D. Bone marrow aspiration positive for anemia.
   E. Blood loss either acute or chronic.
   F. Medical history of kidney disorders.
10. Blood loss either acute or chronic
11. Medical history of kidney disorders.

HESI HINT: Physical symptoms occur as a compensatory mechanism when the body is trying to make up for a deficit somewhere in the system. For instance, cardiac output increases when hemoglobin levels drop below 7 g/dl.

ANALYSIS (NURSING DIAGNOSES)

1. Activity intolerance related to…
2. Anxiety related to…
3. Altered tissue perfusion related to…

NURSING PLANS AND INTERVENTIONS

1. Administer blood products as prescribed. *(See Advanced Clinical Concepts, figure 2-6, Administration of Blood Products)*

2. Alternate periods of activity with periods of rest.
3. Diet teaching to include the following:
   A. Instruct in food selection and preparation to maximize intake.
      1) Iron (red meats, organ meats, whole wheat products, spinach, carrots).
      2) Folic acid (green vegetables, liver, citrus fruits).
      3) Vitamin B_{12} (glandular meats, yeast, green leafy vegetables, milk, and cheese).
   B. Instruct in need for vitamin supplements.
      1) Give iron preparations with meals to decrease gastric irritation.
      2) Administer B_{12} and folic acid orally EXCEPT to clients with pernicious anemia who should receive B_{12} parenterally.
4. If parenteral iron is required, use Z-track method for administration to prevent staining of the skin. *(See figure 3-44, Administration of Iron)*
5. Provide genetic information if client has sickle cell or congenital hemolytic anemia.
6. Sickle cell crisis is precipitated by hypoxia.
   A. Provide pain relief.
   B. Provide adequate hydration.
   C. Teach client to avoid activities that cause hypoxia.
7. Teach the client to report any unusual bleeding to healthcare professional.

ADMINISTRATION OF IRON	
DOS	**DON'TS**
• Use Z-track method of administration. • Use air bubble to avoid withdrawing medication into subcutaneous tissue.	• Do NOT use deltoid muscle. • Do NOT massage injection site.

Figure 3-44

HESI HINT: ONLY use normal saline to flush IV tubing or to run with blood. NEVER add medications to blood products. TWO registered nurses should simultaneously check the physician's prescription, client's identity, and blood bag label.

LEUKEMIA

DESCRIPTION: Malignant neoplasm of the blood-forming organs. *(See figure 3-45, Types of Leukemia)*

1. Leukemia is characterized by an abnormal overproduction of immature forms of any of the leukocytes. There is an interference with normal blood production resulting in decreased erythrocytes and decreased platelets.
   A. Anemia results from decreased RBC production and blood loss.
   B. Immunosuppression occurs because of the large number of IMMATURE white blood cells or profound neutropenia.
   C. Hemorrhage occurs because of thrombocytopenia.
   D. Leukemic invasion of other organ systems occurs such as the liver, spleen, lymph nodes, kidneys, lungs, and brain.
2. Exact etiology of leukemia is unknown but identified precipitating factors include the following:
   A. Genetic abnormalities.
   B. Ionizing radiation (therapeutic or atomic).

   C. Viral infections (human T cells, leukemia virus).
   D. Exposure to certain chemicals or drugs: *(See figure 3-48, Administration of Antineoplastic Chemotherapeutic Agents)*
      1) Benzene.
      2) Alkylating chemotherapeutic agents.
      3) Immunosuppressants.
      4) Chloramphenicol.
      5) Phenylbutazone.
3. Incidence is highest in children 3 to 4 years of age; declines until age 35, then a steady increase occurs.
4. Diagnosis of leukemia is made by biopsy, bone marrow aspiration, lumbar puncture, and frequent blood counts.
5. Leukemia is treated with antineoplastics chemotherapy. *(See figure 3-49, Antineoplastic Chemotherapeutic Agents)*

TYPES OF LEUKEMIA
ACUTE MYELOGENOUS LEUKEMIA
• Inability of leukocytes to mature; those that do are abnormal. • Occurs throughout the life cycle. • Onset is insidious. • Prognosis is poor, 5 year survival of 20%, overall, 50 % for children. • Cause of death tends to be overwhelming infection.
CHRONIC MYELOGENOUS LEUKEMIA

• Results from abnormal production of granulocytic cells.
• Is a bi-phasic disease.
• Chronic stage lasts approximately three years.
• Acute phase tends to last 2 to 3 months.
• Occurs in young to middle age adults.
• Known causes include:
  → Ionizing radiation.
  → Chemical exposure.
• Poor prognosis, 5 year survival rate of 37%.
• Treatment is conservative with oral antineoplastic agents:
  → hydrosyurea (Hydrea: inhibitor or DNA synthesis).
  → interferon (mechanism of action not known.
  → STI-571 (Imatinib or Gleevec) - BCR-ABL-selective inhibitor.

ACUTE LYMPHOCYTIC LEUKEMIA
• Abnormal leukocytes in blood-forming tissue. • Occurs in children (most common childhood cancer). • Favorable prognosis, 80% of children treated live 5 years or longer.
CHRONIC LYMPHOCYTIC LEUKEMIA
• Increased production of leukocytes and lymphocytes and proliferation of cells within the bone marrow, spleen, and liver. • Occurs after the age of 35, often in the elderly. • 5 year survival rate of 73% overall. • Most clients are asymptomatic and are not treated.

Figure 3-45

HESI HINT: A 24-year-old is admitted with large areas of ecchymosis on both upper and lower extremities. She is diagnosed with acute myleogenous leukemia. What are the expected laboratory findings for this client and what is the expected treatment?
Lab: Decreased Hgb, decreased Hct, decreased platelet count, altered WBC (usually quite high).
Treatment: Prevention of infection; prevention and/or control of bleeding; high-protein, high-calorie diet; assistance with ADL; drug therapy.

NURSING ASSESSMENT
1. Tendency to bleed.
   A. Petechiae.
   B. Nosebleeds.
   C. Bleeding gums.
   D. Ecchymosis.
   E. Non-healing skin abrasions.
2. Anemia.
   A. Fatigue.
   B. Pallor.
   C. Headache.
   D. Bone and joint pain.
   E. Hepatosplenomegaly.
3. Infection.
   A. Fever.
   B. Tachycardia.
   C. Lymphadenopathy (swollen lymph nodes).
   D. Night sweats.

E. Skin infection, poor healing.
4. GI distress.
   A. Anorexia.
   B. Weight loss.
   C. Sore throat.
   D. Abdominal pain.
   E. Diarrhea.
   F. Oral lesions, typically thrush.

ANALYSIS (NURSING DIAGNOSES)
1. Potential for infection related to…
2. Potential for injury: bleeding related to…
3. Fatigue related to…
4. Anxiety related to…

NURSING PLANS AND INTERVENTIONS
IMMUNOSUPPRESSED CLIENTS AND/OR CLIENTS
WITH BONE MARROW SUPPRESSION
1. Monitor WBC count daily and inform physician of count.
2. Routinely assess oral cavity and genital area for signs of infection.
3. Monitor vital signs frequently:
   A. Note baseline.
   B. Report fever to physician as requested.
      1) Parameters for reporting tend to be lower than those of postoperative clients.
      2) Usually report temperature elevations of 100.5°F.
4. Administer antibiotics as prescribed maintaining a strict schedule.
5. Notify physician if delay in administration occurs.
   A. Obtain trough and peak blood levels of antibiotics.
      1) Trough: draw blood sample shortly **BEFORE** administration of antibiotic.
      2) Peak: draw blood sample 30 minutes to 1 hour **AFTER**.administration of drug.
   B. Monitor blood levels of antibiotics for therapeutic dose range.
6. Teach client and family the importance of infection control.
   A. **WASH HANDS** using good handwashing technique.
   B. Avoid contact with any infected person.
   C. Avoid crowds.
   D. Maintain daily hygiene to prevent spread of microorganisms.
   E. Avoid eating uncooked foods as they contain bacteria.
   F. Avoid water standing in cups, vases, etc., as these are an excellent source of growth for microorganisms.
7. Institute an oral hygiene regime.
   A. Use soft-bristle toothbrush to avoid bleeding.
   B. Use salt and soda mouth rinse.
   C. Perform oral hygiene after each meal and at bedtime.
   D. Lubricate lips with water-soluble gel.
   E. Avoid lemon-glycerine swabs; they dry oral mucosa.
8. Encourage coughing and deep breathing to prevent stasis of secretions in lungs.
9. Avoid rectal thermometers and suppositories to prevent further bleeding.
10. Monitor fluid status and balance; febrile clients dehydrate rapidly.
    A. Monitor I&O.
    B. Encourage fluid intake of at least 3 liters/day.
11. Encourage mobility to decrease pulmonary stasis.
12. Provide care for invasive catheters and lines. *(See figure 3-47, Care of Intravenous Lines and Catheters)*
    A. Use **strict aseptic** technique for all invasive procedures.

    B. Change dressings 2 to 3 times/week and/or when soiled.
    C. Use catheter line for piggybacking medication depending on the purpose of the line and the fluid

being infused, i.e., NO medications can be piggybacked with an infusion of chemotherapeutic agents.

    D.   Lines can often be used for collecting blood samples thereby avoiding "sticking" the client.

13. Protect the client from bleeding and injury.

    A.   Handle the client gently.

    B.   Avoid needle sticks. Use smallest gauge needle possible, and apply pressure for 10 minutes after needle sticks.

    C.   Encourage use of electric razor only for shaving.

    D.   Instruct client to avoid blowing or picking nose.

    E.   Assess for signs of bleeding.

    F.   Avoid use of salicylates.

HODGKIN'S DISEASE

DESCRIPTION: Malignancy of the lymphoid system.

1. Hodgkin's disease is characterized by a generalized painless lymphadenopathy.
2. Incidence is higher in males and young adults.
3. Etiology is unknown.
4. Prognosis is good: 5-year survival rate of 90%, however, late recurrences after 5 to 10 years are not uncommon.
5. Diagnosis is made by excision of node for biopsy; characteristic cell called Reed-Sternberg.
6. Determination of stage of disease is done by surgical laparotomy. *(See figure 3-46, Four Stages of Hodgkin's Disease)*
7. Treatment:

    A.   Radiotherapy.

    B.   Chemotherapy: nitrogen mustard, Adriamycin, vincristine, Prednisone.

    C.   Splenectomy.

NURSING ASSESSMENT
1. Enlarged lymph nodes (one or more).
2. Anemia, thrombocytopenia, elevated leukocytes, decreased platelets.
3. Fever, increased susceptibility to infections.
4. Anorexia, weight loss.
5. Malaise, bone pain.
6. Night sweats.

ANALYSIS (NURSING DIAGNOSES)
1. Potential for infection related to…
2. Anxiety related to…
3. Altered nutrition: less than body requirements related to…
4. Altered tissue perfusion related to…

NURSING PLANS AND INTERVENTIONS
1. Protect from infection, monitor temperature carefully.
2. Observe for signs of anemia.
3. Provide adequate rest.
4. Provide preoperative and postoperative care for laparotomy and/or splenectomy.
5. Encourage high-nutrient foods.
6. Provide emotional support to client and family.

FOUR STAGES OF HODGKIN'S DISEASE

STAGE I	STAGE II	STAGE III	STAGE IV
Involvement of single lymph node region or a single extralymphatic organ or site.	Involvement of two or more lymph nodes on the same side of the diaphragm or localized involvement of an extralymphatic organ or site.	Involvement of lymph node areas on both sides of the diaphragm to localized involvement of one extra-lymphatic organ, the spleen, or both.	Diffuse involvement of one or more extralymphatic organs with or without lymph node involvement.

Figure 3-46

HESI HINT: Hodgkin's is one of the most curable of all adult malignancies. Emotional support is vital. Career development is often interrupted for treatment. Chemotherapy renders many male clients sterile. May bank sperm prior to treatment, if desired.

CARE OF INTRAVENOUS LINES AND CATHETERS	
TYPES OF IVS AND CATHETERS	**USE AND CARE OF IVS AND CATHETERS**
• CVC (Central venous catheter) • Hickman • Broviac • Single lumen • Triple lumen • Port-a-cath (implanted reservoir, must be accessed with a special needle)	• Stay in place for extended periods of time. • Used for clients who require immunosuppressive therapy and/or are receiving long-term IV therapy. • Uses include: 　→ IV hyperalimentation. 　→ IV antineoplastics chemotherapy. 　→ IV antimicrobial. • Exit sites include: 　→ At the upper chest. 　→ Femoral area. 　→ Antecubital area. • In order to prevent an air embolus when a central line is open to air, position client in Trendelenburg position or have client do a Valsalva maneuver, if no slide clamp on line. • Maintain a patent IV site by flushing with heparin or saline. (The amount of heparin used depends on the size of the lumen, length of tubing, if reservoir exists, i.e., portacath). • Immediately after insertion of a central line, the nurse should auscultate breath sounds. • After insertion of a central line, a chest x-ray must be taken to determine correct placement and detect pneumothorax - observe for unequal expansion of chest wall.

Figure 3-47

ADMINISTRATION OF ANTINEOPLASTIC CHEMOTHERAPEUTIC AGENTS
• Follow OSHA guidelines for administration, as well as decontamination of non-disposable areas/equipment, and self. • Obtain complete and detailed instructions about administration (routine knowledge of procedures for IV administration is not sufficient). • These drugs are toxic to cancer cells and normal cells in both the client and caregiver who are infusing the drugs. • Nurses who are pregnant or are considering becoming pregnant should notify supervisor (many agencies discourage or prohibit such caregivers from administering these drugs). • Wear gloves when handling drugs. • Check the drug with another nurse against physician's order and client's record to ensure that it is the correct medication. • If catheter line is used for infusion, verify line placement and patency with another nurse, i.e., and aspirate a blood return. • If a vesicant (caustic) drug is administered peripherally, stay with the client throughout administration and check IV placement and patency frequently by aspirating a blood return. • If peripheral site is used for infusion, use a new site daily. • Dispose of all IV equipment in the specially provided waste receptacle so that personnel handling trash do not come into contact with vesicant drugs.

Figure 3-48

ANTINEOPLASTIC CHEMOTHERAPEUTIC AGENT			
DRUGS	**INDICATIONS**	**ADVERSE REACTIONS**	**NURSING IMPLICATIONS**
ALKYLATING AGENTS • **cyclophosphamide** (Cytoxan, Neosar) • **mechlorethamine** HCL (Nitrogen Mustard) • **cisplatin** (Platinol) • **busulfan** (Myleran) • **procarbazine** (Matulane) • **decarbazine** (Carboximide, Imidazole)	• Hodgkin's • Leukemia • Neuroblastoma • Retinoblastoma • Multiple myeloma	• Bone marrow suppression • Nausea and vomiting • Cystitis • Stomatitis • Alopecia • Gonadal suppression • Toxic effects occur slowly with high dosage • Toxic to kidneys and ears • Pleural effusion • Seizures	• Use immediately after reconstitution • Avoid vapors in eyes • Vesicant, if comes in contact with skin, flush with water • Check placement of infusing system • Hydrate well before and during treatment with IV fluids and mannitol • Monitor renal functioning and watch for signs of cystitis • Force fluids • Monitor hearing & vision
ANTIMETABOLITES • **fluorouracil** (Adrucil, 5-FU) • **methotrexate sodium** (Mexate) REQUIRES LEUCOVORIN RESCUE to prevent toxic effects • **mercaptopurine/6-MP** (Purinethol) • **cytarabine** (Cytosar-U, ARA-C) • **gemcitabine** (Gemzar)	• Acute lymphocytic leukemia • Acute myelocytic leukemia • Brain tumors • Ovarian, breast, prostatic, testicular cancers	• Nausea and vomiting • Diarrhea • Myelosuppression (bone marrow depression) • Proctitis • Stomatitis • Dermatitis • Renal toxicity • Hepatotoxicity • Anaphylaxis	• Administer antiemetics as needed • When outdoors, wear sunscreen • Toxic to liver and kidney, avoid: • Aspirin • Sulfonamide • Tetracycline • Vitamins containing folic acid • Leucovorin used with methotrexate as antidote for high doses, called "Leucovorin Rescue" • Give allopurinol concurrently with 6-MP to inhibit uric acid production from cell destruction; it increases drug's potency • Monitor liver function
ANTITUMOR ANTIBIOTICS • **dactinomycin** (Actinomycin) • **bleomycin sulfate** (Blenoxane) • **daunorubicin HCL** (Cerubidine) • **mitomycin** (Mutamycin) • **doxorubicin HCL** (Adriamycin) • **idarubicia** (Idamycin)	• Sarcoma • Neuroblastoma • Head and neck tumors • Testicular, ovarian, breast cancer • Hodgkins • Lymphocytic leukemia • Acute myelocytic leukemia	• Bone marrow suppression • Anorexia • Nausea and vomiting • Alopecia • Cardiac toxicity • Vesicant	• Monitor placement and patency of infusing system • Monitor for cardiac dysrhythmia • Inform client that urine turns red • Administer antiemetics as needed

Figure 3-49

MEDICAL SURGICAL NURSING

169

ANTINEOPLASTIC CHEMOTHERAPEUTIC AGENTS (CONTINUED)

DRUGS	INDICATIONS	ADVERSE REACTIONS	NURSING IMPLICATIONS
MISCELLANEOUS ANTINEOPLASTICS **hydroxyurea** (Hydrea) **asparaginase** (Elspar)	• Urea-derived antineoplastic against solid tumors & C.M.L. • Anticancer enzyme against A.L.L	• Drowsiness • Renal dysfunction • N/V, diarrhea • Hepatitis • Myesuppression	• Comfort measures for stomatitis, GI discomforts • Monitor for complications • Maintain adequate hydration
PLANT ALKALOIDS • **vincristine sulfate** (Oncovin) • **vinblastine sulfate** (Velban)	• Acute lymphocytic leukemia • Hodgkin's • Wilms' tumor • Sarcoma • Breast cancer • Testicular cancer	• Bone marrow suppression • Neurotoxic • Weakness • Paresthesia • Jaw pain • Constipation • Stomatitis • Alopecia • Headaches • Minimal nausea and vomiting	• Administer antiemetics as needed • Monitor for neurotoxicity • Check placement and patency of infusing system
MITOTIC INHIBITORS • **palitaxel** (Taxol) • **doxetaxel** (Taxotere)	• Breast cancer • Ovarian cancer • Non-small cell lung cancer • Kaposi's sarcoma	• Decreased WBC and RBC • Hairloss • N/V, diarrhea • Joint, muscle pain	• Monitor for signs and syptoms of infection • Administer antiemetics and antidiarrheals as needed
HORMONAL AGENTS **CORTICOSTEROIDS:** • **prednisone** (Cortalone) • **dexamethasone** (Decadron) **MALE SPECIFIC** • **flutsmide** (Eulexin) • **leuprolide** (Lupron) • **goserelin** (Zolodex) **FEMALE SPECIFIC** • **tamoxifen citrate** (Nolvadex) • **megestrol** (Megace) • **medroxyprogesterone** (Provera)	• Leukemia • Hodgkin's • Breast cancer • Lymphoma • Multiple myeloma • Cerebral edema (due to brain metastasis) • Prostate cancers • Testicular cancers • Breast cancer • Prostatic cancer	• *See Endocrine* • H/A, paresthesias, cardiac arrhythmias, N/V hypoglycemia, neuropathies • Hot flashes • Mild nausea	• *See Endocrine* • Bone pain & voiding problems • Safety with neuropathies • Administer antiemetics as needed

Figure 3-49 (continued)

ANTINEOPLASTIC CHEMOTHERAPEUTIC AGENTS (CONTINUED)

DRUGS	INDICATIONS	ADVERSE REACTIONS	NURSING IMPLICATIONS
ANDROGENS • **testosterone** (Oreton) • **fluoxymesterone** (Halotestin)	• Breast cancer (postmenopausal women)	• Fluid retention • Nausea • Masculinization	• Low-salt diet
TOPOISOMERASE-1 INHIBITORS **ironotecan** (Camptosar) **topotecan** (Hycamptin)	• Used after failure of initial treatment of ovarian, small-cell lung, and colorectal cancers	• Myelosuppression • Moderate N/V • Diarrhea	• Camptosar diarrhea treated with Atropine due to physiologic cause • Give antiemetics per protocol
MONOCLONAL ANTIBODIES **trastuzumab** (Hercaptia) **rifuxamab** (Rituxan)	• Targets specific malignant cells with less damage to healthy cells in non Hodgkins lymphoma, breast cancer	• Fever, chills, infection • N/V, diarrhea • Bronchospasm, dyspnea, ARDS • Hypotension • Ventricular dysfunction CHF	• Pre-medicate with antiemetics • Monitor for identified side effects

Figure 3-49 (continued)

BIOLOGIC RESPONSE MODIFIERS

DRUGS	INDICATIONS	ADVERSE REACTIONS	NURSING IMPLICATIONS
ANTIANEMIC • **epoetin** (Procrit, Epogen)	• Anemia from chronic renal failure, chemotherapy, HIV-related treatments	• Seizures • Hypertension • Pain at injection site	• Do not shake vial; may cause inactivation of medication • Monitor Hct levels • Pain at injection site; give slowly SC
GRANULOCYTE-STIMULATING FACTOR • **filgrastim** (Neupogen)	• Improve immune competence by increasing neutophils	• Medullary bone pain during initial treatment • Pain at injection site	• Monitor WBC/differential; absolute neutrophil count (ANC) • Give SC slowly due to local pain at site • Assess bone pain & medicate with analgesics
THROMBOETIC GROWTH FACTOR • **oprellvekin** (Neumega)	• Stimulates production of megakaryocytes and platelets	• Dizziness, H/A, insomnia, blurred vision, nervousness • Pleural effusion • Vasodilation, cardiac arrhythmias • Bone pain, myalgia • GI upsets • Fluid retention	• Give slowly to reduce pain at injection site • Assess for complications related to fluid retention • Start within 6 to 24 hours of chemotherapy start & continued for 10 to 21 days • Monitor CBC: H&H may decrease; monitor platelets

Figure 3-50

171

BIOLOGIC RESPONSE MODIFIERS (CONTINUED)

DRUGS	INDICATIONS	ADVERSE REACTIONS	NURSING IMPLICATIONS
INTERFERON-B PRODUCTS • **interferon B-1a** (Avonex) • **interferon B-1b** (Betaseron)	• Relapsing Multiple Sclerosis • AIDS • Kaposi's sarcoma • Malignant melanoma • Hepatitis C	• Seizures, H/A, weakness, insomnia, depression, suicidal ideation • Hypertension, chest pain, vasodilation, edema, palpitations • Dyspnea • N/V, elevated liver function studies, GI disorders • Myalgia, flu-like symptoms	• Anticipate discomforts from side effects & initiate relief measures early • Notify physician if evidence of depression • Sunscreen & protective clothing needed for photosensitivity • Do not shake or swirl solution; use soon after reconstitution • Monitor CBC & blood chemistries
INTERLEUKINS • **aldesleukin** (Proleukin, Interleukin-2)	• Metastatic renal cell carcinoma	• Respiratory failure; pulmonary edema • CHF, MI, arrhythmias, stroke • Bowel perforation, hepatomegaly, GI disturbances • Serious electrolyte imbalances • Coagulation disorders • Pancytopenia	• Vigilance in monitoring for serious side effects with stat response
INTERFERON-a PRODUCTS • **interferon-a 2a** (Roferon A) • **interfereon-a 2b** (Intron A)	• 2a: Hairy cell leukemia, Kaposi's sarcoma • 2b: Chronic Hepatitis B&C; K. sarcoma; HC leukemia	• Similar to those of Interferon-B products	• Similar to those of Interferon-B products

Figure 3-50 (continued)

ANTIEMETICS

DRUGS	INDICATIONS	ADVERSE REACTIONS	NURSING IMPLICATIONS
• **prochlorperazine** (Compazine) • **promethazine HCL** (Phenergan)	• Nausea and vomiting	• Drowsiness • Dizziness • Extrapyramidal symptoms • Orthostatic hypotension • Blurred vision • Dry mouth	• Dilute oral solution with juice, etc. • Determine baseline BP prior to administration • Give deep IM • Monitor BP carefully
• **metoclopramide HCL** (Reglan) • **haloperidol** (Haldol)	• Nausea and vomiting	• Drowsiness • Restlessness • Fatigue • Extrapyramidal symptoms	• Caution client of decreased alertness • Avoid alcohol • Discontinue if extrapyramidal symptoms occur

Figure 3-51

ANTIEMETICS (CONTINUED)

DRUGS	INDICATIONS	ADVERSE REACTIONS	NURSING IMPLICATIONS
• **diphenhydramine HCL** (Benadryl)	• Given with Reglan and Haldol to reduce extrapyramidal symptoms	• Sedation • Dizziness • Hypotension • Dry mouth	• Same as above
• **ondansetron HCL** (Zofran)	• Prevention of nausea and vomiting associated with cancer • Postoperative nausea and vomiting	• Headache often requiring analgesic for relief	• Administer tablets 30 minutes prior to chemotherapy and 1 to 2 hours prior to radiation therapy • Dilute IV injection in 50 ml of 5% dextrose or 0.9% NaCl
• **granisetron** (Kytril)	• Nausea & vomiting associated with chemotherapy & abdominal radiation	• Hypertension • CNS stimulation • Elevated liver enzymes	• Assess for extrapyramidal symptoms • Monitor liver enzymes • Give only on day of chemotherapy or radiation treatment and 1 hour before

Figure 3-51 (continued)

GENERAL ONCOLOGY CONTENT

ONCOLOGY TERMS

- **CANCER**: Disease characterized by uncontrolled growth of abnormal cells
- **NEOPLASM**: New formation
- **CARCINOMA**: Malignant tumor arising from epithelial tissue
- **SARCOMA**: Malignant tumor arising from nonepithelial tissue
- **DIFFERENTIATION**: Degree to which neoplastic tissue is different from parent tissue
- **METASTASIS**: Spread of cancer from the original site to other parts of the body
- **ADJUVANT THERAPY**: Supplemental therapy to the primary therapy
- **PALLIATIVE PROCEDURE**: Relieves symptoms without curing the cause

TUMORS IDENTIFIED BY TISSUE OF ORIGIN

Adeno	Glandular tissue
Angio	Blood vessels
Basal cell	Epithelium (sun-exposed areas)
Embryonal	Gonads
Fibro	Fibrous tissue
Lympho	Lymphoid tissue
Melano	Pigmented cells of epithelium
Myo	Muscle tissue
Osteo	Bone
Squamous Cell	Epithelium

Figure 3-52

SEVEN WARNING SIGNS OF CANCER
1. Change in usual bowel and bladder function
2. A sore that does not heal
3. Unusual bleeding or discharge, hematuria, tarry stools, ecchymosis, bleeding mole
4. Thickening or a lump in the breast or elsewhere
5. Indigestion or dysphagia
6. Obvious changes in a wart or mole
7. Nagging cough or hoarseness

Figure 3-53

REVIEW QUESTIONS

HEMATOLOGY/ONCOLOGY

1. **List three potential causes of anemia.**
2. **Write two nursing diagnoses for the client suffering from anemia.**
3. **What is the only intravenous fluid compatible with blood products?**
4. **What actions should the nurse take if a hemolytic transfusion reaction occurs?**
5. **List three interventions for clients with a tendency to bleed.**
6. **Identify two sites, which should be assessed for infection in immunosuppressed clients.**
7. **Name three food sources of vitamin B_{12}.**
8. **Describe care of invasive catheters and lines.**
9. **List three safety precautions for the administration of antineoplastic chemotherapy.**
10. **Describe the use of Leucovorin.**
11. **Describe the method of collecting the trough and peak blood levels of antibiotics.**
12. **What is the characteristic cell found in Hodgkin's disease?**
13. **List four nursing interventions for care of the client with Hodgkin's disease.**
14. **List four topics you would cover when teaching an immunosuppressed client about infection control.**

ANSWERS TO REVIEW QUESTIONS

1. Diet lacking in iron, folate and/or vitamin B_{12}; use of salicylates, thiazides, diuretics; exposure to toxic agents such as lead or insecticides.
2. Activity intolerance and altered tissue perfusion.
3. Normal saline.
4. Turn off transfusion. Take temperature. Send blood being transfused to lab. Obtain urine sample. Keep vein patent with normal saline.
5. Use a soft toothbrush, avoid salicylates, do not use suppositories.
6. Oral cavity and genital area.
7. Glandular meats (liver), milk, green leafy vegetables.
8. Use strict aseptic technique. Change dressings 2 to 3 times/week or when soiled. Use caution when piggybacking drugs; check purpose of line and drug to be infused. Use lines for obtaining blood samples to avoid "sticking" client when possible.
9. Double check order with another nurse. Check for blood return prior to administration to ensure that medication does not go into tissue. Use a new IV site daily for peripheral chemotherapy. Wear gloves when handling the drugs, and dispose of waste in special containers to avoid contact with toxic substances.
10. Leucovorin is used as an antidote with methotrexate to prevent toxic reactions.
11. Collection of trough: draw blood 30 minutes prior to administration of antibiotic. Collection of peak: draw blood 30 minutes after administration of antibiotic.
12. Reed-Sternberg.
13. Protect from infection. Observe for anemia. Encourage high-nutrient foods. Provide emotional support to client and family.
14. Handwashing technique. Avoid infected persons. Avoid crowds. Maintain daily hygiene to prevent spread of microorganisms.

REPRODUCTIVE SYSTEM

BENIGN TUMORS OF THE UTERUS: LEIOMYOMAS (FIBROIDS, MYOMAS, FIBROMYOMAS, FIBROMAS)
DESCRIPTION: Benign tumors arising from the muscle tissue of the uterus.

1. Benign tumors are more common in black women than white women.
2. Benign tumors are more common in women who have never been pregnant.
3. Most common symptom is abnormal uterine bleeding.
4. Tend to disappear after menopause.
5. Rarely become malignant.
6. Intervention for severe symptoms is hysterectomy.
   A. Vaginal hysterectomy.
   B. Abdominal hysterectomy.

NURSING ASSESSMENT

1. Menorrhagia (hypermenorrhea: profuse or prolonged menstrual bleeding).
2. Dysmenorrhea (extremely painful menstrual periods).
3. Uterine enlargement.
4. Low back pain and pelvic pain.

> **HESI HINT:** Menorrhagia (profuse or prolonged menstrual bleeding) is the most important factor relating to benign uterine tumors. Assess for signs of anemia.

UTERINE PROLAPSE, CYSTOCELE, AND RECTOCELE

DESCRIPTION: Uterine prolapse is downward displacement of the uterus. Cystocele is the relaxation of the anterior vaginal wall with prolapse of the bladder. Rectocele is the relaxation of the posterior vaginal wall with prolapse of the rectum.

1. Preventive measures:
   A. Postpartum perineal exercises.
   B. Spaced pregnancies.
   C. Weight control.
2. Surgical intervention:
   A. Hysterectomy.
   B. Anterior and posterior vaginal repair (A&P repair).
3. Nonsurgical Intervention (for uterine prolapse):
   A. Kegel exercises
   B. Knee-chest position
   C. Pessary use

> **HESI HINT:** What is the anatomical significance of a prolapsed uterus? When the uterus is displaced, it impinges on other structures in the lower abdomen. The bladder, rectum, and small intestine can protrude through the vaginal wall.

NURSING ASSESSMENT

1. Predisposing conditions:

   A. Multiparity.
   B. Pelvic tearing during childbirth.
   C. Vaginal muscle weakness associated with aging.
   D. Obesity.
2. Symptoms associated with uterine prolapse:
   A. Dysmenorrhea.
   B. Dragging sensation in pelvis and back.
   C. Dyspareunia
3. Symptoms associated with cystocele:
   A. Incontinence, or stress incontinence (dribbling with coughing or sneezing or any activity that increases intra-abdominal pressure).
   B. Urinary retention.
   C. Bladder infections (cystitis).
4. Symptoms associated with rectocele:
   A. Constipation.
   B. Hemorrhoids.
   C. Sense of pressure or need to defecate.

ANALYSIS (NURSING DIAGNOSES)

1. Pain related to…
2. Knowledge deficit related to…
3. Alteration in self-concept related to…

NURSING PLANS AND INTERVENTIONS
HYSTERECTOMY

1. Provide pre- and postoperative care. *(See Advanced Clinical Concepts: Perioperative Care)*
2. Administer enema and douche as prescribed pre-op.
3. Note amount and character of vaginal discharge. Postoperatively, there should be less than one saturated pad in 4 hours.
4. Avoid rectal thermometers or tubes, especially when A&P repair has been performed.
5. Check extremities for warmth and/or tenderness as indicators of thrombophlebitis.
6. Pain management postoperatively:
   A. Assess character of pain and determine appropriate analgesic.
   B. Administer analgesics as needed and determine effectiveness.
7. Encourage ambulation as soon as possible.
8. Monitor urinary output (Foley catheter is usually inserted in surgery).
9. After catheter removal, assess voiding patterns, catheterize q6 to 8 hours if unable to void.
10. Observe incision for bleeding.
11. Note abdominal distention may be a sign of gas (flatus) or internal bleeding.
12. Gradually increase diet from liquids to

general.

13. Provide stool softeners prior to first bowel movement and thereafter as needed.
14. Instruct client in follow-up care:
    A. Limit tampon use.
    B. Avoid douching.
    C. Refrain from intercourse until approved by physician (usually 3 to 6 weeks).
    D. Avoid heavy lifting (6 to 8 lbs) or heavy housework for 4 to 6 weeks postoperatively.
15. Maintain adequate fluid intake (3 liters/day).
16. Notify physician of complications.
    A. Elevated temperature above 101°F.
    B. Redness, pain, or swelling of suture line.
17. Encourage verbalization of feelings, especially with significant other.

CANCER OF THE CERVIX

DESCRIPTION: Of cancers occurring in the cervix, 95% are squamous cell in origin.
1. Cancer of the cervix is easily detected early with the Papanicolaou test.
2. The precursor to cancer of the cervix is dysplasia.
3. Cancer of the cervix is subdivided into three stages.
    A. Early dysplasia can be treated in a variety of ways including:
       1) Cryosurgery.
       2) Electrocautery.
       3) Laser.
       4) Conization.
       5) Hysterectomy.

> **HESI HINT:** Laser therapy or cryosurgery is used to treat cervical cancer when the lesion is small and localized. Invasive cancer is treated with radiation, conization, hysterectomy, or pelvic exenteration (a drastic surgical procedure where the uterus, ovaries, fallopian tubes, vagina, rectum, and bladder are removed in an attempt to stop metastasis). Chemotherapy is not useful with this type of cancer.

    B. Early carcinoma can be treated with:
       1) Hysterectomy.
       2) Intracavity radiation.
    C. Late carcinoma (the tumor size and stage of invasion of surrounding tissues

increases), treatment often includes:
       1) External beam radiation along with hysterectomy.
       2) Antineoplastic chemotherapy is of limited use for cancers arising from squamous cells.
       3) Pelvic exenteration.

> **HESI HINT:** New American College of Obstetricians and Gynecologists recommentations (2003): Pap smears should begin within 3 years of having intercourse or no later than age 21, whichever comes first. Should be done annually until age 30 and then may be done every 2 to 3 years if a woman has 3 consecutive normal results. After age 70 may stop if woman has 3 consecutive normal and no abnormal pap smears in last 10 years. Women at high risk should have annual screenings.

CARE OF THE CLIENT WITH RADIATION IMPLANTS

1. Radiation implants are used to treat disease by delivering high-dose radiation directly to the affected tissue.
2. The nurse must take certain precautions for protection of self as well as the client and visitors.
3. Follow specific guidelines provided by the agency. General care guidelines provided by the agency. General care guidelines include:
    A. Remind the client that she is not radioactive; only the implants contain radioactivity.
    B. Remind the client that her isolation time is limited; isolation is not necessary indefinitely.
4. Assign to a private room and place a "Caution: Radioactive Material" sign on the door.
5. Do not permit pregnant caretakers or pregnant visitors into the room.
6. Discourage visits by small children.
7. Keep a lead-lined container in the room for disposal of the implant should it become dislodged.
8. Client should remain in bed with as little movement as possible.
9. Be aware that ALL client secretions have the potential of being radioactive.
10. Wear latex gloves when handling potentially contaminated secretions. (Remember Universal Precautions!!)

11. Wear a radiation badge when providing care to clients with radiation implants.
    A. Badge is not to be worn out of doors.
    B. Badge is checked at regular intervals by health officials.
12. Provide nursing care in an efficient but caring manner.
    A. Plan care to limit overall time in the client's room.
    B. When in the room, stand at the greatest distances away from the client to minimize exposure.
    C. Stop by to check on the client from the door frequently.
13. Keep all supplies and equipment the client might need within reach.

OVARIAN CANCER

DESCRIPTION: Cancer of the ovaries can occur at all ages including infancy and childhood. Early diagnosis is difficult because no useful screening test exists at present.

NURSING ASSESSMENT
1. Asymptomatic in early stages.
2. Laparotomy is primary tool for diagnosis and staging of the disease - ovarian cancer is surgically staged, rather than clinically staged.
3. Advanced clinical manifestations include:
    A. Pelvic discomfort.
    B. Low back pain.
    C. Weight change.
    D. Abdominal pain.
    E. Nausea and vomiting.
    F. Constipation.
    G. Urinary frequency.

HESI HINT: Ovarian cancer is the leading cause of death from gynecologic cancers in the U.S. Growth is insidious, so it is not recognized until it is at an advanced stage.

ANALYSIS (NURSING DIAGNOSES)
1. Anticipatory grieving related to…
2. Pain related to…
3. Self-care deficit related to…

NURSING PLANS AND INTERVENTIONS
1. Care required for any major abdominal surgery following laparotomy.
2. Teach client and family about disease and follow-up treatment.
3. Offer supportive care to client and family throughout diagnosis and treatment.

HESI HINT: The major emphasis in nursing management of cancers of the reproductive tract is early detection.

BREAST CANCER

DESCRIPTION: Cancer originating in the breast.
1. Breast cancer is the leading cancer in women in the United States.
2. One in eight women will develop breast cancer in their lifetime.
3. Early detection is important to successful treatment.
4. Men can develop breast cancer. They account for <1% of reported cases.
5. Of all breast cancers, 90 to 95% are discovered through breast self-examination.
6. Risk factors include:
    A. Positive family history.
    B. Menarche before 12 years of age and/or menopause after age 50.
    C. Nulliparous, or those with first child after age 30.
    D. History of uterine cancer.
    E. Daily alcohol intake.
    F. Highest incidence in those age 40 to 49 and over 65.
7. Breast cancer is generally adenocarcinoma, originating in epithelial cells and occurs in the ducts or lobes.
8. Tumors tend to be located in the upper outer quadrant of the breast and more often in the left breast than the right.
9. Early detection is important.
    A. Every woman should perform a breast self-examination monthly, preferably as soon as menstrual bleeding ceases.

HESI HINT: The importance of teaching female clients how to do a self-breast examination cannot be overemphasized. Early detection is related to positive outcomes.

    B. Mammography is very helpful with early detection of cancer of the breast.
        1) Baseline mammogram at approximately 35 to 50 years of age.
        2) Mammogram every 1 to 2 years for women in their 40s.

3) Annual mammogram for women over 50 years of age.
4) Advise not to use lotions, talc powder, or deodorant under arms prior to procedure (may mimic calcium deposits on x-ray).
C. Physical examination by a professional skilled in examination of the breast should be done annually.

10. Tumors less than 4 cm. are deemed curable.
11. Larger tumors require much more aggressive treatment (cure is difficult).
12. Definitive diagnosis of cancer of the breast is made with biopsy.
13. Common sites of metastasis (spread) are the axillary, supraclavicular, or mediastinal lymph nodes followed by metastases to the lungs, liver, brain, and spine.
14. Bone metastasis is extremely painful.
15. Treatment is dependent on the stage of disease.
   A. Mastectomy is commonly performed.
   B. Adjuvant treatment consists of radiation (either external beam or implants), antineoplastic chemotherapy, and hormonal therapy.

HESI HINT: The presence or absence of hormone receptors is paramount in selecting clients for adjuvant therapy.

NURSING ASSESSMENT
1. Hard lump (not freely moveable and not painful).
2. Dimpling of skin.
3. Retraction of nipple.
4. Alterations in contour of breast.
5. Change in skin color.
6. Change in skin texture (peau d'orange).
7. Discharge from nipple.
8. Pain and ulcerations (late signs).
9. Diagnostic tests include:
   A. Mammogram.
   B. Biopsy and frozen section.

ANALYSIS (NURSING DIAGNOSES)
1. Altered body image related to…
2. Anticipatory grieving related to…
3. Pain related to…
4. Self-care deficit related to…

NURSING PLANS AND INTERVENTIONS

1. Assess lesion.
   A. Location.
   B. Size.
   C. Shape.
   D. Consistency.
   E. Fixation to surrounding tissues.
   F. Lymph node involvement.
2. Preoperative:
   A. Explore client's expectations of surgery and what the surgical site will look like postoperatively.
   B. Discuss skin graft if one is possible and cosmetic reconstruction that might be implemented with mastectomy or at a later time.
3. Postoperative:
   A. Monitor bleeding, check under dressing, HemoVac, and under client's back (bleeding will run to back).
   B. Position arm on operative side on a pillow, slightly elevated.
   C. Avoid BP measurements, injections, and venipuncture in affected arm.
   D. Instruct client to avoid injury such as burns or scrapes to affected arm.
   E. Encourage hand activity by squeezing a small rubber ball.
   F. Encourage client to perform activities that will use arm, like brushing hair.
   G. Teach post-mastectomy exercises (wall climbing with affected arm and rope turning).
4. Encourage client to verbalize concerns:
   A. Cancer.
   B. Death.
   C. Loss of breast.
5. Encourage client to discuss operation, diagnosis, feelings, concerns, and fears.
6. Be with client when she first looks at the operative site; offer emotional support.
7. Arrange for Reach-to-Recovery visit, Y-me (MD prescription required).
8. Recognize the grief process.
   A. Allow client to cry, withdraw, etc.
   B. Help client to focus on the future while allowing discussions of loss.
9. If reconstruction was not discussed preoperatively, encourage client to discuss or explore these options postoperatively.
10. Discuss use of temporary and/or permanent prosthesis.

TESTICULAR CANCER

MEDICAL SURGICAL NURSING

DESCRIPTION: Cancer of the testes is the leading cause of death from cancer in males 15 to 35 years of age. If untreated, death usually occurs within 2 to 3 years. If detected and treated early, there is a 90 to 100% chance of cure.

NURSING ASSESSMENT
1. Early signs are subtle and usually go unnoticed.
2. Feeling of heaviness or dragging in lower abdomen and groin.
3. Lump or swelling (painless).
4. Late signs include:
    A. Low back pain.
    B. Weight loss.
    C. Fatigue.

ANALYSIS (NURSING DIAGNOSES)
1. Knowledge deficit related to …
2. Altered body image related to …
3. Anticipatory grieving related to …

> **HESI HINT:** Men whose testes have not descended into the scrotum or whose testes descended after age 6 are at high risk for developing testicular cancer. The most common symptom is the appearance of a small, hard lump about the size of a pea on the front or side of the testicle. Manual testicular examination should be done by all males after age 14. It should be done after a shower by gently palpating the testes and cord to look for a small lump. Swelling may also be a sign of testicular cancer.

NURSING PLANS AND INTERVENTIONS
1. Postoperative care following orchidectomy:
    A. Observe for hemorrhage.
    B. Active movement may be contraindicated.
2. Care for clients receiving radiation therapy.
3. Encourage genetic counseling (sperm banking is often recommended prior to surgery).
4. Counsel that sexual functioning is usually not affected because the remaining testis undergoes hyperplasia, producing sufficient testosterone to maintain sexual functioning. Though ejaculatory ability may be decreased, orgasm is still possible.

ANALYSIS (NURSING DIAGNOSES)
1. Knowledge deficit related to…
2. Altered body image related to…

3. Bowel incontinence related to…
4. Anticipatory grieving related to…

NURSING PLANS AND INTERVENTIONS
1. Teach the importance of early detection.
2. Provide preoperative bowel preparation to prevent fecal contamination of operative site.
    A. Enemas and cathartics.
    B. Sulfasalazine (Azulfidine) or neomycin.
    C. Clear fluids only the day before surgery to prevent fecal contamination of operative site.
3. Provide postoperative care:
    A. Monitor for urine leaks, hemorrhage, and signs of infection.
    B. Provide support dressing or supportive underwear to perineal incision.
    C. Use donut cushion to relieve pressure on incision site while sitting.
    D. *Avoid* rectal manipulation (rectal thermometers, rectal tubes, and hard suppositories).
    E. Provide low-residue diet until wound healing is advanced.
    F. Institute measures to prevent bowel action in the first postoperative week to prevent contamination of incision.

CANCER OF THE PROSTATE
DESCRIPTION: Prostate cancer rarely occurs before 40 years of age, but it is the second leading cause of death from cancer in American men. High-risk groups include those with a history of multiple sexual partners, STDs, or certain viral infections.

NURSING ASSESSMENT
1. Asymptomatic if confined to gland.
2. Symptoms of urinary obstruction.
3. With metastasis: low back pain, fatigue, aching in legs, and hip pain.
4. Elevated prostate-specific antigen (PSA).
    A. PSA test should be conducted prior to a digital rectal exam so that manipulation of the prostate does not give a false positive reading.
    B. Serial blood screening should be done to observe trends. A rise in PSA or consistently high PSA is more reliable than a single assay.
    C. PSA levels can rise with inflammation,

benign hypertrophy, or irritation, as well as in response to cancer.

5.   Elevated prostatic acid phosphatase (PAP).
6.   Digital rectal examination (DRE) reveals palpable nodule.
7.   Transrectal ultrasound (TRUS) visualizes nonpalpable tumors.
8.   Definitive diagnosis is made by biopsy.

SEXUALLY TRANSMITTED DISEASES (STDs)

DESCRIPTION: Diseases which may be transmitted during intimate sexual contact.
1.   STDs are the most prevalent communicable diseases in the United States.
2.   Most cases of STDs occur in adolescent and young adults.

HESI HINT: STDs in infants and children usually indicate sexual abuse and should be reported. The nurse is legally responsible to report suspected cases of child abuse.

NURSING ASSESSMENT
(See figure 3-54, Sexually Transmitted Diseases)

ANALYSIS (NURSING DIAGNOSES)
1.   Knowledge deficit related to…
2.   Anxiety related to…
3.   Anticipatory grieving related to…

SEXUALLY TRANSMITTED DISEASES		
STD	SYMPTOMS	TREATMENT
TREPONEMA PALLIDUM, SYPHILIS Laboratory Diagnosis: VDRL, FTA-ABS	**Primary** (Local): up to 90 days post exposure • Chancre (red, painless lesions with indurated border) • Highly infectious **Secondary** (Systemic): 6 weeks to 6 months post-exposure • Influenza type symptoms • Generalized rash which affects palms of hands and soles of feet • Lesions contagious **Tertiary:** 10 to 30 years post-exposure • Cardiac and Neurologic destruction	penicillin G IM (usually 2.4 to 4.8 million units)
NEISSERIA GONORRHOEAE, GONORRHEA Laboratory Diagnosis: Smears, Cultures	• Females: majority are asymptomatic • Males: dysuria, yellowish-green urethral discharge, urinary frequency	• ceftriaxone sodium plus doxycycline hyclate • spectinomycin HCL plus doxycycline hyclate
CHILAMYDIA TRACHOMATIS, CHLAMYDIA Laboratory Diagnosis: Tissue culture Chamydiazine Microtrak	• Females: many asymptomatic, but may exhibit dysuria, urgency, vaginal discharge • Males: leading cause of nongonococcal urethritis	• doxycycline hyclate or tetracycline HCL
TRICHOMONAS VAGINALS TRICHOMONLASIS Laboratory Diagnosis: Wet Slide	• Females: green, yellow, or white frothy foul-smelling vaginal discharge with itching. • Males: asymptomatic	• metronidazole (Flagyl) (male partners to be treated to prevent re-infection)

Figure 3-54

SEXUALLY TRANSMITTED DISEASES (CONTINUED)		
STD	**SYMPTOMS**	**TREATMENT**
CANDIDA ALBICANS, CANDIDIASIS Laboratory Diagnosis: Viral Culture	• Females: odorless, white or yellow, cheesy discharge • Males: asymptomatic	• miconazole nitrate (Monistat) • clotrimazole (Gyne-Lotrimin) • nystatin (Mycostatin)

HERPES SIMPLEX VIRUS 2, HERPES	• Vesicles in clusters which rupture and leave painful erosions that cause painful urination
	• Characterized by remissions and exacerbations
		• acyclovir (Zovirax) partially controls symptoms
		• Palliative care
		  → Viscous lidocaine topically to ease pain
		  → Keep lesions clean and dry

HUMAN PAPPILLAMAVIRUS (HPV)	• Multiple strains (>70), some of which are implicated in cervical cancer • Alarming rate increase in adolescent population • Lesions may be small, wart-like or clustered • May be flat or raised	• Applied medications such as podopyllin (contraindicated in pregnancy) • Trichoracetic acid (TCA) • Laser • Cryotherapy (freezing)
HUMAN IMMUNODEFICIENCY VIRUS (HIV), AIDS	*(See HIV in Advanced Clinical Concepts)*	

Figure 3-54 (continued)

HESI HINT: Chlamydia is the most reported communicable disease in the United States.

NURSING PLANS AND INTERVENTIONS
1. Use a nonjudgmental approach; be straightforward when taking history.
2. Reassure client that all information is strictly confidential. Obtain a complete sexual history which needs to include:
  A. The client's sexual orientation.
  B. Sexual practices.
    1) Penile-vaginal.
    2) Penile-anal.
    3) Penile-oral.
    4) Oral-vaginal.
    5) Anal-oral.
  C. Type of protection (barrier) used.
  D. Contraceptive practices.
  E. Previous history of STDs.
3. Develop teaching plan and include the following:

A. Signs and symptoms of STDs.
B. Mode of transmission of STDs. (Remember not all persons practice sex in the same manner).
C. Sexual contact should be avoided with anyone while infected.
D. Provide concise written instructions about treatment; request a return verbalization of these instructions to ensure the client has "heard" the instructions and understands them.
4. Encourage client to provide information regarding ALL sexual contacts.
5. Report incidents of STDs to appropriate health agencies/departments.
6. Instruct women of childbearing age about risks to newborn.
  A. Gonorrheal conjunctivitis.
  B. Neonatal herpes.
  C. Congenital syphilis.
  D. Oral candidiasis.

MEDICAL SURGICAL NURSING

> **HESI HINT:** Pelvic inflammatory disease (PID) involves one more of the pelvic structures. The infection can cause adhesions and eventually result in sterility. Manage the pain associated with PID with analgesics and warm sitz baths. Bedrest in a semi-Fowler's position may increase comfort and promote drainage. Antibiotic treatment is necessary to reduce inflammation and pain.

7. Teach "safer sex."
   A. Reduce the number of sexual contacts.
   B. Avoid sex with those who have multiple partners.
   C. Examine genital area and avoid sexual contact if anything abnormal is present.
   D. Wash hands and genital area before and after sexual contact.
   E. Use a latex condom as a barrier.
   F. Use water-based lubricants rather than oil-based lubricants.
   G. Use a vaginal spermicidal gel.
   H. Avoid douching before and after sexual contact; douching increases risk of infections because the body's normal defenses are reduced or destroyed.
   I. Seek attention from Healthcare provider immediately should symptoms occur.

> **HESI HINT:** A client comes into the clinic with a chancre on his penis. What is the usual treatment? IM dose of penicillin (such as Benzathine penicillin G 2.4 million units). Obtain a sexual history, including the names of his sex partners, so that they can receive treatment.

REVIEW QUESTIONS
REPRODUCTIVE SYSTEM

1. What are the indications for a hysterectomy in the client who has fibromas?
2. List the symptoms and conditions associated with cystocele.
3. What are the most important nursing interventions for the postoperative client who has had a hysterectomy with an A&P repair?
4. Describe the priority nursing care for the client who has had radiation implants.
5. What screening tool is used to detect cervical cancer? What are the American Cancer Society's recommendations for women ages 30 to 70 with three consecutive normal results?
6. Cite two nursing diagnoses for a client undergoing a hysterectomy for cervical cancer.
7. What are the three most important tools for early detection of breast cancer? How often should these tools be used?
8. Describe three nursing interventions to help decrease edema post mastectomy.
9. Name three priorities to include in a discharge plan for the client who has had a mastectomy.
10. What is the most common cause of nongonococcal urethritis?
11. What is the causative organism for syphilis?
12. Malodorous, frothy, greenish-yellow vaginal discharge is characteristic of which STD?
13. Which STD is characterized by remissions and exacerbations in both males and females?
14. Outline a teaching plan for the client with an STD.

ANSWERS TO REVIEW QUESTIONS

1. Severe menorrhagia leading to anemia, severe dysmenorrhea requiring narcotic analgesics, severe uterine enlargement causing pressure on other organs, severe low back and pelvic pain.
2. Symptoms include incontinence/stress incontinence, urinary retention, and recurrent bladder infections. Conditions associated with cystocele include multiparity, trauma in childbirth, and aging.
3. Avoid rectal temps and/or rectal manipulation; manage pain; and encourage early ambulation.
4. Do not permit pregnant visitors or pregnant caretakers in room. Discourage visits by small children. Confine client to room. Nurse must wear radiation badge. Nurse limits time in room. Keep supplies and equipment within client's reach.
5. Pap smear. Women ages 30 to 70 with 3 consecutive normal results may have pap smears every 2 to 3 years.
6. Altered body image related to uterine removal. Pain related to postoperative incision.

7. Breast self-exam monthly; mammogram baseline at age 35 followed by exams every 1 to 2 years in 40s and every year after age 50; physical examination by a professional skilled in examination of the breast.
8. Position arm on operative side on pillow. Avoid BP measurements, injections, or venipunctures in operative arm. Encourage hand activity and use.
9. Arrange for Reach-to-Recovery visit. Discuss the grief process with the client. Have physician discuss with client the reconstruction options.
10. Chlamydia trachomatis.
11. Treponema pallidum (spirochete bacteria).
12. Trichomonas vaginalis.
13. Herpes simplex Type II.
14. Signs and symptoms of STD. Mode of transmission. Avoid sex while infected. Provide concise written instructions regarding treatment and request a return verbalization to ensure the client understands. Teach "safer sex" practices.

BURNS

DESCRIPTION: Tissue injury or necrosis caused by transfer of energy from a heat source to the body.
1. Categories:
   A. Thermal.
   B. Radiation.
   C. Electrical.
   D. Chemical.
2. Tissue destruction results from:
   A. Coagulation.
   B. Protein denaturation.
   C. Ionization of cellular contents.
3. Critical systems affected include:
   A. Respiratory.
   B. Integumentary.
   C. Cardiovascular.
   D. Renal.
   E. Gastrointestinal.
   F. Neurologic.
4. Severity determined by **burn depth**:
   A. First Degree:
      1) Superficial partial-thickness, e.g., sunburn.
      2) Leaves skin pink or red.
      3) Dry.
      4) Painful (relieved by cooling).
      5) Slight edema.
   B. Second Degree:
      1) Deep partial-thickness destruction

of epidermis and upper layers of dermis.
      2) Injury to deeper portions of the dermis.
      3) Painful (sensitive to touch and cold air).
      4) Appears red or white, weeps fluid, blisters.
      5) Hair follicles remain intact i.e., hair does not pull out easily.
      6) Very edematous.
      7) Blanching followed by capillary refill.
      8) Heals without surgical intervention, usually does not scar.
   C. Third Degree
      1) Full-thickness involves total destruction of dermis and epidermis.
      2) Skin cannot regenerate.
      3) Requires skin grafting.
      4) Underlying tissue (fat, fascia, tendon, bone) may be involved.
      5) Wound appears dry and leathery as eschar develops.
      6) Painless.
5. Severity is determined by extent of **surface area burned**:
   A. Rules of nines: head and neck 9%, upper extremities 9% each, lower extremities 18% each, front trunk 18%, back trunk 18%, perineal area 1% (for adults). *(See figure 3-55, Rule of Nines)*
   B. Lund and Browder chart: critical body areas are face, hands, feet, and perineum. *(See figure 3-56, Lund and Browder Chart)*
6. Three stages of burn care:
   A. Stage I/Emergent Phase.
      1) Begins at the time of injury and concludes with the restoration of capillary permeability which typically reverses 48 to 72 hours following the injury.
      2) Characterized by fluid shift from intravascular to interstitial and shock. Focus of care is to preserve vital organ functioning.
      3) Expect to administer large volumes of fluid in this phase.
   B. Stage II/Acute Phase.

1) Occurs from beginning of diuresis to near completion of wound closure.
2) Characterized by fluid shift from interstitial to intravascular.

C. Stage III/Rehabilitation Phase.
1) Occurs from major wound closure to return to optimal level of physical and psychosocial adjustment (approximately 5 years).
2) Characterized by grafting and rehabilitation specific to the client's needs.

NURSING ASSESSMENT

1. Absence of bowel sounds indicating paralytic ileus.
2. Radically decreased urinary output in the first 72 hours after injury with increased specific gravity.
3. Radically increased urinary output (diuresis) 72 hours to two weeks after initial injury.
4. Signs of inadequate hydration.
    A. Restlessness.
    B. Disorientation.
    C. Decreased urinary volume, urinary sodium, and increased urine specific gravity.
5. Signs of inhalation burn.
    A. Singed nasal hairs.
    B. Circumoral burns.
    C. Conjunctivitis.
    D. Sooty or bloody sputum.
    E. Hoarseness.
    F. Asymmetry of chest movements with respirations and use of accessory muscles indicative of pneumonia.
    G. Rales, wheezing and rhonchi denoting smoke inhalation.
6. Description of physiological responses to burns. *(See figure 3-57, Physiological Responses to Burns)*
7. Preexisting conditions/illnesses which may influence recovery.

HESI HINT: ABCS OF ASSESSMENT
- **AIRWAY**
- **BREATHING**
- **CIRCULATION**

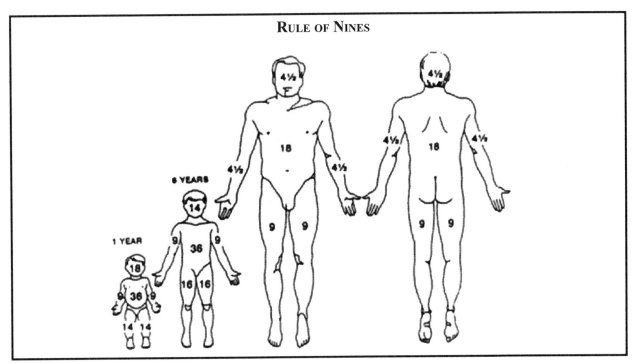

RULE OF NINES

Figure 3-55

LUND AND BROWDER CHART						
AREA	**1 YEAR**	**1 TO 4 YEARS**	**5 TO 9 YEARS**	**10 TO 14 YEARS**	**15 YEARS**	**ADULT**
Head	19	17	13	11	9	7
Neck	2	2	2	2	2	2
Anterior Trunk	13	13	13	13	13	13
Posterior Trunk	13	13	13	13	13	13
Right Buttock	2 ½	2 ½	2 ½	2 ½	2 ½	2 ½
Left Buttock	2 ½	2 ½	2 ½	2 ½	2 ½	2 ½
Genitalia	1	1	1	1	1	1
Right Upper Arm	4	4	4	4	4	4
Left Upper Arm	4	4	4	4	4	4
Right Lower Arm	3	3	3	3	3	3
Left Lower Arm	3	3	3	3	3	3
Right Hand	2 ½	2 ½	2 ½	2 ½	2 ½	2 ½
Left Hand	2 ½	2 ½	2 ½	2 ½	2 ½	2 ½
Right Thigh	5 ½	6 ½	8	8 ½	9	9 ½
Left Thigh	5 ½	6 ½	8	8 ½	9	9 ½
Right Leg	5	5	5 ½	6	6 ½	7
Left Leg	5	5	5 ½	6	6 ½	7
Right Foot	3 ½	3 ½	3 ½	3 ½	3 ½	3 ½
Left Foot	3 ½	3 ½	3 ½	3 ½	3 ½	3 ½

Figure 3-56

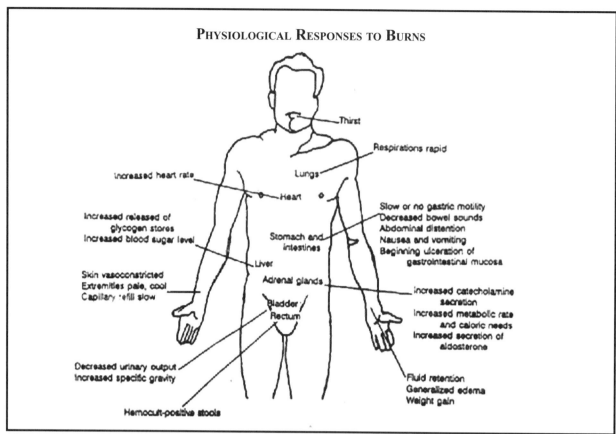

PHYSIOLOGICAL RESPONSES TO BURNS

Thirst

Respirations rapid

Lungs

Increased heart rate

Heart

Increased released of glycogen stores
Increased blood sugar level

Stomach and intestines

Liver

Skin vasoconstricted
Extremities pale, cool
Capillary refill slow

Adrenal glands

Bladder
Rectum

Slow or no gastric motility
Decreased bowel sounds
Abdominal distention
Nausea and vomiting
Beginning ulceration of gastrointestinal mucosa

Increased catecholamine secretion
Increased metabolic rate and caloric needs
Increased secretion of aldosterone

Decreased urinary output
Increased specific gravity

Fluid retention
Generalized edema
Weight gain

Hemocult-positive stools

Figure 3-57

ANALYSIS (NURSING DIAGNOSES)

1. Ineffective airway clearance related to…
2. Impaired gas exchange related to…
3. Decreased cardiac output related to…
4. Fluid volume deficit related to…
5. Inadequate tissue perfusion related to…
6. Impaired skin integrity related to…
7. Pain related to…
8. Altered body image related to…
9. Altered nutrition, less than body requirements related to…
10. Potential for infection related to…
11. Decreased mobility related to…

NURSING PLANS AND INTERVENTIONS

EMERGENT PHASE: Efforts are directed toward stabilization with ongoing assessment.

1. Provide admission care.
    A. Extinguish source of burn (burning may continue with clothing attached to skin).
        1) Thermal: remove clothing, cool burns by immersion in tepid water, apply dry sterile dressings.
        2) Chemical: flush with water or saline.
        3) Electrical: separate client from electrical source.
    B. Provide an open airway; intubation may be necessary if laryngeal edema is a risk.
    C. Determine baseline data: vital signs, blood gases, weight.
    D. Determine depth and extent of burn.
    E. Administer tetanus toxoid.
    F. Initiate fluid and electrolyte therapy: Ringer's Lactate with electrolytes and colloids adjusted according to lab results and fluid resuscitation formula used.

> **HESI HINT:** Massive volumes of IV fluids are given. It is not uncommon to give over 1,000 cc/hour during various phases of burn care. Hemodynamic monitoring must be closely observed to be sure the client is supported with fluids but is not overloaded.

    G. Insert NG tube to prevent vomiting, abdominal distention, or gastric aspiration.
    H. Administer IV pain medication as prescribed.
2. Monitor hydration status.
    A. Record urinary output hourly (30 to 100 ml/hour is normal range).

B. Maintain IV fluids titrated to keep urine output at 30 to 100 ml/hour.

C. Accurately record I&O.

D. Weigh daily.

E. Observe for signs of inadequate hydration.
  1) Restlessness.
  2) Disorientation.
  3) Hypothermia.
  4) Decreased urine output.

3. Monitor respiratory functioning.
A. Provide care for the intubated client.
B. Suction endotrach or nasotrach.
C. Monitor ABGs.
D. Observe for cyanosis, disorientation.
E. Administer O_2.
F. Encourage use of incentive spirometer, coughing, and deep breathing.

4. Provide wound care.
A. Use strict aseptic technique.

HESI HINT: Infection is a life-threatening risk for those with burns.

B. Debridement and dressing changes according to client's condition.
C. Change dressings in minimum time (very painful), premedicate.
D. Maintain room temperature above 90° F, humidified, and free of drafts.
E. Monitor body temperature frequently; have hyperthermia blankets available.

5. Assess for paralytic ileus.
A. Absence of bowel sounds.
B. Nausea and vomiting.
C. Abdominal distension.

6. Assist with management of pain.
A. Administer analgesics intravenously.
B. Teach distraction/relaxation techniques.
C. Teach use of guided imagery.

7. Assess for circulatory compromise in burns that constrict body parts. Prepare client for escharotomy.

ACUTE PHASE: Characterized by fluid shift from interstitial to intravascular (diuresis begins); occurs from 72 hours to two weeks after initial injury to near completion of wound closure.

1. Provide infection control including the following:
A. Maintain protective isolation of entire burn unit.
B. Cover hair at all times.
C. Wear masks during dressing changes.
D. Use sterile technique for hydrotherapy, dressing change, and debridement.
E. Administer IV antibiotics if indicated.
F. Live plants and flowers are prohibited.

2. Splint and position client to prevent contractures. Avoid use of pillows with neck burns.

3. Perform range of motion (ROM); it is painful.
A. Administer pain medication immediately prior to performing ROM.
B. Perform active ROM for 3 to 5 minutes frequently during day.
C. Mobilize as soon as possible using splints designed for the client.
D. Encourage active ROM when up and about.

4. Provide fluid therapy; may use colloids to keep fluid in vascular space.
A. Monitor serum chemistries at all times.
B. Keep an IV site available; a heparin lock is helpful.
C. Maintain strict I&O.
D. Encourage oral intake of fluids.

5. Provide adequate nutrition.
A. Provide high-calorie (up to 5000 calories/day), high-protein, high-carbohydrate diet.
B. Give nutritional supplements via NG tube feeding at night if caloric intake is inadequate.
C. Keep accurate calorie counts.
D. Administer all medications with either milk or juice.
E. Weigh daily.

6. Provide burn/wound care.
   A. Cleansing per agency routine (daily or up to three times a day) in hydrotherapy or shower.
   B. Wet to dry dressing changes two to three times a day to remove eschar.

HESI HINT: Dressing changes are VERY PAINFUL! Medicate client prior to procedure.

   C. Apply silver sulfadiazine (Silvadene) or mafenide acetate (Sulfamylon) to burn as prescribed. *(See figure 3-58, Topical Antimicrobial Agents)*
   D. Cover (closed method) or leave open (open method) according to agency policy or physician's presciption.
   E. Prepare client for grafting when eschar has been removed.
   F. Prepare client for autografts (use of client's own skin for grafting).
   G. Use heat lamp to donor site following graft to allow the area to reepithelize.

HESI HINT: Pre-existing conditions that might influence burn recovery are age, chronic illness (diabetes, cardiac problems, etc.), physical disabilities, disease, medications used routinely, and drug and/or alcohol abuse.

TOPICAL ANTIMICROBIAL AGENTS			
DRUGS	**INDICATIONS**	**ADVERSE REACTIONS**	**NURSING IMPLICATIONS**
mafenie acetate (Sulfamylon)	• Treatment of burns • Usually used with OPEN method of wound care	• Painful • Causes mild acidosis	• Administer pain medication PRIOR to dressing changes • Penetrates wound rapidly
silver sulfadiazine (Silvadene)	• Treatment of burns • Usually used with OPEN method of wound care • Used to avoid acid-base complications • Keeps eschar soft making debridement easier	• Penetrates wound slowly	• Administer pain medication PRIOR to dressing change • Is soothing to the burn
nitrofurazone (Furacin)	• Treatment of burns • Used to prevent infections • Interferes with bacterial enzymes	• Allergic contact dermatitis • May see super infections	• Administer pain medication PRIOR to dressing change • Monitor for signs of infection

Figure 3-58

REHABILITATION PHASE: Characterized by the absence of infection risk.
1. Ongoing discharge planning.
2. May return home when the danger of infection has been eliminated.
3. High-protein fluids with vitamin supplement.
4. Pressure dressings such as Jobst garments may be worn continuously to prevent hypertrophic scarring and contractures.

REVIEW QUESTIONS

BURNS

1. **List four categories of burns.**
2. **Burn depth is a measure of severity. Describe the characteristics of superficial partial-thickness, deep partial-thickness, and full-thickness burns.**
3. **Describe fluid management in the emergent phase, acute phase, and rehabilitation phase of the burned client.**
4. **Describe pain management of the burned client.**
5. **Outline admission care of the burned client.**
6. **Nutritional status is a major concern when caring for a burned client. List three specific dietary interventions used with burned clients.**
7. **Describe the method of extinguishing each of the following burns: thermal, chemical, and electrical.**
8. **List four signs of an inhalation burn.**
9. **Why is the burned client allowed NO "free" water?**
10. **Describe an autograft.**

ANSWERS TO REVIEW QUESTIONS

1. Thermal, radiation, chemical, electrical.
2. Superficial partial-thickness: 1st degree = pink to red skin (i.e., sunburn), slight edema, and pain relieved by cooling. Deep partial-thickness: 2nd degree = destruction of epidermis and upper layers of dermis; white or red, very edematous, sensitive to touch and cold air, hair does not pull out easily. Full-thickness: 3rd degree = total destruction of dermis and epidermis; reddened areas do not blanch with pressure, not painful, inelastic, waxy white skin to brown, leathery eschar.
3. Stage I (Emergent Phase): Replacement of fluids is titrated to urine output. Stage II (Acute Phase): Maintain patent infusion site in case supplemental IV fluids are needed; heparin lock is helpful; may use colloids. Stage III (Rehabilitation Phase): No extra fluids are needed, but high-protein drinks are recommended.
4. Administer pain medication, especially prior to dressing wound (usually Morphine 10 mg.). Teach distraction/relaxation techniques. Teach use of guided imagery.
5. Provide a patent airway as intubation may be necessary. Determine baseline data. Initiate fluid and electrolyte therapy. Administer pain medication. Determine depth and extent of burn. Administer tetanus toxoid. Insert NG tube.
6. High-calorie, high-protein, high-carbohydrate diet. Medications with juice or milk; NO "free" water. Tube feeding at night. Maintain accurate, daily calorie counts. Weigh client daily.
7. Thermal: remove clothing, immerse in tepid water. Chemical: flush with water or saline. Electrical: separate client from electrical source.
8. Singed nasal hairs, circumoral burns; sooty or bloody sputum, hoarseness, and pulmonary signs including: asymmetry of respirations, rales, or wheezing.
9. Water may interfere with electrolyte balance. Client needs to ingest food products with highest biological value.
10. Use of client's own skin for grafting.

GROWTH AND DEVELOPMENT

DESCRIPTION: Growth and development follows an orderly yet individual pattern. *(See figure 4-1, Birth to One Year)* Nurses should assess growth and the emergence of developmental skills in all pediatric clients. Knowledge of cognitive abilities allows a nurse to adapt teaching to the level of the child. Knowledge of appropriate toys and interests of children at different ages enables the nurse to use play to facilitate the child's development and minimize problems caused by the hospitalization.

BIRTH TO ONE YEAR	
DEVELOPMENTAL MILESTONES	**NURSING IMPLICATIONS**
• Birth weight doubled by 6 months, tripled by 12 months. • Birth length increased by 50% at 12 months. • Posterior fontanel closes by 8 weeks. • Social smile at 2 months. • Turns head to locate sounds at 3 months. • Moro reflex disappears around 4 months. • Achieves steady head control at 4 months. • Turns completely over at 5 to 6 months. • Plays peek-a-boo after 6 months. → 9 mos. • Transfers objects hand to hand at 7 months. • Develops stranger anxiety at 7 to 9 months. • Sits unsupported at 8 months. • Crawls at 10 months. • Fine pincer grasp appears at 10 to 12 months. • Waves bye-bye at 10 months. • Walks with assistance at 10 to 12 months. • Says a few words in addition to "mama" or "dada" at 12 months. • Explores environment by motor and oral means.	• During hospitalization, the infant's emerging skills may disappear. • If the parents are not able to be with the infant, the baby may be inconsolable due to separation anxiety. • The nurse should encourage and plan to have the parents be part of the infant's care. • The infant's schedule from home should be respected. • Preparation or teaching should be directed to the family. However, the nurse should always speak to the infant, and console the infant especially while performing painful or stressful procedures. • Toys for hospitalized infants include mobiles, rattles, squeaking toys, picture books, balls, colored blocks, and activity boxes.
Erikson's theory: Developing a sense of trust vs mistrust	

Figure 4-1

HESI HINT: NCLEX-RN® questions often focus on growth and development milestones. Do not believe the following are the only ones tested. However, these are frequently tested content areas:

• When does birth length double?	Answer: By 4 years
• When does the child sit unsupported?	Answer: 8 months
• When does a child achieve 50% of adult height?	Answer: 2 years
• When does a child throw a ball overhand?	Answer: 18 months
• When does a child speak 2 to 3 word sentences?	Answer: 2 years
• When does a child use scissors?	Answer: 4 years
• When does a child tie his/her shoes?	Answer: 5 years

• Be aware that a girl's growth spurt during adolescence begins earlier than boys (as early as 10 years old).
• Temper tantrums are common in the toddler, i.e., considered "normal," or average behavior.
• Be aware that adolescence is a time when the child forms his/her identity and that rebellion against family values is common for this age group.

HESI HINT: Normal growth and development knowledge is used to evaluate interventions and therapy. For example, "What behavior would indicate that thyroid hormone therapy for a 4-month-old is effective?" You must know what milestones are accomplished by a 4-month-old. One correct answer would be "has steady head control" which is an expected milestone for a 4-month-old and indicates that replacement therapy is adequate for growth.

TODDLER (1 TO 3 YEARS)

DEVELOPMENTAL MILESTONES	NURSING IMPLICATIONS
• Birth weight quadruples by 30 months. • Achieves 50% of adult height by 2 years. • Growth velocity slows. • Appears to be bowlegged and potbellied. • All primary teeth (20) are present. • Anterior fontanel closes by 12 to 18 months. • Throws a ball overhand at 18 months. • Kicks a ball at 24 months. • Feeds self with spoon and cup at 2 years. • Daytime toilet training can usually be started around 2 years. • Two to three word sentences at 2 years. • Three to four word sentences at 3 years. • States own first and last name by 2½ to 3 years. • Temper tantrums common. *Ritualism, parallel play, give choices, food on the run.* **Erikson's theory: Developing a sense of autonomy** *vs. shame/doubt*	• Give simple, brief explanations before procedures. • During hospitalization, enforced separation from parents is the greatest threat to the toddler's psychological and emotional integrity. • Security objects or favorite toys from home should be provided for toddler. • Teach parents to explain their plans to child, e.g., "I will be back after your nap." • Respect the child's routine. • Expect regression, e.g., bedwetting. • Toys for the hospitalized toddler include board and mallet, push/pull toys, toy telephone, stuffed animals, and storybooks with pictures. Toddlers benefit from being taken to the hospital playroom, as mobility is very important to their development. • Toddlers are learning to name body parts and are concerned about their bodies. • Very basic explanations should be given to toddlers about procedures. • Support autonomy by giving choices.

Figure 4-2

PRESCHOOL CHILD (3 TO 5 YEARS)

DEVELOPMENTAL MILESTONES	NURSING IMPLICATIONS
• Each year gains about 5 lbs. and grows 2½ to 3 inches. • Stands erect with more slender posture. • Learns to run, jump, skip, and hop. • Three-year-olds ride a tricycle. • Handedness is established. • Uses scissors at 4 years. • Ties shoelaces at 5 years. • Learns colors, shapes. • Visual acuity approaches 20/20. • Thinking is egocentric and concrete. • Uses sentences of 5 to 8 words. • Learns sexual identity (curiosity and masturbation common). • Imaginary playmates and fears are common. • Aggressiveness at 4 years is replaced by more independence at 5 years. *magical thinking* **Erikson's theory: Developing a sense of initiative** *vs. guilt*	• Nursing care for hospitalized preschoolers needs to emphasize understanding of the child's egocentricity. Explain that he/she did not cause the illness and that painful procedures are not a punishment for misdeeds. • The child's questions need to be answered at their level. Use simple words that will be understood by the child. • Therapeutic play or medical play to allow the child to act out their experiences is helpful. • Fear of mutilation from procedures is common. A Band-Aid® may be quite helpful to restore body integrity. • Toys and play for the hospitalized preschooler include coloring books, puzzles, cutting and pasting, dolls, building blocks, clay, and toys that allow the preschooler to work out hospitalization experiences. • The preschooler needs preparation for procedures. He or she needs to understand what is and what is not going to be "fixed." Simple explanations and basic pictures are helpful. Let child handle equipment or models of the equipment.

Figure 4-3

HESI HINT: Use facts and principles related to growth and development in planning teaching interventions. For example: "What task could a 5-year-old diabetic boy be expected to accomplish by himself?" One correct answer would be to pick the injection sites. This is possible for a preschooler to do and gives the child some sense of control.

(handwritten top:) Learn to read

SCHOOL-AGE CHILD (6 TO 12 YEARS)

DEVELOPMENTAL MILESTONES	NURSING IMPLICATIONS
• Each year gains 4 to 6 lbs. and about 2 inches in height. • Girls may experience menarche. • Loss of primary teeth and eruption of most permanent teeth will occur. • Fine and gross motor skills mature. • Able to write script at 8 years. • Dresses self-completely. • Egocentric thinking is replaced by social awareness of others. • Learns to tell time and understands past, present, and future. • Learns cause and effect relationships. • Socialization with peers becomes important. • Molars (6-year) erupt. *(handwritten:)* Fear losing control, follow rules. **Erikson's theory: Developing a sense of industry**	• The hospitalized school-age child may need more support from parents than they wish to admit. • Maintaining contact with peers and school activities is important during hospitalization. • Explanation of all procedures is important. They can learn from verbal explanations, pictures, books, or from handling equipment. • Privacy and modesty are important, and should be respected during hospitalization, e.g., close curtains during procedures, allow privacy during baths, etc. • Participation in care and planning with staff fosters a sense of involvement and accomplishment. • Toys for the hospitalized school-age child include board games, card games, and hobbies, such as stamp collecting, puzzles, and video games. *(handwritten:)* baseball card collection.

Figure 4-4   *(handwritten:)* VS. inferiority   understands death.   *(handwritten right:)* bicycle safety.

HESI HINT: School-age children are in Erikson's stage of industry, meaning they like to do and accomplish things. Peers are also becoming important for this age child.

ADOLESCENCE (12 TO 19 YEARS)

DEVELOPMENTAL MILESTONES	NURSING IMPLICATIONS
• Girls' growth spurt during adolescence begins earlier than boys (may begin as early as 10 for girls). • Boys catch up around 14 and continue to grow. • Girls finish growth around 15, boys around 17. • Secondary sex characteristics develop. • Adult-like thinking begins around 15. They can problem solve and use abstract thinking. • Family conflicts develop. *(handwritten:)* Puberty, reach adult height. fear of losing control peers more important than family. **Erikson's theory: Developing a sense of identity** *(handwritten:)* VS. role confusion	• Hospitalization of adolescents disrupts school and peer activities; they need to maintain contact with both. • Should room with other adolescents. • Illness, treatments, or procedures which alter the adolescent's body image can be viewed as devastating by the adolescent. • Teaching about procedures should include time without parents present. When parents are present, direct questions to the adolescent, not the parent. • Many hospitals require the adolescent's consent to treatment as well as the parents' to demonstrate that the adolescent understands the medical plan. • For prolonged hospitalizations, adolescents need to maintain identity, e.g., their own clothing, posters, visitors. A teen room or teen night is very helpful. Parents rooming-in is discouraged. • Some assessment questions should be asked without parents' presence. • When teaching adolescent needs, the focus should be on "here and now, i.e., how will this affect me today?"

Figure 4-5   *(handwritten:)* eat lots of junk food. Drive @ this age. Takes Risks

HESI HINT: Age groups concepts of bodily injury:
• **Infants:** After 6 months, their cognitive development allows them to remember pain.
• **Toddlers:** Fear intrusive procedures.
• **Preschoolers:** Fear body mutilation.
• **School age:** Fear loss of control of their body.
• **Adolescent:** Major concern is change in body image.

(side tab:) PEDIATRIC NURSING

PAIN ASSESSMENT AND MANAGEMENT IN THE PEDIATRIC CLIENT

DESCRIPTION: Historically, pain in the pediatric population has been unrecognized and/or undertreated. Research has shown that children, including neonates and infants, experience pain. Untreated pain may lead to complications such as delayed recovery, alterations in sleep patterns, and alterations in nutrition.

Pain assessment is often referred to as the fifth vital sign.

NURSING ASSESSMENT

1. Verbal report by the child. Children as young as 3 years of age are able to report the location and degree of pain they are experiencing.
2. Observe for non-verbal signs of pain such as grimacing, irritability, restlessness, and difficulty with sleeping and/or feeding.
3. Include the child's parents in the assessment.
4. Observe for physiologic responses to pain such as increased heart rate, increased respiratory rate, diaphoresis, and decreased oxygen levels.
5. Physiologic responses to pain are most often seen in response to acute pain, rather than in response to chronic pain.

ANALYSIS (NURSING DIAGNOSES)

1. Alteration ion comfort related to …
2. Anxiety related to …
3. Alteration in sleep pattern related to …
4. Alteration in feeding pattern related to …

NURSING PLANS AND INTERVENTIONS

1. Use a pain rating scale appropriate for the child's age and developmental level.
   A. Faces Pain Scale (Wong & Baker, 1996) and the Poker Chip Scale (Hester & Barcus, 1986) can be utilized by children of preschool age and older.
   B. Numeric Pain Scale can be used by children 9 years of age and older.
   C. Documentation of the child's self-report of pain is essential to effectively treating the child's pain.
   D. Non-verbal child can be assessed using the FLACC pain assessment tool (Merkel et al., 1997). This tool has the nurse evaluate the child's facial expression, leg movement, activity, cry, and consolability.
2. Non-pharmacologic Interventions
   A. Utilize based on the child's age and developmental level.
   B. Infants may respond best to pacifiers, holding and rocking.
   C. Toddler and preschoolers may respond best to distraction. Distraction may be through books, music, television, bubble blowing.
   D. School-agers and adolescents may utilize guided imagery.
   E. Other interventions may include massage, application of heat/cold, and deep breathing exercises.
3. Pharmacologic Interventions
   A. Prior to administering a pain medication to the pediatric client, verify that the prescribed dose is safe for the child, based on the child's weight.
   B. Monitor the child's vital signs following administration of opioid medications.
   C. Children as young as 5 years of age may be taught to use a patient-controlled analgesia (PCA) pump.
   D. Children may deny pain if they fear receiving an IM injection.

CHILD HEALTH PROMOTION

DESCRIPTION: Immunization of children against communicable diseases is one of the greatest accomplishments of modern medicine. Childhood mortality and morbidity rates have greatly decreased. Protection against disease should begin in infancy according to the recommendations of the American Academy of Pediatrics and the United States Public Health Service. *(See figure 4-6, Recommended Immunization Schedule; and figure 4-7, Vaccines)*

RECOMMENDED CHILDHOOD AND ADOLESCENT IMMUNIZATION SCHEDULE
UNITED STATES, 2006*

AGE ▶ VACCINE ▼	Birth	1 mo	2 mos	4 mos	6 mos	12 mos	15 mos	18 mos	24 mos	4 to 6 yrs	11 to 12 yrs	13 to 14 yrs	15 yrs	16-18 yrs
Hepatitis B[1]	HepB	HepB		*HepB[1]*	HepB				HepB Series					
Diphtheria, Tetanus, Pertussis[2]			DTaP	DTaP	DTaP		DTaP			DTaP	Tdap	Tdap		
H. Influenzae Type B[3]			Hib	Hib	*Hib[3]*	Hib								
Inactivated Poliovirus			IPV	IPV	IPV					IPV				
Measles, Mumps, Rubella[4]						MMR				MMR	MMR			
Varicella[5]						Varicella				Varicella				
Meningococcal[6]							Vaccines within broken line are for selected populations			MPSV4	MCV4	MCV4 MCV4		
Pneumoccal[7]			PCV	PCV	PCV	PCV				PVC	PPV			
Influenza[8]					Influenza (yearly)					Influenza (yearly)				
Hepatitis A[9]						HepA Series				HepA Series				

This schedule indicates the recommended ages for routine administration of currently licensed childhood vaccines, as of December 1, 2005, for children through age 18 years. Any dose not administered at the recommended age should be administered at any subsequent visit, when indicated and feasible.

[gray box] Indicates age groups that warrant special effort to administer those vaccines not previously administered. Additional vaccines might be licensed and recommended during the year. Licensed combination vaccines may be used whenever any components of the combination are indicated and other components of the vaccine are not contraindicated and if approved by the Food and Drug Administration for that dose of the series. Providers should consult respective Advisory Committee on Immunization Practices (ACIP) statements for detailed recommendations. Clinically significant adverse events that follow vaccination should be reported through the Vaccine Adverse Event Reporting System (VAERS). Guidance about how to obtain and complete a VAERS form is available at http://www.vaers.hhs.gov or by telephone, 800-822-7967.

Footnotes 1-9, see website. (http://www.cdc.gov/nip/acip/)

[box] Range of recommended ages

[box] Catch-up immunization

PEDIATRIC NURSING

Figure 4-6

VACCINES	
TYPE OF VACCINE	**DESCRIPTION**
MMR VACCINE Measles, Mumps, Rubella (MMR) Offers protection against these three diseases.	• Generally administered at 12 to 15 months of age and repeated at 4 to 6 years or by 11 to 12 years. • In times of measles epidemic, it is possible to give measles protection at 6 months and repeat the MMR at 15 months. • Measles vaccine is contraindicated for persons with history of anaphylactic reaction to neomycin or eggs, those with known altered immunodeficiency, and pregnant women. May give to those with HIV and breastfeeding women. • Administer subcutaneously at separate sites. • Child may have a light transient rash 2 weeks after administration of vaccine.
HESI HINT: Pertinent history should be obtained prior to administering certain immunizations because reactions to previous immunizations or current health conditions may contraindicate current immunizations: • **DPT:** History of seizures, neurological symptoms after previous vaccine, or systematic allergic reactions. • **MMR:** History of anaphylactic reaction to eggs or neomycin.	
DTAP VACCINE Diphtheria, Pertussis, Tetanus Offers protection against these diseases.	• Beginning at age two months, administer three doses at two-month intervals. • Booster doses given at 15 to 18 months; and at 4 to 6 years. • Administer intramuscularly (separate site from other vaccine). • Not given to children past the 7th birthday; they receive Td which contains full strength protection against tetanus and lesser strength diphtheria protection • When pertussis vaccine is contraindicated, give DT, full strength diphtheria and tetanus without pertussis vaccine, until 7th birthday. • Contraindications to pertussis vaccine include: → Encephalopathy within 7 days of previous dose of DTP. → History of seizures. → Neurologic symptoms after receiving the vaccine. → Systemic allergic reactions to the vaccine. • Parents should be instructed to begin acetaminophen (Tylenol) administration after the immunization (normal dosage is 10 to 15 mg/kg). • Instruct parents to immediately report any side effects of the immunization to the primary caregiver.
HESI HINT: Pertussis fatalities continue to occur in unimmunized infants in the U.S.	
POLIO VACCINE **Inactive Polio Vaccine (IPV)**	• Recommended for all persons under 18 years. • Administer at 2 months of age and again at 4 months of age. Boosters given at 6 to 18 months, and 4 to 6 years. • Administer IPV subcutaneously or IM at separate site. • IPV is contraindicated for those with history of anaphylactic reaction to neomycin or streptomycin. • May give with all other vaccines.

Figure 4-7

VACCINES (CONTINUED)	
TYPE OF VACCINE	DESCRIPTION
HIB (HAEMOPHILUS INFLUENZA TYPE B) VACCINE Offers protection against bacteria that causes serious illness (epiglottitis, bacterial meningitis, septic arthritis) in small children or those with chronic illnesses such as sickle cell anemia.	• Three conjugate vaccines have been recommended for administration to infants. PRP-OPMs and be given beginning as early as 2 months of age. DaTP/Hib combinations should not be used as primary immunizations at ages 2, 4, or 6 months • Vaccines have different series administration schedules; the schedules cover children up through 5 years. • Children at high risk who were not immunized previously should be immunized after 5 years. • Administer intramuscularly. • No contraindications.
HEPATITIS B Offers protection against hepatitis B. Typically, given to all newborns prior to hospital discharge. Vaccinate all children 0 to 18 years of age.	• Contraindicated for persons with anaphylactic reaction to common baker's yeast. • Administer IM at 0 to 2 months, 1 to 4 months, and 6 to 18 months of age. • ***See note at bottom of Recommended Childhood Immunization Table, Figure 4-6.***
VARICELLA Offers protection against chickenpox. School entry requirement in 33 states. Safe for children with asymptomatic HIV infection.	• Administer at 12 to 18 months of age (must be at least 12 months). • Give MMR and varicella on same day or >30 days apart (separate site). • ***See note at bottom of Recommended Childhood Immunization Table, Figure 4-6.***

TUBERCULOSIS (TB) SKIN TESTING
Offers SCREENING for exposure to TB.
	• Screening usually done using one of the following:
	  → Mantoux test with PPD (tuberculin purified protein derivative) injected intradermally on the forearm; standard method for identifying infection with *M. tuberculosis*.
	  → Tine test (OT, Old Tuberculin) which consists of 4 prongs pressed into the forearm. These multiple puncture tests are unreliable and should not be used to determine the presence of a TB infection.
	• A positive reaction represents exposure to *M. tuberculosis*.
	• Screening can be initiated at 12 months.

HESI HINT: Subcutaneous injection, rather than intradermal, invalidates the Mantoux test.

Figure 4-7 (continued)

HESI HINT: The common cold is not a contraindication for immunization.

HESI HINT: Following immunization, what teaching should the nurse provide to the parents?
• Irritability, fever (<102°F), redness and soreness at injection site for 2 to 3 days are normal side effects of DPT and IPV administration.
• Call health care provider if seizures, high fever, or high-pitched crying occur.
• A warm washcloth on the thigh injection site and "bicycling" the legs with each diaper change will decrease soreness.
• Acetaminophen (Tylenol) is administered orally every 4 to 6 hours (10 to 15 mg/Kg).

PEDIATRIC NURSING

The nursing care of children with communicable diseases is virtually the same regardless of the particular disease. *Figure 4-8* describes commonly occurring communicable diseases in children and the nursing care for children with these diseases.

COMMON CHILDHOOD COMMUNICABLE DISEASES	
DISEASE	**DESCRIPTION**
RUBEOLA (Measles)	• A highly contagious, viral disease that can lead to neurologic problems or death. • Transmitted by direct contact with droplets from infected persons. • It is contagious mainly during the prodromal period which is characterized by fever and upper respiratory symptoms. • Classic symptoms include the following: → Photophobia. → Koplik's spots on the buccal mucosa. → Confluent rash that begins on the face and spreads downward.
VARICELLA ZOSTER (Chicken Pox)	• Viral disease characterized by skin lesions. • Lesions begin on the trunk and spread to the face and proximal extremities. • Progresses through macular, popular, vesicular, and pustular stages. • Transmitted by direct contact, droplet spread, or freshly contaminated objects. • Communicability end when scabs have formed.
RUBELLA (German Measles)	• Common viral disease which has teratogenic effects on fetus during the first trimester of pregnancy. • Transmitted by droplet and direct contact with infected person. • Discrete red maculopapular rash starts on face and rapidly spreads to entire body. • Rash disappears within 3 days.
PERTUSSIS (Whooping Cough)	• An acute, infectious respiratory disease usually occurring in infancy. • Pertussis is caused by a gram-negative bacillus. • Begins with upper respiratory symptoms. • Paroxysmal stage of the disease is characterized by prolonged coughing and crowing or whooping upon inspiration; lasts from 4 to 6 weeks. • Transmitted by direct contact, droplet spread, or freshly contaminated objects. • It is treated with erythromycin. • Complications include pneumonia, hemorrhage, and seizures.
NURSING CARE FOR CHILDREN WITH COMMUNICABLE DISEASES	
• Isolate child during period of communicability. • Treat fever with NON-ASPIRIN product. • Report occurrence to the health department. • Prevent child from scratching skin, i.e., cut nails, apply mittens, and provide soothing baths. • Administer Diphenhydramine HCL (Benadryl) as prescribed for itching. • **WASH HANDS** after caring for child and handling secretions or child's articles.	

Figure 4-8

NUTRITIONAL ASSESSMENT

DESCRIPTION: A profile of the child's and family's eating habits.

1. Iron deficiency occurs most frequently in children 12 to 36 months old, in adolescent females, and in females during their childbearing years.
2. The vitamins most often consumed in less than appropriate amounts by preschool and school-age children are:
   A. Vitamin A
   B. Vitamin C
   C. Vitamin B_6
   D. Vitamin B_{12}

NURSING PLANS AND INTERVENTIONS

4. Determine dietary history
   A. The 24-hour recall: ask the family to recall all food and liquid intake for the past 24 hours.
   B. Food diary: ask the family to keep a 3-day record (2 weekdays and 1 weekend day) of all food and liquid intake.
   C. Food frequency record: provide a questionnaire and ask family to record information regarding the number of times per day, week, or month a child consumes items from the four food groups.
5. Perform a clinical examination.
   A. Assess skin, hair, teeth, gums, lips, tongue, and eyes.
   B. Use of anthropometry: measurement of height, weight, head circumference in young children, proportion, skinfold thickness, and arm circumference.
      1) Height and head circumference reflect past nutrition.
      2) Weight, skinfold thickness, and arm circumference reflect present nutritional status (especially protein and fat reserves).
      3) Skinfold thickness provides a measurement of the body's fat content (one-half of the body's total fat stores are directly beneath the skin).
   C. Obtain biochemical analysis.
      1) Plasma, blood cells, urine, or tissues from liver, bone, hair, or fingernails can be used to determine nutritional status.
      2) Hgb, Hct, albumin, creatinine, and nitrogen laboratory testing are common laboratory procedures used to determine nutritional status.
6. Implement appropriate nursing interventions, including client/family teaching to correct identified nutritional deficits. (See figure 4-9, Nutritional Assessment)

PEDIATRIC NURSING

NUTRITIONAL ASSESSMENT

NUTRIENT	SIGNS OF DEFICIENCY	FOOD SOURCES	
IRON	• Anemia • Pale conjunctiva • Pale skin color • Atrophy of papillae on tongue • Brittle, ridged, spoon-shaped nails • Thyroid edema	• Iron-fortified formula • Infant high-protein cereal	• Infant rice cereal • Liver • Beef • Pork • Eggs
VITAMIN B₂ (RIBOFLAVIN)	• Redness and fissuring of eyelid corners; burning, itching, tearing eyes; photophobia • Tongue is magenta color, glossitis • Seborrheic dermatitis, delayed wound healing	• Prepared infant formula • Liver • Cow's milk • Cheddar cheese • Enriched cereals	• Some green leafy vegetables (broccoli, green beans, spinach)
VITAMIN A (RETINOL)	• Dry, rough skin • Dull cornea; soft cornea; Bitot's spots • Night blindness • Defective tooth enamel • Retarded growth; impaired bone formation • Decreased thyroxine formation	• Liver • Sweet potatoes • Carrots • Spinach • Peaches • Apricots	
VITAMIN C (ASCORBIC ACID)	• Scurvy • Receding gums that are spongy and prone to bleeding • Dry, rough skin, petechiae • Decreased wound healing • Increased susceptibility to infection • Irritable, anorectic, apprehensive	• Strawberries • Oranges and orange juice • Tomatoes • Broccoli • Cabbage • Cauliflower • Spinach	
VITAMIN B₆ (PYRIDOXINE)	• Scaly dermatitis • Weight loss • Anemia • Irritability • Convulsions • Peripheral neuritis	• Meats, especially liver • Cereals (wheat and corn) • Yeast • Soybeans	• Peanuts • Tuna • Chicken • Bananas

HESI HINT:
• **Teach proper cooking and storage to preserve potency, i.e., cook vegetables in small amount of liquid.**
• **Store milk in opaque container.**

Figure 4-9

DIARRHEA

DESCRIPTION: Increased number or decreased consistency of stools.

1. Diarrhea can be a serious or FATAL illness, especially in infancy.
2. Causes include, but are not limited to the following:
   A. Infections: bacterial, viral.
   B. Malabsorption problems.
   C. Inflammatory diseases.
   D. Dietary factors.
3. Conditions associated with diarrhea:
   A. Dehydration.
   B. Metabolic acidosis.
   C. Shock.

NURSING ASSESSMENT

1. Usually occurs in infants.
2. History of exposure to pathogens, contaminated food, dietary changes.
3. Signs of dehydration:
   A. Poor skin turgor.
   B. Absence of tears.
   C. Dry mucous membranes.
   D. Weight loss (5 to 15%).
   E. Depressed fontanel.
   F. Decreased urinary output, increased specific gravity.
4. Laboratory signs of acidosis:
   A. Loss of bicarbonate (serum pH <7.33).
   B. Loss of sodium and potassium through stools.
   C. Elevated Hct.
   D. Elevated BUN.
5. Signs of shock:
   A. Decreased blood pressure.
   B. Rapid, weak pulse.
   C. Mottled to gray skin color.
   D. Changes in mental status.

ANALYSIS (NURSING DIAGNOSES)

1. Alteration in bowel elimination: diarrhea related to...
2. Potential fluid volume deficit related to...

NURSING PLANS AND INTERVENTIONS

1. Assess hydration status and vital signs frequently.
2. Monitor intake and output.
3. Do NOT take temperature rectally.
4. Rehydrate as prescribed with fluids and electrolytes.
5. Calculate IV hydration to include maintenance and replacement fluids.
6. Collect specimens to aid in diagnosis of cause.
7. Check stools for pH, glucose, and blood.
8. Administer antibiotics as prescribed.
9. Check urine for specific gravity.
10. Institute careful isolation precautions, WASH HANDS.
11. Teach home care of child with diarrhea:
    A. Oral rehydration solution such as Pedialyte or Lytren.
    B. May temporarily need lactose-free diet.
    C. Children should not receive anti-diarrheals,, e.g., Imodium A-D.
    D. Do not give grape juice, orange juice, apple juice, cola, or gingerale. These solutions have high osmolality.

> **HESI HINT:** Add potassium to IV fluids ONLY with adequate urine output.

BURNS

DESCRIPTION: Tissue injury caused by heat, electricity, chemicals, or radiation.

1. Second leading cause of accidental death in children under 15 (second to automobile accidents).
2. Estimated that 75% of burns are preventable.
3. Children under age 2 have a higher mortality rate due to:
   A. Greater body surface area.
   B. Greater fluid volume (proportionate to body size).
   C. Less effective cardiovascular responses to volume shifts.
4. In childhood, a partial-thickness burn is considered a major burn if it involves more than 25% of body surface.
5. A full-thickness burn is considered major if it involves more than 10% of body surface.
6. Because of the changing proportions of the child, especially the infant, the rule of nines cannot be used to assess the percent of burn. *(See Medical Surgical figure 3-55, Rule of Nines)*
7. An assessment tool, such as the Lund-Browder chart that takes into account the changing proportions of the child, should be used.
8. Fluid needs should be calculated from the time of the burn.
9. The formula for calculating fluid replacement and maintenance is based on child's body surface area and should include

volume for burn losses and maintenance.
10. Adequacy of fluid replacement is determined by evaluating urinary output.

> **HESI HINT:** Urinary output for infants and children should be 1 to 2 ml/kg/hour.

11. Specific gravity should be less than 1.025.
12. *See Medical Surgical Nursing, Burns.*

CHILD ABUSE

DESCRIPTION: Includes physical and mental injury, sexual abuse, and emotional and physical neglect. A national problem from which 3,000 to 5,000 children die each year. *(See Psychiatric Nursing, Abuse)*

POISONINGS

DESCRIPTION: Ingesting, inhaling, or absorbing a toxic substance.
1. Poisoning, particularly by ingestion, is a frequent cause of childhood injury or illness.
2. Most poisonings occur in children under the age of six, with a peak at age two.
3. The exploratory behavior, curiosity, and oral-motor activity of early childhood place the child at risk for poisonings.
4. Ninety percent of poisonings occur in the home.

NURSING ASSESSMENT
1. Child found near the source of the poison.
2. G.I. disturbance: nausea, abdominal pain, diarrhea, vomiting.
3. Burns of mouth, pharynx.
4. Respiratory distress.
5. Seizures, changes in level of consciousness.
6. Cyanosis.
7. Shock.

ANALYSIS (NURSING DIAGNOSES)
1. Potential for injury: poisoning related to…
2. Knowledge deficit about home safety related to…

NURSING PLANS AND INTERVENTIONS
1. Identify the poisonous agent **quickly!**
2. Assess the child's respiratory, cardiac, and neurologic status.
3. Instruct parent to bring any emesis, stool, etc., to the emergency room.
4. Determine the child's age and weight.

> **HESI HINT:** Use of syrup of ipecac is no longer recommended by the American Academy of Pediatrics. Teach parents that it is NOT recommended to induce vomiting in any way as it may cause more damage.

5. Poison removal or care may require gastric lavage, activated charcoal, or naloxone HCL (Narcan).
6. Teach home safety:
   A. Poison-proof/child-proof the home:
      1) Identify location of poisons: under the sink (cleaning supplies, drain cleaners, bug poisons); medicine cabinets; storage rooms (paints, varnishes); garages (antifreeze, gasoline); poisonous plants (philodendron, dieffenbachia).
      2) Put locks on cabinets.
      3) Use safety containers: do NOT place poisonous materials in other, non-safe containers.
      4) Discard unused medications.
      5) Make sure child is always under adult supervision.
   B. Post phone number for local Poison Control Center by telephone.
   C. Examine the environment from the child's viewpoint (the height that a two to five-year-old can reach).
9. Refer to community health nurse or child welfare agency if necessary.

REVIEW QUESTIONS
CHILD HEALTH PROMOTION
1. **List two contraindications for live virus immunization.**
2. **List three classic signs and symptoms of measles.**
3. **List the signs and symptoms of iron deficiency?**
4. **Identify food sources for Vitamin A.**
5. **What disease occurs with vitamin C deficiency?**
6. **What measurements reflect present nutritional status?**
7. **List the signs and symptoms of dehydration in an infant.**
8. **List the laboratory findings that can be expected in a dehydrated child.**
9. **How should burns in children be assessed?**

10. How can the nurse BEST evaluate the adequacy of fluid replacement in children?

11. How should a parent be instructed to "child proof" a house?

12. What interventions should the nurse do FIRST in caring for a child who has ingested a poison?

1. Immunocompromised child or a child in a household with an immunocompromised individual.

2. Photophobia, confluent rash that begins on the face and spreads downward, and Koplik's spots on the buccal mucosa.

3. Anemia, pale conjunctiva, pale skin color, atrophy of papillae on tongue, brittle/ridged/spoon-shaped nails, and thyroid edema.

4. Liver, sweet potatoes, carrots, spinach, peaches, and apricots.

5. Scurvy.

6. Weight, skinfold thickness, and arm circumference.

7. Poor skin turgor, absence of tears, dry mucous membranes, weight loss, depressed fontanel and decreased urinary output.

8. Loss of bicarbonate/decreased serum pH, loss of sodium (hyponatremia), loss of potassium (hypokalemia), elevated Hct, and elevated BUN.

9. Use the Lund-Browder chart, which takes into account the changing proportions of the child's body.

10. Monitor urine output.

11. Lock all cabinets, safely store all toxic household items in locked cabinets, and examine the house from the child's point of view.

12. Assess the child's respiratory, cardiac, and neurological status.

RESPIRATORY DISORDERS

IMPORTANT SIGNS FOR CHILDREN			
NORMAL PULSE AND RESPIRATORY RATES FOR CHILDREN			
AGE	PULSE	RESPIRATIONS	NURSING IMPLICATIONS
NEWBORN	100 to 160	30 to 60	These ranges are averages only and vary with the sex, age, and condition of child. Always note if the child is crying, febrile, or in some distress.
1 to 11 months	100 to 150	25 to 35	
1 to 3 years (toddler)	80 to 130	20 to 30	
3 to 5 years (preschooler)	80 to 120	20 to 25	
6 to 10 years (school age)	70 to 110	18 to 22	
10 to 16 years (adolescent)	60 to 90	16 to 20	

SIGNS OF RESPIRATORY DISTRESS IN CHILDREN	
CARDINAL SIGNS OF RESPIRATORY DISTRESS • Restlessness • Increased respiratory rate • Increased pulse rate • Diaphoresis OTHER SIGNS OF RESPIRATORY DISTRESS • Flaring nostrils • Retractions • Grunting • Adventitious breath sounds (or absent breath sounds) • Use of accessory muscles, head bobbing • Alterations in blood gases: decreased Po_2, elevated Pco_2 • Cyanosis and pallor	NURSING IMPLICATIONS • Pediatric client will often go into respiratory failure before cardiac failure. • The nurse should know the signs of respiratory distress

Figure 4-10

ASTHMA

DESCRIPTION: An inflammatory reactive airway disease that is often chronic.
1. The airways become edematous.
2. Airways become congested with mucus.
3. Smooth muscles of bronchi and bronchioles constrict.
4. Air trapping occurs in the alveoli.

NURSING ASSESSMENT
1. History of asthma in the family.
2. History of allergies.
3. Home environment contains pets or other allergens.
4. Tight cough (non-productive cough).
5. Breath sounds: course, EXPIRATORY WHEEZING, rales, crackles.
6. Chest diameter enlarges (late sign/symptom).
7. Increased number of school days missed during past 6 months.
8. Signs of respiratory distress. *(See figure 4-10, Important Signs for Children)*

ANALYSIS (NURSING DIAGNOSES)
1. Impaired gas exchange related to…
2. Ineffective breathing pattern related to…

NURSING PLANS AND INTERVENTIONS
1. Monitor carefully for increasing respiratory distress.
2. Administer rapid-acting bronchodilators and steroids for acute attacks.
3. Maintain hydration (oral fluids or IV).
4. Monitor blood gas values for signs of respiratory acidosis. *(See Advanced Clinical Concepts, Fluid and Electrolyte Balance)*
5. Administer oxygen and/or nebulizer therapy as prescribed.
6. Monitor pulse oximetry as prescribed (usually >95% is normal).
7. Monitor Theophylline levels (10 to 20 mcg/ml desired level). Beta-adrenergic agonists – 2nd generation sympathomimetic agents (e.g., albuterol, Intal, Xopenex, or Pulmicort) most commonly used. *(See figure 3-3, Bronchodilators/Corticosteroids, and figure 4-11, Adrenergics)*
8. Cromolyn sodium used prophylactically to prevent inflammatory response.
9. Teach home care program:
    A. Identify precipitating factors.
    B. Reduce allergens in the home.
    C. Use of metered-dose inhaler.
    D. Home monitoring of peak expiratory flow rate.
    E. Breathing exercises.
    F. Monitor drug actions, dosages, and side effects.
    G. How to manage acute episode and when to seek emergency care.
10. Refer child/family for emotional/psychological counseling.

CYSTIC FIBROSIS

DESCRIPTION: An atuosomal recessive disease that causes dysfunction of the exocrine glands.
1. Tenacious mucus production obstructs vital structures.
2. Multiple problems result from the exocrine dysfunction:
    A. Lung insufficiency (most critical problem).
    B. Pancreatic insufficiency.
    C. Increased loss of sodium and chloride in sweat.

NURSING ASSESSMENT
1. Usually Caucasian infant/child.
2. Meconium ileus at birth (10 to 20% of cases).
3. Recurrent respiratory infection.
4. Pulmonary congestion.
5. Steatorrhea (excessive fat, greasy stools).
6. Foul-smelling bulky stools.
7. Delayed growth and poor weight gain.
8. Skin tastes "salty" when kissed (caused by excessive secretions from sweat glands).
9. Later: cyanosis, nail bed clubbing, CHF.

ANALYSIS (NURSING DIAGNOSES)
1. Ineffective airway clearance related to…
2. Altered nutrition: less than body requirements related to…

NURSING PLANS AND INTERVENTIONS
1. Monitor respiratory status.
2. Assess for signs of respiratory infection.
3. Administer IV antibiotics as prescribed, manage vascular access.
4. Administer pancreatic enzymes (Cotazym-S, Pancrease) (infants with applesauce, rice or cereal, and with an older child take with food).
5. Administer fat-soluble vitamins (A, D, E, K) in water-soluble form.
6. Administer oxygen/nebulizer treatments as prescribed. *(See figure 4-12, Respiratory Client)*

7. Evaluate effectiveness of respiratory treatments.
8. Teach family percussion and postural drainage techniques.
9. Dietary recommendations would be high calories, high protein, high fat (more calories per volume), and moderate to low carbohydrates (to avoid an increase in CO_2 drive).

> **HESI HINT:** Child needs 150% of the usual calorie intake for normal growth and development.

10. Provide age appropriate activities.
11. Refer family for genetic counseling.

EPIGLOTTITIS

DESCRIPTION: Severe, life-threatening infection of the epiglottis.
1. Epiglottitis progresses rapidly, causing acute airway obstruction.
2. The organism usually responsible for epiglottitis is *Haemophilus influenzae (H. influenzae,* primarily type B).

NURSING ASSESSMENT
1. Sudden onset.
2. Restlessness.
3. High fever.
4. Sore throat, dysphagia.
5. Drooling.
6. Muffled voice.
7. Child assumes upright sitting position with chin out and tongue protruding ("tripod" position).

ANALYSIS (NURSING DIAGNOSES)
1. Ineffective breathing pattern related to…
2. Anxiety related to…

NURSING PLANS AND INTERVENTIONS
1. Encourage prevention with Hib vaccine.
2. Maintain child in upright sitting position.
3. Prepare for intubation or tracheostomy.
4. Administer IV antibiotics as prescribed.
5. Prepare for hospitalization in ICU.
6. Restrain as needed to prevent extubation.
7. Prevention: *H. Influenzae* type B *(See figure 4-6, Recommended Immunization Schedule)*

> **HESI HINT:** Do not examine the throat of a child with epiglottitis due to the risk of completely obstructing the airway, i.e., do not put a tongue blade or any object in the throat.

BRONCHIOLITIS

DESCRIPTION: A viral infection of the bronchioles characterized by thick secretions.
1. Bronchiolitis is usually caused by respiratory syncytial virus (RSV) and is found to be readily transmitted by close contact with hospital personnel, families, and other children.
2. Bronchiolitis occurs primarily in young infants.

NURSING ASSESSMENT
1. History of upper respiratory symptoms.
2. Irritable, distressed infant.
3. Paroxysmal coughing.
4. Poor eating.
5. Nasal congestion.
6. Nasal flaring.
7. Prolonged expiratory phase of respiration.
8. Wheezing, rales can be auscultated.
9. Deteriorating condition that is often indicated by shallow, rapid respirations.

ANALYSIS (NURSING DIAGNOSES)
1. Impaired gas exchange related to…
2. Ineffective airway clearance related to…

NURSING PLANS AND INTERVENTIONS
1. Isolate child (isolation of choice for RSV is contact isolation).
2. Assign nurses to clients with RSV who have NO responsibility for any other children (to prevent transmission of the virus).
3. Monitor respiratory status; observe for hypoxia.
4. Clear airway of secretions using a bulb syringe for suctioning.
5. Provide care in mist tent; administer oxygen as prescribed.
6. Maintain hydration (oral and IV fluids).
7. Monitor antiviral agent, ribavirin aerosol, if prescribed.
8. Evaluate response to respiratory therapy treatments.
9. Synagis (palivizumab) may be given to provide passive immunity against RSV in high-risk children (less than 2 years of age with a history of prematurity, lung disease, or congenital heart disease).

OTITIS MEDIA

DESCRIPTION: Inflammatory disorder of the middle ear.

1. Otitis media may be suppurative or serous.
2. Anatomic structure of the ear predisposes young child to ear infections.
3. There is a risk of conductive hearing loss if untreated or incompletely treated.

NURSING ASSESSMENT

1. Fever, pain, infant may pull at ear.
2. Enlarged lymph nodes.
3. Discharge from ear (if drum is ruptured).
4. Upper respiratory symptoms.
5. Vomiting, diarrhea.

ANALYSIS (NURSING DIAGNOSES)

1. Potential for infection related to…
2. Alteration in comfort: pain related to…

NURSING PLANS AND INTERVENTIONS

1. Administer antibiotics if prescribed.
2. Reduce body temperature (can be very high with risk of seizures).
   A. Tepid baths.
   B. Acetaminophen (Tylenol) if prescribed.
3. Position child on affected side.
4. Comfort measure: warm compress on affected ear.
5. Teach home care.
   A. Finish all prescribed antibiotics.
   B. Encourage follow-up visit.
   C. Monitor for hearing loss.
   D. Teach preventive care (smoking and bottle feeding in supine position are predisposing factors).

TONSILLITIS

DESCRIPTION: Inflammation of the tonsils.

1. Tonsillitis may be viral or bacterial.
2. Tonsillitis may be related to strep infection.
3. If related to strep, treatment is **VERY IMPORTANT** because of the risk of developing acute glomerulonephritis or rheumatic heart disease.

NURSING ASSESSMENT

1. Sore throat.
2. Fever.
3. Enlarged tonsils (may have purulent discharge on tonsils).
4. Breathing may be obstructed (tonsils touching called "kissing tonsils").
5. Throat culture to determine viral or bacterial etiology.

ANALYSIS (NURSING DIAGNOSES)

1. Impaired swallowing related to…
2. Potential for injury related to…

NURSING PLANS AND INTERVENTIONS

1. Collect throat culture if prescribed.
2. Instruct parents in home care:
   A. Encourage warm saline gargles.
   B. Provide ice chips.
   C. Administer antibiotics if prescribed.
   D. Manage fever with acetaminophen.
3. Provide surgical care if indicated:
   A. Preoperative teaching and assessment.
   B. Monitor for signs of postoperative bleeding.
      1) Frequent swallowing.
      2) Vomiting fresh blood.
      3) Clearing throat.
   C. Encourage soft foods and oral fluids (avoid red fluids, which mimic signs of bleeding). **NO straws**.
   D. Comfort measure: ice collar will help with pain and with vasoconstriction.
   E. Highest risk of hemorrhage is first 24 hours and 5 to 10 days AFTER surgery.

ADRENERGICS			
DRUGS	INDICATIONS	ADVERSE REACTIONS	NURSING IMPLICATIONS
epinephrine HCL (SusPhrine)	• Rapid-acting bronchodilator • Drug of choice for acute asthma attack	• Tachycardia • Hypertension • Tremors • Nausea	• Give sub-Q, IV, nebulizer • May be repeated in 20 minutes
theophylline (Theo-Dur)	• Bronchodilator, used in asthma to reverse bronchospasm	• Tachycardia • Irritability • Palpitations • Hypotension • Nausea, vomiting	• Auscultate lungs before and after administration • Monitor blood levels

Figure 4-11

HESI HINT: When calculating a pediatric dosage, the nurse must often change the child's weight from pounds to kilograms. HINT: weight expressed in kilograms should *always* be a smaller number than weight expressed in pounds.

RESPIRATORY CLIENT
ADMINISTRATION OF OXYGEN

- Oxygen Hood: Used for infants.
- Nasal prongs: Provides low to moderate concentrations of oxygen.
- Tents: Provide mist and oxygen. Monitor child's temperature. Keep edges tucked in. Keep child dry.

MEASUREMENT OF OXYGENATION

- Pulse oximetry measures oxygen saturation (SaO_2) of arterial hemoglobin non-invasively via a sensor that is usually attached to the finger or toe.
- Nurse should be aware of the alarm parameters signaling decreased SaO_2 (usually <95%).
- Blood gas evaluation is usually monitored in respiratory clients through arterial sampling.
- Norms: PO_2: 83 to 100; PCO_2: 35 to 45 for infants and children (not newborns).

Figure 4-12

PEDIATRIC NURSING

REVIEW QUESTIONS

RESPIRATORY DISORDERS

1. **Describe the purpose of bronchodilators.**
2. **What are the physical assessment findings for a child with asthma?**
3. **What nutritional support should be provided for the child with cystic fibrosis?**
4. **Why is genetic counseling important for the cystic fibrosis family?**
5. **List seven signs of respiratory distress in a pediatric client.**
6. **Describe the care of a child in a mist tent.**
7. **What position does the child with epiglottitis assume?**
8. **Why are IV fluids important for the child with an increased respiratory rate?**
9. **Children with chronic otitis media are at risk for developing what problem?**
10. **What is the most common postoperative complication following a tonsillectomy? Describe the signs and symptoms of this complication.**

ANSWERS TO REVIEW QUESTIONS

1. Reverse bronchospasm.
2. Expiratory wheezing, rales, right cough, and signs of altered blood gases.
3. Pancreatic enzyme replacement, fat-soluble vitamins, and a moderate-to-low-carbohydrate, high-protein, moderate-fat diet.
4. The disease is autosomal recessive in its genetic pattern.
5. Restlessness, tachycardia, tachypnea, diaphoresis, flaring nostrils, retractions, and grunting.
6. Monitor child's temperature. Keep tent edges tucked in. Keep clothing dry. Assess child's respiratory status. Look at child inside tent.
7. Upright, sitting, with chin out and tongue protruding ("tripod" position).
8. The child is at risk for dehydration and acid/base imbalance.
9. Hearing loss.
10. Hemorrhage; frequent swallowing, vomiting fresh blood, and clearing throat.

Cardiovascular Disorders

Congenital Heart Disorders

Description: Heart anomalies that develop in utero and manifest at birth or shortly thereafter.

1. Congenital heart disorders occur in 4 to 10 children per 1000 live births.
2. May be categorized as:
   A. Acyanotic (VSD, ASD, PDA, Coarctation of Aorta, AS):
      1) Left to right shunts or increased pulmonary blood flow.
      2) Obstructive defects.
   B. Cyanotic (Tetralogy of Fallot, TA, TGV):
      1) Right to left shunts or decreased pulmonary blood flow.
      2) mixed blood flow.
3. May use hemodynamic classification:
   A. Increased pulmonary blood flow defects (ASD, VSD, PDA).
   B. Obstructive defects (Coarctation of Aorta, AS).
   C. Decreased pulmonary blood flow defects (Tetralogy of Fallot).
   D. Mixed defects (TGV, TA).

Acyanotic Heart Defect

Ventricular Septal Defect (VSD) (Increased Pulmonary Blood Flow)

1. Hole between the ventricles.
2. Oxygenated blood from left ventricle is shunted to right ventricle and re-circulated to the lungs.
3. Small defects may close spontaneously.
4. Large defects cause Eisenmenger's syndrome or congestive heart failure and require surgical closures.

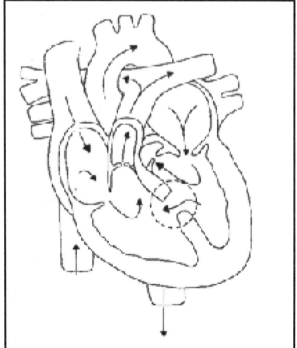

Figure 4-13

Atrial Septal Defect (ASD)
(Increased Pulmonary Blood Flow)

1. Hole between the atria.
2. Oxygenated blood from the left atrium is shunted to the right atrium and lungs.
3. Most defects do not seriously compromise children.
4. Surgical closure is recommended before school age. It can lead to significant problems such as congestive heart failure or atrial dysrhythmias later in life if not corrected. *(See figure 4-14)*

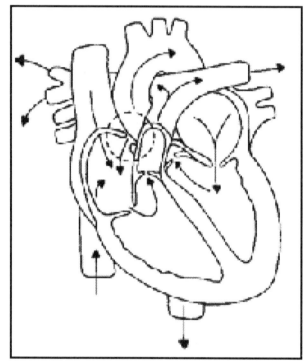

Figure 4-14

PEDIATRIC NURSING

PATENT DUCTUS ARTERIOSUS (PDA)
(INCREASED PULMONARY BLOOD FLOW)

1. Abnormal opening between the aorta and pulmonary artery.
2. Usually closes within 72 hours after birth.
3. If it remains patent, oxygenated blood from the aorta returns to pulmonary artery.
4. Increased blood flow to the lungs causes pulmonary hypertension.
5. May require medical intervention with indomethacin (Indocin) administration or surgical closure. *(See figure 4-15)*

COARCTATION OF THE AORTA (OBSTRUCTION OF BLOOD FLOW FROM VENTRICLES)

1. An obstructive narrowing of the aorta.
2. The most common sites: aortic valve and aorta near ductus arteriosus.
3. Common finding: hypertension in the upper extremities and decreased or absent pulses in the lower extremities.
4. May require surgical correction. *(See figure 4-16)*

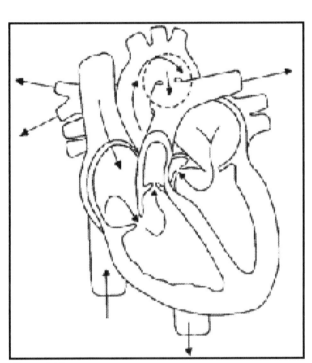

Figure 4-15

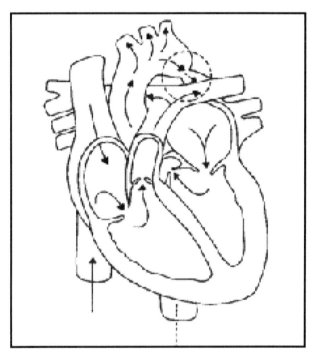

Figure 4-16

AORTIC STENOSIS (AS) (Obstruction of Blood Flow From Ventricles)

1. An obstructive narrowing immediately before, at, or after the aortic valve (It is most commonly valvular).
2. Oxygenated blood flow from the left ventricle into systemic circulation is diminished.
3. Symptoms are due to low cardiac output.
4. May require surgical correction.
   (See figure 4-17)

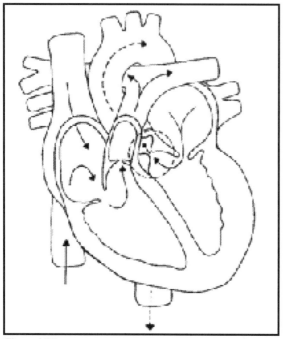

Figure 4-17

TRADITIONAL THREE T'S OF CYANOTIC HEART DISEASE

1. Transposition of the Great Arteries: pulmonary artery leaves the left ventricle and the aorta exits from the right ventricle.
2. Tetralogy of Fallott: a combination of four defects. (1) a ventricular septal defect (VSD); (2) an aorta placed over and above the ventricular septal defect (overriding aorta); (3) pulmonary stenosis (PS) that obstructs right ventricular outflow; and (4) right ventricular hypertrophy. The severity of the pulmonary stenosis is related to the degree of right ventricular hypertrophy and the extent of shunting.
3. Truncus Arteriosus: one artery (truncus), rather than two arteries (aorta and pulmonary artery), arises from both ventricles.

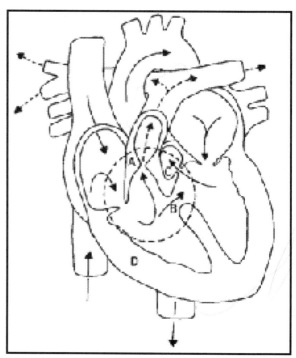

Figure 4-18

TETRALOGY OF FALLOT (TOF)
(DECREASED PULMONARY BLOOD FLOW) *(See figure 4-18)*

1. Consists of four defects:
   A. Pulmonary stenosis (PS).
   B. Ventricular-septal defect (VSD).
   C. Overriding aorta.
   D. Right ventricular hypertrophy.
2. Cyanosis occurs because unoxygenated blood is pumped into the systemic circulation.
3. Decreased pulmonary circulation due to the pulmonary stenosis.
4. Child experiences "tet" spells, or hypoxic episodes; relieved by child squatting or being placed in knee-chest position.
5. Requires staged surgery to correct.

> **HESI HINT:** Polycythemia is common in children with cyanotic defects.

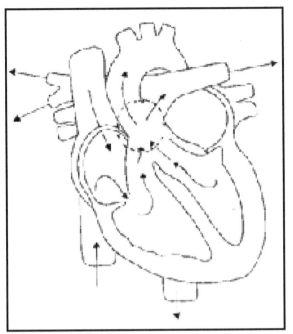

Figure 4-19

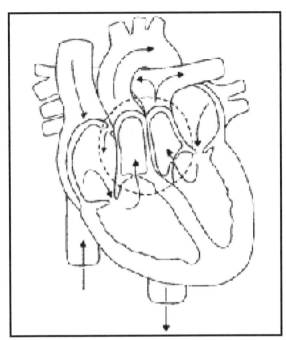

Figure 4-20

TRUNCUS ARTERIOSUS *(See figure 4-19)*

1. Pulmonary artery and aorta do not separate.
2. One main vessel receives blood from the left and right ventricles all together.
3. Blood mixes in right and left ventricles through a large ventricular septal defect (USD), resulting in cyanosis.
4. Increase pulmonary resistance results in increased cyanosis.
5. This congenital defect requires surgical correction; only the presence of the large VSD allows for survival at birth.

TRANSPOSITION OF THE GREAT VESSELS
(MIXED BLOOD FLOW)

1. The great vessels are reversed.
2. The pulmonary circulation arises from the left ventricle and the systemic circulation arises from the right ventricle.
3. This is incompatible with life unless coexisting VSD, ASD and/or PDA is present.
4. The diagnosis is a MEDICAL EMERGENCY. The child will receive prostaglandin E (PGE) to keep ductus open. *(See figure 4-20)*

CARE OF CHILDREN WITH CHD
NURSING ASSESSMENT
Congenital Heart Disease Manifestations

1. Murmur (present or absent; thrill, or rub).
2. Cyanosis, clubbing of digits (usually after age 2).
3. Poor feeding, poor weight gain - FTT.
4. Frequent regurgitation.
5. Frequent respiratory infections.
6. Activity intolerance, fatigue.

Assess for the following:

1. Heart rate and rhythm and heart sounds.
2. Pulses (quality and symmetry).

> **HESI HINT:** For normal cardiac rates in children, see Respiratory in this chapter. The heart rate of a child will increase with crying or fever.

3. Blood pressure (upper and lower extremities).
4. History of maternal infection during pregnancy.

ANALYSIS (NURSING DIAGNOSES)

1. Decrease in cardiac output related to…
2. Activity intolerance related to…
3. Alteration in growth and development related to…

NURSING PLANS AND INTERVENTIONS

1. Provide care for the child with cardiovascular dysfunction.
   A. Maintain nutritional status; feed small, frequent feedings. Provide high-calorie formula.

211

    B.   Maintain hydration (polycythemia increases risk for thrombus formation).
    C.   Maintain neutral thermal environment.
    D.   Plan frequent rest periods.
    E.   Organize activities to disturb child only as indicated.
    F.   Administer digoxin/diuretics as prescribed.
    G.   Monitor for signs of deteriorating condition or Congestive Heart Failure (CHF).
    H.   Teach family the need for prophylactic antibiotics prior to any dental or invasive procedures due to risk of endocarditis.

2.   Assist with diagnostic tests and support family during diagnosis.
    A.   EKG.
    B.   Echocardiography.

3.   Prepare family and child for cardiac catheterization (conducted when surgery is probable or as an intervention for certain procedures).
    A.   Risks of catheterization are similar to those for a child undergoing cardiac surgery:
        1)   Arrhythmias.
        2)   Bleeding.
        3)   Perforation.
        4)   Phlebitis.
        5)   Arterial obstruction at the entry site.
    B.   Child requires reassurance and close monitoring post catheterization.
        1)   Vital signs.
        2)   Pulses.
        3)   Incision site.
        4)   Cardiac rhythm.
    C.   Prepare family and child (as able) for surgical intervention if necessary.

4.   Prepare child as appropriate for age.
    A.   Show to ICU.
    B.   Explain chest tubes, IVs, monitors, dressings, and ventilator.
    C.   Show family/child waiting area for families.
    D.   Use a doll or simple drawing for explanations.
    E.   Provide emotional support.

HESI HINT: Basic difference between cyanotic and acyanotic defects:
- **Acyanotic:** Has abnormal circulation, however, all blood entering the systemic circulation is oxygenated.
- **Cyanotic:** Has abnormal circulation with unoxygenated blood entering systemic circulation.

CHF: Congestive heart failure is more often associated with acyanotic defects.

CONGESTIVE HEART FAILURE (CHF)
DESCRIPTION: Condition in which the heart is unable to effectively pump the volume of blood that is presented to it.

HESI HINT: CHF is a common complication of congenital heart disease. It reflects the increased workload of the heart resulting from shunts or obstructions. The two objectives in treating CHF are to reduce the workload of the heart and increase cardiac output.

NURSING ASSESSMENT
1.   Tachypnea, shortness of breath.
2.   Tachycardia.
3.   Difficulty feeding.
4.   Cyanosis.
5.   Grunting, wheezing, pulmonary congestion.
6.   Edema (face, eyes of infants), weight gain.
7.   Diaphoresis (especially head).
8.   Hepatomegaly.

ANALYSIS (NURSING DIAGNOSES)
1.   Decreased cardiac output related to…
2.   Impaired gas exchange related to…

NURSING PLANS AND INTERVENTIONS
1.   Monitor vital signs frequently and report signs of increasing distress.
2.   Assess respiratory functioning frequently.
3.   Elevate head of bed or use infant seat.
4.   Administer oxygen therapy as prescribed.
5.   Administer digoxin and diuretics as prescribed. *(See figure 4-21, Managing Digoxin)*
6.   Weigh frequently (may be every shift for infants).
7.   Maintain strict I&O, weigh diapers (1gm=1cc).
8.   Report any unusual weight gains.
9.   Provide low-sodium diet or formula.
10.   Gavage feed infants if unable to get adequate nutrition by mouth.
11.   Continue care for infant or child with a congenital defect as indicated.
12.   See Nursing Plans and Interventions, Cyanotic Heart Defects.

HESI HINT: When frequent weighings are required, weigh client on the same scale at same time of day so that accurate comparisons can be made.

MANAGING DIGOXIN	
ADMINISTRATION	**TOXICITY**
• Prior to administering, nurse MUST take child's apical pulse to assess for bradycardia. Hold dose if pulse is below normal heart rate for child's age. • Therapeutic blood levels of digoxin are 0.8 to 2.0 ng/ml (nanograms). • Teach families safe home administration of digoxin: → Administer on a regular basis; Do NOT skip or make up doses. → Give one hour before or two hours after meals. Do NOT mix with formula or food. → Take child's pulse prior to administration and know when to call the caregiver. → Keep in safe place, e.g., a locked cabinet.	• Nurse must be acutely aware of the signs of digoxin toxicity. A small child or infant cannot describe feeling bad or nauseated. • Vomiting is an early, common sign of toxicity. This symptom is often overlooked because infants often "spit-up." • Other GI symptoms include: anorexia, diarrhea, and abdominal pain. • Neurologic signs include: fatigue, muscle weakness, and drowsiness. • Hypokalemia can increase digoxin toxicity.

Figure 4-21

RHEUMATIC FEVER

DESCRIPTION: An inflammatory disease.

1. Rheumatic fever is the most common cause of ACQUIRED heart disease in children. It usually affects the aortic and mitral valves of the heart.
2. Rheumatic fever is associated with an antecedent beta hemolytic strep infection.
3. Rheumatic fever is a collagen disease that injures heart, blood vessels, joints, and subcutaneous tissue.

NURSING ASSESSMENT

1. Chest pain, shortness of breath (carditis).
2. Tachycardia, even during sleep.
3. Migratory large joint pain.
4. Chorea (irregular, involuntary movements).
5. Rash (Erythema marginatum).
6. Subcutaneous nodules over bony prominences.
7. Fever.
8. Lab findings:
   A. Elevated ESR (erythrocyte sedimentation rate).
   B. Elevated ASO titer (antistreptolysin O).

ANALYSIS (NURSING DIAGNOSES)

1. Alteration in cardiac output related to ...
2. Potential for injury related to ...

NURSING PLANS AND INTERVENTIONS

1. Monitor vital signs.
2. Assess for increasing signs of cardiac distress.
3. Encourage bed rest (as needed during febrile illness).
4. Assist with ambulation.
5. Reassure child/family that chorea is temporary.
6. Administer prescribed medications
   A. Penicillin or erythromycin.
   B. Aspirin for anti-inflammatory and anticoagulant actions.
7. Teach home care program:
   A. Explain the necessity for prophylactics.
      1) Antibiotics taken either orally or IM. Oral penicillin, b.i.d.
      2) IM Penicillin G, each month. *(See figure 4-22 Anti-Infective)*
   B. Inform dentist and other health care providers of diagnosis so they can evaluate the necessity for prophylactic antibiotics.

ANTI-INFECTIVE			
DRUGS	**INDICATIONS**	**ADVERSE REACTIONS**	**NURSING IMPLICATIONS**
penicillin G (Bicillin)	• Prophylaxis for recurrence of rheumatic fever	• Allergic reactions ranging from rashes to anaphylactic shock and death	• Penicillin G is released very slowly over several weeks giving sustained levels of concentration • Have emergency equipment available wherever medication is administered • ALWAYS determine existence of allergies to penicillin and cephalosporins, check chart/ record and inquire of client/family

Figure 4-22

REVIEW QUESTIONS

CARDIOVASCULAR DISORDERS

1. **Differentiate between a right to left and left to right shunt in cardiac disease.**
2. **List the four defects associated with Tetralogy of Fallott.**
3. **List the common signs of cardiac problems in an infant.**
4. **What are the two objectives in treating congestive heart failure?**
5. **Describe nursing interventions to reduce the workload of the heart.**
6. **What position would best relieve the child experiencing a "tet" spell?**
7. **What are common signs of digoxin toxicity?**
8. **List five risks of cardiac catheterization.**
9. **What cardiac complications are associated with rheumatic fever?**
10. **What medications are used to treat rheumatic fever?**

ANSWERS TO REVIEW QUESTIONS

1. A left to right shunt moves oxygenated blood back through the pulmonary circulation. A right to left shunt bypasses the lungs and delivers unoxygenated blood to the systemic circulation causing cyanosis.
2. VSD, overriding aorta, pulmonary stenosis and right ventricular hypertrophy.
3. Poor feeding, poor weight gain, respiratory distress/infections, edema and cyanosis.
4. Reduce the workload of the heart and increase cardiac output.
5. Small, frequent feedings or gavage feedings. Plan frequent rest periods. Maintain a neutral thermal environment. Organize activities to disturb child only as indicated.
6. Knee-chest position, or squatting.
7. Diarrhea, fatigue, weakness, nausea and vomiting. The nurse should check for bradycardia prior to administration.
8. Arrhythmia, bleeding, perforation, phlebitis, and obstruction of the arterial entry site.
9. Aortic valve stenosis and mitral valve stenosis.
10. Penicillin, erythromycin, and aspirin.

Neuromuscular Disorders

Down Syndrome
DESCRIPTION: The most common chromosomal abnormality in children.
1. Down syndrome is evidenced by various physical characteristics and mental retardation.
2. Down syndrome results from a trisomy of chromosome 21.
3. Down syndrome is associated with maternal age over 35 as well as paternal age.

Nursing Assessment
1. Common physical characteristics:
    A. Flat, broad nasal bridge.
    B. Inner epicanthal eye folds.
    C. Upward, outward slant of eyes.
    D. Protruding tongue.
    E. Short neck.
    F. Transverse palmar crease (Simian).
    G. Hyperextensible and lax joints (hypotonia).
2. Common associated problems:
    A. Cardiac defects.
    B. Respiratory infections.
    C. Feeding difficulties.
    D. Delayed developmental skills.
    E. Mental retardation.

Analysis (Nursing Diagnoses)
1. Alteration in growth and development related to…
2. Potential alteration in parenting related to…

Nursing Plans and Interventions
1. Assist and support parents during the diagnostic process.
2. Assess and monitor growth and development.
3. Teach use of bulb syringe for suctioning nares.
4. Teach signs of respiratory infection.
5. Assist family with feeding problems.
6. Feed to back and side of mouth.
7. Monitor for signs of cardiac difficulty or respiratory infection.
8. Refer family to early intervention program.
9. Refer to other specialists as indicated: nutritionist, speech therapist, physical therapist, and occupational therapist.

> **HESI HINT:** The nursing goal in caring for children with Down syndrome is to help the child reach his/her OPTIMAL level of functioning.

Cerebral Palsy (CP)
DESCRIPTION: A nonprogressive injury to the motor centers of the brain causing neuromuscular problems of spasticity or dyskinesia (involuntary movements).
1. Associated problems may include mental retardation and seizures.
2. Etiology includes:
    A. Anoxic injury before, during, or after birth.
    B. Maternal infections.
    C. Kernicterus.
    D. Low birth weight (major risk factor).

Nursing Assessment
1. Persistent neonatal reflexes (Moro, tonic neck) after 6 months.
2. Delayed developmental milestones.
3. Apparent early preference for one hand.
4. Poor suck, tongue thrust.
5. Spasticity (may be described as "difficulty with diapering" by mother/caregiver).
6. Scissoring of legs is a common characteristic of spastic cerebral palsy (legs are extended and crossed over each other, feet are plantar flexed).
7. Involuntary movements.
8. Seizures.

Analysis (Nursing Diagnoses)
1. Alteration in growth and development related to…
2. Potential alteration in nutrition: less than body requirements related to…

Nursing Plans and Interventions
1. Identify CP through follow-up of high-risk infants such as premature infants.
2. Refer to community-based agencies.
3. Coordinate with physical therapist, occupational therapist, speech therapist, nutritionist, orthopedic surgeon, and neurologist.

> **HESI HINT:** Feed infant or child with cerebral palsy using nursing interventions aimed at preventing aspiration. Position child upright and support the lower jaw.

4. Support family through grief process at diagnosis and throughout the child's life. Caring for severely affected children is very challenging.
5. Administer anticonvulsant medications such as Dilantin if prescribed.
6. Administer diazepam (Valium) for muscle spasms if prescribed.

Attention Deficit Disorder/ Attention Deficit Hyperactivity Disorder

DESCRIPTION: It is classified under DSM-IV. However, recent studies indicate that these disorders are neurological. *(See Psychiatric Nursing)*

Spina Bifida

DESCRIPTION: A malformation of the vertebrae and spinal cord resulting in varying degrees of disability and deformity.

1. Spina bifida occulta is a defect of vertebrae only. No sac is present and it is usually a benign condition, although bowel and bladder problems may occur.
2. With meningocele and myelomeningocele, a sac is present at some point along the spine.
3. Meningocele contains only meninges and spinal fluid and has less neurological involvement than a myelomeningocele.
4. Myelomeningocele is more severe than meningocele because the sac contains spinal fluid, meninges, and nerves.
5. The severity of neurologic impairment is determined by the anatomic level of the defect.
6. All children with a history of spina bifida should be screened for latex allergies.
7. Prevention: folic acid 0.4 mg at least 3 months prior to pregnancy.

Nursing Assessment

1. Spina bifida occulta: dimple with/without hair tuft at base of spine.
2. Presence of sac in myelomeningocele is usually lumbar or lumbosacral.
3. Flaccid paralysis and limited or no feeling below the defect.
4. Head circumference at variance with norms on growth grids.
5. Associated problems.
   A. Hydrocephalus (90% with myelomeningocele).
   B. Neurogenic bladder, poor anal sphincter tone.
   C. Congenital dislocated hips.
   D. Club feet.
   E. Skin problems associated with anesthesia below the defect.
   F. Scoliosis.

Analysis (Nursing Diagnoses)

1. Potential for infection related to...
2. Alteration in urinary elimination patterns related to ...

3. Impaired physical mobility related to...

Nursing Plans and Interventions

1. Preoperative:
   A. Keep sac free of stool and urine.
   B. Cover sac with moist sterile dressing.
   C. Elevate foot of bed and position on abdomen with legs abducted.
   D. Measure head circumference at least every 8/hours/every shift; check fontanel.
   E. Assess neurological function.
   F. Monitor for signs of infection.
   G. Empty bladder using Credé's method, or catheterize if needed.
   H. Promote parent-infant bonding.
2. Postoperative:
   A. Same as preoperative.
   B. Assess incision for drainage/infection.
   C. Assess neurological function.
3. Long-term care:
   A. Teach family catheterization program when child is young.
   B. Help older children to learn self-catheterization.
   C. Administer Pro-Banthine or Urecholine as prescribed to improve continence.
   D. Develop bowel program:
      1) High-fiber diet.
      2) Increased fluids.
      3) Regular fluids.
      4) Suppositories, as needed.
   E. Assess skin condition frequently.
   F. Assist with ROM exercises, ambulation, and bracing, if client is able.
   G. Coordinate with team members: neurologist, orthopedist, urologist, physical therapist, and nutritionist.
4. Support independent functioning of child.
5. Assist family to make realistic developmental expectations of child.

Hydrocephalus

DESCRIPTION: A condition characterized by an abnormal accumulation of cerebral spinal fluid (CSF) within the ventricles of the brain.

1. Usually caused by an obstruction in the flow of CSF between the ventricles.
2. Hydrocephalus is most often associated with spina bifida; can be a complication of meningitis.

NURSING ASSESSMENT

1. Older children show classic signs of increased intracranial pressure (ICP):
   A. Change in level of consciousness (LOC).
   B. Irritability.
   C. Vomiting.
   D. Headache on awakening.
   E. Motor dysfunction.
   F. Unequal pupil response.
   G. Seizures.
   H. Decline in academics.
   I. Change in personality.
2. Signs of increased ICP in infants:
   A. Irritable, lethargic.
   B. Increasing head circumference.
   C. Bulging fontanels.
   D. Widening suture lines.
   E. "Sunset" eyes.
   F. High-pitched cry.

ANALYSIS (NURSING DIAGNOSES)

1. Alteration in growth and development related to…
2. Potential for injury related to…

NURSING PLANS AND INTERVENTIONS

1. Prepare infant/family for diagnostic procedures.
2. Monitor for signs of increased ICP.
3. Maintain seizure precautions.
4. Elevate head of bed.
5. Prepare parents for surgical procedure.
   A. Shunt is inserted into ventricle.
   B. Tubing is tunneled through skin to peritoneum where it drains excess CSF.
6. Postoperative care:
   A. Assess for signs of shunt malfunction.
   B. Assess for signs of infection (meningitis).
   C. Monitor I&O closely.

7. Teach home care program:
   A. Watch for signs of increased ICP or infection.
   B. Child will eventually outgrow shunt and show symptoms of difficulty.
   C. Child will need shunt revision.
   D. Anticipatory guidance for potential problems with growth and development.

SEIZURES

DESCRIPTION: An uncontrolled electrical discharge of neurons in the brain.

1. Seizures are more common in children under age two.
2. Seizures can be associated with immaturity of the central nervous system (CNS), fevers, infections, neoplasms, cerebral anoxia, and metabolic disorders.
3. Seizures are categorized as generalized or partial.
   A. Generalized seizures are:
      1) Tonic-clonic (grand mal); consciousness is lost.
         a) Tonic phase – generalized stiffness of entire body.
         b) Clonic phase – spasm followed by relaxation.
      2) Absence (petit mal); momentary loss of consciousness, posture is maintained; has minor face, eye, hand movements.
   B. Partial seizures arise from a specific area in the brain and cause limited symptoms. Examples: focal and psychomotor seizures.

NURSING ASSESSMENT

1. Tonic-Clonic (grand mal):
   A. Aura (a warning sign of impending seizure).
   B. Loss of consciousness.
   C. Tonic phase is characterized by generalized stiffness of entire body.
   D. Apnea, cyanosis.
   E. Clonic phase is characterized by spasms followed by relaxation.
   F. Pupils dilated and nonreactive to light.

G. Incontinence.

H. Post-seizure: disoriented, sleepy.

2. Absence seizures (petit mal):

A. Usually occur between 4 to 12 years.

B. Lasts 5 to 10 seconds.

C. Child appears inattentive "day-dreaming."

D. Poor performance in school.

> **HESI HINT:** Medication noncompliance is the most common cause of increased seizure activity.

ANALYSIS (NURSING DIAGNOSES)

1. Potential for injury: trauma related to …

2. Medication noncompliance related to …

NURSING PLANS AND INTERVENTIONS

1. Maintain airway during seizure: turn on side to aid ventilation.

2. Do not restrain.

3. Protect from injury during seizure and support head (avoid neck flexion).

4. Document seizure, noting all data in assessment.

5. Maintain seizure precautions:

A. Reduce environmental stimuli as much as possible.

B. Pad side rails or crib rails.

C. Have suction equipment and oxygen quickly accessible.

D. Tape oral airway to the head of the bed.

> **HESI HINT:** Do NOT use tongue blade, padded or not, during a seizure. It can cause traumatic damage to mouth/oral cavity.

6. Support during diagnostic tests: EEG, CT scan.

7. Support during work-up for infections such as meningitis.

8. Administer anticonvulsant medications as prescribed.

A. For tonic-clonic seizures: phenytoin (Dilantin), carbamazepine (Tegretol), Phenobarbital (Luminal), and Cerebyx (fosphenoiton)-IV.

B. For absence seizures: ethosuximide (Zarontin), valproic acid (Depakene). *(See figure 4-23, Anticonvulsants)*

9. Monitor therapeutic drug levels.

10. Teach family about drug administration: dosage, action, and side effects.

ANTICONVULSANTS			
DRUGS	**INDICATIONS**	**ADVERSE REACTIONS**	**NURSING IMPLICATIONS**
phenobarbital (Luminal)	• Tonic-clonic and partial seizures • Is the longest acting of common barbiturates • Usually combined with other drugs	• Drowsiness • Nystagmus • Ataxia • Paradoxical excitement	• Therapeutic levels; 15 to 40 mcg/ml • Avoid rapid IV infusion • Monitor BP during IV infusion
phenytoin (Dilantin)	• Tonic-clonic and partial seizures	• Gingival hyperplasia • Dermatitis • Ataxia • Nausea, anorexia • Bone marrow depression • Nystagmus	• Therapeutic levels 10 to 20 mcg/ml • Monitor any drug interactions • Meticulous oral hygiene • Monitor CBC • Report to MD if any rash develops • For IV administration, flush IV before and after with normal saline ONLY • Do not administer with milk

Figure 4-23

DRUGS	INDICATIONS	ADVERSE REACTIONS	NURSING IMPLICATIONS
fosphenytoin sodium (Cerebyx)	• Generalized convulsive status epilecticus • Prevention/treatment of seizures during neurosurgery • Short-term parenteral replacement for phenytoin oral (Dilantin)	• Rapid IV infusion (greater than rate of 15 mg PE/minute) can cause hypotension • Severe: ataxia, CNS toxicity, confusion, gingival hyperplasia, irritability, lupus erythematosus, nervousness, nystagmus, paradoxical excitement, Stevens-Johnson syndrome, toxic epidural necrosis	• Used for short-term parenteral (IV infusion or IM injection) only • Should always be prescribed and dispensed in phenytoin sodium equivalents (P.E.) • Prior to IV infusion, dilute in D_5W or NS to administer solution of 1.5 to 25 mgPE/ml • Infuse at IV rate of no more than 150 mgPE/minute
valproic acid (Depakene)	• Absence seizures • Myoclonic seizures	• Hepatotoxicity especially in children under two years old • Prolonged bleeding times • GI disturbances	• Monitor liver function studies • Potentiates phenobarbital and Dilantin altering blood levels • Therapeutic levels: 50 to 100 mcg/ml
carbamazepine (Tegretol)	• Tonic-clonic, mixed seizures • Drowsiness • Ataxia	• Hepatitis • Agranulocytosis	• Monitor liver function tests while on therapy • Therapeutic level: 6 to 12 mcg/ml
lamotrigine (Lamictal)	• Partial seizures • Tonic-clonic seizures • Absence seizures	• Dizziness • Headache • Nausea • Rash	• Withhold drug if rash develops • Do not discontinue abruptly
clonazepam (Klonopin)	• Absence seizures • Myoclonic seizures	• Drowsiness • Hyperactivity • Agitation • Increased salivation	• Therapeutic levels 20 to 80 mcg/ml • Do not abruptly discontinue drug • Monitor liver functions tests, CBC, and renal function tests periodically

Figure 4-23 (continued)

BACTERIAL MENINGITIS

DESCRIPTION: Bacterial inflammatory disorder of the meninges that covers the brain and spinal cord.

1. Meningitis is usually caused by Haemophilus influenza, Type B (less prevalent), Streptococcus pneumoniae, or Neisseria meningitis.
2. The usual source of bacterial invasion is from the middle ear or nasopharynx.
3. Other sources of bacteria from wounds include fractures of the skull, lumbar punctures, or shunts.
4. Exudate covers brain, and cerebral edema occurs.
5. Lumbar puncture shows:
   A. Increased WBC.
   B. Decreased glucose.
   C. Elevated protein.
   D. Increased ICP.
   E. Positive culture for meningitis.

NURSING ASSESSMENT
1. Older children:
   A. Classic signs of increased ICP *(See Hydrocephalus).*
   B. Fever, chills.
   C. Neck stiffness, opisthotonos.
   D. Photophobia.
   E. Positive Kernig's sign (inability to extend leg when thigh is flexed anteriorly at hip.
   F. Positive Brudzinski's sign (neck flexion causes adduction and flexion movements of lower extremities).

2. Infants:
   A. Absence of classic signs.
   B. Ill, with generalized symptoms.
   C. Poor feeding.
   D. Vomiting, irritability.
   E. Bulging fontanel (an important sign).
   F. Seizures.

ANALYSIS (NURSING DIAGNOSES)

1. Alteration in sensory-perceptual related to ...
2. Potential for injury: trauma related to ...

NURSING PLANS AND INTERVENTIONS

1. Administer antibiotics (usually Ampicillin, penicillin, and/or Chloramphenicol) and antipyretics as prescribed.
2. Isolate for at least 24 hours.
3. Monitor vital signs and neuro signs.
4. Keep environment quiet and darkened to prevent over stimulation.
5. Implement seizure precautions.
6. Position for comfort: head of the bed slightly elevated, with client on side if prescribed.
7. Measure head circumference daily in infants.
8. Monitor I&O closely.
9. Hib vaccine to protect against *H. Influenzae* infection. *(See figure 4-7, Vaccines)*

> **HESI HINT:** Monitor hydration status and IV therapy carefully. With meningitis, there may be inappropriate ADH secretions causing fluid retention (cerebral edema) and dilutional hyponatremia.

REYE'S SYNDROME

DESCRIPTION: Acute, rapidly progressing encephalopathy and hepatic dysfunction.
1. Etiology includes antecedent viral infections such as influenza or chicken pox.
2. Etiology is often associated with aspirin usage.
3. Disease is staged by the clinical manifestations to reflect the severity of the condition.

NURSING ASSESSMENT

1. Usually occurs in school-age children.
2. Lethargy, rapidly progressing to deep coma (marked cerebral edema).
3. Vomiting.
4. Elevated SGOT/AST, SGPT/ALT, LDH, serum ammonia, decreased PT.
5. Hypoglycemia.

ANALYSIS (NURSING DIAGNOSIS)

1. Alteration in fluid volume: excess related to...
2. Ineffective breathing pattern related to...

NURSING PLANS AND INTERVENTIONS

1. Provide critical care early in syndrome.
2. Monitor neurological status: frequent noninvasive assessments and invasive ICP monitoring.
3. Maintain ventilation.
4. Monitor cardiac parameters, i.e., invasive cardiac monitoring system.
5. Administer Mannitol, if prescribed, to increase blood osmolality. *(See figure 4-24, Diuretic)*
6. Monitor I&O accurately.
7. Care for Foley catheter.
8. Provide family with emotional support.

BRAIN TUMORS

DESCRIPTION: The second most common cancer in children.
1. Most pediatric brain tumors are infratentorial, making them difficult to excise surgically.
2. Tumors usually occur close to vital structures.
3. Gliomas are the most common childhood brain tumor.

NURSING ASSESSMENT

1. Headache.

> **HESI HINT:** Headache upon awakening is the most common presenting symptom of brain tumors.

2. Vomiting (usually in the morning) often without nausea.
3. Loss of concentration.
4. Change in behavior or personality.
5. Vision problems, tilts head.
6. In infants: widening sutures, increasing frontal occipital circumference, tense fontanel.

ANALYSIS (NURSING DIAGNOSES)

1. Alteration in cerebral tissue perfusion related to...
2. Potential for injury: trauma related to...
3. Potential for infection (postoperative) related to...

NURSING PLANS AND INTERVENTIONS

1. Identify baseline neurological functioning.
2. Support child/family during diagnostic work-up and treatment.
3. If surgery is treatment of choice, provide preoperative teaching:
   A. Explain that head will be shaved.

B. Describe ICU, dressings, IVs, etc.
C. Identify child's developmental level and plan teaching accordingly.
4. Assess family's response to the diagnosis and treat family appropriately.
5. After surgery, position client as prescribed by the healthcare provider.

> **HESI HINT:** Most postoperative clients with infratentorial tumors are prescribed to lie flat and turn to either side. A large tumor may require that the child NOT be turned to the operative side.

6. Monitor IV fluids and output carefully. Over-hydration can cause cerebral edema and increased ICP.
7. Administer steroids and osmotic diuretics as prescribed. *(See figure 4-24, Diuretic)*
8. Support child/family to promote optimum functioning post-op.

> **HESI HINT:** Suctioning, coughing, straining, and/or turning causes increased ICP.

DIURETIC			
DRUGS	**INDICATIONS**	**ADVERSE REACTIONS**	**NURSING IMPLICATIONS**
mannitol (Osmitrol)	Osomotic diuretic used to reduce: • Cerebral edema • Postoperative swelling or trauma	• Circulatory overload • Confusion • Hypokalemia • Hyponatremia	• Use in-line filter for IV administration and avoid extravasation • Monitor I&O • Lasix may also be prescribed

Figure 4-24

MUSCULAR DYSTROPHY

DESCRIPTION: An inherited disease of the muscles, causing muscle atrophy and weakness.
1. Most serious and most common of the dystrophies is Duchenne muscular dystrophy, an X-linked recessive disease affecting primarily males.
2. Duchenne muscular dystrophy appears in early childhood (ages 3 to 5 years). It rapidly progresses causing respiratory or cardiac complications and death, usually by 25 years of age.

NURSING ASSESSMENT
1. Waddling gait, lordosis.
2. Increasing clumsiness, muscle weakness.
3. Gowers' sign: difficulty rising to standing position has to "walk" up legs using hands.
4. Pseudohypertrophy of muscles (especially noted in calves) due to fat deposits.
5. Muscle degeneration, especially the thigh and fatty infiltrates (detected with muscle biopsy). Cardiac muscle is also involved.
6. Delayed cognitive development.
7. Elevated CPK and SGOT/AST.
8. Later in disease, scoliosis, respiratory difficulty, and cardiac difficulties occur.
9. Child is eventually wheelchair dependent and then confined to bed.

ANALYSIS (NURSING DIAGNOSES)
1. Impaired physical mobility related to…
2. Disturbance in self-concept related to…

NURSING PLANS AND INTERVENTIONS
1. Provide supportive care.
2. Provide exercises (active and passive).
3. Prevent exposure to respiratory infection.
4. Encourage a balanced diet to avoid obesity.
5. Support family's grieving process.
6. Support participation with Muscular Dystrophy Association.
7. Coordinate with health care team: physical therapist, occupational therapist, nutritionist, neurologist, orthopedist, and geneticist.

PEDIATRIC NURSING

REVIEW QUESTIONS

NEUROMUSCULAR DISORDERS

1. **What are the physical features of a child with Down syndrome?**
2. **Describe "scissoring."**
3. **What are two nursing priorities for a newborn with myelomeningocele?**
4. **List the signs and symptoms of increased ICP in older children.**
5. **What teaching should parents of a newly shunted child receive?**
6. **State the three main goals in providing nursing care for a child experiencing a seizure.**
7. **What are the side effects of Dilantin?**
8. **Describe the signs and symptoms of a child with meningitis.**
9. **What antibiotics are usually prescribed for bacterial meningitis?**
10. **How is a child usually positioned after brain tumor surgery?**
11. **Describe the function of an osmotic diuretic.**
12. **What nursing interventions increase intracranial pressure?**
13. **Describe the mechanism of inheritance for Duchenne muscular dystrophy.**
14. **What is "Gowers' sign?"**

ANSWERS TO REVIEW QUESTIONS

1. Simian creases of palms, hypotonia, protruding tongue, and upward/outward slant of eyes.
2. A common characteristic of spastic cerebral palsy in infants. The legs are extended and crossed over each other, the feet are plantar flexed.
3. Prevention of infection of the sac and monitoring for hydrocephalus (measure head circumference; check fontanel; assess neurological functioning).
4. Irritability, change in LOC, motor dysfunction, headache, vomiting, unequal pupil response, and seizures.
5. Signs of infection and increased ICP. *(See signs of Increased ICP and Meningitis)*. Shunt should not be pumped. Child will need revisions due to growth. Provide guidance for growth and development.
6. Maintain patent airway, protect from injury, and observe carefully.
7. Gingival hyperplasia of the gums, dermatitis, ataxia, GI distress.
8. Fever, irritability, vomiting, neck stiffness, opisthotonos, positive Kernig's sign, positive Brudzinski's sign. Infant does not show all classic signs, but is very ill.

9. Ampicillin, penicillin, and/or Chloramphenicol.
10. Flat on his/her side.
11. Osmotic diuretics remove water from the CNS to reduce cerebral edema.
12. Suctioning and positioning/turning.
13. Duchenne muscular dystrophy is inherited as an X-linked recessive trait.
14. Gowers' sign is an indicator of muscular dystrophy. The child has to "walk" up legs using hands to stand.

RENAL DISORDERS

ACUTE GLOMERULONEPHRITIS (AGN)

DESCRIPTION: An immune complex response to an antecedent beta-hemolytic streptococcal infection of skin or pharynx. Antigen-antibody complexes become trapped in the membrane of the glomeruli causing inflammation and decreased glomerular filtration.

NURSING ASSESSMENT
1. Recent streptococcal infection.
2. Mild to moderate edema (often confined to face).
3. Irritable, lethargic.
4. Hypertension.
5. Dark-colored urine (hematuria).
6. Slight to moderate proteinuria.
7. Elevated antistreptolysin (ASO) titer, elevated BUN and creatinine.

ANALYSIS (NURSING DIAGNOSES)
1. Alteration in fluid volume: excess, related to…
2. Potential for injury: trauma, related to…

NURSING PLANS AND INTERVENTIONS
1. Provide supportive care.
2. Monitor vital signs (especially BP) frequently.
3. Monitor I&O closely.
4. Weigh daily.
5. Provide low-sodium diet with NO added salt; low potassium, if oliguric.
6. Encourage bed rest during acute phase (usually 4 to 10 days).
7. Administer antihypertensives if prescribed.
8. Monitor for seizures (hypertensive encephalopathy).
9. Monitor for signs of congestive heart failure (CHF).
10. Monitor for signs of renal failure (uncommon).

HESI HINT: Decreased urinary output is FIRST sign of renal failure.

NEPHROTIC SYNDROME

DESCRIPTION: A disorder in which the basement membrane of the glomeruli becomes permeable to plasma proteins. Most often idiopathic in nature.

1. Usually occurs between ages 2 to 3 years.
2. Course may have exacerbations and remissions over several years.
3. *See figure 4-25, A Comparison of Acute Glomerulonephritis (AGN) and Nephrotic Syndrome*.

NURSING ASSESSMENT

1. Edema which begins insidiously becomes severe and generalized.
2. Lethargy.
3. Anorexia.
4. Pallor.
5. Frothy-appearing urine.
6. Massive proteinuria.
7. Decreased serum protein (Hypoproteinemia).
8. Elevated serum lipids.

ANALYSIS (NURSING DIAGNOSES)

1. Alteration in fluid volume: excess, related to…
2. Alteration in nutrition: less than body requirements related to…

NURSING PLANS AND INTERVENTIONS

1. Provide supportive care.
2. Monitor temperature, assess for signs of infection.
3. Protect from persons with infections.
4. Provide skin care (edematous areas are vulnerable).
5. Maintain bed rest during edematous phase.
6. Administer steroids such as Prednisone and cholinergics such as Urecholine as prescribed. *(See figure 4-27, Medications Used with Renal Disorders)*
7. Monitor I&O.
8. Measure abdominal girth daily.
9. Administer Cytoxan if prescribed (used if non-responsive to Prednisone).
10. Provide small, frequent feedings of a normal protein, low-salt diet. Will often receive IV albumin followed by diuretic.
11. Teach home care:
    A. Weigh child daily.
    B. Medication side effects.
    C. Signs of relapse. *(See Nursing Assessment Data Collection)*
    D. Prevention of infection.

A COMPARISON OF ACUTE GLOMERULONEPHRITIS (AGN) AND NEPHROTIC SYNDROME

VARIABLE	ACUTE GLOMERULONEPHRITIS (AGN)	NEPHROTIC SYNDROME
ETIOLOGY	Follows streptococcal infection	Usually idiopathic
EDEMA	Mild, usually around eyes	Severe, generalized
BLOOD PRESSURE	Elevated	Normal
URINE	Dark, tea-colored (hematuria) Slight/moderate proteinuria	Dark, frothy yellow Massive proteinuria
BLOOD	Normal serum protein Positive ASO titer	Decreased serum protein Negative ASO titer

Figure 4-25

URINARY TRACT INFECTION (UTI)

DESCRIPTION: A bacterial infection anywhere along the urinary tract (most are ascending).

NURSING ASSESSMENT

1. In infants:
    A. Vague symptoms.
    B. Fever.
    C. Irritability.
    D. Poor food intake.
    E. Diarrhea, vomiting, jaundice.
    F. Strong-smelling urine.
2. In older children:
    A. Urinary frequency.
    B. Hematuria.
    C. Enuresis.
    D. Dysuria.
    E. Fever.
3. Urine cultures often reveal presence of *E. coli*.

ANALYSIS (NURSING DIAGNOSES)

1. Alteration in urinary elimination patterns related to…
2. Knowledge deficit about medications related to…

NURSING PLANS AND INTERVENTIONS

1. Suspect and assess for UTI in infants who are ill.
2. Assess for recurrent urinary tract infections. In infants and young boys, UTI may indicate structural abnormalities of the urinary system.
3. Collect clean, voided or catheterized specimen, as prescribed. *(See figure 4-26, Collection of Urine Specimens)*
4. Administer antibiotics as prescribed.
5. Teach home program:
   A. Finish all prescribed medication.
   B. Follow-up specimens are needed.
   C. Avoid bubble baths.
   D. Increase acidic oral fluids; e.g., apple, cranberry juices.
   E. Void frequently.
   F. Clean genital area from front to back.
   G. Symptoms of recurrence. *(See Nursing Assessment Data Collection)*

VESICOURETERAL REFLEX

DESCRIPTION: Results from valvular malfunction and back flow of urine into the ureters (and higher) from the bladder. Severe cases are associated with hydronephrosis.

NURSING ASSESSMENT

1. Recurrent UTI.
2. Reflux common with neurogenic bladder.
3. Reflux noted on VCUG (voiding cystourethrogram).

ANALYSIS (NURSING DIAGNOSES)

1. Potential for infection related to…
2. Potential for injury: trauma related to…

NURSING PLANS AND INTERVENTIONS

1. Teach home program for prevention of UTI.
2. Teach family the importance of medication compliance, which usually leads to resolution of mild cases.
3. Provide support for children and families requiring surgery.
4. Explain the goal of ureteral reimplantation: stop reflux and prevent kidney damage.
5. Monitor postoperative urinary drainage (may be suprapubic and/or urethral).
   A. Measure output from EACH catheter.
   B. Assess dressing/incision for drainage.
   C. Restrain child's hands as necessary.
6. Maintain hydration with IV or oral fluids.
7. Manage pain relief postoperative:
   A. Surgical pain.
   B. Bladder spasms.

WILMS' TUMOR
(NEPHROBLASTOMA)

DESCRIPTION: A malignant renal tumor.
1. Wilms' tumor is embryonic in origin.
2. This tumor is encapsulated.
3. Occurs in young, preschool children.
4. With early detection, surgery, adjuvant chemotherapy, as well as radiation therapy postoperative, the prognosis is good.

NURSING ASSESSMENT

1. Mass in the flank area, confined to MIDLINE.
2. Parents often discover mass when bathing child.
3. Fever.
4. Pallor, lethargy.
5. Elevated BP (excess renin secretion).
6. Hematuria (rare).

ANALYSIS (NURSING DIAGNOSES)

1. Potential for injury: trauma related to…
2. Fear related to…

NURSING PLANS AND INTERVENTIONS

1. Support family during diagnostic period.
2. Protect child from injury; place a sign on bed stating, "NO ABDOMINAL PALPATION."
3. Prepare family and child for imminent nephrectomy.
4. Provide postoperative care.
   A. Monitor for increased BP.
   B. Monitor kidney function: I&O, urine specific gravity.
   C. Provide care for abdominal surgery client.
      1) Maintain NG tube.
      2) Check for bowel sounds.
   D. Support child/family during chemotherapy and/or radiation therapy.

HYPOSPADIAS

DESCRIPTION: Congenital defect of uretheral meatus in males. Urethera opens on ventral side of penis behind the glans.

NURSING ASSESSMENT

1. Abnormal placement of meatus.
2. Altered voiding stream.
3. Presence of chordee.
4. Undescended testes and inguinal hernia may occur concurrently.

ANALYSIS (NURSING DIAGNOSES)

1. Alteration in pattern of urinary elimination related to…
2. Potential disturbance in self-concept related to…

NURSING PLANS AND INTERVENTIONS

1. Prepare child and family for surgery (no circumcision prior to surgery).
2. Assess circulation to tip of penis postoperatively.
3. Monitor urinary drainage after urethroplasty.
    A. Foley catheter.
    B. Suprapubic tube.
    C. Urethral stent.
4. Restrain child's arms and legs as necessary.
5. Maintain hydration (IV and oral fluids).
6. Teach home care:
    A. Care of catheters.
    B. How to empty drainage bag.
    C. Prevention of catheter displacement or blockage.
    D. Increase oral fluids.
    E. Signs of infection.

COLLECTION OF URINE SPECIMENS

METHOD	DESCRIPTION FOR CHILDREN/INFANTS
CLEAN CATCH	• Best obtained using a urine bag to catch the specimen. • Apply from side to side or back to front. Diaper should be applied over the bag. • Check child frequently to note urination.
CATHETERIZATION	• Sterile feeding tube is often used to catheterize small children and infants.
STERILE SPECIMEN	• In small infants it is best collected by the physician performing a bladder tap. Urine is aspirated through a needle inserted directly into bladder. The nurse is responsible for making sure infant is appropriately hydrated and restrained during the procedure.

Figure 4-26

MEDICATIONS USED WITH RENAL DISORDERS

DRUGS	INDICATIONS	ADVERSE REACTION	NURSING IMPLICATIONS
bethanechol chloride (Urecholine)	• Cholinergic used to treat: → Urinary retention → Neurogenic bladder → Gastric reflux	• Orthostatic hypotension • Flushing • Asthmatic reaction • GI distress	• ***Do not give IV or IM (may cause circulatory collapse)*** • Monitor vital signs • Preferably give on empty stomach
prednisone (Deltasone)	• Adrenocorticosteriod used to treat: → Immunosupression (acts as an anti-inflammatory) → Edema (promotes diuresis in nephrotic syndrome)	• Mood changes • Increased susceptibility to infection • Cushingoid appearance (moon face and buffalo hump) • Acne • GI distress • Thrombocytopenia • Edema • Potassium loss • ***Growth failure in children***	• In children, every other day administration is best to avoid growth failure when drug is taken long term • Discontinuing this drug requires tapering dose • Avoid live virus vaccines in children receiving prednisone

Figure 4-27

MEDICATIONS USED WITH RENAL DISORDERS (CONTINUED)

DRUGS	INDICATIONS	ADVERSE REACTION	NURSING IMPLICATIONS
oxybutymin (Ditropan) **tolterodine** (Detrol)	• Genitourinary smooth muscle relaxants (antispasmodics) used to treat: → Uninhibited neurogenic bladder → Reflex urogenic bladder which are characterized by voiding symptoms of urgency, frequency, nocturia, and incontinence	• Increased susceptibility to urinary tract infection (UTI) • GI distress • Dry eyes • Dry mouth • Vision changes • Dizziness • Chest pain • Drowsiness	• Administered orally; available in extended-release forms • Do not administer with other medications which have anticholinergic effects • May exacerbate reflux esophagitis • Contraindicated in clients with untreated glaucoma or any GI narrowing (GI obstruction may occur). • Safety for use with children has not been established

Figure 4-27 (continued)

REVIEW QUESTIONS

RENAL DISORDERS

1. Compare the signs and symptoms of acute glomerulonephritis (AGN) with nephrosis.
2. What antecedent event occurs with acute glomerulonephritis?
3. Compare the dietary interventions for acute glomerulonephritis and nephrosis.
4. What is the physiologic reason for the lab finding of hypoproteinemia in nephrosis?
5. Describe safe monitoring of prednisone administration and withdrawal.
6. What interventions can be taught to prevent urinary tract infections in children?
7. Describe the pathophysiology of vesicoureteral reflux.
8. What are the priorities for a client with Wilms' tumor?
9. Explain why hypospadias correction is done before the child reaches preschool age.

ANSWERS TO REVIEW QUESTIONS

1. AGN: gross hematuria, recent strep infection, hypertension, and mild edema. Nephrosis: severe edema, massive proteinuria, frothy-appearing urine, anorexia.
2. Beta-hemolytic strep infection.
3. AGN: low-sodium diet with no added salt. Nephrosis: high-protein, low-salt diet.
4. Hypoproteinemia occurs because the glomeruli are permeable to serum proteins.
5. Long-term prednisone should be given every other day. Signs of edema, mood changes, and GI distress should be noted and reported. The drug should be tapered, not discontinued suddenly.
6. Avoid bubble baths, void frequently; drink adequate fluids especially acidic fluids such as apple or cranberry juice, and clean genital area from front to back.
7. A malfunction of the valves at the end of the ureters allowing urine to reflux out of the bladder into the ureters and possibly the kidneys.
8. Protect the child from injury to the encapsulated tumor. Prepare the family/child for surgery.
9. Preschoolers fear castration, are achieving sexual identity, and acquiring independent toileting skills.

GASTROINTESTINAL DISORDERS
CLEFT LIP AND/OR PALATE

DESCRIPTION: Malformations of the face and oral cavity which seem to be multi-factorial in inheritance.

1. Cleft lip is readily apparent.
2. Cleft palate may not be identified until the infant has difficulty with feeding.
3. Initial closure of cleft lip is performed when infant weighs approximately 10 pounds and has an Hgb of 10 g/dl.
4. Closure of palate defect is usually performed at 1 year of age to minimize speech impairment.

NURSING ASSESSMENT
1. Failure of fusion of the lip and/or palate.
2. Difficulty sucking and swallowing.
3. Parent reaction to facial defect.

ANALYSIS (NURSING DIAGNOSES)
1. Alteration in nutrition: less than body requirements related to…
2. Alteration in parenting related to…

NURSING PLANS AND INTERVENTIONS
1. Promote family bonding and grieving during newborn period.
2. Inform family that successful corrective surgery is available.
3. In newborn period, assist with feeding.
   - A. Feed in upright position.
   - B. Feed slowly with frequent bubbling.
   - C. Use soft, large nipples, lamb's nipple, prosthetic palate, or rubber-tipped asepto syringe.
   - D. Support mother breastfeeding if possible.
4. Provide postoperative care:
   - A. Maintain patent airway and proper positioning.
     1) Cleft lip – on side or upright in infant seat (not prone).
     2) Cleft palate – on side or abdomen.
     3) Remove oral secretions carefully.
   - B. Protect surgical site:
     1) Apply elbow restraints.
     2) Minimize crying to prevent strain on lip suture line.
     3) Maintain "Logan Bow" to lip if applied.
   - C. Provide care for restrained child.
     1) Remove one restraint at a time and do range of motion exercises.
     2) Provide age appropriate stimulation.
   - D. Resume feeding as prescribed. Cleanse suture site after feeding – formula sitting on suture line may impede healing, lead to infection.
   - E. Encourage family participation in care and feeding.
5. Usually for cleft palate, coordinate long-term care with other team members: plastic surgeon, ENT specialist, nutritionist, speech therapist, orthodontist, pediatrician, nurse.

> **HESI HINT:** Typical parent/family reactions to a child with an obvious malformation such as cleft lip/palate are guilt, disappointment, grief, sense of loss, and anger.

ESOPHAGEAL ATRESIA WITH TRACHEOESOPHAGEAL FISTULA (TEF)

DESCRIPTION: Congenital anomaly in which the esophagus does not fully develop.

1. Most common: upper esophagus ends in a blind pouch with the lower part of the esophagus connected to the trachea.
2. This condition is a **CLINICAL AND SURGICAL EMERGENCY**.

NURSING ASSESSMENT
1. Three Cs of TEF in the newborn:
   - A. Choking.
   - B. Coughing.
   - C. Cyanosis.
2. Excess salivation.
3. Respiratory distress.
4. Aspiration pneumonia.

ANALYSIS (NURSING DIAGNOSES)
1. Potential for aspiration related to…
2. Alteration in nutrition: less than body requirements related to…

NURSING PLANS AND INTERVENTIONS
1. Provide preoperative care:
   - A. Monitor respiratory status.
   - B. Remove excess secretions (suction is usually continuous to blind pouch).
   - C. Elevate infant into anti-reflux position of 30 degrees.
   - D. Provide oxygen as prescribed.
   - E. NPO.

F.   Administer IV fluids as prescribed.
2.   Provide postoperative care:
   A.   NPO.
   B.   Administer IV fluids.
   C.   Monitor I&O.
   D.   Provide gastrostomy tube care and feedings as prescribed.
   E.   Provide pacifier to meet developmental needs.
   F.   Monitor child for postoperative stricture of the esophagus.
3.   Promote parent-infant bonding for high-risk infant.

PYLORIC STENOSIS

DESCRIPTION: A narrowing of the pyloric sphincter. The circular muscle of the pylorus hypertrophies to twice the normal size.

NURSING ASSESSMENT
1.   Usually occurs in first-born males.
2.   Vomiting (free of bile) usually begins after 14th day of life and becomes projectile.
3.   Hungry, fretful infant.
4.   Weight loss, failure to gain weight.
5.   Dehydration with decreased sodium and potassium.
6.   Metabolic alkalosis (decreased serum chloride, increased pH and bicarbonate or CO_2 content).
7.   Palpable olive-shaped mass in upper right quadrant of the abdomen.
8.   Visible peristaltic waves.

ANALYSIS (NURSING DIAGNOSES)
1.   Alteration in nutrition: less than body requirements related to…
2.   Fluid volume deficit: actual, related to…

HESI HINT: Children with cleft lip/palate and those with pyloric stenosis both have a nursing diagnosis "alteration in nutrition; less than body requirements."
- Cleft lip/palate is related to decreased ability to suck.
- Pyloric stenosis is related to frequent vomiting.

NURSING PLANS AND INTERVENTIONS
1.   Preoperative care:
   A.   Assess for dehydration.
   B.   Administer IV fluids and electrolytes as prescribed.
   C.   Weigh daily, monitor I&O.
   D.   Provide small, frequent feedings if prescribed.
2.   Prepare family for surgery by teaching that:
   A.   Hypertrophied muscle will be split.
   B.   Prognosis is excellent.
3.   Postoperative care:
   A.   Continue IV fluids as prescribed.
   B.   Provide small oral feedings with electrolyte solutions or glucose (usually 4 to 6 hours postoperative).
   C.   Position on RIGHT side in semi-Fowler's after feeding.
   D.   Burp frequently – do not want stomach to become distended and put pressure on surgical site.
   E.   Weigh daily, monitor I&O.

INTUSSUSCEPTION

DESCRIPTION: Telescoping of one part of the intestine into another part of the intestine, usually the ileum into the colon (called ileocolic).
1.   Partial to complete bowel obstruction occurs.
2.   Blood vessels become trapped in the telescoping bowel, causing necrosis.

NURSING ASSESSMENT
1.   Child under one year of age.
2.   Acute, intermittent abdominal pain.
3.   Screaming with legs drawn up to abdomen.
4.   Vomiting.
5.   "Currant jelly" stools (mixed with blood and mucus).
6.   Sausage-shaped mass in upper right quadrant, while lower right quadrant is empty (Dance sign).

ANALYSIS (NURSING DIAGNOSES)
1.   Alteration in tissue perfusion: bowel related to…
2.   Potential fluid volume deficit related to…

NURSING PLANS AND INTERVENTIONS
1.   Monitor carefully for shock or bowel perforation.
2.   Administer IV fluids as prescribed.
3.   Monitor I&O.
4.   Prepare family for emergency intervention.
5.   Prepare child for barium enema (which provides hydrostatic reduction). Two out of three cases respond to this treatment; if not, surgery is necessary.
6.   Provide postoperative care for infants who require abdominal surgery.

CONGENITAL/AGANGLIONIC MEGACOLON

(HIRSCHSPRUNG'S DISEASE)

DESCRIPTION: Congenital absence of autonomic parasympathetic ganglion cells in a distal portion of the colon and rectum.

1. Lack of peristalsis in the area of the colon where the ganglion cells are absent.
2. Fecal contents accumulate above the aganglionic area of the bowel.
3. Correction usually involves a series of surgical procedures:
   A. A temporary colostomy.
   B. Later, a reanastomosis and closure of the colostomy.

NURSING ASSESSMENT

1. Suspicion in newborn who fails to pass meconium within 24 hours.
2. Distended abdomen, chronic constipation alternating with diarrhea.
3. Nutritionally deficient child.
4. Enterocolitis may occur as an emergency event.
5. Ribbon-like stools in the older child.

ANALYSIS (NURSING DIAGNOSES)

1. Alteration in bowel elimination: constipation and/ or diarrhea related to…
2. Alteration in nutrition: less than body requirements related to…

NURSING PLANS AND INTERVENTIONS

1. Provide preoperative care.
   A. Begin preparation for abdominal surgery.
   B. Provide bowel cleansing program as prescribed.
   C. Insert rectal tube if prescribed.
   D. Observe for symptoms of bowel perforation:
      1) Abdominal distention – measure abdominal girth.
      2) Vomiting.
      3) Increased abdominal tenderness.
      4) Irritability.
      5) Dyspnea and cyanosis.
   E. Initiate preoperative teaching regarding colostomy.
2. Provide postoperative care:
   A. Check vital signs, axillary temperature.

   B. Administer IV fluids as prescribed.
   C. Monitor I&O.
   D. Care for NG tube with connection to intermittent suction.
   E. Check abdominal/perineal dressings.
   F. Assess bowel sounds.
3. Prepare family for home care:
   A. Teach care of temporary colostomy.
   B. Teach skin care.
   C. Refer family to enterostomal therapist and social services.
4. Prepare child and family for closure of temporary colostomy.
5. After closure, encourage family to be patient with child when toileting.
6. Begin toilet training after age two.

ANORECTAL MALFORMATIONS

DESCRIPTION: Congenital malformation of the anorectal section of the GI tract (imperforate anus).

1. Often associated with a fistula.
2. May also be associated with urinary tract anomalies.
3. Type and level of rectal anomaly determines surgical procedure and degree of bowel control possible.

NURSING ASSESSMENT

1. An unusual appearing anal dimple.
2. Newborn who does not pass meconium stool within 24 hours.
3. Meconium appearing from perineal fistula or in urine.

ANALYSIS (NURSING DIAGNOSES)

1. Alteration in bowel elimination related to…
2. Knowledge deficit about bowel or colostomy home program related to…

NURSING PLANS AND INTERVENTIONS

1. Determine newborn's first temperature, typically using a rectal thermometer to assess for imperforate anus.
2. Assess newborn for passage of meconium.

PEDIATRIC NURSING

3. Assist family's ability to cope with diagnosis.
4. Provide preoperative care to infant:
   A. Assess vital signs.
   B. Administer IV fluids (NPO).
   C. Monitor I&O.
5. Provide postoperative care for anal reconstruction.
   A. Keep perineal site clean.
   B. Position side-lying prone with hips elevated (decreased pressure on perineal sutures).
   C. Provide colostomy care if needed.
6. Home care:
   A. Teach home care of colostomy if necessary.
   B. With high-level defects, long-term follow-up is required.
   C. Toilet training is delayed and full continence may not be achieved.

REVIEW QUESTIONS
GASTROINTESTINAL DISORDERS
1. **Describe feeding techniques for the child with cleft lip or palate.**
2. **List the signs and symptoms of esophageal atresia with TEF.**
3. **What nursing actions are initiated for the newborn with suspected esophageal atresia with TEF?**
4. **Describe the postoperative nursing care for an infant with pyloric stenosis.**
5. **Describe why a barium enema is used to treat intussusception.**
6. **Describe the preoperative nursing care for a child with Hirschsprung's disease.**
7. **What care is needed for the child with a temporary colostomy?**
8. **What are the signs of anorectal malformation?**
9. **What are the priorities for a child undergoing abdominal surgery?**

ANSWERS TO REVIEW QUESTIONS
1. Lamb's nipple, or prosthesis. Feed child upright with frequent bubbling.
2. Choking, coughing, cyanosis, and excess salivation.
3. NPO immediately and suction secretions.
4. Maintain IV hydration and provide small, frequent oral feedings of glucose and/or electrolyte solutions within 4 to 6 hours.

Gradually increase to full strength formula. Position on right side in semi-Fowler's position after feeding.
5. A barium enema reduces the telescoping of the intestine through hydrostatic pressure without surgical intervention.
6. Check vital signs and take axillary temperatures. Provide bowel cleansing program and teach about colostomy. Observe for bowel perforation; measure abdominal girth.
7. Family needs education about skin care and appliances. Referral to an enterostomal therapist is appropriate.
8. A newborn who does not pass meconium within 24 hours, meconium appearing from a fistula or in the urine, or an unusual appearing anal dimple.
9. Maintain fluid balance (I&O, NG suction, monitor electrolytes), monitor vital signs, care of drains if present, assess bowel function, prevent infection of incisional area and other postoperative complications, and support child/family with appropriate teaching.

HEMATOLOGICAL DISORDERS

IRON DEFICIENCY ANEMIA
DESCRIPTION: Hemoglobin levels below normal range because of the body's inadequate supply, intake, or absorption of iron.
1. Iron deficiency anemia is the leading hematological disorder in children.
2. The need for iron is greater in children than adults due to accelerated growth.
3. Anemia may be caused by the following:
   A. Inadequate stores during fetal development.
   B. Deficient dietary intake.
   C. Chronic blood loss.
   D. Poor utilization of iron by the body.

NURSING ASSESSMENT
1. Pallor, paleness of mucous membranes.
2. Tiredness, fatigue.
3. Usually seen in infants 6 to 24 months old (times of growth spurt). Toddlers and female adolescents most affected.
4. Overweight "milk baby."
5. Dietary intake low in iron.
6. Milk intake greater than 32 oz/day.
7. Pica habit (eating nonfood substances).

8. Lab values:
    A. Decreased hemoglobin (Hgb).
    B. Low serum iron level.
    C. Elevated total iron binding capacity (TIBC).

HESI HINT: REMEMBER the Hgb norms.
- **Newborn:** 14 to 24 g/dl
- **Infant:** 10 to 15 g/dl
- **Child:** 11 to 16 g/dl

ANALYSIS (NURSING DIAGNOSES)
1. Alteration in tissue perfusion related to…
2. Activity intolerance related to…

NURSING PLANS AND INTERVENTIONS
1. Support child's need to limit activities.
2. Provide rest periods.
3. Administer oral iron (ferrous sulfate) as prescribed.

HESI HINT: TEACH FAMILY ABOUT ADMINISTRATION OF ORAL IRON:
- **Give on empty stomach (as tolerated for better absorption).**
- **Give with citrus juices (vitamin C) for increased absorption.**
- **Use dropper or straw to avoid discoloring teeth.**
- **Stools will become tarry.**
- **Iron can be fatal in severe overdose; keep away from children. Do not give with dairy products.**

---

4. Teach family nutritional facts concerning iron deficiency.
    A. Limit milk intake to less than 32 oz/day.
    B. Dietary sources of iron:
        1) Meat.
        2) Green, leafy vegetables.
        3) Fish.
        4) Liver.
        5) Whole grains.
        6) Legumes.
        7) For infants: iron-fortified cereals and formula.
    C. Teach appropriate nutrition for age.
5. Be aware of family's income and cultural food preferences.
6. Refer to nutritionist.
7. Refer to Women, Infants and Children's nutrition program, if available to family.

HEMOPHILIA
DESCRIPTION: Inherited bleeding disorder.
1. Transmitted by an X-linked recessive chromosome (mother is the carrier, her sons may express the disease).
2. A normal individual has between 50 and 200% factor activity in blood; the hemophiliac has from 0 to 25% activity.
3. The affected individual usually is missing either Factor VIII (classic, 75% of cases) or Factor IX.

NURSING ASSESSMENT
1. Male child. First "red flag" may be prolonged bleeding following circumcision.
2. Prolonged bleeding with minor trauma.
3. Hemarthrosis (most frequent site of bleeding).
4. Spontaneous bleeding into muscles and tissues (less severe cases have fewer bleeds).
5. Loss of motion in joints.
6. Pain.
7. Lab values:
    A. PTT is prolonged.
    B. Factor assays less than 25%.

ANALYSIS (NURSING DIAGNOSES)
1. Potential for injury: trauma, related to…
2. Knowledge deficit about home care related to…

NURSING PLANS AND INTERVENTIONS
1. Administer fresh frozen plasma, cryoprecipitate of fresh plasma, or lyophilized (freeze dried) concentrate as prescribed.
2. Administer pain medication as prescribed (analgesics containing *no* aspirin).
3. Follow blood precautions: risk of hepatitis.
4. Teach child/family home care:
    A. Recognize early signs of bleeding into joints.
    B. Local treatment for minor bleeds (pressure, splinting, ice).
    C. Administration of factor replacement.
    D. Dental hygiene: soft toothbrushes.
    E. Protective care: soft toys, padded bed rails.
    F. Wear medic alert identification.
5. Refer family for genetic counseling.
6. Support child/family during periods of growth and development when increased risk for bleeding occurs (i.e., learning to walk, tooth loss)

HESI HINT: Inherited bleeding disorders (hemophilia and sickle cell anemia) are often used to test knowledge of genetic transmission patterns. Remember:
- Autosomal recessive: Both parents must be heterozygous, or carriers of the recessive trait, for the disease to be expressed in their offspring. With each pregnancy, there is a 1:4 chance of the infant having the disease. However, all children of such parents CAN get the disease – NOT 25% of them. This is the transmission for sickle cell anemia, cystic fibrosis, and phenylketonuria (PKU).
- X-linked recessive trait: The trait is carried on the X chromosome, therefore, usually affects male offspring, e.g., hemophilia. With each pregnancy of a woman who is a carrier there is a 25% chance of having a child with hemophilia. If the child is male, he has a 50% chance of having hemophilia. If the child is female, she has a 50% chance of being a carrier.

SICKLE CELL ANEMIA

DESCRIPTION: Inherited autosomal recessive disorder of hemoglobin.
1. Occurs primarily in blacks and persons of eastern Mediterranean descent. One in 12 black persons is a carrier of the heterozygous gene HgbAS. Therefore, the risk of two black parents having a child with sickle cell disease is 0.7%.
2. Usually appears after 6 months of age.
3. Hemoglobin S (HgbS) replaces all or part of the normal hemoglobin, which causes the red blood cells to sickle when oxygen is released to the tissues.
   A. Sickled cells cannot flow through capillary beds.
   B. Dehydration promotes sickling.

HESI HINT: Hydration is very important in treatment of sickle cell disease because it promotes hemodilution and circulation of red cells through the blood vessels.

4. An HgbS has a less than normal lifespan (less than 40 days), which leads to chronic anemia.
5. Tissue ischemia causes widespread pathological changes in spleen, liver, kidney, bones, and central nervous system.

HESI HINT: Important terms:
- Heterozygous gene (HgbAS) sickle cell trait
- Homozygous gene (HbSS) sickle cell disease
- Abnormal hemoglobin (HGBS) disease and trait

NURSING ASSESSMENT
1. Black child, usually over 6 months of age.
2. Parents with sickle cell trait or sickle cell anemia.
3. Lab diagnosis: Hgb electrophoresis (differentiates TRAIT from disease).
4. Frequent infections (nonfunctional spleen).
5. Tiredness.
6. Chronic hemolytic anemia.
7. Delayed physical growth.
8. Vaso-occlusive crisis is the classic sign.
   A. Fever.
   B. Severe abdominal pain.
   C. Hand-foot syndrome (infants): painful edematous hands and feet.
   D. Arthralgia.
9. Leg ulcers (adolescents).
10. Cerebral vascular accidents (increased risk with dehydration).

ANALYSIS (NURSING DIAGNOSES)
1. Alteration in comfort: acute pain related to…
2. Potential for infection related to…
3. Knowledge deficit concerning crisis prevention related to…

NURSING PLANS AND INTERVENTIONS
1. Teach family prevention of crisis (hypoxia).
   A. Avoid strenuous exercise.
   B. Avoid high altitudes.
   C. Avoid infection and seek care at first sign of infection.
   D. Use of prophylactic penicillin if prescribed.
   E. Keep child well hydrated (more than 125 ml/kg/day).
   F. Enuresis is a complication of treatment and disease; do not withhold fluids at night.
2. For child hospitalized with a vaso-occlusive crisis:
   A. Administer IV fluids (one to two times maintenance) and electrolytes, as

prescribed, to increase hydration and treat acidosis.

- B. Monitor I&O.
- C. Administer blood products as prescribed.
- D. Administer analgesics including parenteral morphine for severe pain as prescribed.
- E. Use warm compresses – not ice.
- F. Administer prescribed antibiotics to treat infection.

3. Administer pneumococcal vaccine, meningococcal vaccine, and Haemophilus B vaccine as prescribed.
4. Administer hepatitis B vaccine as prescribed (for child at risk from transfusions).
5. Refer family for genetic counseling.
6. Support child/family experiencing chronic disease.

HESI HINT: Supplemental iron is not given to clients with sickle cell anemia. The anemia is not caused by iron deficiency. Folic acid is given orally to stimulate RBC synthesis.

ACUTE LYMPHOCYTIC LEUKEMIA

DESCRIPTION: A cancer of the blood-forming organs.

1. Acute lymphocytic leukemia accounts for about 80% of childhood leukemia.
2. Noted by the presence of lymphoblasts (immature lymphocytes) replacing normal cells in the bone marrow.
3. Blast cells are also seen in the peripheral blood count.
4. Acute lymphocytic leukemia is classified by whether it is:
   - A. T lymphocyte.
   - B. B lymphocyte.
   - C. Null cell (neither T cell or B cell).
5. Over 75% of children with acute lymphocytic leukemia have null cell, which has the best prognosis.
6. Signs and symptoms of leukemia result from replacement of normal cells by leukemic cells in the bone marrow and extramedullary sites.
7. Treatment has four phases:
   - A. Induction.
   - B. Sanctuary.
   - C. Consolidation.
   - D. Maintenance.

NURSING ASSESSMENT

1. Pallor, tiredness, weakness, lethargy due to anemia.
2. Petechia, bleeding, bruising due to thrombocytopenia.
3. Infection, fever due to neutropenia.
4. Bone joint pain due to leukemic infiltration of bone marrow.
5. Enlarged lymph nodes; hepatosplenomegaly.
6. Headache and vomiting (signs of central nervous system involvement).
7. Anorexia, weight loss.
8. Lab data: bone marrow aspiration reveals 80-90% immature blast cells.

ANALYSIS (NURSING DIAGNOSES)

1. Potential for infection related to…
2. Fear related to…
3. Knowledge deficit about disease process and chemotherapy related to…

NURSING PLANS AND INTERVENTIONS

1. Recommend private room.
2. Reverse isolation if prescribed.
3. Provide child with age-appropriate explanations for diagnostic tests, treatments, and nursing care.
4. Examine child for infection of skin, needle stick site, dental problems.
5. Administer blood products as prescribed.
6. Administer antineoplastic chemotherapy.
7. Monitor for side effects of chemotherapeutic agents. *(See Medical Surgical Nursing, Figure 3-49, Antineoplastic Chemotherapeutic Agents)*
   - A. Vincristine (Induction).
   - B. L-asparaginase (Induction).
   - C. Methotrexate (Sanctuary and Maintenance).
   - D. Mercaptopurine (6-MP) (Maintenance).

HESI HINT: Have epinephrine and oxygen readily available to treat anaphylaxis when administering l-asparaginase.

---

8. Provide care directed toward managing side effects and toxic effects of antineoplastic agents.
   - A. Administer antiemetics as prescribed.
   - B. Monitor fluid balance.
   - C. Monitor for signs of infection.
   - D. Monitor for signs of bleeding.
   - E. Monitor for cumulative toxic

effects of drugs: hepatic toxicity, cardiac toxicity, renal toxicity, and neurotoxcity.

    F.   Provide oral hygiene.

    G.   Provide small, appealing meals; increase calories and protein; refer to nutritionist.

    H.   Promote self-esteem and positive body image if child has alopecia, severe weight loss, or other disturbance in body image.

    I.   Provide care to prevent infection.

9. Provide emotional support for family in crisis.

10. Encourage family and child's input and control in plans and treatment.

> **HESI HINT:** Prednisone is frequently used in combination with antineoplastic drugs to reduce the mitosis of lymphocytes. Allopurinol, a xanthine-oxidase inhibitor, is also administered to prevent renal damage from uric acid build up during cellular lysis.

REVIEW QUESTIONS
HEMATOLOGICAL DISORDERS

1. **Describe what information families should be given when a child is receiving oral iron preparations.**

2. **List dietary sources of iron.**

3. **What is the genetic transmission pattern of hemophilia?**

4. **Describe the sequence of events in a vaso-occlusive crisis in sickle cell anemia.**

5. **Explain why hydration is a priority in treating sickle cell disease.**

6. **What should families and clients do to avoid triggering sickling episodes?**

7. **Nursing interventions and medical treatment for the child with leukemia are based on what three physiological problems?**

ANSWERS TO REVIEW QUESTIONS

1. Give oral iron on an empty stomach and with vitamin C. Use straws to avoid discoloring teeth. Tarry stools are normal. Increase dietary sources of iron.

2. Meat, green leafy vegetables, fish, liver, whole grains, legumes.

3. It is an X-linked recessive chromosomal disorder, transmitted by the mother and

expressed in male children.

4. A vaso-occlusive crisis is caused by clumping of red blood cells which block small blood vessels; therefore, the cells cannot get through the capillaries, causing pain and tissue/organ ischemia. Lowered oxygen tension affects the HgbS, which causes sickling of the cells.

5. Hydration promotes hemodilution and circulation of the red cells through the blood vessels.

6. Keep child well hydrated. Avoid known sources of infections. Avoid high altitudes. Avoid strenuous exercise.

7. Anemia (decreased erythrocytes). Infection (neutropenia). Bleeding thrombocytopenia (decreased platelets).

METABOLIC AND ENDOCRINE DISORDERS

CONGENITAL HYPOTHYROIDISM

DESCRIPTION: A congenital condition resulting from inadequate thyroid tissue development in utero. Mental retardation and growth failure occur if it is not detected and treated in early infancy.

NURSING ASSESSMENT
NEWBORN SCREENING: LOW T_4 (THYROXINE) AND HIGH TSH (THYROID STIMULATING HORMONE).

1. Symptoms in the newborn:

    A.   Long gestation (over 42 weeks).

    B.   Large hypoactive infant.

    C.   Delayed meconium passage.

    D.   Feeding problems (poor suck).

    E.   Prolonged physiologic jaundice.

    F.   Hypothermia.

2. Symptoms in early infancy:

    A.   Large protruding tongue.

    B.   Coarse hair.

    C.   Lethargic, sleepy.

    D.   Flat expression.

    E.   Constipation.

> **HESI HINT:** An infant with hypothyroidism is often described as a "good, quiet baby" by the parents.

ANALYSIS (NURSING DIAGNOSES)

1. Alteration in growth and development related to...

2. Knowledge deficit about medication program related to...

NURSING PLANS AND INTERVENTIONS
1. Perform newborn screening programs before discharge.
2. Assess newborn for signs of congenital hypothyroidism.
3. Teach family replacement therapy with thyroid hormone.
   A. Life long need.
   B. Give single dose in morning.
   C. Teach family to check pulse daily before giving thyroid medication.
   D. Signs of overdose include rapid pulse, irritability, fever, weight loss, diarrhea.
   E. Signs of underdose include lethargy, fatigue, constipation and poor feeding.
   F. Necessary for periodic thyroid testing.

PHENYLKETONURIA (PKU)

DESCRIPTION: An autosomal recessive disorder in which the body cannot metabolize the essential amino acid, phenylalanine.
1. The build-up of serum phenylalanine leads to CNS damage, most notably mental retardation.
2. Decreased melanin (produces light skin and blond hair).

NURSING ASSESSMENT
1. Newborn screening using the Guthrie test is positive when serum phenylalanine is 4 mg/dl.
2. Frequent vomiting, failure to gain weight.
3. Irritability, hyperactivity.
4. Musty urine odor.

HESI HINT: Early detection of hypothyroidism and phenylketonuria is essential in preventing mental retardation in infants. Knowledge of normal growth and development is important, since a lack of attainment can be used to detect the existence of these metabolic/ endocrine disorders and attainment can be used for evaluating the treatment's effect.

ANALYSIS (NURSING DIAGNOSES)
1. Alteration in growth and development related to...
2. Knowledge deficit about disease and diet related to...

NURSING PLANS AND INTERVENTIONS
1. Perform newborn screening at birth and again within three weeks of age.
2. Teach family dietary management.
   A. Stress importance of strict adherence to prescribed low-phenylalanine diet.
   B. Provide special formulas for infants: Lofenalac, PKU 1.
   C. Provide Phenyl-free (milk substitute) after age 2 years.
   D. Avoid dietary sources high in phenylalanine: high-protein foods, e.g., meat, milk, diary products, and eggs.
   E. Offer foods low in phenylalanine: vegetables, fruits, juices, cereals, breads, and starches.
   F. Work with nutritionist.
   G. Diet must be maintained at least until brain growth is complete (age 6 to 8 years).
3. Refer for genetic counseling.

HESI HINT: Nutrasweet™ (aspartame) contains phenylalanine and should not therefore, be given to a child with phenylketonuria.

DIABETES MELLITUS OR TYPE I DIABETES (IDDM)

DESCRIPTION: A metabolic disorder in which the insulin-producing cells of the pancreas are nonfunctioning as a result of some insult. *(See Medical Surgical Nursing for Additional Data)*
1. Heredity, viral infections, and autoimmune processes are implicated in diabetes mellitus.
2. Diabetes causes altered carbohydrate, protein, and fat metabolism.
3. Insulin replacement dietary management and exercise are the treatments.

NURSING ASSESSMENT
1. Classic three "Ps":
   A. Polydipsia.
   B. Polyphagia.
   C. Polyuria, enuresis (bedwetting) in previously continent child.
2. Irritability, fatigue.
3. Weight loss.
4. Abdominal complaints, nausea, and vomiting.
5. Usually occurs in school-age children, but can occur even in infancy.
6. *See Medical Surgical Nursing, figure 3-32, Hypoglycemia and Hyperglycemia Signs and Symptoms.*

1. Alteration in nutrition: less than body requirements related to…
2. Knowledge deficit about home program for diabetes related to…

> **HESI HINT:** Diabetes mellitus (DM) in children was typically diagnosed as insulin dependent diabetes (Type I) until recently. A marked increase in Type II DM has occurred recently in the U.S., particularly among Native-American, African-American, and Hispanic children and adolescents. Adolescence frequently causes difficulty with management since growth is rapid and the need to be like peers makes compliance difficult. Remember to consider the child's age, cognitive level of development, and psychosocial development when answering NCLEX-RN® questions.

NURSING PLANS AND INTERVENTIONS

1. Assist with diagnosis (fasting blood sugar greater than 120 mg/dl glucose).
2. If child is in ketoacidosis, provide care for seriously ill child (may be unconscious).
   A. Monitor vital signs and neuro status.
   B. Monitor blood glucose, pH, serum electrolytes.

> **HESI HINT:** When child is in ketoacidosis, administer regular insulin IV as prescribed in normal saline.

   C. Administer IV fluids, insulin, and electrolytes as prescribed.
   D. Assess hydration status.
   E. Maintain strict I&O.
3. Initiate home teaching program as soon as possible involving child and family.
   A. Insulin administration.
      1) Child usually receives two daily injections.
      2) Before breakfast dose is usually the larger dose.
      3) Use rapid-acting and intermediate-acting insulin.
   B. Dietary management (carbohydrate counting preferred):
      1) Meals and snacks.
      2) Growth and exercise needs.
      3) Basic four food groups, no concentrated sweets.
      4) Refer to nutritionist.

   C. Exercise:
      1) Regular, planned activity.
      2) Diet modification; snacks before or during exercise.
   D. Home glucose monitoring and urine testing.
   E. Signs and symptoms of hyperglycemia and hypoglycemia.
4. Initiate program for school-age child, as appropriate:
   A. Identify issues specific to school:
      1) P.E. class/exercise.
      2) Scheduled meal times and snacks.
      3) Cooperation with teachers and school nurse.
      4) Need to be like peers.
   B. School-age child should be responsible for most management.
   C. Wear medic alert ID bracelet.

> **HESI HINT:** There has been an increase in the number of children diagnosed with Type II diabetes. The increasing rate of obesity in children is thought to be a contributing factor. Other contributing factors include lack of physical activity and a family history of Type II diabetes.

REVIEW QUESTIONS
METABOLIC AND ENDOCRINE DISORDERS

1. How is congenital hypothyroidism diagnosed?
2. What are the symptoms of congenital hypothyroidism in early infancy?
3. What are the outcomes of untreated congenital hypothyroidism?
4. What are the metabolic effects of PKU?
5. What two formulas are prescribed for infants with PKU?
6. List foods high in phenylalanine content.
7. What are the three classic signs of diabetes?
8. Differentiate signs of hypoglycemia and hyperglycemia.
9. Describe the nursing care of a child with ketoacidosis.
10. Describe developmental factors that would impact the school-age child with diabetes.
11. What is the relationship between hypoglycemia and exercise?

1. Newborn screening revealing a low T4 and high TSH.
2. Large protruding tongue, coarse hair, lethargy, sleepiness, and constipation.
3. Mental retardation and growth failure.
4. CNS damage, mental retardation, and decreased melanin.
5. Lofenalac and PKU 1.
6. Meat, milk, dairy products, and eggs.
7. Polydipsia, polyphagia, and polyuria.
8. Hypoglycemia: tremors, sweating, headache, hunger, nausea, lethargy, confusion, slurred speech, anxiety, tingling around mouth, nightmares. Hyperglycemia: Polydipsia, Polyuria, Polyphagia, blurred vision, weakness, weight loss, and syncope.
9. Provide care for an unconscious child, administer regular insulin IV in normal saline, monitor blood gas values, and maintain strict I&O.
10. Need to be like peers. Assuming responsibility for own care. Modification of diet, snacks, and exercise in school.
11. During exercise, insulin uptake is increased and the risk of hypoglycemia occurs.

SKELETAL DISORDERS

FRACTURES

DESCRIPTION: Traumatic injury to bone.
1. Fractures can be classified according to types:
   A. Complete fractures: bone fragments completely separate.
   B. Incomplete fractures: bone fragments remain attached (e.g., greenstick, bends, buckle).
   C. Comminuted fractures: bone fragments from the fractured shaft break free and lie in the surrounding tissue. This type of fracture is rare in children.
2. Fractures that occur in the epiphyseal plate (growth plate) may affect growth of the limb.

HESI HINT: Fractures in older children are common as they fall during play and are involved in motor vehicle accidents.
- Spiral fractures (caused by twisting) and fractures in infants may be related to child abuse.
- Fractures involving the epiphyseal plate (growth plate) can have serious consequences in terms of growth of the affected limb.

NURSING ASSESSMENT
1. General condition:
   A. Visible bone fragments.
   B. Pain.
   C. Swelling.
   D. Contusions.
   E. Child guarding or protecting the extremity.
2. May be able to use fractured extremity due to intact periosteum.
3. The five "Ps" (may indicate the presence of ischemia).
   A. Pain.
   B. Pallor.
   C. Pulselessness.
   D. Paresthesia.
   E. Paralysis.

ANALYSIS (NURSING DIAGNOSES)
1. Potential alteration in tissue perfusion: peripheral, related to…
2. Alteration in comfort: acute pain related to…

NURSING PLANS AND INTERVENTIONS
1. Obtain baseline data and frequently perform neurovascular assessments.
   A. **PULSES**: Check pulses distal to the injury to assess circulation.
   B. **COLOR**: Check injured extremity for pink, brisk, capillary refill.
   C. **MOVEMENT** and **SENSATION**: Check injured extremity for nerve impairment; compare symmetry to uninjured extremity (child may guard injury).
   D. **TEMPERATURE**: Check extremity for warmth.
   E. **SWELLING**: Check for an increase in swelling (elevate extremity to prevent swelling).
   F. **PAIN**: Monitor for severe pain, which is not relieved by analgesics.
2. Report abnormal assessment **PROMPTLY**! Compartment syndrome may occur which results in permanent damage to nerves and

PEDIATRIC NURSING

vasculature of the injured extremity due to compression.

3. Maintain traction if prescribed. Note bed position, type of traction, weights, pulleys, pins, pin sites, adhesive strips, ace wraps, splints, and casts.
   A. Skin traction: force applied to skin:

> **HESI HINT:** Skin traction for fracture reduction should NOT be removed unless prescribed by healthcare provider.

   1) Buck's extension traction: lower extremity, legs extended, no hip flexion.
   2) Dunlop traction: two lines of pull on the arm.
   3) Russell traction: two lines of pull on the lower extremity, one perpendicular, one longitudinal.
   4) Bryant's traction: both lower extremities flexed 90° at hips (rarely used because extreme elevation of lower extremities causes decreased peripheral circulation).

   B. Skeletal traction: pin or wire applies pull directly to the distal bone fragment.
   1) 90 degree – 90 degree traction: 90 degree flexion of hip and knee; lower extremity is in a boot cast. Can also be used on upper extremities. *(See figure 4-28, 90° – 90°)*
   2) Dunlop traction may be used as skeletal traction.

> **HESI HINT:** Pin sites can be sources of infection. Monitor for signs of infection. Cleanse and dress pin sites as prescribed.

4. Maintain child in proper body alignment, restrain if necessary.
5. Monitor for problems of immobility.
6. Provide age appropriate play/toys.
7. Prepare child for cast application, use age appropriate terms when explaining procedures.
8. Provide routine cast care following application; petal cast edges.
9. Teach home cast care to family:
   A. Neurovascular assessment of casted extremity.
   B. Do not get cast wet.
   C. Do not stick anything under cast.
   D. Keep small objects, toys, and food out of cast.
   E. Modify diapering and toileting to prevent cast soilage.
   F. Hip spica: may use Bradford frame under small child to help with toileting; **DO NOT** use abduction bar to turn child.
   G. Follow-up care with healthcare provider.

> **HESI HINT:** Skeletal disorders affect the infant's or child's physical mobility, and typical NCLEX-RN® questions focus on appropriate toys or activities for the child who is on bedrest and/or immobilized.

90 ° - 90 ° Traction 90 ° Flexation of Hip and Knee
(Can also be used on upper extremeties)

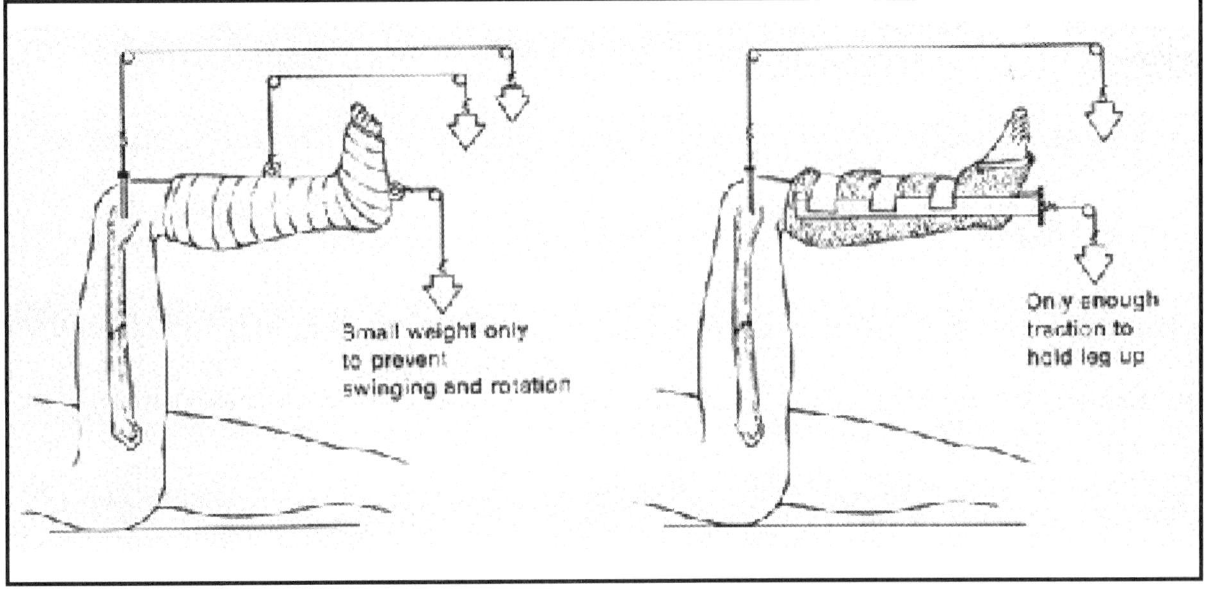
Small weight only
to prevent
swinging and rotation
Only enough
traction to
hold leg up

Figure 4-28

Congenital Dislocated Hip

(Developmental Dysplasia of HIP)

Description: Abnormal development of the femoral head in the acetabulum.

1. Conservative treatment consists of splinting.
2. Surgical intervention is necessary if splinting is not successful.

Nursing Assessment

1. Infant
   A. Positive Ortolani sign ("clicking" with abduction).
   B. Unequal folds of skin on buttocks and thigh.
   C. Limited abduction of affected hip.
   D. Unequal leg lengths.
2. Older child:
   A. Limp on affected side.
   B. Trendelenburg sign.

Analysis (Nursing Diagnoses)

1. Impaired physical mobility related to…
2. Knowledge deficit regarding home care related to…

Nursing Plans and Interventions

1. Perform newborn assessment at birth.
2. Apply abduction device/splint (Pavlik harness; Frejka or Von Rosen splint) as prescribed. Therapy involves positioning legs in flexed, abducted position.
3. Teach parents home care:
   A. Application/removal of device (worn 24 hours/day).
   B. Skin care and bathing (physician may allow parents to remove device for bathing).
   C. Diapering.
   D. Follow-up: care frequent adjustments due to growth.
4. Provide care for infant in Bryant's traction (used if splinting is ineffective).
   A. Maintain hips in 90° flexion.
   B. Elevate buttocks off bed.
   C. Monitor circulation to feet.
   D. Meet developmental needs for immobilized infant.
   E. Incorporate family in care.
   F. Prepare family for spica cast application.
5. Provide nursing care for a child requiring surgical correction.
   A. Preoperative teaching of child and family including cast application.
   B. Postoperative care:
      1) Assess vital signs.
      2) Check cast for drainage and bleeding.
      3) Perform neurovascular assessment of extremities.
      4) Promote respiratory hygiene.
      5) Administer narcotic analgesics. (Demerol/Morphine) either IV (preferred) or IM. ***(See figure 4-30, Medications Used with Skeletal Disorders)***

PEDIATRIC NURSING

6) Teaching family cast care when child gets home.

SCOLIOSIS

DESCRIPTION: Lateral curvature of the spine.
1. If severe, it can cause respiratory compromise.
2. Surgical correction with spinal fusion or instrumentation may be required if conservative treatment is ineffective.

NURSING ASSESSMENT
1. Occurs most frequently in adolescent females (10 to 15 years old).
2. Elevated shoulder or hip.
3. Head and hips not aligned.
4. While bending forward, a rib hump is apparent. (Ask child to bend forward from the hips with arms hanging free and examine child for a curve of the spine, rib hump, and hip asymmetry).

ANALYSIS (NURSING DIAGNOSES)
1. Impaired physical mobility related to…
2. Disturbances in self-concept: body image, related to…

NURSING PLANS AND INTERVENTIONS
1. Screen all adolescent children, especially females, during "growth spurt."
2. Prepare child/family for conservative treatment such as use of brace.
   A. Teach application of Milwaukee brace:
      1) Wear 23 hours/day.
      2) Wear T-shirt under brace to decrease skin irritation.
      3) Check skin for areas of irritation or breakdown.
   B. Suggest clothing modifications to camouflage brace.
   C. Reinforce prescribed exercise regime for back and abdominal muscles.
   D. Plan with adolescent to increase self-concept.
   E. Teach family that severe, untreated scoliosis can cause respiratory difficulty.

3. Prepare child/family for surgical correction if required.
   A. Teach child and family log-rolling technique.
   B. Practice respiratory hygiene.
   C. Orient to ICU.
   D. Discuss "postoperative tubes": Foley, NG tube, and chest tube (if anterior fusion is performed).
   E. Describe postoperative pain management; patient-controlled analgesic (PCA) may be used.
   F. Obtain a baseline neurological assessment.
4. Provide postoperative care:
   A. Perform frequent neurological assessments.
   B. Log-roll for five days. *(See figure 4-29, Log Rolling)*
   C. Administer IV fluids and analgesics as prescribed.
   D. Oral hygiene (client NPO).
   E. Monitor NG tube and bowel sounds.
   F. Assist with ambulation, provide body jacket; progressively ambulate.
   G. Teach child/family that body jacket will be worn for several months until the bone fusion is stable.
   H. Determine the need for a homebound teacher.
   I. Encourage child's participation in care to promote self-esteem.

JUVENILE RHEUMATOID ARTHRITIS (JRA)

DESCRIPTION: Chronic inflammatory disorder of the joint synovium.
1. Single or multiple joints may be involved.
2. May also have systemic presentation.
3. Occurs between ages 2 to 5 years and 9 to 12 years.

NURSING ASSESSMENT
1. Joint swelling and stiffness (usually large joints).
2. Painful joints.
3. Generalized symptoms; fever, malaise, and rash.
4. Periods of exacerbations and remissions.
5. Varying severity: may be mild and self-limiting or severe and disabling.
6. Lab data: Latex fixation test (usually negative), and elevated ESR.

7. Poorest prognosis:
   A. Positive rheumatoid factor.
   B. Polyarticular systemic onset.

ANALYSIS (NURSING DIAGNOSES)
1. Impaired physical mobility related to…
2. Alteration in comfort: chronic pain related to…

NURSING PLANS AND INTERVENTIONS
1. Plan home program of prescribed exercise, splinting, and activity.
2. Assist with identifying adaptations in routine, e.g., Velcro fasteners, frequent rest periods, etc.
3. Support maintaining school schedule and activities appropriate for age.
4. Teach medication regimen: combination drugs are used. *(See Medical Surgical Nursing)*
   A. Nonsteroidal, anti-inflammatory drugs:
      1) Aspirin.
      2) Tolmetin sodium.
      3) Ibuprofen.
      4) Naproxen.
   B. Antirheumatic drugs (Gold salts). *(See figure 4-30, Medications Used with Skeletal Disorders)*
   C. Corticosteroids (prednisone).
   D. Cytotoxic drugs (Cyclophosphamide, methotrexate).
5. Teach child/family side effects and toxic effects of prescribed drugs.
6. Inform child/family that optimum anti-inflammatory effects from drugs may take a month to achieve.
7. Encourage periodic eye exams for early detection of iridocyclitis to prevent vision loss.
8. Encourage family to allow child's independence.

> **HESI HINT:** Corticosteroids are used short term in low doses during exacerbations. Long-term use is avoided due to side effects and their adverse effect on growth.

LOG ROLLING
• Usually requires two or more persons depending on the size of the client.
• Client is carefully moved on a draw sheet to the side of the bed away from which they are to be turned (moved to the left if they are to face to the right).
• Client is then turned in a simultaneous motion (log-rolled), maintaining the spine in a straight position.
• Pillows are arranged for support and comfort, and they assist the client to maintain alignment.

Figure 4-29

MEDICATIONS USED WITH SKELETAL DISORDERS			
DRUGS	**INDICATIONS**	**ADVERSE REACTIONS**	**NURSING IMPLICATIONS**
meperidine HCL (Demerol)	• Narcotic analgesic used to treat acute pain	• Respiratory depression • Nausea • Vomiting	• Do not give if client has increased intracranial pressure • Has duration of action of 2 to 4 hours (shorter than codeine or morphine)
infliximab (Remicade) **methocarbamol** (Robaxin) **cyclobenzaprine** (Flexeril)	• Non narcotics to treat pain, stiffness, and discomfort	• Fever • Chills • Dizziness • Nausea • Drowsiness (robaxin) • Chest pain • Allergic response: rash, difficulty breathing, etc.	• Review History: heart disease (all) – thyroid disorders or use of MAOI's (Flexeril) • Remicade use can worsen TB

Figure 4-30

REVIEW QUESTIONS

SKELETAL DISORDERS

1. List normal findings in a neurovascular assessment.
2. What is compartment syndrome?
3. What are the signs and symptoms of compartment syndrome?
4. Why are fractures of the epiphyseal plate a special concern?
5. How is skeletal traction applied?
6. What discharge instructions should be included for a child with a spica cast?
7. What are the signs and symptoms of congenital dislocated hip in infants?
8. How would the nurse conduct scoliosis screening?
9. What instructions should the child with scoliosis receive about the Milwaukee brace?
10. What care is indicated for a child with juvenile rheumatoid arthritis?

ANSWERS TO REVIEW QUESTIONS

1. Warm extremity, brisk capillary refill, free movement, normal sensation of the affected extremity, and equal pulses.
2. Damage to nerves and vasculature of an extremity due to compression.
3. Abnormal neurovascular assessment: cold extremity, severe pain, inability to move the extremity, and poor capillary refill.
4. Fractures of the epiphyseal plate (growth plate) may affect the growth of the limb.
5. Skeletal traction is maintained by pins or wires applied to the distal fragment of the fracture.
6. Check circulation. Keep cast dry. Do not stick anything under cast. Prevent cast soilage during toileting or diapering. DO NOT TURN with abductor bar.
7. Unequal skin folds of the buttocks, ortolani sign, limited abduction of the affected hip, and unequal leg lengths.
8. Ask the child to bend forward from the hips with arms hanging free. Examine the child for a curve of the spine, rib hump, and hip asymmetry.
9. Wear the brace 23 hours per day. Wear T-shirt under brace. Check skin for irritation. Perform back and abdominal exercises. Modify clothing. Encourage the child to maintain normal activities as able.
10. Prescribed exercise to maintain mobility, splinting of affected joints, and teaching medication management and side effects of drugs.

Anatomy and Physiology of Reproduction

The Menstrual Cycle

Description: Composed of four (4) phases. The normal cycle is 21 to 45 days in length. The mean age for menarche (first menstruation) in the U.S. is 12.87 years or 1 to 3 years after breast budding. Pregnancy can occur from the very first menstrual cycle. Most women have ovulatory cycles within 24 months after menarche.

PHASES OF THE MENSTRUAL CYCLE	
PHASE	**DESCRIPTION**
MENSTRUAL PHASE	Days 1 to 5 of cycle. Shedding of the endometrium occurs as uterine bleeding, approximately 50 to 60 cc (<2 ounces).
HESI HINT: The menstrual phase varies in length for most women.	
PROLIFERATIVE (FOLLICULAR) PHASE	Day 5 to ovulation. Endometrium is restored under primary hormone influence of estrogen. In this pre-ovulatory phase, FSH (follicle stimulating hormone) is secreted by the anterior pituitary. Pre-ovulatory surge of LH (luteinizing hormone) affects one follicle and ovulation occurs.
SECRETORY (LUTEAL) PHASE	Ovulation to approximately 3 days before menstrual cycle. Estrogen levels level off and progesterone levels increase.
ISCHEMIC PHASE	If fertilization did not occur, the corpus luteum degenerates and estrogen and progesterone levels drop off causing the endometrium to become "blood starved," leading to menstruation.
HESI HINT: From ovulation to the beginning of the next menstrual cycle is usually exactly 14 days. In other words, ovulation occurs 14 days *before* the next menstrual period.	

Figure 5-1

HESI HINT: Sperm lives approximately 3 days and eggs live about 24 hours. A couple must avoid unprotected intercourse for several days before the anticipated ovulation and for 3 days after ovulation in order to prevent pregnancy.

FACTORS AFFECTING FERTILIZATION	
INDICATIONS OF OVULATION	**CONDITIONS FOR FERTILIZATION**
• Slight drop in temperature one day prior to ovulation with a one-half to one-degree rise in temperature at ovulation, that remains elevated for approximately 10 to 12 days. • Cervical mucus is abundant, watery, clear, and more alkaline. • Cervical os dilates slightly, softens, and rises in the vagina. • Spinnbarkeit (egg-white stretchiness of cervical mucus). • Ferning under microscope.	• Postcoital test demonstrates live, motile, normal sperm present in cervical mucus. • Fallopian tubes patent. • Endometrial biopsy indicates adequate progesterone and secretory endometrium. • Semen is supportive to pregnancy: 2 ml semen; at least 20 million sperm/cc; >60% normal; and >50% motile (moving forward).

Figure 5-2

IMPLANTATION AND FETAL DEVELOPMENT

IMPLANTATION	FETAL DEVELOPMENT	DESCRIPTION
• Fertilization takes place in ampulla (outer 1/3) portion of the Fallopian tube. • Zygote (fertilized ovum) takes 3 to 4 days to enter the uterus. • Takes 7 to 10 days to complete the process of nidation (implantation).	• Zygote • 12 to 14 days after fertilization	From the time the ovum is fertilized until it is implanted in the uterus.
	• Embryo • 3 to 8 weeks after fertilization	During this period, embryo is most vulnerable to teratogens: viruses, drugs, radiation, or infections can cause MAJOR congenital anomalies.
	• Fetus • 9 weeks from fertilization to term (38+ weeks)	Teratogen influence during fetal period results in fewer major anomalies.

Figure 5-3

MATERNAL PHYSIOLOGIC CHANGES DURING PREGNANCY

1. Pregnancy length is counted from the first day of last menstrual period (LMP).
   A. 280 days (approximately).
   B. 40 weeks.
   C. 10 lunar months (perfect 28-day months).
   D. 9 calendar months.
2. Pregnancy is divided into three 13 week trimesters:
   A. First trimester: from the first day of LMP through 13 weeks.
   B. Second trimester: 14 weeks through 26 weeks.
   C. Third trimester: 27 weeks to 40 weeks.

> **HESI HINT:** Because some women experience implantation bleeding or spotting, they do not know they are pregnant.

FETAL/MATERNAL CHANGES 8 WEEKS

FETAL DEVELOPMENT	MATERNAL CHANGES
• Rapid development • Heart begins to pump blood • Limb buds are well developed • Facial features discernible • Major divisions of brain discernible • Ears develop from skin folds • Tiny muscles are formed beneath this skin embryo • Weighs 2 grams	• Nausea persists up to 12 weeks • Uterus changes from pear to globular shape • Hegar's sign (softening of the isthmus of cervix) • Goodell's sign (softening of cervix) • Cervix flexes • Leukorrhea increases • Ambivalence about pregnancy may occur • No noticeable weight gain • Chadwick's sign appears (bluing of vagina) appears as early as 4 weeks gestation.

NURSING INTERVENTIONS

Teach prevention of nausea:
• Eat dry crackers before getting out of bed in the morning
• Eat small, frequent meals, avoid fatty foods, and avoid skipping meals.

Teach safety:
• Avoid hot tubs, saunas, and steam rooms throughout pregnancy (increases risk of neural tube defects in first trimester; hypotension may cause fainting)

Prepare for pregnancy:
• Discuss attitudes toward pregnancy
• Discuss value of early pregnancy classes that focus on what to expect during pregnancy
• Provide information about childbirth preparation classes
• Include father/family in preparation for childbirth (Expectant fathers experience many of the same feelings/ conflicts experienced by the expectant mother

Figure 5-4

FETAL/MATERNAL CHANGES 12 WEEKS (CONTINUED)	
FETAL DEVELOPMENT	**MATERNAL CHANGES**
• Embryo becomes a fetus • Heart discernible by ultrasound • Lower body develops • Sex determinable • Kidneys produce urine • Fetus weighs 19 to 28 grams (<1 ounce)	• Uterus rises ABOVE pelvic brim • Braxton Hicks contractions possible (continue throughout pregnancy) • Potential for UTI increases (exists throughout pregnancy) • Weight gain 2 ½ to 4 lbs. during first trimester • Placenta: fully functioning and producing hormones
NURSING INTERVENTIONS	
Teach prevention of UTI: • Adequate fluid intake, 3 liters/day • Void frequently (every 2 hours while awake) • Void before and after intercourse • Wipe from front to back **Discuss nutrition and exercise:** • Increase caloric intake by 300 calories/day • Stress value of regular exercise **Discuss possible effects of pregnancy on sexual relationship** • Recognize father's role as he labors to incorporate the parental role into his self-identity	

FETAL/MATERNAL CHANGES 20 WEEKS	
FETAL DEVELOPMENT	**MATERNAL CHANGES**
• Vernix protects body • Lanugo (fine hair) covers body, protects body • Eyebrows, eyelashes, head hair develop • Fetus sleeps, sucks, and kicks • Fetus weighs 200 to 400 grams (11 to 14 ounces)	• Fundus reaches level of umbilicus • Breasts begin secreting colostrums, areola darken • Amniotic sac holds approximately 400 ml fluid • Postural hypotension may occur • Fetal movement felt (quickening) pregnancy becomes "real" • Nasal stuffiness may begin • Leg cramps may begin • Varicose veins may develop • Constipation may develop
NURSING INTERVENTIONS	
Teach comfort measures: • Sit with feet elevated when possible • Avoid pressure on lower thighs • Use of support stockings may be helpful • Dorsiflect foot to relieve leg cramps • Apply heat to muscles affected by cramps • Cool-air vaporizer or saline nasal spray may help with nasal stuffiness **Teach measures to avoid constipation** • Eat raw fruits, vegetables, cereals with bran • Drink 3 liters fluid/day • Exercise frequently	

Figure 5-4 (continued)

FETAL/MATERNAL CHANGES 28 WEEKS (CONTINUED)

FETAL DEVELOPMENT	MATERNAL CHANGES
• Fetus can breathe, swallow, regulate temperature • Surfactant forms in lungs • Baby can hear • Eyelids open • Period of greatest fetal weight gain begins • Fetus weighs 1100 grams (2 ½ pounds)	• Fundus halfway between umbilicus and xiphoid process • Thoracic breathing replaces abdominal breathing • Fetal outline palpable • Woman becomes more introspective and concentrates interest on the unborn child • Heartburn may begin • Hemorrhoids may develop

NURSING INTERVENTIONS

Treatment of hemorrhoids:
• Sitz baths
• Gentle reinsertion of hemorrhoids with lubricated fingertip
• Suppositories as prescribed
• Topical anesthetic agents
• Stool softeners as prescribed

Teach comfort measures:
• Elevate legs when sitting
• Assume side-lying position when resting

Teach measures to avoid heartburn:
• Eat small, frequent meals
• Avoid fatty foods
• Avoid lying down after meals
• Antacids may be prescribed
• Avoid sodium bicarbonate

Prepare for delivery and parenthood:
• Discuss mother's/father's/family's expectations of labor and delivery
• Discuss mother's/father's/family's expectations of caring for an infant
• Start childbirth preparation classes

FETAL/MATERNAL CHANGES 32 WEEKS

FETAL DEVELOPMENT	MATERNAL CHANGES
• Brown fat deposits develop beneath skin to insulate baby following birth • Fetus is 15 to 17 inches in length • Begins storing iron, calcium, and phosphorus • Fetus weighs 1800 to 2200 grams (4 to 5 pounds)	• Fundus reaches xiphoid process • Breasts full and tender • Urinary frequency returns • Swollen ankles may occur • Sleeping problems may develop • Dyspnea may develop

NURSING INTERVENTIONS

Teach measures to decrease edema:
• Elevate legs 1 to 2 times/day for approximately one hour
• Use naturally-occurring diuretics, e.g., watermelon or 2 Tbsp. lemon juice/1 cup water

Teach comfort measures:
• Wear well-fitting supportive bra
• Maintain proper posture
• Use semi-Fowler's position at night for dyspnea

Prepare for childbirth:
• Review signs of labor
• Discuss plans for other children (if any)
• Discuss plans for transportation to agency
• Assess father's (family member's) role during childbirth

Figure 5-4 (continued)

MATERNITY NURSING

FETAL/MATERNAL CHANGES 38 WEEKS	
FETAL DEVELOPMENT	**MATERNAL CHANGES**
• Fetus occupies entire uterus; activity is restricted • Maternal antibodies are transferred to fetus (provides immunity for approximately 6 months, until infant's own immune system can take over) • L/S ratio 2:1 • Fetus weighs 3200+ grams (7+ pounds)	• Lightening occurs • Placenta weighs approximately 20 oz. • Mother eager for birth, may have burst of energy • Backaches increase • Urinary frequency increases • Braxton Hicks contractions intensify (cervix and lower uterine segment prepare for labor
NURSING INTERVENTIONS	
Teach safety measures: • Wear low-heeled shoes or flats • Avoid heavy lifting • Sleep on side to relieve bladder pressure; urinate frequently **Prepare for delivery:** • Continue pelvic tilt exercises • Pack a suitcase for delivery • Encourage couple to tour labor and delivery area • Discuss postpartum: circumcision, rooming-in, possibility of postpartum "blues," birth control, need for adequate rest, father's role	

Figure 5-4 (continued)

ANTEPARTUM NURSING CARE

PSYCHOSOCIAL RESPONSES TO PREGNANCY	
FIRST TRIMESTER	• Ambivalence: whether pregnancy is planned or unplanned, ambivalence is normal. • Financial worries about increased responsibility are normal. • Career concerns.
SECOND TRIMESTER	• Quickening occurs. • Pregnancy becomes real. • Pregnant woman accepts pregnancy. • Ambivalence wanes.
THIRD TRIMESTER	• Pregnant woman becomes introverted and self-absorbed. • Pregnant woman begins to ignore partner (may strain the relationship).
THROUGHOUT PREGNANCY	• Wide mood swings occur. • Pregnant woman is ultra-sensitive. • Strained relationship occurs with partner.

Figure 5-5

HESI HINT: Look for signs of maternal-fetal bonding DURING pregnancy. For example: talking to fetus in utero, massaging abdomen, nicknaming fetus are all healthy psychosocial activities.

ACTIVITIES DURING FIRST PRENATAL VISIT
1. Obtain history:
   A. Medical history.
   B. Obstetric history.
   C. History of current pregnancy.

HESI HINT: For many women, BATTERING (emotional or physical abuse) BEGINS during pregnancy. Women should be assessed for abuse in private, AWAY from the male partner, by a nurse who knows local resources and how to determine the safety of the client.

2. Determine gravidity and parity:

A. Gravida: refers to the number of times one has been pregnant regardless of the outcome.

B. Para: refers to the number of **deliveries** (not children) that have occurred after 20 weeks gestation.

C. When calculating parity, multiple births only count as ONE.

D. Pregnancy losses occurring before 20 weeks are counted as abortions (whether spontaneous or voluntary terminations), and only add to a client's gravidity.

E. A fetus born dead after 20 weeks is STILL added to the parity count.

> **HESI HINT:** Practice determining gravidity and parity: A women who is 6 weeks pregnant has the following maternal history:
> • Has a 2-year-old, healthy daughter.
> • Had a miscarriage at 10 weeks, 3 years ago.
> • Had an elective abortion at 6 weeks, 5 years ago. With this pregnancy, she is a gravida 4, para 1 (only 1 delivery after 20 weeks gestation).

3. Physical exam, including pelvic exam.

4. Calculate gestational age: EDB (estimated date of birth) using Nagele's Rule:

A. Count back 3 months from the first day of the last normal menstrual period and add 7 days.

B. For example: if LMP was March 23, EDB would be December 30

.

> **HESI HINT:** Practice calculating EDB (estimated date of birth). If the first day of a woman's last normal menstrual period was October 17, what is her EDB using Nägele's Rule? July 24. Count back three months and add seven days (always give February 28 days).

5. Vital signs:

A. BP should rise no more than 30 points systolic and 15 points diastolic from previous baseline normal. Average BP is 90 to 140 systolic and 60 to 90 diastolic.

B. Average pulse is 60 to 90 beats/minute.

C. Average respiration is 16 to 24 breaths/minute.

D. Average temperature is 97° to 100ºF.

6. Schedule future office visits.

A. Low-risk client's schedule includes:
1) Every month until 28 weeks.
2) Every 2 weeks from 28 weeks until 36 weeks.
3) Every week from 36 weeks until delivery.

B. High-risk client's schedule is determined by client's needs; visits are scheduled as needed.

7. Obtain laboratory data. *(See Appendices, A: Normal Lab Values)*

A. Hgb, pregnant values >11.

B. Hct, pregnant values >33.

> **HESI HINT:** At approximately 28 to 32 weeks gestation, the maximum plasma volume increase of 25 to 40% occurs, resulting in normal hemodilution of pregnancy and Hct values of 32 to 42%. High Hct values may look "good," but in reality represent pregnancy-induced hypertension and a depleted vascular space.

C. WBC and differential.

D. Hgb electrophoresis (sickle cell).

E. Pap smear and cytology (gonorrhea and chlamydia).

F. Antibody screens.
1) HIV.
2) Hepatitis B.
3) Toxoplasmosis.
4) Rubella (>1:8=immunity).
5) Syphilis (RPR, VDRL).
6) Cytomegalovirus.

G. Tuberculin skin testing (PPD).

H. Rh and blood type.

I. Urinalysis.

> **HESI HINT:** Hgb/Hct data can be used to evaluate nutritional status. Example: A 22-year-old primigravida at 12 weeks gestation has a Hgb of 9.6 g/dl and a Hct of 31%. She has gained 3 pounds during the first trimester. A weight gain of 3.5 to 5 pounds during the first trimester is recommended and this client is anemic. Supplemental iron and a diet higher in iron are needed.
> **Foods High in Iron:**
> • Fish and red meats.
> • Cereal and yellow vegetables.
> • Green leafy vegetables and citrus fruits.
> • Egg yolks and dried fruits.

ACTIVITIES DURING SUBSEQUENT VISITS

1. Check urine for:
   A. Albumin: no more than a trace for a normal finding (related to preeclampsia).
   B. Glucose: no more than 1+ for a normal finding (related to gestational diabetes).
2. Graph weight gain.
   A. 2 to 4 pounds in the first trimester is considered normal.
   B. 0.9 pound per week thereafter (>2 lbs/wk related to preeclampsia-edema).
   C. Total weight gain during the pregnancy should be between 25 to 35 pounds.
3. Check fundal height. *(See figure 5-6, Fundal Height Assessment)*
   A. 12 to 13 weeks: fundus rises out of symphysis.
   B. 20 weeks: at umbilicus.
   C. 24 weeks: fundal height is measured in cm, with the number of cm above the symphysis equal to the number of weeks gestation, after 24 weeks gestation.

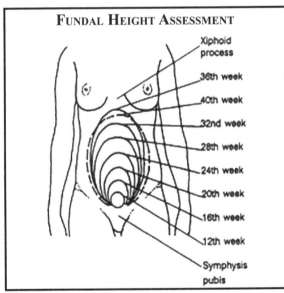

FUNDAL HEIGHT ASSESSMENT

Figure 5-6

HESI HINT: As pregnancy advances, the uterus presses on abdominal vessels (vena cava and aorta). Teach the woman that a side-lying position increases perfusion to uterus, placenta, and fetus. Recent research indicates that the knee-chest position is best for increasing perfusion and that the side-lying position (either left or right side-lying) is the second most desirable position to increase perfusion. Prior to this research, the left side-lying position was usually encouraged.

4. Check fetal heart rate.
   A. 10 to 12 weeks detectable using Doppler.
   B. 15 to 20 weeks detectable by using fetoscope.
   C. 110 to 160 beats per minute (BPM) is normal range.

HESI HINT: Fetal well-being is determined by assessing fundal height, fetal heart tones/rate, fetal movement and uterine activity (contractions). Changes in fetal heart rate are the first and most important indicator of compromised blood flow to the fetus, and these changes require action! Remember, the normal FHR is 110 to 160 BPM.

5. Teach the importance of continuing prenatal care.
6. Anticipatory guidance: first trimester
   A. Discomforts such as nausea, fatigue and urinary frequency subside after 13 weeks.
   B. Sleep needs increase to 8 hrs/day.
   C. Plan rest periods.
   D. May exercise as long as is able to converse easily while exercising. If not, **slow down**.
   E. May work if no hazardous chemical/toxin exposure.
   F. May bathe until membranes rupture (usually within hours of delivery).
   F. May travel by car, but will need frequent breaks and must wear seat belt.
   G. Airtravel: policies vary by airline. Remain well hydrated. Move about frequently to minimize risk of thrombophlebitis
   H. Best to ingest **No** medications and **No** alcohol, and to **STOP SMOKING**.
7. Anticipatory guidance: second trimester
   A. Sexual needs/desires may change for better/worse. Encourage communication with partner regarding adjustments.
   B. Have regular check-ups/dental hygiene (gum hypertrophy common). Delay x-rays and major dental work if possible.
8. Anticipatory guidance: third trimester:
   A. Schedule childbirth classes.
   B. Urinary frequency and dyspnea return.

C. Review interventions for leg cramps (dorsiflect foot), nasal stuffiness, varicose veins, and constipation.

D. Teach safety related to balance.

E. Position with pillows for comfort.

F. Round ligament pain will occur.

G. Instruct client to come to hospital when contractions are occurring regularly 5 minutes apart.

H. Provide information on feeding methods.

I. Encourage choosing a pediatrician/ clinic.

J. Reinforce nutritional needs because third trimester is a period of rapid fetal growth.

K. Teach the risks/symptoms of preterm labor.

HESI HINT: Danger Signs During Pregnancy Teach clients to immediately report any of the following danger signs. Early intervention can optimize maternal and fetal outcome.
Possible indications of preeclampsia/eclampsia:
• Visual disturbances.
• Swelling of face, fingers, or sacrum.
• Severe, continuous headache.
• Persistent vomiting.
Signs of infection:
• Chills.
• Temperature over 100.4°F.
• Dysuria.
• Pain in abdomen.
• Fluid discharge from vagina (anything other than normal leukorrhea).
• Change in fetal movement and/or increased FHR.

NUTRITION

NURSING ASSESSMENT

1. Diet.
   A. Ask client to recall diet for last 24 hrs.
   B. Use a questionnaire to determine individual deficiencies.
   C. Determine skinfold anthropometric measurement to assess percent of body fat.
   D. Note symptoms of malnutrition:
      1) Glossitis.
      2) Cracked lips.
      3) Dry, brittle hair.
2. Dental caries, periodontitis.
3. Weight (those who weigh less than 100 lbs or over 200 lbs are at risk).

ANALYSIS (NURSING DIAGNOSES)

1. Alteration in nutrition < or > body requirements related to…
2. Knowledge deficit related to…

NURSING PLANS AND INTERVENTIONS

1. Teach minimum nutritional increases.
   A. Increase of 300 calories above basal and activity needs.
   B. Increase protein by 30 gm/day.
   C. Increase intake of iron (30+ mg) and folic acid (800 to 1,000 mcg) with diet and supplementation.
   D. Increase intake of vitamin A, vitamin C, and calcium with diet.

HESI HINT: Most providers prescribe prenatal vitamins to ensure that the client receives an adequate intake of vitamins. However, only the healthcare provider can prescribe prenatal vitamins. It is the nurse's responsibility to teach about proper diet and taking prescribed vitamins, if prescribed by the healthcare provider.

   E. Drink a total of 8 to 10 glasses of fluid/ day; 4 to 6 glasses should be water.
2. Relate recommended weight gain by trimester to fetal growth/fetal health.
   A. Record weight at each visit, using graph.
   B. Maintain steady weight gain of 0.9 lb/ week in 2nd and 3rd trimester.
3. Provide a copy of daily food guide to post on refrigerator (consider cultural food patterns in choices given). Include the following:
   A. 3 servings from dairy group (milk, cheese).
   B. 5 servings of protein (meats, eggs, legumes).
   C. 5 servings of vegetables (green, deep yellow, are good sources of vitamin C.
   D. 6 servings of breads/cereals.
   E. 4 servings of fruit.
4. Advise regarding vitamin and iron supplementation.
5. Explain that poor nutrition can lead to anemia, preterm labor, obesity, and intrauterine growth restriction.

HESI HINT: It is recommended that pregnant women drink one quart of milk/day. This will ensure that the daily calcium needs are met and help to alleviate the occurrence of leg cramps.

REVIEW QUESTIONS

ANATOMY & PHYSIOLOGY OF REPRODUCTION

ANTEPARTUM NURSING CARE

1. State the objective signs that signify ovulation.
2. Ovulation occurs how many days before the next menstrual period?
3. State three ways to identify the chronological age of a pregnancy (gestation).
4. What maternal position provides optimum fetal maternal/placental perfusion during pregnancy?
5. Name the major discomforts of the first trimester and one suggestion for amelioration of each.
6. If the first day of a woman's last normal menstrual period was May 28, what is the estimated date of birth (EDB) using Nägele's Rule?
7. At twenty weeks gestation, the fundal height would be _____, the fetus would be weigh approximately _____ and look like _____.
8. State the normal psychosocial responses to pregnancy in the second trimester.
9. Hemodilution of pregnancy peaks at _____ weeks and results in a/an _____ in a woman's Hct.
10. State three principles relative to the PATTERN of weight gain in pregnancy.
11. During pregnancy a woman should add _____ calories to her diet, and drink ____ of milk/day.
12. Fetal heart rate can be auscultated by Doppler at _____ weeks gestation.
13. Describe the schedule for prenatal visits for a low-risk pregnant woman.

ANSWERS TO REVIEW QUESTIONS

1. Abundant, thin, clear cervical mucus; spinnbarkeit (egg-white stretchiness) of cervical mucus; open cervical os; slight drop in BBT and then 0.5 to 1.0 degree F. rise; ferning under the microscope.
2. 14 days.
3. 10 lunar months, 9 calendar months consisting of 3 trimesters of 3 months each, 40 weeks, 280 days.
4. The knee-chest position, but the ideal position of COMFORT for the mother which supports fetal/ maternal/placental perfusion is the side-lying position off the abdominal vessels (vena cava, aorta).
5. Nausea and vomiting: crackers before rising. Fatigue: teach the need for rest periods/naps and 7 to 8 hours sleep at night.
6. Count back three months and add seven days: March 7**Always give February 28 days.**
7. At the umbilicus; 300 to 400 grams; a "baby" with hair, lanugo and vernix, but without any subcutaneous fat.
8. Ambivalence wanes and acceptance of pregnancy occurs; pregnancy becomes "real;" signs of maternal-fetal bonding occur.
9. 28 to 32 weeks, decrease.
10. Total gain should average 24 to 30 pounds. Gain should be consistent throughout pregnancy. An average of 0.9 lb/week should be gained in the second and third trimester.
11. 300; 1 quart.
12. 10 to 12.
13. Once a month until 28 weeks, every two weeks from 28 to 36 weeks, then once a week until delivery.

MATERNITY NURSING

251

FETAL/MATERNAL ASSESSMENT TECHNIQUES

DESCRIPTION: Techniques used to obtain data regarding fetal and maternal physiological status.

Maternal risk factors include, but are not limited to:
1. Age under 17 or over 34.
2. High parity >5.
3. Pregnancy (3 months since last delivery).
4. Hypertension, preeclampsia in current pregnancy.
5. Anemia, history of hemorrhage, or current hemorrhage.
6. Multiple gestation.
7. Rh incompatibility.
8. History of dystocia or previous operative delivery.
9. Under 60 inches (5 feet) of height.
10. Malnutrition (15% under ideal weight) or extreme obesity (20% over ideal weight).
11. Medical disease in pregnancy (diabetes, hyperthyroidism, hyperemesis, clotting disorders, such as thrombocytopenia).
12. Infection in pregnancy: TORCH diseases, influenza, HIV, Chlamydia, human papilloma virus (HPV).
13. History of family violence, lack of social support.
14. Various techniques are used to determine fetal/maternal well-being. *(See figure 5-7, Ultrasonography; figure 5-8, Chorionic Villi Sampling (CVS); figure 5-9, Amniocentesis; figure 5-10, Variables Measured with Fetal Monitoring; figure 5-11, Non-Stress Test (NST); figure 5-12, Contraction Stress Test (CST) or Oxytocin Challenge Test (OCT); and figure 5-13, Fetal pH Blood Sampling)*

> **HESI HINT:** In some states, the screening for neural tube defects through either maternal serum AFP levels or amniotic fluid AFP levels is mandated by state law. This screening test is highly associated with both false positives and false negatives.

ULTRASONOGRAPHY	
Description: High frequency sound waves beamed on the pregnant abdomen; echoes are returned to a machine, which records the "objects" location and size.	
Used in the first trimester to determine: • Number of fetuses • Presence of fetal cardiac movement/rhythm • Uterine abnormalities • Assessment of gestational age	Used in the 2nd and 3rd trimester to determine: • Fetal viability/gestational age • Size/date discrepancies • Amniotic fluid volume • Placental location/maturity • Uterine anomalies/abnormalities • Used routinely with amniocentesis
FINDINGS	**NURSING CARE**

• Fetal heart activity as early as 6 to 7 weeks gestation.
• Serial evaluation of biparietal diameter and limb length can differentiate between wrong dates and true intrauterine growth restriction (IUGR).
• Biophysical profile (BPP) for fetal well-being:
  → Five variables assessed; fetal breathing movements, gross body movements, fetal tone, reactivity of fetal heart rate, and amniotic fluid volume.
  → A score of 2 or 0 can be obtained on each variable. An overall score of 10 designates that the fetus is "well" the day of the exam.
	• Instruct woman to drink 3 to 4 glasses of water prior to coming for exam and not to urinate. When the fetus is very small (in the first-second trimesters), the client's bladder must be full for exam in order for uterus to be supported for imaging. (A full bladder is not needed if ultrasound is done transvaginally instead of abdominally).
	• Position woman with pillows under neck and knees to keep pressure off bladder, late in the third trimester, place wedge under right hip to displace uterus to the left.
	• Position display so woman can watch if she wishes.
	• Have bedpan or bathroom immediately available.

	COMPLICATIONS: • No known complications • Controversy regarding routine use of ultrasound in pregnancy

Figure 5-7

CHORIONIC VILLI SAMPLING (CVS)

Description: Removal of small piece of villi between 8 to 12 weeks gestation under ultrasound guidance. Cannot replace amniocentesis completely since no sample of amniotic fluid can be obtained (for alpha-fetoprotein or Rh disease testing).

FINDINGS	NURSING CARE
• Determines genetic diagnosis early in the first trimester • Results obtained in one week	• Informed consent needed before procedure • Place woman in lithotomy position using stirrups • Warn of slight sharp pain upon catheter insertion • Results should NOT be given over the phone
	COMPLICATIONS: • Spontaneous abortion (5%) • Controversy regarding fetal anomalies (limb)

Figure 5-8

AMNIOCENTESIS

Description: Removal of amniotic fluid sample from uterus as early as 14 to 16 weeks.

• Used to determine:
  → Fetal genetic diagnosis (usually in the first trimester)
  → Fetal maturity (last trimester)
  → Fetal well-being
• Performed when uterus rises out of symphysis at 13 weeks and amniotic fluid has formed
• Usually takes 10 days to 2 weeks to develop cultured cell karyotype. Therefore, could be well into 2nd trimester before diagnosis is made, making choice for abortion more dangerous

FINDINGS	NURSING CARE
Genetic Disorders: • Karyotype: determines Down syndrome (trisomy 21), other trisomies, and sex chromatin (sex-linked disorders). • Biochemical analysis: determines over 60 types of metabolic disorders (Tay-Sachs). • Alpha-fetoprotein (AFP): elevations may be associated with neutral tube defects, low levels may indicate trisomy 21. Fetal Maturity: • L/S ratio (lecithin/sphingomyelin): 2:1 ratio indicates fetal lung maturity unless mother is diabetic, has Rh disease, or fetus is septic. • L/S ratio and presence of Phosphatidylglycerol (PG): most accurate determination of fetal maturity. PG present after 35 weeks gestation. • Lung maturity is the best predictor of extra-uterine survival. • Creatinine: renal maturity indicator > 1.8. • Orange-staining cells: lipid-containing exfoliating sebaceous gland maturity; >20% stained orange=35 weeks or more. Fetal Well-Being: • Bilirubin Delta OD assessment in mother previously sensitized to the fetal Rh+ RBC and having antibodies to the Rh+ circulating cells. Done at 24 weeks gestation. • Meconium in amniotic fluid may indicate fetal stress.	• Obtain baseline vital signs and FHR. • Place client in supine position with hands across chest. • If prescribed, shave area and scrub with Betadine (povidone/iodine). • Draw maternal blood sample for comparison with post-procedure blood sample to determine maternal bleeding. • Provide emotional support, explain procedure, stay with the client (do not leave alone). • Label samples; if bilirubin test is prescribed, darken room and immediately cover the tubes with aluminum foil or use opaque tubes. • After specimen is drawn, wash abdomen, assist woman to empty bladder. A full bladder can irritate the uterus and cause contractions. • Monitor FHR for 1 hr. after procedure and assess for uterine contractions/irritability. • Instruct woman to report any contractions, change in fetal movement, or fluid leaking from vagina.
	COMPLICATIONS: • Spontaneous abortion (1%) • Fetal injury • Infection

Figure 5-9

VARIABLES MEASURED WITH FETAL MONITORING

CONTRACTIONS	• Depicts the beginning, peak, and end of each contraction • Duration (length) of each contraction from beginning to end • Frequency: beginning of one contraction to beginning of another. Must measure at least 3 to 5 contractions. • Intensity: strength not measured by external monitoring, measured in mmHg by internal (intrauterine) monitoring. Range from 30 (mild) to 70 (strong) mmHg at peak
BASELINE FETAL HEART RATE	• The range of FHR (average 110 to 160 BPM) between contractions, monitored over a 10 minute period • The balance between parasympathetic and sympathetic impulses usually produces no observable changes in the FHR during uterine contractions (with a HEALTHY fetus, HEALTHY placenta, and GOOD uteroplacental perfusion)

NURSING ACTIONS BASED ON FETAL HEART RATE

FHR	DESCRIPTION
Baseline FHR: Normal Rhythmicity Average FHR 110-160 BPM	• The FHR results from the balance between the parasympathetic and the sympathetic branches of the autonomic nervous system • The most important indicator of fetal central nervous system health
Baseline Variability: Normal Irregularity of Cardiac Rhythm	• Short-term variability (STV): change in FHR from one beat to the next → Fetal scalp electrode (internal monitoring) is necessary to evaluate STV → If STV is PRESENT, the fetus is NOT experiencing cerebral asphyxia, therefore its presence is a reassuring sign • Long-term variability (LTV): averages 6 to 10 changes per minute, i.e., heart rate may average 140 BPM, but change from 137 to 149 during that minute → LTV can be evaluated with external or internal monitoring
NURSING ACTIONS	• Assess contractions using monitor strip • Assess FHR for normal baseline range and variability
Periodic Changes: FHR changes in relation to uterine contractions	• Accelerations: → Caused by sympathetic fetal response → Occur in response to fetal movement → Indicative of a reactive, healthy fetus • Early decelerations: → Benign pattern caused by parasympathetic response (head compression) → Heart rate slowly and smoothly decelerates at beginning of contraction and returns to baseline at end of contraction
NURSING ACTIONS FOR EARLY DECELERATIONS	• No nursing interventions required except to monitor for progress of labor • Document the processes of labor

EARLY DECELERATIONS – UNIFORM SHAPE

Figure 5-10

NON-REASSURING WARNING SIGNS	
FHR	**DESCRIPTION**
Variability: absent or minimal Short-term variability is absent. Long-term variability is minimal (3 to 5 changes/min)	• Hypoxia (asphyxia) • Acidosis • Maternal drug ingestion (narcotics, CNS depressants such as $MgSO_4$) • Fetal sleep
Bradycardia Baseline FHR is below 110 BPM (assessed between contractions) lasting for 10 minutes (to differentiate from a periodic change)	• Late manifestation of fetal hypoxia • Medication induced (narcotics, $MgSO_4$) • Maternal hypotension • Fetal heart block • Prolonged umbilical cord compression
Tachycardia Baseline FHR above 160 BPM (assessed between contractions) lasting for 10 minutes)	• Early sign of fetal hypoxia • Fetal anemia • Dehydration • Maternal infection/maternal fever • Maternal hyperthyroid disease (hyper) • Medication induced (atropine, ritodrine, terbutaline, hydroxyzine)
NURSING ACTIONS FOR DECREASED VARIABILITY, BRADYCARDIA, AND TACHYCARDIA	• Treat based on cause
Variable deceleration pattern	• Most common periodic pattern • Occurs in 40% of all labors and is caused mainly by cord compression but can also indicate rapid fetal descent Characterized by an abrupt transitory decrease in the FHR that is VARIABLE in duration, depth of fall, and timing relative to the contraction cycle • Occasional variable is usually benign
NURSING ACTIONS FOR VARIABLE DECELERATIONS	• Change maternal position • Simulate fetus if indicated • Discontinue oxytocin if infusing • Administer oxygen at 10 liters by tight face mask • Perform a vaginal exam to check for cord prolapse • Report findings to physician and document

Variable Decelerations – Variable Shape

Figure 5-10 (continued)

MATERNITY NURSING

NON-REASSURING/OMINOUS SIGNS (CONTINUED)	
FHR	**DESCRIPTION**
SEVERE VARIABLE DECELERATIONS	• FHR below 70 BPM lasting longer than 30 to 60 seconds • Slow return to baseline • Decreasing or absent variability
LATE DECELERATIONS	• Ominous/potentially disastrous, NON-reassuring sign • Indicative of uteroplacental insufficiency (UPI) • The shape of the deceleration is uniform and the FHR returns to baseline after the contraction is over • Depth of deceleration does not indicate severity, rarely falls below 100 BPM
NURSING ACTIONS FOR SEVERE VARIABLE/LATE DECELERATIONS	• Immediately turn client to side • Check scalp stimulation for accelerations (a non-compromised fetus will demonstrate accelerations with scalp compression) • Administer O₂ at 10 liters by tight face mask • Assist with fetal blood sampling if indicated • Maintain intravenous line and, if possible, elevate legs to increase venous return • Correct any underlying hypotension (by increasing IV rate or with prescribed medications • Determine presence of FHR variability • Notify healthcare provider • Document pattern and response to each nursing action

Late Decelerations – Uniform Shape

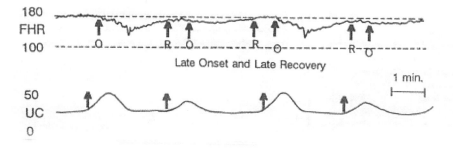

Late Onset and Late Recovery

HESI HINT: Early decelerations, caused by head compression and fetal descent, usually occur between 4 and 7 cm and in the 2ⁿᵈ stage. Check for labor progress if early decelerations are noted.

HESI HINT: If cord prolapse is detected, the examiner should position the mother to relieve pressure on the cord (i.e., knee-chest position) or push the presenting part off the cord until IMMEDIATE Cesarean delivery can be accomplished.

HESI HINT: Late decelerations indicate uteroplacental insufficiency and are associated with conditions such as postmaturity, preeclampsia, diabetes mellitus, cardiac disease, and abruptio placentae.

HESI HINT: When deceleration patterns (late or variable) are associated with decreased or absent variability and tachycardia, the situation is OMINOUS (potentially disastrous) and requires immediate intervention and fetal assessment.

HESI HINT: A decrease in uteroplacental perfusion results in late decelerations; cord compression results in a pattern of variable decelerations. Nursing interventions should include changing maternal position, discontinuing Pitocin infusion, administering oxygen, and notifying the healthcare provider.

Figure 5-10 (continued)

MATERNITY NURSING

NON-STRESS TEST (NST)

DESCRIPTION	NURSING CARE
• Used to determine fetal well-being in high-risk pregnancy, especially useful in post-maturity (notes response of the fetus to his/her own movement. • A healthy fetus will usually respond to own movement by FHR acceleration of 15 beats lasting for at least 15 seconds after the movement. • The fetus that responds with the 15/15 acceleration is considered "reactive" and healthy.	• Apply fetal monitor, ultrasound, and tocodynamometer to maternal abdomen. • Give mother hand-held event marker and instruct her to push the button whenever fetal movement is felt or recorded "FM" on the fetal heart rate strip. • Monitor client for 20 to 30 minutes observing for reactivity. • Suspect fetus sleeping if no fetal movement. Stimulate fetus acoustically or physically, or have mother move fetus around and begin test again.

Figure 5-11

CONTRACTION STRESS TEST (CST) OR OXYTOCIN CHALLENGE TEST (OCT)

DESCRIPTION	NURSING CARE
• The fetus is challenged with the "stress" of labor by inducing uterine contractions, and the fetal response to physiologically decreased oxygen supply during uterine contractions is noted. • An unhealthy fetus will develop non-reassuring fetal heart rate patterns in response to uterine contractions: late decelerations indicative of uteroplacental insufficiency (UPI). • Contractions can be induced by nipple stimulation or by infusing a dilute solution of oxytocin intravenously.	• Assess for contraindications: prematurity, placenta previa, hydramnios, multiple gestation, and previous uterine classical scar, rupture of membranes. • Place external monitors on abdomen (FHR ultrasound monitor, and tocotransducer). • Record a 20-minute baseline strip to determine fetal well-being (reactivity) and presence/absence of contractions. • To assess for fetal well-being, a recording of at least 3 contractions in 10 minutes must be obtained. • If nipple stimulation attempted, have woman apply warm, wet washcloths to nipples and roll the nipple of one breast for 10 minutes. Begin rolling both breast nipples if contractions do not begin in 10 minutes. Proceed with oxytocin infusion if unsuccessful with nipple stimulation. • Piggyback oxytocin (10 units of Pitocin) to main IV line. Begin at 0.5 mu/minute and increase by 0.5 mu/minute every 20 minutes to achieve 3 firm contractions, each lasting 40 seconds, over a period of 10 minutes. • A negative test suggests **fetal well-being**, i.e., no occurrence of late decelerations.

Figure 5-12

> **HESI HINT:** The danger of nipple stimulation lies in controlling the "dose" of oxytocin stimulated from the posterior pituitary. The chance of hyper-stimulation or tetany (contractions over 90 seconds or contractions with less than 30 seconds in between) is increased.

MATERNITY NURSING

FETAL pH BLOOD SAMPLING

DESCRIPTION	NURSING CARE
• This technique is only performed in the intrapartum period when the fetal blood from the presenting part (breech or scalp) can be taken, i.e., when membranes are ruptured and the cervix is dilated 2 to 3 cm. • Used to determine true acidosis when non-reassuring fetal heart rate is noted (late decelerations, severe variable decelerations unresponsive to treatment, decreased variability unrelated to non-asphyxial causes, tachycardia unrelated to maternal variables). • Because fetal blood gas values vary rapidly with transient circulatory changes, this is usually done only in tertiary centers with the capabilities of repetitive sampling and rapid results.	• Client in lithotomy position at end of labor bed and prepare with perineal cleansing and sterile draping. • Nurse assists the healthcare provider with sterile supplies and provides ice in cup or emesis basin to carry pipette filled with blood to unit pH machine or to lab.

Figure 5-13

BIOPHYSICAL PROFILE (BPP)

DESCRIPTION	NURSING CARE

• Ultrasonography used to evaluate fetal health by assessing five variables.
  → Fetal breathing movements (FBM).
  → Gross body movements (FM).
  → Fetal tone (FT).
  → Reactive fetal heart rate (non-stress test).
  → Qualitative amniotic fluid volume (AFV).
• Each variable receives 2 points for a normal response or 0 points for an abnormal or absent response.
	• Prepare client for procedure.
	• Inform client of purpose for exam.
	• Provide psychological support, especially if testing will continue throughout the pregnancy.
	• Advise client that a low score may indicate fetal compromise which would warrant more detailed investigation

Figure 5-14

MATERNITY NURSING

> **HESI HINT:** Percutaneous umbilical blood sampling (PUBS) can be done during pregnancy under ultrasound for prenatal diagnosis and therapy. Hemoglobinopathies, clotting disorders, sepsis, and some genetic testing can be done using this method.

> **HESI HINT:** The most important determinant of fetal maturity for extra-uterine survival is the L/S ratio (2:1 or higher).

REVIEW QUESTIONS
FETAL/MATERNAL ASSESSMENT TECHNIQUES

1. Name five maternal variables associated with diagnosis of a high-risk pregnancy.
2. Is one ultrasound examination useful in determining the presence of intrauterine growth retardation (IUGR)?
3. What does the biophysical profile (BPP) determine?
4. List 3 necessary nursing actions prior to an ultrasound exam for a woman in the first trimester of pregnancy.
5. State the advantage of CVS over amniocentesis.
6. Why are serum or amniotic AFP levels done prenatally?
7. What is the most important determinant of fetal maturity for extrauterine survival?
8. Name the 3 most common complications of amniocentesis.
9. Name the four periodic changes of the fetal heart rate, their causes, and one nursing treatment for each.
10. What is the most important indicator of fetal autonomic nervous system integrity/health?
11. Name four causes of decreased FHR variability.
12. State the most important action to take when a cord prolapse is determined.
13. What is a "reactive" non-stress test?
14. What are the dangers of the nipple-stimulation stress test?
15. Normal fetal scalp pH in labor is _____ and values below _____ indicate true acidosis.

ANSWERS TO REVIEW QUESTIONS

1. Age (under 17 years or over 34 years of age), parity (over 5), <3 months between pregnancies, diagnosis of preeclampsia, diabetes mellitus, or cardiac disease.
2. No, serial measurements are needed to determine IUGR.
3. Fetal well-being.
4. Have client fill bladder. Do not allow client to void. Position supine with uterine wedge.
5. Can be done between 8 to 12 weeks gestation with results returned within one week, which allows for decision about termination while still in first trimester.
6. To determine if alpha-fetoprotein levels are elevated which may indicate the presence of neural tube defects; or low levels, which may indicate trisomy 21.
7. L/S ratio (lung maturity, lung surfactant development).
8. Spontaneous abortion, fetal injury, infection.
9. *Accelerations*: caused by burst of sympathetic activity; they are reassuring and require no treatment. *Early decelerations*: caused by head compression, are benign and caution the nurse to monitor for labor progress and fetal descent. *Variable decelerations*: caused by cord compression; change of position should be tried first. *Late decelerations*: are caused by UPI (uteroplacental insufficiency) and should be treated by placing client on her side and administering O_2.
10. Fetal heart rate variability.
11. Hypoxia, acidosis, drugs, fetal sleep.
12. Examiner should position mother to relieve pressure on the cord or push the presenting part off the cord with fingers until emergency delivery is accomplished.
13. FHR acceleration of 15 beats per minute for 15 seconds in response to fetal movement.
14. The inability to control "oxytocin" dosage and the chance of tetany/hyperstimulation.
15. 7.25 to 7.35, 7.2.

INTRAPARTUM NURSING CARE

DESCRIPTION: Begins with true labor and consists of four stages.

Stage I: From the beginning of regular contractions or rupture of membranes to 10 centimeters of dilatation and effacement. *(See figure 5-15, First Stage of Labor)*

Stage II: 10 centimeters to delivery.
Stage III: Delivery of the placenta.
Stage IV: First 1 to 4 hours following delivery (recovery).

FIRST STAGE OF LABOR		
PHASE	**DESCRIPTION**	**PSYCHOLOGICAL/PHYSICAL RESPONSES**
LATENT	• From beginning of true labor until 3 to 4 centimeters cervical dilation	• Mildly anxious, conversant • Able to continue usual activities • Contractions mild, initially 10 to 20 minutes apart, 15 to 20 seconds duration; later 5 to 7 minutes apart, 30 to 40 seconds duration
ACTIVE	• From 4 to 7 centimeters cervical dilation	• Increased anxiety • Increased discomfort • Unwillingness to be left alone • Contractions moderate to severe, 2 to 3 minutes apart, 30 to 60 seconds duration
TRANSITION	• From 8 to 10 centimeters cervical dilation	• Changed behavior • May have sudden nausea, hiccups • Extreme irritability and unwillingness to be touched although desirous of companionship • Contractions severe, 1½ minutes apart, 60 to 90 seconds duration

Figure 5-15

HESI HINT: Be able to differentiate true labor from false labor.

True Labor:
- Pain in lower back that radiates to abdomen.
- Accompanied by regular, rhythmic contractions.
- Contractions that intensify with ambulation.
- Progressive cervical dilation and effacement.

False Labor:
- Discomfort is localized in abdomen.
- No lower back pain.
- Contractions decrease in intensity and/or frequency with ambulation.

NURSING ASSESSMENT

1. Prodromal labor signs include the following:
   A. Lightening (fetus drops into true pelvis).
   B. Braxton Hicks contractions (practice contractions).
   C. Cervical softening and slight effacement.
   D. Bloody show or expulsion of mucous plug.
   E. Burst of energy, "nesting instinct."
2. Determine the following:
   A. Gravidity and parity: parity >5=grand multiparity.
   B. Gestational age: 37 to 42 weeks=term gestation.
   C. FHR: best heard over fetal back. *(See figure 5-16, Leopold's Maneuvers)*
   D. Maternal vital signs.
   E. Contraction frequency, intensity, and duration.
3. Perform vaginal exam to determine:
   A. Fetal presentation and position.
   B. Cervical dilatation, effacement, position, and consistency.
   C. Fetal station. *(See figure 5-17, Vaginal Exam)*
4. Assess the client for:
   A. Status of membranes (ruptured or intact).

LEOPOLD'S MANEUVERS

DESCRIPTION: Abdominal Palpations used to determine fetal presentation, lie, position, and engagement.

- With client in supine position, place both cupped hands over fundus and palpate to determine whether breech (soft, immovable, large) or vertex (hard, moveable, small).
- Place one hand firmly on side and palpate with other hand to determine presence of small parts or fetal back. (Fetal heart rate is heard best through fetal back.)
- Facing client, grasp the area over the symphysis with the thumb and fingers and press to determine the degree of descent of the presenting part. (A ballottable or floating head can be rocked back and forth between the thumb and fingers.)
- Facing the client's feet, outline the fetal presenting part with the palmar surface of both hands to determine the degree of descent and attitude of the fetus. (If cephalic prominence is located on the same side as small parts, assume the head is flexed.)

Figure 5-16

B. Urine glucose and albumin data.
C. Comfort level.
D. Labor/delivery preparation.
E. Presence of support person.
F. Presence of true or false labor.

ANALYSIS (NURSING DIAGNOSES)

1. Knowledge deficit about labor/delivery related to...
2. Alteration in comfort: acute pain related to...
3. Anxiety related to...

HESI HINT: Know normal findings for clients in labor:
- Normal FHR in labor: 110 to 160 BPM
- Normal maternal BP: <140/90
- Normal maternal pulse: <100 BPM
- Normal maternal temperature: <100.4°F
- Slight elevation is often due to dehydration and the work of labor. Anything higher indicates infection and must be reported immediately.

NURSING PLANS AND INTERVENTIONS

1. Determine fetal heart rate (auscultation schedule).
   A. FHR q30 minutes in early latent stage.
   B. FHR q15 to 30 minutes in mid-active stage.
   C. FHR q15 minutes in transition stage.
2. Assess maternal vital signs.

A. Take BP, **between contractions**, in side-lying position at least every hour unless abnormal (BP increases during contractions).

B. Take temperature q4 hours until membranes rupture, then every hour.

3. Explain all activities and procedures to mother and support person.

4. Determine birth plan and desires for:
   A. Analgesia and anesthesia.
   B. Delivery situation.

HESI HINT: Admission Procedures
• **Vulvar/ perineal shave (may not be done).**
Enema:
• **Enema may be refused by woman due to pre-labor diarrhea or recent, large bowel movement.**
• **An enema should not be administered to a client in active labor.**
• **If head is floating, watch for cord prolapse.**

---

5. Assess urine q8 hours unless abnormal. Normal findings:
   A. Protein (<trace).
   B. Glucose (1+ or less).

6. Assess contractions when assessing fetal heart rate.
   A. Frequency: time contractions from beginning of one contraction to beginning of the next (measured in minutes apart).
   B. Duration: length of the entire contraction (from beginning to end).
   C. Strength: intensity of strongest part (peak) of contraction. Measured by clinical estimation of indentability of the fundus (use gentle pressure of fingertips to determine):
      1) Very indentable (mild).
      2) Moderately indentable (moderate).
      3) Unindentable (firm).
   D. Norms:
      Contraction frequency, duration, and intensity vary with the stage of labor.

VAGINAL EXAM

Preceded by antiseptic cleansing with client in modified lithotomy position.

- Wear sterile gloves.
- Exams are not done routinely. Sharply curtailed after membranes rupture to prevent infection.
- Exams are done:
  - → Prior to analgesia/anesthesia.
  - → To determine progress of labor.
  - → To determine if 2nd stage pushing can begin.

Purpose of vaginal exam is to determine:

- Cervical dilatation: cervix opens from 0-10 centimeters.
- Cervical effacement: cervix is taken up into the upper uterine segment; expressed in percent from 0-100%; cervix is "shortened" from 3 cm to <0.5 cm in length; often called "thinning of the cervix" (misnomer).
- Cervical position: cervix can be directly anterior and palpated easily or posterior and difficult to palpate.
- Cervical consistency: firm to soft.

Fetal Station:

- Location of presenting part in relation to mid-pelvis or ischial spines. Expressed as cm above or below the spines.
  - → Station 0 is ENGAGED.
  - → Station –2 is 2 cm above the ischial spines.

Fetal Presentation:

- Part of the fetus that presents to the inlet.
  - → Vertex (head, cephalic).
  - → Shoulder (acromion).
  - → Breech (buttocks).
  - → Other variations include: brow (sinciput), chin (mentum).

Fetal Position:

- The relationship of the point of reference (occiput sacrum, acromion) on the fetal presenting part (vertex, breech, shoulder) to the mother's pelvis. Most common is LOA (left occiput anterior). The point of reference on the vertex (occiput) is pointed up toward the symphysis and directed toward the left side of the maternal pelvis.

Fetal Lie:

- The relationship of the long axis (spine) of the fetus to the long axis (spine) of the mother. It can be either longitudinal (up and down), transverse (perpendicular), or oblique (slanted).

Fetal Attitude:

- Relationship of the fetal parts to one another.
- Flexion or extension.
- Flexion is desired so that the smallest diameters of the presenting part move through the pelvis.

Figure 5-17

7. If membranes or bag of waters (BOW) ruptured:
   A. Nitrazine paper turns black or dark blue.
   B. Vaginal fluid "ferns" under microscope.
   C. Note color, amount of amniotic fluid.
   D. Allow woman to ambulate during labor only if the FHR is within a normal range and if the fetus is engaged (zero station). If fetus is not engaged, there is an increased risk for a prolapsed cord to occur.
8. Begin graph of labor progress (Friedman's graph). *(See figure 5-18, Friedman's Graph)*
   A. Prolonged latent phase lasts >20 hours in primigravida, >14 hours in multipara.
   B. Primigravidas dilate an average of 1.2 cm/hr in the mid-active phase, multioparas 1.5 cm/hr.

> **HESI HINT:** Meconium-stained fluid is yellow-green or gold-yellow and may indicate fetal stress.

9. Take client to bathroom or offer bedpan at least every two hours during labor. **(Full bladder can impede labor progress.)**
10. Assist woman with use of psychoprophylactic coping techniques such as breathing exercises and effleurage (abdominal massage).

> **HESI HINT:** Breathing techniques such as deep chest, accelerated, and cued are not prescribed by the stage and phase of labor, but by the discomfort level of the laboring woman. If coping is decreasing, switch to a new technique.

11. Provide mouth care, ice chips, and hard candy as needed for dry mouth.

> **HESI HINT:** Hyperventilation results in respiratory alkalosis due to blowing off too much CO_2.
> Symptoms include:
> • Dizziness.
> • Tingling of fingers.
> • Stiff mouth.
> Have woman breathe into her cupped hands or a paper bag in order to rebreathe CO_2.

12. Maintain asepsis in labor by frequent perineal care, changing of linen and underpads.
13. Allow sips of clear fluid if NO general anesthesia is anticipated.
14. Offer anesthesia/analgesia in mid-active phase of labor.
    A. If given too early, it will retard the progress of labor.
    B. If given too late, narcotics increase the risk of neonatal respiratory depression.
15. Monitor fetus continuously if **any** high-risk situation occurs.
16. Notify healthcare provider if any of the following occur:
    A. Labor progress is retarded.
    B. Maternal vital signs are abnormal.
    C. Fetal distress noted.

SECOND STAGE OF LABOR

DESCRIPTION: Heralded by the involuntary need to push, 10 centimeters of cervical dilation, rapid fetal descent, and birth.
1. The second stage of labor averages one hour for the primigravida, 15 minutes for the multipara.
2. The addition of abdominal force to the uterine contraction force enhances the cardinal movements of the fetus: engagement, descent, flexion, internal rotation, extension, restitution, and external rotation.

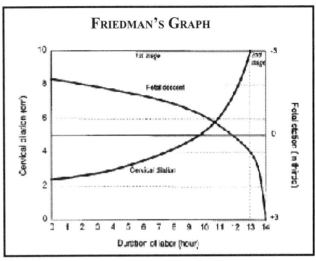

Figure 5-18: An example of Friedman's graph.

NURSING ASSESSMENT
1. Assess BP and pulse q5 to 15 minutes.
2. Determine FHR with every contraction.
3. Observe perineal area for the following:
   A. Increase in bloody show.
   B. Bulging perineum and anus.
   C. Visibility of the presenting part.
4. Palpate bladder for distention.
5. Assess amniotic fluid for color and consistency.

ANALYSIS (NURSING DIAGNOSES)
1. Alteration in comfort: acute pain related to…
2. Potential for injury related to…
3. Knowledge deficit (specify) related to…

NURSING PLANS AND INTERVENTIONS
1. Document maternal BP and pulse q15 minutes between contractions.
2. Check FHR with each contraction or by continuous fetal monitoring.
3. Continue comfort measures: mouth care, linen change, positioning.
4. Decrease outside distractions.
5. Teach mother positions such as squatting, side-lying, or high-Fowler's/lithotomy for pushing.
6. Teach mother to hold breath for NO LONGER than 5 seconds during pushing.
7. Teach mother to exhale when pushing or use "gentle" pushing technique (pushes down on vagina, while constantly exhaling through open mouth, followed by deep breath).

MATERNITY NURSING

> **HESI HINT:** Determine cervical dilation before allowing client to push. Cervix should be completely dilated (10 cm) before the client begins pushing. If pushing starts too early, the cervix can become edematous and never fully dilate.

8. If delivering in another room/setting:
    A. Transfer multipara at 8 to 9 centimeters, +2 station.
    B. Transfer primigravida at 10 centimeters with presenting part visible between contractions AND during contractions.
9. Set up delivery table including bulb syringe, cord clamp, and sterile supplies.
10. Perform perineal cleansing.
11. At crowning, put gentle counter pressure against the perineum. Do not allow rapid delivery over woman's perineum.
12. Make sure client and support person can visualize delivery if so desired. If sibling(s) present, make sure closely accompanied by support person giving explanations that his/her mom is OK.
13. Record EXACT delivery time (complete delivery of baby).

THIRD STAGE OF LABOR

DESCRIPTION: From complete expulsion of the baby to complete expulsion of the placenta.
1. Average length of 3rd stage of labor is 5 to 15 minutes.
2. The longer the third stage of labor, the greater the chance for uterine atony or hemorrhage to occur.

NURSING ASSESSMENT
1. Signs of placental separation:
    A. Lengthening of umbilical cord outside vagina.
    B. Gush of blood.
    C. Uterus changes from oval (discoid) shaped to globular.
2. Mother describes "full" feeling in vagina.
3. Continued firm uterine contractions.

ANALYSIS (NURSING DIAGNOSES)
1. Potential for fluid volume deficit related to…
2. Anxiety related to…

NURSING PLANS AND INTERVENTIONS

> **HESI HINT:** Give the oxytocin after the placenta is delivered because the drug will cause the uterus to contract. If the oxytocic drug is administered before the placenta is delivered, it may result in a retained placenta, which predisposes the client to hemorrhage and infection.

1. Place hand under drape and palpate fundus of uterus for firmness and placement at or below the umbilicus. At signs of placental separation, instruct mother to push gently.
2. Take maternal BP before and after placental separation.
3. Check patency and site integrity of infusing IV.
4. Administer oxytocic medication immediately after delivery of the placenta. *(See figure 5-19, Uterine Stimulants)*
5. Observe for blood loss and ask physician for estimate of blood loss (EBL). 500 cc
6. Dry and suction infant, perform Apgar assessment, place blanket on mother's abdomen or allow skin-to-skin contact with mother after delivery.
7. Place stockinette cap on newborn's head or cover head to prevent heat loss.
8. Allow father/support person to hold infant during repair of episiotomy.
9. Allow sibling(s) if present to hold new family member.
10. Gently cleanse vulva and apply sterile perineal pad.

> **HESI HINT:** Application of Perineal Pads After Delivery
> • Place two on perineum.
> • DO NOT touch inside of pad.
> • DO apply from front to back, being careful not to drag pad across the anus.

11. Remove both legs simultaneously if legs are in stirrups.
12. Provide clean gown and warm blanket.
13. Lock bed before moving mother and raise side rails during transfer.

MATERNITY NURSING

UTERINE STIMULANTS			
DRUGS	**INDICATIONS**	**ADVERSE REACTIONS**	**NURSING IMPLICATIONS**
oxytocin synthetic (Pitocin, Syntocinon)	• Uterine atony	• Severe afterpains in multipara • Hypertension	• Give immediately after delivery of placenta to avoid "trapped" placenta • 10 to 20 units added to remaining IV fluid (at least 500cc) • May stimulate let-down milk reflex and flow of milk when engorged
methylergonovine maleate (Methergine)	• Uterine atony	• Hypertension	• Usual dose: 0.2 mg IM followed by tabs of 0.2 mg q4 to 6 hours • Use with caution in clients with elevated BP or preeclampsia • Take BP **prior** to administration and if 140/90 or above, **withhold** and notify physician.
prostaglandin F$_2$ $\propto$ (Hemabate)	• Uterine atony	• Headache • Nausea and vomiting • Fever • Bronchospasm wheezing	• Contraindicated for clients with asthma • Dose 0.25 IM q15 to 90 minutes; up to 8 doses. May be given intramyometrially by provider • Check temperature q1 to 2 hours • Auscultate breath sounds frequently

Figure 5-19

HESI HINT: Methergine is NOT given to clients with hypertension due to its vasoconstrictive action. Pitocin is given with caution to those with hypertension.

FOURTH STAGE OF LABOR

DESCRIPTION: The fourth stage of labor is the first one to four hours after delivery of placenta.

NURSING ASSESSMENT

1. Review antepartum and labor and delivery records for possible complications.
   A. Postpartum hemorrhage.
   B. Uterine hyperstimulation.
   C. Uterine over-distension.
   D. Dystocia.
   E. Antepartum hemorrhage.
   F. Magnesium sulfate therapy.
   G. Bladder distension.
2. Routine postpartum physical assessment.
3. Maternal/infant bonding.

ANALYSIS (NURSING DIAGNOSES)

1. Potential fluid volume deficit related to…
2. Potential for injury related to…
3. Potential alteration in parenting related to…

NURSING PLANS AND INTERVENTIONS

1. Maintain bedrest for at least 2 hours to prevent orthostatic hypotension.
2. Assess BP, pulse, and respirations q15 min. x1hr.

then q30 min. until stable (BP<140/90, pulse <100, and respiration <24).
3. Assess temperature at beginning of 4th stage and prior to discharge to postpartum room. If above >100.4°F report to physician and monitor hourly.
4. Assess fundal firmness and height, bladder, lochia, and perineum q15 min. x1hr., then q30 min x2 hrs.
   A. **Fundus**: firm, midline, at or below the umbilicus. Massage if soft or boggy. Suspect full bladder if above umbilicus and up to the right side of abdomen.

HESI HINT: FULL BLADDER is one of the most common reasons for uterine atony and/or hemorrhage in the first 24 hours after delivery. If the nurse finds the fundus soft, boggy, and displaced above and to the right of the umbilicus, what action should be taken first? First, perform fundal massage; then have the client empty her bladder. Recheck fundus q15 minutes x4 (1 hour); q30 minutes x 2 hours.

   B. **Lochia**: rubra (red), moderate, and clots <2 to 3 cm. Suspect undetected laceration if fundus firm and bright red blood continues to trickle. Always check perineal pad AND under buttocks.

C. **Perineum**: intact, clean, and slightly edematous. Suspect hematomas if very tender, discolored, or pain is disproportionate to vaginal delivery.

5. Report to healthcare provider:
   A. Abnormal vital signs.
   B. Uterus does not become firm with massage.
   C. Second perineal pad soaked in 15 minutes.
   D. Signs of hypovolemic shock: pale, clammy, tachycardia, light-headed, hypotension.
6. Monitor infusion of intravenous Pitocin. (Check healthcare provider prescription/hospital policy).
7. Change perineal pads and cleanse vulva/perineum with each change.
8. Prevent discomfort of afterpains.
   A. Keep bladder empty. Catheterize only if absolutely necessary.
   B. Place warm blanket on abdomen.
   C. Administer analgesics as prescribed (usually codeine, acetaminophen, or ibuprofen).

> **HESI HINT:** If narcotic analgesics (codeine, meperidine) are given, raise side rails and place call light within reach. Instruct client not to get out of bed or ambulate without assistance. Caution client about drowsiness as a side effect.

9. Offer PO fluids when alert and able to swallow.
10. Apply ice pack to perineum to minimize edema especially if 3rd or 4th degree episiotomy, or if lacerations are present.
11. Apply witch hazel compresses for comfort.

> **HESI HINT:** A 1st degree tear involves only the epidermis. A 2nd degree tear involves dermis, muscle, and fascia. A 3rd degree tear extends into the anal sphincter, and a 4th degree extends up the rectal mucosa. Tears cause pain and swelling. Avoid rectal manipulations.

12. Support parental emotional needs and promote bonding.
    A. Allow extended time with newborn.
    B. Openly share in the joy and excitement of childbirth as well as grieve with parents experiencing loss.
    C. Encourage initiation of breastfeeding.
    D. Provide a warm, darkened environment so newborn will open eyes.
    E. Withhold eye prophylaxis for up to two hours.

F. Perform newborn admission/routine procedures in room with parents.

NEWBORN CARE (DELIVERY ROOM)

DESCRIPTION: Care provided to newborn, usually performed by the nurse.

NURSING ASSESSMENT
1. Maternal history/labor data indicating potential problems with newborn.
2. Apgar scores.
3. Findings of brief physical examination performed in delivery room.

ANALYSIS (NURSING DIAGNOSES)
1. Potential ineffective airway clearance related to…
2. Potential for injury related to…

NURSING PLANS AND INTERVENTIONS
1. Immediately dry infant under warmer or skin to skin with mother, suction mouth and nose with bulb syringe, keep head slightly lower than body, and assess airway status.
   A. Assess for 5 symptoms of respiratory distress:
      1) Retractions.
      2) Tachypnea (rate >60).
      3) Dusky color/circumoral cyanosis.
      4) Expiratory grunt.
      5) Flaring nares.
   B. Do not hyperextend the newborn neck at any time (may close glottis). Place infant in "sniff" position (neck slightly extended as if sniffing the air) to open airway.

> **HESI HINT:** If it was documented that the fetus passed meconium in utero or the nurse noted LATE passage of meconium in delivery room, the neonate MUST be attended by a pediatrician, neonatologist, and/or nurse practitioner to determine, through endotracheal tube observation and suction, the presence of meconium below the cords. It can result in pneumonitis/meconium aspiration syndrome, which will necessitate a sepsis workup including a chest x-ray early in the transitional newborn period.

2. Obtain Apgar score at 1 and 5 minutes. *(See figure 5-20, Apgar Assessment)*
3. Continue to allow maternal/parent contact if

newborn is stable.

4. Keep neonate's head covered.
5. Do quick gestational age assessment. *(See figure 5-21, Gestational Age Assessment)*
   A. Sole creases.
   B. Breast tissue bud.
   C. Skin, vessels, and peeling.
   D. Genitalia.
   E. Resting posture.
6. Examine cord for presence of 3 vessels (2 arteries, 1 vein) and document.
7. Make sure cord blood is collected for analysis and sent to lab.
   A. Rh.
   B. Blood type.
   C. Hct.
   D. Possible cord blood gases.
8. Document passage of meconium or urine after delivery.

9. Place two identibands on neonate and one on mother.
10. Obtain newborn footprints and maternal thumb/fingerprint. Follow institutional policy regarding identification procedures.
11. Perform brief physical exam of newborn.
    A. Check for gross anomalies: spina bifida, hydrocephaly, and cleft lip/palate.
    B. Elicit several reflexes: Moro (startle).
    C. Examine cord clamp for closure, no oozing of blood from cord; again check for presence of 3 vessels.
12. May instill eye prophylaxis in delivery room. *(See figure 5-22, Newborn Prophylactic Eye Care)*
13. If parents desire "open eye" bonding period, delay eye prophylaxis until later. The Center for Disease Control (CDC) states a delay of up to 2 hours is safe.

APGAR ASSESSMENT	

- Performed at exactly 1 and 5 minutes after birth.
- Cannot just eyeball, must have hands-on examination.
- Score:
  - → 7 to 10 Good
  - → 4 to 6   Needs moderate resuscitative efforts
  - → 0 to 3   Severe need for resuscitation

HESI HINT: Do NOT wait until a 1 minute Apgar is assigned to begin resuscitation of the compromised neonate.

FIVE CRITERIA	SCORING
Heart rate	Absent = 0, Under 100 = 1, 100 or > = 2
Respiratory effort	No cry = 0, Weak cry = 1, Vigorous cry = 2
Muscle tone	Flaccid = 0, Some flexion = 1, Total flexion = 2
Reflex irritability	No response to foot tap = 0, Slight response to foot tap (grimace) = 1, Quick foot removal = 2
Color	Dusky, cyanotic = 0, Acrocyanotic = 1, Totally pink = 2

Figure 5-20

HESI HINT: Apgar scores of 6 or < at 5 minutes require an additional Apgar assessment at 10 minutes.

GESTATIONAL AGE ASSESSMENT	
28 WEEKS	• No nipple bud. • Testes in the inguinal canal or labia majora widely separated with labia minora prominent open and equal in size. • Vernix (cheesy coating) over the entire body. • Lanugo (fine, downy hair) over the entire body. • Full extension of extremities in resting posture.
40 WEEKS	• Raised nipple with a tissue bud underneath. • Descended testes with large rugae (folds) on the scrotum. • Labia majora large and covering the minora. • Vernix only in the creases. • Lanugo perhaps only over the shoulders. • Hypertonic flexion of extremities in resting posture.

Figure 5-21

NEWBORN PROPHYLACTIC EYE CARE			
DRUGS	**INDICATIONS**	**ADVERSE REACTIONS**	**NURSING IMPLICATIONS**
OINTMENTS **Erythromycin** **Tetracycline**	• Prevention of ophthalmia neonatorum and Chlamydia trachomatis conjunctivitis	• Most commonly used agents • None known, except puffy eyes from manipulation	• Place a thin line of ointment along the entire lower lid in conjunctival sac • Use only one tube per baby and DISCARD • Manipulate upper lid to ensure complete eye coverage • After one minute, may wipe excess from around eye
SILVER NITRATE	• Prevention of ophthalmia neonatorum from gonorrhea exposure through the birth canal in a vaginal delivery	• Chemical conjunctivitis (red, puffy eyes) • Staining of skin if contact occurs	• Eye prophylaxis is mandatory in the United States • May not kill other organisms such as Chlamydia • Instill 2 gtts. in lower conjunctival sac making sure drops spread over entire eye • DO NOT irrigate eyes following instillation

Figure 5-22

LABOR WITH ANALGESIA/ANESTHESIA

1. Analgesia/anesthesia in labor is usually withheld until the mid-active phase.
   A. If given in the early latent phase of the first stage of labor, it may retard the progress of labor.
   B. If given late in transition or in 2nd stage, it may depress the newborn (some narcotic analgesics).
2. Most drugs used for systematic pain relief/ relaxation cause CNS depression, which can slow labor and harm fetus.
3. Regional blocks (epidural, caudal, and subarachnoid) cause a temporary interruption of nerve impulses (especially pain) but also **cause vasodilation in area below block, causing pooling of blood and hypotension.**

NURSING ASSESSMENT

1. Acute pain experienced in active labor.
2. Birth plan; includes use of analgesic/anesthetic agents.
3. Decreased coping and increased anxiety.
4. Assess the client and obtain the following data:
   A. Vital signs and fetal heart rate.
   B. Labor progress, i.e., cervical dilatation and effacement, fetal position and lie.
   C. Last time and amount of food/fluids ingested.
   D. Lab values (Hgb, Hct, clotting time).
   E. Hydration status.
   F. Signs/symptoms of infection.

ANALYSIS (NURSING DIAGNOSES)

1. Alteration in comfort: acute pain related to…
2. Ineffective individual coping related to…
3. Potential for injury to mother/fetus related to…

NURSING PLANS AND INTERVENTIONS
Administration of analgesic drugs in labor.

1. Document baseline maternal vital signs and fetal heart rate prior to administration of narcotics or sedatives. *(See figure 5-23, Analgesics)*
2. Assess phase/stage of labor.
3. Obtain physician's order for medication.
4. Determine client/family desires regarding analgesics and verbally praise informed choice.
5. Do NOT give PO medications. Labor retards gastrointestinal activity and absorption.
6. Administer medications IV when possible, IM if necessary.

> **HESI HINT:** IV administration of analgesics is preferred to IM for the client in labor because the onset and peak occurs more quickly and duration of the drug is shorter. KNOW the following:
> **IV ADMINISTRATION**
> • Predictable onset: 5 minutes.
> • Peak: 30 minutes.
> • Duration: 1 hour.
> **IM ADMINISTRATION**
> • Onset: within 30 minutes.
> • Peak: 1 to 3 hours after injection.
> • Duration: 4 to 6 hours.

7. Push IV bolus into line **slowly**, at the beginning of a contraction, i.e., give medication during contraction, when uterine blood vessels are constricted, so less reaches the fetus.
8. Explain the purpose of the drug to the laboring woman, but **do not** promise results.
9. After drug administration:
    A. Record the woman's response and level of pain relief.
    B. Monitor maternal vital signs, FHR, and characteristics of uterine contractions q15 minutes for one hour after administration.
    C. Monitor bladder for distention/ retention (medication can decrease perception of bladder filling).
    D. Decrease environmental stimuli; darken room, reduce number of visitors, turn off TV.
    E. Note time between drug administration and birth of baby on delivery record.
    F. If baby delivers during PEAK drug absorption time, notify pediatrician and/or neonatologist for delivery room assistance and possible use of NARCAN for neonate. *(See figure 5-23, Analgesics)*

10. General anesthesia is rarely used in today's obstetric units. It might be used in emergency deliveries or when regional block anesthesia is contraindicated or refused.
    A. Administer drugs to reduce gastric secretions such as cimetidine (Tagamet) or clear (non-particulate) antacids to neutralize gastric acid. (The most common cause of maternal death is aspiration of gastric contents into the lung.)

> **HESI HINT:** Tranquilizers (ataractics and/or phenothiazines) Phenergan, Vistaril, are used in labor as analgesic-potentiating drugs to decrease the amount of narcotic needed and to decrease maternal anxiety.

> **HESI HINT:** Agonist narcotic drugs (Demerol, morphine) produce narcosis and have a higher risk for maternal/fetal respiratory depression. Antagonist drugs (Stadol, Nubain) have less respiratory depression but MUST be used with caution in a mother with preexisting narcotic dependency since withdrawal symptoms occur immediately.

    B. Assist with speedy delivery. (General anesthesia may depress fetus if delivery is not accomplished quickly.)
    C. Assess closely for uterine atony; check fundal firmness and uterine contraction. (General anesthesia is associated with postpartum uterine atony.)

MATERNITY NURSING

ANALGESICS			
DRUGS	**INDICATIONS**	**ADVERSE REACTIONS**	**NURSING IMPLICATIONS**
meperidine HCL (Demerol, Pethidine) **fentanyl** (Sublimaze) **morphine sulfate** (MS Contin)	• Opioid agonists • Narcotic used to produce analgesia, euphoria, and sedation in labor • Analgesia during labor	• Respiratory depression • Fetal narcosis/ distress • Hypotension • Fetus receives normeperidine which is linked to fetal compromise • Itching • Urinary retention • Respiratory depression	• Store in narcotic's cabinet • Record use accurately • Do NOT administer if respirations < 12/ minute • Have narcotic antagonist available (NARCAN) • Monitor respirations, pulse, BP, closely • *(See figure 5-59, Narcotic Analgesics)*
butorphanol tartrate (Stadol) **nalbuphine** (Nubain)	• Opioid agonist/ antagonists • Provision of analgesia in labor • Narcotic analgesic	• Woman with preexisting narcotic dependency will experience withdrawal symptoms immediately (abstinence syndrome)	• Give IV or IM • Obtain drug history before administration • Monitor respirations, pulse
naloxone HCL (Narcan)	• Narcotic antagonist used to counteract narcotic effects on mother/fetus	• Decreased respirations rarely occur	• Monitor respirations closely since drug action is shorter than the narcotic (may need to readminister) • Pain returns after administration to mother • Can be administered to newborn after delivery (0.01 mg/kg body weight) to counteract narcotic depression

Figure 5-23

REGIONAL BLOCK ANESTHESIA

1. Local anesthesia.
   A. Used for pain relief during episiotomy, and perineal repair.
   B. Safe for mother and infant.
2. Regional blocks.
   A. Used for relief of perineal and uterine pain.
   B. Usually safe for mother and infant unless severe hypotension occurs.
   C. Types of regional blocks:
      1) Pudendal block: given in 2nd stage to deaden pudendal nerve plexus which deadens perineum and vagina
         a) Has NO effect on pain of uterine contractions.
         b) Safe for mother and baby.
      2) Peridural (epidural, caudal) block: given in 1st or 2nd stage of labor and blocks nerve impulses from T10 to S5, thereby deadening pain of contractions.
         a) Used in conjunction with local or pudendal for delivery; or a **delivery dose** is given to deaden perineum for delivery.
         b) May be given in single dose or continuously through catheter threaded into epidural space.
         c) Moderately associated with hypotension, which can cause maternal and fetal distress.
         d) Epidural block associated with prolonged 2nd stage due to decreased effectiveness of pushing.
      3) Intradural (subarachnoid, spinal) block; given in 2nd stage of labor to deaden uterine and perineal pain.
         a) Rapid onset, but highly associated with maternal hypotension which can cause maternal and fetal distress.
         b) Client must remain flat for 6 to 8 hours after delivery.
3. Contraindications to subarachnoid and peridural blocks include the following:
   A. Client's refusal or fear.
   B. Anticoagulant therapy or presence of bleeding disorder.
   C. Presence of antepartum hemorrhage causing acute hypovolemia.

D. Infection or tumor at injection site.
E. Allergy to –caine drugs.
F. CNS disorders, previous back surgery, or spinal anatomic abnormality.

HESI HINT: Pudendal block and sub-arachnoid (saddle block) are used only for second stage of labor. Peri/epidural may be used for all stages of labor.

NURSING ASSESSMENT

1. No contraindications to regional block anesthesia.
2. Experiencing severe pain.
3. Possible need for Cesarean delivery.
4. BP before block >100/70.
5. Status of maternal-fetal unit.

ANALYSIS (NURSING DIAGNOSES)

1. Potential alteration in tissue perfusion (mother and fetus) related to…
2. Potential for injury to fetus/client related to…
3. Potential urinary retention related to…

NURSING PLANS AND INTERVENTIONS

1. Ensure that the healthcare provider has explained procedures, the risks, benefits, and alternatives.
2. Pre-hydrate client to counteract possible hypotension; 500 to 1000 ml. IV fluid (isotonic) infused over 20 to 30 minutes before initiation of regional block.
3. Place client in a modified Sims' position or sitting on side of bed with head flexed.
4. Ask client to describe symptoms after test dose of medication is given.
   A. Metallic taste in mouth/ringing in ears denotes possible injection of medication into blood stream.
   B. Nausea/vomiting is one of first signs of hypotension.

HESI HINT: The first sign of block effectiveness is usually warmth and tingling of ball/big toe of foot.

5. Determine BP q1 to 2 minutes for 15 minutes after injection of anesthetic drug and initiate continuous fetal monitoring.
6. Determine BP q15 minutes during continuous regional block infusion.

7. Assist client to keep bladder empty.
8. Assess level of pain relief with sharp/dull technique and record return of pain sensation.
9. Report return of pain sensation, incomplete anesthesia, or uneven anesthesia to anesthesiologist.
10. If hypotension occurs, DO the following:
    A. Immediately turn client to left side.
    B. Increase intravenous infusion.
    C. Begin O_2 at 10 L/min by facemask.
    D. Notify healthcare provider stat and have ephedrine available at bedside.
    E. Assess FHR.
11. Assist client in pushing technique once complete dilatation is achieved.

HESI HINT: Discontinue continuous infusion at end of Stage I or during transition to increase pushing effectiveness.

HESI HINT: Regional Block Anesthesia and Fetal Presentation
- Internal rotation is harder to achieve when the pelvic floor is relaxed by anesthesia resulting in persistent occiput posterior position of fetus.
- Monitor for fetal position. REMEMBER, mother cannot tell you she has back pain, which is the cardinal sign of persistent posterior fetal position.
- Regional blocks, especially epidural and caudal, often result in assisted (forceps or vacuum) delivery due to the inability to push effectively in 2nd stage.

HESI HINT: Nerve block anesthesia (spinal or epidural) during labor blocks motor as well as nerve fibers. Vasodilation below the level of the block results in blood pooling in the lower extremities and maternal hypotension. Approximately 20 minutes prior to nerve block anesthesia, the client should be hydrated with 500 to 1000 cc of lactated ringers IV. Monitor maternal vital signs and FHR q5 to 15 minutes. If hypotension occurs – turn the client to her side, administer O_2 at 10L/min by facemask, and increase IV rate.

REVIEW QUESTIONS

INTRAPARTUM

1. List five prodromal signs of labor the nurse might teach the client.
2. How is true labor discriminated from false labor?
3. State two ways to determine if the membranes have truly ruptured (ROM).
4. Are psychoprophylactic breathing techniques prescribed for use by the stage and phase of labor?
5. Identify two reasons to withhold anesthesia and analgesia until the mid-active phase of Stage I labor.
6. Hyperventilation often occurs to the laboring client. What results from hyperventilation and what actions should the nurse take to relieve the condition?
7. Describe maternal changes that characterize the transition phase of labor.
8. When should a laboring client be examined vaginally?
9. Define cervical effacement.
10. Where is the fetal heart rate best heard?
11. Normal fetal heart rate in labor is _____.
    Normal maternal BP in labor is _____.
    Normal maternal pulse in labor is _____.
    Normal maternal temperature in labor is ____.
12. List four nursing actions for the second stage of labor.
13. List three signs of placental separation.
14. When should the postpartum dosage of Pitocin be administered? Why is it administered?
15. State one contraindication to the use of ergot drugs (Methergine).
16. State five symptoms of respiratory distress in the newborn.
17. If meconium was passed in utero, what action must the nurse take in the delivery room?
18. What score is considered a "good" Apgar score?
19. What is the purpose of eye prophylaxis for the newborn?
20. What is the danger associated with regional blocks?
21. What is the major cause of maternal death when general anesthesia is administered?
22. Why are PO medications avoided in labor?
23. State the best way to administer IV drugs in labor.
24. When is it dangerous to administer butorphanol (Stadol), an agonist/antagonist narcotic?
25. Hypotension often occurs after the laboring client receives a regional block. What is one of the first signs the nurse might observe?
26. State three actions the nurse should take when hypotension occurs in a laboring client.
27. The fourth stage is defined as:
28. What actions can the nurse take to assist in preventing postpartum hemorrhage?
29. To promote comfort, what nursing interventions are used for a 3rd degree episiotomy, which extends into the anal sphincter?
30. What nursing interventions are used to enhance maternal-infant bonding during the fourth stage of labor?
31. List three nursing interventions to ease the discomfort of afterpains.
32. List symptoms of a full bladder, which might occur in the fourth stage of labor.
33. What action should the nurse take first when a soft, boggy uterus is palpated?
34. What are the symptoms of hypovolemic shock?
35. How often should the nurse check the fundus during the fourth stage of labor?

ANSWERS TO REVIEW QUESTIONS

1. Lightening, Braxton Hicks contractions, increased bloody show, loss of mucous plug, burst of energy, and nesting behaviors.
2. True labor: regular, rhythmic contractions that intensify with ambulation, pain in the abdomen sweeping around from the back, and cervical changes. False labor: irregular rhythm, abdominal pain (not in back) that decreases with ambulation.
3. Nitrazine testing: paper turns dark blue or black. Demonstration of fluid "ferning" under microscope.
4. No, clients should use these techniques according to their discomfort level and change techniques when one is no longer working for relaxation.
5. If given too early, can retard labor; if given too late, can cause fetal distress.
6. Respiratory alkalosis occurs which is caused by blowing off CO_2 and is relieved by breathing into a paper bag or cupped hands.

MATERNITY NURSING

272

7. Irritability, unwillingness to be touched but does not want to be left alone, nausea and vomiting, and hiccupping.

8. Vaginal exams should be done prior to analgesia/ anesthesia, to rule out cord prolapse, to determine labor progress if it is questioned, and to determine when pushing can begin.

9. The taking up of the lower cervical segment into the upper segment; shortening of the cervix expressed in percent from 0 to 100% or complete effacement.

10. Through the fetal back in vertex, OA positions.

11. 110 to 160 BPM. <140/90. <100 BPM. <100.4°F.

12. Make sure cervix is completely dilated before pushing is allowed. Assess FHR with each contraction. Teach woman to hold breath for no longer than 5 seconds. Teach pushing technique.

13. Gush of blood, lengthening of cord, and globular shape of uterus.

14. Give immediately after placenta is delivered to prevent postpartum hemorrhage/atony.

15. Hypertension.

16. Tachypnea, dusky color, flaring nares, retractions, and grunting.

17. Arrange for immediate endotracheal tube observation to determine the presence of meconium below the vocal cords (prevents pneumonitis/meconium aspiration syndrome).

18. 7 to 10.

19. Prevent ophthalmia neonatorum, which results from exposure to gonorrhea in vagina.

20. Hypotension resulting from vasodilation below the block, which pools blood in periphery reducing venous return.

21. Aspiration of gastric contents.

22. Gastric activity slows or stops in labor, decreasing absorption from PO route; may cause vomiting.

23. At beginning of contraction, push a little medication in while uterine blood vessels are constricted, thereby reducing dose to fetus.

24. When the client is an undiagnosed drug abuser of narcotics, it can cause immediate withdrawal symptoms.

25. Nausea.

26. Turn client to left side. Administer O$_2$ by mask at 10 L/min. Increase speed of intravenous infusion (if it does not contain medication).

27. The first one to four hours after delivery of placenta.

28. Massage the fundus (**gently**) and keep the bladder emptied.

29. Ice pack, witch hazel compresses, and no rectal manipulation.

30. Withhold eye prophylaxis for up to two hours. Perform newborn admission/routine procedures in room with parents. Encourage early initiation of breastfeeding. Darken room to encourage newborn to open eyes.

31. Keep bladder empty. Provide a warm blanket to abdomen. Administer analgesics prescribed by healthcare provider.

32. Fundus above umbilicus, dextroverted (to the right side of abdomen), increased bleeding (uterine atony).

33. Perform fundal massage.

34. Pallor, clammy skin, tachycardia, lightheadedness, and hypotension.

35. q15 minutes x 4 (1 hour), q30 minutes x 2 hours if normal.

MATERNITY NURSING

Normal Puerperium

(Postpartum)

Description: Period after pregnancy and delivery (usually 6 weeks) when the body returns to the non-pregnant state. *(See figure 5-24, Normal Puerperium Changes)*

1. Care in this period is focused on wellness and family integrity.
2. Teaching must be initiated early to cover the physical self-care needs and emotional needs of the mother, infant, and family.

NORMAL PUERPERIUM CHANGES	
REPRODUCTIVE SYSTEM	**ANATOMIC & PHYSIOLOGIC CHANGES**

UTERUS	• Myometrial contractions occur for 12 to 24 hours post delivery due to high oxytocin levels (prominent in multiparas, breastfeeding clients, and women who experienced over distension of the uterus)
	• Involution occurs (1 to 2 cm/day)
	  → First day: at, or 1 to 2 cm above umbilicus
	  → 7 to 10 days: decreases to 12 weeks size, slides back under symphysis pubis
	• Placenta site contracts and heals without scarring

CERVIX	• Becomes parous with a transverse slit • Heals within 6 weeks
VAGINA	• Rugae (folds) reappear within 3 weeks • Walls thin and dry

BREASTS	• Non-lactating
	  → Nodules palpable
	  → Engorgement may occur 2 to 3 days PP
	• Lactating
	  → Milk sinuses (lumps) palpable
	  → Colostrum (yellowish fluid) expressed first, then milk (bluish-white)
	  → May feel warm, firm, tender for 48 hours

CARDIOVASCULAR SYSTEM	**ANATOMIC & PHYSIOLOGICAL CHANGES**
AT DELIVERY	• Maternal vascular bed reduced by 15% • Pulse may decrease to 50 (normal puerperal bradycardia) • These changes are hypothesized to result in client "shivering" • BP and P should quickly return to pre-pregnant levels
FIRST 72 HOURS	• 24 to 48 hours postpartum, cardiac output remains elevated (returns to non-pregnant levels in 2 to 3 weeks) • Plasma loss >RBC loss; reverses hemodilution of pregnancy (Hct rises) • Diaphoresis (especially at night) helps restore normal plasma volume
HEMATOLOGICAL SYSTEM	• Hct rises • WBC count elevated (12,000 up to 25,000) • Difficult to use white count for determination of infection • Blood-clotting factors elevated; increases risk of thromboembolism
URINARY SYSTEM	• Diuresis occurs; excretes up to 3000 cc/day of urine • Bladder distention and incomplete emptying common • Persistent dilatation of ureter/renal pelvis increase risk of UTI • Urine glucose, creatinine, and BUN levels normal after 7 days
GASTROINTESTINAL SYSTEM	• Excess analgesia/anesthesia may decrease peristalsis • No bowel movements expected for 2 to 3 days
INTEGUMENTARY SYSTEM	• Chloasma and hyper-pigmentation areas (linea nigra, areolae) regress; some areas may remain permanently darker • Palmar Erythema declines quickly • Spider nevi fade, some in legs may remain

Figure 5-24

MATERNITY NURSING

NORMAL PUERPERIUM CHANGES	
REPRODUCTIVE SYSTEM	ANATOMIC & PHYSIOLOGIC CHANGES
MUSCULOSKELETAL SYSTEM	• Pelvic muscles regain tone in 3 to 6 weeks • Abdominal muscles regain tone in 6 weeks unless diastasis recti (separation of rectus abdominis muscles) occurs

Figure 5-24 (continued)

HESI HINT: Normal leukocytosis of pregnancy averages 12,000 to 15,000 mm³. The first 10 to 12 days post-delivery, values of 25,000 mm³ are common. Elevated WBC and the normal elevated ESR may confuse interpretation of acute postpartal infections. For example, if the nurse assesses a client's temperature to be 101°F on the client's second postpartum day, what assessments should be made before notifying the physician? Assess fundal height and firmness, perineal integrity, check for a positive Homan's sign and other symptoms of thromboembolism, pulse, respirations, and blood pressure, client's subjective description of symptoms, i.e., burning on urination, pain in leg, excessive tenderness of uterus.

HESI HINT: Client/family teaching is a common area for NCLEX-RN® questions. Remember, when teaching the first step is to assess the client's (parent's) level of knowledge and identify their readiness to learn. Client teaching regarding lochia changes, perineal care, breastfeeding, sore nipples are commonly tested content.

NURSING ASSESSMENT
1. Review prenatal, antepartum, L&D, and early postpartum records for status, lab data, and possible complications.
2. Review newborn record for Apgar scores, sex, possible complications, and relevant psychosocial information (adoption, single parent, etc.).
3. Assess postpartum status: vital signs, fundal height and firmness, lochia, urination, perineum, bowel sounds, presence of thrombophlebitis.
4. Assess maternal/infant bonding and identify teaching needs of mother/family.

ANALYSIS (NURSING DIAGNOSES)
1. Alteration in comfort: pain related to…
2. Potential for infection related to…
3. Urinary retention related to…
4. Knowledge deficit (specify) related to…
5. Potential for low self-esteem related to…

NORMAL POSTPARTAL VITAL SIGNS	
VITAL SIGN	DESCRIPTION
TEMPERATURE	May rise to 100.4°F due to dehydrating effects of labor: ANY higher elevation may be due to infection and must be reported.
PULSE	May decrease to 50 (normal puerperal bradycardia). Pulse >100 may indicate excessive blood loss or infection.
BLOOD PRESSURE	Should be normal; suspect hypovolemia if it decreases, preeclampsia if it increases.
RESPIRATIONS	Rarely change: if respirations increases significantly, suspect pulmonary embolism, uterine atony, and/or hemorrhage.

Figure 5-25

NURSING PLANS AND INTERVENTIONS
1. Monitor vital signs q4 hrs. x 24 hrs. then q8 hrs.
2. Check fundal height and firmness:
   A. On the first postpartum day (first day following birth), the top of the fundus is located approximately 1 cm below the umbilicus. *(See figure 5-26, Postpartum Fundal Height)*
   B. Should be midline and firm immediately after delivery.
   C. Massage if soft, and/or boggy by stabilizing back of uterus before applying pressure; teach mother procedure but advise against over-stimulation, which can lead to atony.
   D. Teach normalcy of afterpains.
3. Assess and document lochia:
   A. Lochia rubra: blood-tinged discharge including shreds of tissue and deciduas; lochia rubra lasts 2 to 3 days PP.
   B. Lochia serosa: pale pinkish to brownish discharge lasting one week PP.
   C. Lochia alba: thicker, whitish-yellowish discharge with leukocytes and degenerated cells; lochia alba lasts up to 4 weeks PP.

D. Subinvolution: placental site does not heal, lochia persists with brisk periods of lochia rubra, and a D&C may be necessary.
E. Document amount:
    1) Scant: <1 inch on pad.
    2) Small: <4 inch stain on pad.
    3) Moderate: <6 inch stain on pad.
    4) Heavy: saturated pad within 1 hour.
    5) Clots should be <2 to 3 cm.
    6) Odor: fleshy, not foul.

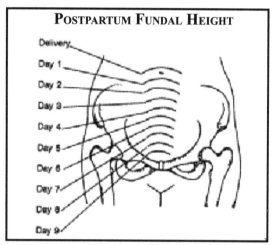

POSTPARTUM FUNDAL HEIGHT

Delivery
Day 1
Day 2
Day 3
Day 4
Day 5
Day 6
Day 7
Day 8
Day 9

Figure 5-26

F. Teach client normal lochia changes.
    1) Flow increases with ambulation and breastfeeding.
    2) Expect color changes.

4. Assess perineum/episiotomy site:
    A. Place in lateral Sims' position, don gloves, and use flashlight to increase visualization.
    B. Check for redness, edema, intactness, and presence of hematomas; teach self-inspection with mirror.
    C. Teach hygiene and comfort and healing measures.
        1) Change pad as needed and with every voiding/defecation.
        2) Wipe perineum front to back.
        3) Good handwashing technique.
        4) Ice packs, sitz baths, peri bottle lavage, and topical application of anesthetic spray or pads. *(See figure 5-27, Postpartum Teaching)*
5. Examine breasts:
    A. Assess nipples for cracks, fissures, redness, and/or tenderness.
    B. Assess breasts for engorgement.
    C. Palpate breasts for lumps/nodules.
    D. Determine motivation to breast or bottle-feed.
    E. If not breastfeeding, teach non-pharmacologic measures for milk suppression: supportive bra or binder, ice packs, and avoid breast stimulation.
    F. Teach breast self-exam. *(See figure 5-27, Postpartum Teaching)*

MATERNITY NURSING

276

POSTPARTUM TEACHING

BREAST SELF-EXAM

- Begin with inspection in a mirror. Place both hands at sides and observe; then look again with hands overhead and bending forward. Assess for:
  → Change in size and shape.
  → Dimpling, puckering, scaling, redness, swelling of any part of breast.
- Lie flat with right hand under head and pillow or towel under right shoulder.
  → Use left hand to palpate using concentric circles around right breast, feeling for lumps, nodules or thickening.
  → Repeat with left breast.

EPISIOTOMY CARE
- Perineal Care
- Fill bottle with warm water, and if prescribed, an ounce of povidone/iodine solution.
- Lavage perineum with several squirts and blot dry instead of rubbing; avoid anal area.

Figure 5-27

HESI HINT: Client should void within 4 hours of delivery. Monitor closely for urine retention. Suspect retention if voiding is frequent and <100 cc per voiding.

HESI HINT: Women often have a syncopal spell (faint) on the first ambulation after delivery (usually related to vasomotor changes, orthostatic hypotension). The astute nurse will check for client's Hgb and Hct for anemia and the blood pressure, sitting and lying for orthostatic hypotension.

6. Assist mother/infant with breastfeeding. *(See figure 5-28, Teaching Breastfeeding)*
7. Assess bladder and urine output:
   A. Palpate for spongy, full feeling over symphysis.
   B. Check urge to void when bladder palpated.
   C. Assist to ambulate for first void (possible orthostatic hypotension) measure if possible.
   D. Run warm water over perineum or place spirit of peppermint in bedpan to relax urethra if necessary.
   E. Catheterize ONLY if necessary.
   F. Teach symptoms of UTI: dysuria, frequency, and urgency.
   G. Promote retoning of perineal muscles by Kegel exercises.

HESI HINT: Kegel Exercises: increase integrity of introitus and improve urine retention. Teach client to alternate contraction and relaxation of the pubococcygeal muscles.

TEACHING BREASTFEEDING

TOPICS TO INCLUDE	DATA RELATED TO TOPICS
ADVANTAGES OF BREASTFEEDING	• Low cost • Distinct immunologic advantages for newborn
MILK PRODUCTION	• Stimulated by the decrease in postpartum estrogen production which allows release of prolactin from the pituitary • Prolactin responsible for milk production
LET-DOWN REFLEX (MILK EJECTION)	• Caused by action of oxytocin released from posterior pituitary which stimulates myoepithelial cells around milk ducts/sinuses • Initiated by breast stimuli or even the mere presence or cry of the neonate
BREAST SIZE	• Has no relationship to successful breastfeeding
INVERTED AND RETRACTED NIPPLES	• Women with inverted or retracted nipples can wear shields which may help the infant latch onto the nipple

Figure 5-28

TEACHING BREASTFEEDING (CONTINUED)	
TOPICS TO INCLUDE	DATA RELATED TO TOPICS
DIET DURING BREASTFEEDING/ LACTATION	• Avoid dieting • Add 500 calories to pre-pregnant intake • Drink 2 quarts (8 glasses) of non-caffeinated beverages daily
AVOID	• Smoking and the intake of drugs, alcohol, and caffeine • Stress, most common reason for decreased milk supply
ENCOURAGE	• Rest
CARE OF BREAST AND NIPPLES	• Newborn should remain on first breast 10 minutes, switch to second breast and suckle until satisfied. (No longer recommended to limit breastfeeding time to 2 to 3 minutes first day, 5 minutes second, etc.) • Use warm water, not drying soap on nipples • Let nipples air dry for 15 minutes 2 to 3 times daily • Breast creams should not be routinely used. Colostrum may be expressed and rubbed on nipples
ENGORGEMENT	• Nurse more frequently and manually expresses milk to soften areola before feeding • Wear supportive bra • Take warm/hot showers (water over breasts promotes milk flow) • Watch for symptoms of mastitis (commonly occurs when breasts are not emptied) • If desired to wean, give up one feeding every week.
INCORRECT POSITIONING	• Incorrect positioning of baby on breast is most common reason for sore nipples • Make sure baby has as much of areola as possible in mouth • Break suction with insertion of little finger into baby's mouth

Figure 5-28 (continued)

8. Assess bowel/anal area:
   A. Inspect for hemorrhoids; describe size and number.
   B. Administer antihemorrhoidal cream, ointment, or suppositories as prescribed.
   C. Auscultate bowel sounds; check abdominal distension.
   D. Document flatus and/or bowel movement.
   E. Encourage early ambulation.
   F. Encourage increased fluids and use of roughage/bulk in diet.
   G. Administer stool softeners (Colace), enemas, or suppositories (Dulcolax) as prescribed. *(See figure 5-30, Postpartum Drugs)*
   H. Avoid rectal manipulation if 3rd or 4th degree episiotomy was performed.
9. Prevent thrombophlebitis.
   A. Encourage early ambulation.
   B. Encourage foot paddling and ankle rolling after general anesthesia.
   C. Check for positive Homan's sign.

> **HESI HINT:** Assess for thromboembolism: Examine legs of PP client daily for pain, warmth, and tenderness or a swollen vein which is tender to touch. Client may or may not exhibit a positive Homan's sign (dorsiflexion of foot causes compression of tibial veins and pain if thrombus is present).

10. Determine the need for RhoGAM. *(See figure 5-30, Postpartum Drugs)*
11. Determine the need for a rubella vaccine.
12. Assess maternal psychological adaptation. (Reva Rubin identified three distinct emotional stages after delivery).
    A. **Taking-in:** dependency behaviors for 24 to 48 hours; asking for help on simplest of tasks.
    B. **Taking-hold:** less focus on physical discomforts, beginning confidence with infant care taking. Not uncommon for mother to feel inadequate caring for infant; the astute nurse will not "take over" but will praise efforts of parents. At this time new parents are usually most receptive to teaching about infant care.
    C. **Letting-go:** total separation of newborn

from self; confident in care taking activities of self and newborn.

13. Assess maternal/infant-bonding behaviors.
    A. Eye contact between mother/neonate.
    B. Exploration of infant from head to toe.
    C. Stroking, kissing, and fondling the neonate.
    D. Smiling, talking, singing to the neonate.
    E. Use of claiming expressions, e.g., "He's got my feet."
    F. Absence of negative statements such as, "She just doesn't like me."
    G. Naming the newborn quickly.

14. Promote maternal/infant-bonding.
    A. Ensure mother is comfortable: provide pain relief, hygiene, and adequate rest.
    B. If possible, have baby room-in; include family in teaching; praise and reinforce all positive parenting behaviors.
    C. Teach about neonatal behavioral traits.
    D. Assure normalcy of comparing idealized child to looks/sex of real child but prevent long-term disappointment by encouraging verbalization of those feelings now.
    E. Teach responses to cues from the baby.
       1). Pick baby up when crying (reciprocity).
       2). Soothe with calm, interactive responses until baby returns to quiet, active state (synchrony).
    F. Encourage verbalization of feelings; offer support in non-judgmental manner.

HESI HINT: "Postpartum blues" are usually normal, especially 5 to 7 days after delivery (unexplained tearfulness, feeling "down," and a decreased appetite). Encourage use of support persons to help with housework for first two postpartum weeks. Refer to community resources.

15. Notify healthcare provider or clinic promptly of:
    A. Heavy, vaginal bleeding with clots.
    B. Temperature of 100.4°F or higher lasting 24 hours or longer.
    C. A red, warm lump in breast.
    D. Pain on urination.
    E. Tenderness in calf.

16. Teach self-care for discharge:
    A. Continue perineal care and pad changes.
    B. Encourage balanced diet and fluid intake.
    C. Rest/nap when newborn does.

17. Warn about sibling rivalry, especially if a toddler is at home (age 18 months to 3 years).
    A. Sibling may regress.
    B. Bring "present" to toddler from the newborn, and encourage mother to hug toddler.
    C. Plan time alone with sibling(s).
    D. Abstain from sexual intercourse until lochia has ceased. First sexual experience may not be pleasant due to vaginal dryness.

18. Assist client with choice of contraceptive method. Teach use, risks, and technique prior to discharge. *(See figure 5-29, Methods of Contraception)*

METHODS OF CONTRACEPTION	
METHOD	**USE, RISK, AND TECHNIQUE**
DIAPHRAGM	• Use with spermicide • Must be fitted by a nurse practitioner/doctor • Must be left in place 6 hours after intercourse • Refit if excessive weight gain or loss • Check device for integrity • Can irritate urethra
CERVICAL CAP	• Use with spermicide • Contraindicated if cervical anomalies exist • Associated with cervical changes • Pap smear recommended 3 months after use
CONDOM (WITH SPERMICIDE)	• Use condom with spermicide to increase effectiveness • Recommended if any suspicion of STD • Withdraw penis while erect or condom may fall off • Petroleum jelly can deteriorate rubber, use water-soluble jelly

Figure 5-29

METHODS OF CONTRACEPTION (CONTINUED)	
METHOD	**USE, RISK, AND TECHNIQUE**

SYMPTOTHEMAL PTO-THEMAL OR FERTILITY AWARENESS	• Teach signs of ovulation
	    → Cervical mucus assessment
	    → Basal body temperature assessment
	    → Mittelschmerz (abdominal pain in the region of an ovary during ovulation)

IUD (INTRAUTERINE DEVICE)	• Contraindications: diabetes, anemia, abnormal pap, history of pelvic infections • High association with dysmenorrhea and infection
ORAL CONTRACEPTIVES	• Estrogen in pills prevents pituitary secretion of FSH, preventing ovulation • Woman still menstruates • Lowest failure rate of methods • CONTRAINDICATIONS: history of coagulation problems, thromboembolism, liver disease, reproductive cancer, coronary artery disease • Compliance is a problem since pill has to be taken every day • If 1 pill is missed, take it as soon as remembered and take the next one at the usual time • If 2 pills are missed, take 2 pills for 2 days and use alternate method of contraception for next 7 days • If more than 2 pills are missed in the third week, or 3 or more pills missed at any time, quit pills for that cycle and use alternate method of contraception. Resume pills on fifth day of menstruation
TRANSDERMAL CONTRACEPTIVE PATCH	• Mechanism of action, efficacy, contraindications, and side effects are similar to those of oral contraceptives • Delivers continuous levels of progesterone and estradiol • Can be applied to lower abdomen, upper outer arm, buttock, or upper torso (except the breasts) • Apply on the same day once a week for 3 weeks, followed by one week without patch
NORPLANT (LEVONORGESTREL IMPLANT)	• Sustained-release subdermal progestin-only contraceptive • Consist of six thin, flexible capsules made of soft silastic tubing • Placed in a fan like pattern just beneath the skin of the upper arm • Effective within 24 hours after insertion; effective for approximately 5 years • Efficacy is not dependent on client compliance once inserted • Reversible with return to previous level of fertility after removal • Side effects include: menstrual pattern changes, headache, nervousness • Works by suppression of ovulation as well as by thickening cervical mucus • **Efficacy challenged - not available in U.S.** Two-rod implant approved by FDA
DEPO-PROVERA	• IM injection of 100 mg q3 months for contraception • Administered during the first five days of menstrual cycle • New mothers may be given the injection during the postpartum period; before discharge • Efficacy of 99% • Protection from pregnancy is immediate after injection • Most women experience weight gain and irregular or unpredictable menstrual bleeding (after one year's use many women stop having menstrual periods altogether) • Monitor for signs and symptoms of thrombophlebitis • CONTRAINDICATIONS: history of breast cancer, stroke, blood clots, liver disease • Side effects include nervousness, dizziness, GI disturbances, headaches and fatigue; may also increase risk of osteoporosis

Figure 5-29 (continued)

MATERNITY NURSING

POSTPARTUM DRUGS

DRUGS	INDICATIONS	ADVERSE REACTIONS	NURSING IMPLICATIONS
bisocodyl (Dulcolax suppository)	• Constipation	• Abdominal cramping	• Insert suppository into anus past internal rectal sphincter • Since it is a contact laxative stimulating rectal mucosa directly, there may be some burning • Usually effective in 15 minutes to one hour
docusate sodium (Colace)	• Constipation • Painful defecation due to 4th degree tear	• Abdominal cramping	• Encourage increased fluid intake • Results usually occur within 1 to 3 days of continual use

rhoGAM (Rh$_o$(D) immune globulin)	• Prevention of Rh isoimmunization with next pregnancy	• None known	• Given to Rh negative women after miscarriage, abortion, or any procedure or complication that increases the risk of maternal-fetal blood exchange (amniocentesis, PUBs, abdominal trauma)
			• Routinely given at 28 weeks gestation to Rh negative mothers with a negative antibody titer.
			• Given postpartally to Rh negative mother after delivery or abortion when fetus is Rh positive
			• It is never given to an infant or father
			• Must be given within 72 hours of delivery
			• Always given IM
			• Is a blood product:
			  → Must be checked by 2 nurses
			  → Return syringe to lab with label
			  → Not given to a mother with positive indirect Coombs; she is already sensitized to fetal cells and has developed antibodies

Rubella vaccine	• Rubella titer of ≤ 1:8 or enzyme immunoassay (EIA) of ≤ 0.8	• Transient benign arthralgia • Transient rash • Hypersensitivity if allergic to duck eggs	• Given subcutaneously before hospital discharge to non-immune women • May breastfeed • Do not give if woman or other family members are immunocompromised • Requires informed consent • Teach about contraception - women should avoid pregnancy for 2 to 3 months after immunization

Figure 5-30

HESI HINT: Remember, RhoGAM is given to a Rh-negative mother who delivers a Rh-positive fetus and has a negative direct Coombs. If the mother has a positive Coombs, there is no need to give RhoGAM since the mother is already sensitized.

HESI HINT: Because Rh Immune Globulins suppress the immune system, the client who receives both Rho GAM and the Rubella vaccine should be tested for rubella immunity at 3 months.

MATERNITY NURSING

REVIEW QUESTIONS

NORMAL PUERPERIUM (POSTPARTUM)

1. A nurse discovers a postpartum client with a boggy uterus, displaced above and to the right of the umbilicus. What nursing action is indicated?

2. Which women experience afterpains more than others?

3. Upon admission to the postpartum room, 3 hours after delivery, a client has a temperature of 99.5°F. What nursing actions are indicated?

4. A client feels faint on the way to the bathroom. What nursing assessments should be made?

5. What factor places the postpartum client at risk for thromboembolism?

6. A breastfeeding mother complains of very tender nipples. What nursing actions should be taken?

7. Three days postpartum, a lactating mother has full, warm, taut, tender breasts. What nursing actions should be taken?

8. What information should be given to a client regarding resumption of sexual intercourse after delivery?

9. A woman has decided to take birth control pills as her contraceptive method. What should she do if she misses taking the pill two consecutive days?

10. A woman asks why she is urinating so much in the postpartum period. The nurse bases the response on what information.

11. A woman's white blood count returns 17,000; she is afebrile and has no symptoms of infection. What nursing action is indicated?

12. What is the most common cause of uterine atony in the first 24 hours postpartum?

13. What is the purpose of giving docusate sodium (Colace) to the postpartum client?

14. What should the fundal height be at three days postpartum for a woman who has had a vaginal delivery?

15. List three signs of positive bonding between parents and newborn.

ANSWERS TO REVIEW QUESTIONS

1. Perform immediate fundal massage. Ambulate to the bathroom or use bedpan to empty bladder because cardinal signs of bladder distension are present.

2. Breastfeeding women, multiparas, and women who experienced over distension of the uterus.

3. Probably elevated due to dehydration and work of labor; force fluids and retake temperature in an hour; notify physician if above 100.4°F.

4. Assess BP sitting and lying, assess Hgb and Hct for anemia.

5. Increased clotting factors.

6. Have her demonstrate infant position on breast (incorrect positioning often causes tenderness). Leave bra open to air-dry nipples for 15 minutes 3x daily. Express colostrum and rub on nipples.

7. She is engorged; have newborn suckle frequently; use measures to increase milk flow; warm water, breast massage and supportive bra.

8. Avoid until postpartum exam. Use water-soluble jelly. Expect slight discomfort due to vaginal changes.

9. Take two pills for two days and use an alternate form of birth control.

10. Up to 3,000 cc per day can be voided due to the reduction of the 40% plasma volume increase during pregnancy.

11. Continue routine assessments; normal leukocytosis occurs during postpartal period because of placental site healing.

12. A full bladder.

13. To soften the stool in mothers with 3rd or 4th degree episiotomies, hemorrhoids, or Cesarean section delivery.

14. Three fingerbreaths/cm below the umbilicus.

15. Calling infant by name, exploration of newborn head-to-toe, en face position.

THE NORMAL NEWBORN

During the immediate transitional period (first 6 to 8 hours of life) and early newborn period (first few days of life) the nurse assesses, plans, and provides nursing interventions based on the outcomes of the individual newborn exam.

NURSING ASSESSMENT

1. Review L&D report of neonatal history to determine risks during newborn transition caused by medical and obstetric complications:
   A. Cesarean delivery missing vaginal squeeze.
   B. Prematurity or postmaturity.
   C. Diabetic mother.
   D. Prolonged rupture of membranes (ROM) >24 hours: sepsis workup.
   E. Rh+ isoimmunization (+ direct Coombs).
   F. Traumatic/forceps delivery.

2. Review L&D report of neonatal history to

determine risks during newborn transition caused by drugs/anesthesia in labor/delivery:

A. Magnesium Sulfate in labor: Hypermagnesemia in neonate caused depressed respirations, hypocalcemia, and hypotonia.

B. Narcosis (late administration of narcotic analgesics); causes decreased respirations and hypotonia.

3. Review L&D report of neonatal history to determine risks during newborn transition caused by degree of birth asphyxia:

A. Asphyxia in labor: documented late decelerations, decreased variability, severe variable decelerations.

B. Apgar scores at 1 and 5 minutes.

4. Review significant social history: mother with STD, single parent, language barrier, substance abuse, and lack of support system.

5. Assess vital signs q30 minutes x 2 hours, then q1 hour x 5 hours. *(See figure 5-31, Newborn Vital Sign Norms)*

6. Measure the neonate. *(See figure 5-32, Physical Measurement)*

7. Perform a Physical Examination of the newborn.

(See figure 5-33, Physical Exam of the Newborn)

8. Perform Neuromuscular Assessment. The absence of expected reflexes requires investigation into birth trauma/asphyxia or CNS anomaly. *(See figure 5-34, Neuromuscular Assessment)*

9. Perform a systematic Gestational Age Assessment. *(See figure 5-35, Gestational Age Assessment)* Plot measurements on percentile scale to determine if small, average, or large for gestational age.

10. Perform a Behavioral Assessment using the Brazelton's Neonate Behavioral Assessment Scale to evaluate newborn's behavioral uniqueness.

A. Waiting 2-3 days to perform gives neonate a chance to rid body of effects of analgesia/anesthesia/trauma of birth.

B. Measures six categories: habituation, orientation, motor activity, self-quieting ability, social behaviors, sleep/awake states.

C. Performing test with parents present familiarizes them with their newborn's uniqueness and may provide them cues on the best ways to respond to newborn.

NEWBORN VITAL SIGN NORMS		
VITAL SIGN	**NORMAL**	**NURSING IMPLICATIONS**
RESPIRATIONS	Rate: 30-60 breaths per minute	• Remember the ABCs (airway, breathing, circulation) • Count one full minute by observing abdomen or auscultating breath sounds. • Note 5 symptoms of respiratory distress: → Tachypnea → Cyanosis → Flaring nares → Expiratory grunt → Retractions
HEART RATE	110 to 160 BPM; may fall as low as 100 during sleep, as high as 180 during crying	• Auscultate for one full minute at the PMI (point of maximal impulse): 3rd to 4th intercostal space
TEMPERATURE	Range 97.7 to 99.4°F, 36.5 to 37.5°C	• Measure axillary for 5 minutes • Rectal temps may perforate rectum; if taken rectally, insert only ¼ to ½ inch for 5 minutes and hold legs firmly to prevent trauma
BLOOD PRESSURE	Average 80/50	• NOT usually measured unless problems in circulation assessed

Figure 5-31

PHYSICAL MEASUREMENTS

ASSESSMENT	NORMAL	NURSING IMPLICATIONS
WEIGHT	Average 7 lbs. 8 oz. (Majority weigh between 2700 gm and 4000 gm; 6 to 9 lbs.)	• Weigh at birth and daily with neonate completely naked • Normally lose 5 to 15% (average 10%) of birth weight in first week of life; Document weight carefully
LENGTH	Average range: 18 to 21 inches, 46 to 52.5 cm	• Measured from crown to rump and rump to heel, or from crown to heel at birth
HEAD CIRCUMFERENCE	Average range: 33 to 35 cm (Normally, 2 cm larger than chest circumference)	• Place tape measure above eyebrows and stretch around fullest part of occiput, at posterior fontanel (FOC is designation for frontal-occipital circumference)
CHEST CIRCUMFERENCE	Average range: 31to 33 cm	• Stretch tape measure around scapulae and over nipple line

Figure 5-32

HESI HINT: PHYSICAL ASSESSMENT
A detailed physical assessment is performed by the nurse or physician. Regardless of who performs the physical assessment, the nurse must know normal versus abnormal variations of the newborn. Observations must be recorded and the physician notified regarding abnormalities.

PHYSICAL EXAM OF THE NEWBORN

NORMAL	ABNORMAL	RATIONALE
GENERAL APPEARANCE • Awake • Flexed extremities • Moves all extremities • Strong, lusty cry • Obvious presence of subcutaneous fat • No obvious anomalies	• Little subcutaneous fat	• Intrauterine growth problems • Fetal stress
	• Frog position	• Prematurity
	• Flaccid	• Asphyxia • Prematurity
	• Hard to arouse	• Sepsis • CNS problems • Asphyxia
	• High-pitched cry	• CNS damage/anomalies • Hypoglycemia • Drug withdrawal
INTEGUMENT • Smooth, elastic turgor and subcutaneous fat, superficial peeling after 24 hours; rarely are veins visible • Milia, vernix in creases • Lanugo, mottling • Harlequin's sign (pink/red skin on one side of body) • Erythema toxicum (pink papular rash is normal) • Mongolian spots • Telangiectatic nevi (stork bites)	• Extreme desquamation	• Postmaturity
	• Many visible veins	• Prematurity
	• Meconium staining	• Fetal distress
	• Cyanosis	• Heart disease • Asphyxia
	• Jaundice (within 24 hrs)	• Blood incompatibilities • Sepsis • Drug reactions
	• Vesicles	• Herpes, syphilis
	• Café-au-lait spots	• Neurofibromatosis

Figure 5-33

PHYSICAL EXAM OF THE NEWBORN (CONTINUED)		
NORMAL	**ABNORMAL**	**RATIONALE**
HEAD • Round or slightly molded • Caput succedaneum (edema over occiput) • Open, flat anterior & posterior fontanels, slightly separated sutures or overlapping due to molding	• Bulging fontanelle	• Increased ICP
	• Sunken fontanelle	• Dehydration
	• Widely-separated sutures	• Hydrocephalus
	• Premature suture closure	• Genetic disorders
	• Cephalhematoma	• Blood under periosteum due to trauma

HESI HINT: It is difficult to differentiate between caput succedaneum (edema under the scalp) and cephalhematoma (blood under the periosteum). The caput crosses suture lines and is usually present at birth, while the cephalhematoma does NOT cross suture lines and manifests a few hours after birth. The danger of cephalhematoma is increased hyperbilirubinemia due to excess RBC breakdown.

EYES • Symmetrically placed • Pseudo-strabismus • Chemical conjunctivitis (from eye prophylaxis) • Clear cornea • White-blue sclera • Subconjunctival hemorrhage from pressure • Absence of tears • Doll's eye movement (slight Nystagmus)	• Purulent discharge	• Gonorrhea/chlamydia
	• Brushfield's spots in iris	• Down syndrome
	• Absence of red reflex	• Congenital cataracts
	• Epicanthal folds	• Down syndrome
	• Setting sun sign	• CNS disorders
	• Absent glabellar reflex (blink)	• CNS or neuromuscular problem
EARS • Pinna at, or above level of line drawn from outer canthus of eye • Well-formed and firm with instant recoil if folded against head	• Low set	• Down syndrome
	• Unformed, soft	• Prematurity
	• Preauricular sinus	• Possible renal anomaly
NOSE • In midline • Appears flattened • Nose breather • Occasional sneezing	• Short, upturned small philtrum (creases under nose)	• Fetal Alcohol Syndrome
	• Nasal flaring	• Respiratory distress
	• Grunting	• Respiratory distress • Choanal atresia (obstruction between nares and pharynx)
	• Snuffles	• Syphilis
	• Excessive sneezing	• Drug withdrawal
MOUTH AND CHIN • Symmetrical movement • Intact lip/palate • Epstein pearls • Mobile tongue • Sucking pads in cheeks • Presence of rooting, sucking, swallowing, and gagging reflexes	• Asymmetry	• Facial nerve injury (Bell's Palsy)
	• Cleft lip	• Genetic disorder
	• White plaques on cheeks, tongue	• Monilia infection/thrush
	• Absence of protective reflexes	• Prematurity • CNS disorders
	• Excessive drooling	• Esophageal atresia

Figure 5-33 (continued)

PHYSICAL EXAM OF THE NEWBORN (CONTINUED)		
NORMAL	ABNORMAL	RATIONALE
NECK • Short • ROM • Nonpalpable thyroid • Ability to lift head momentarily	• Limited range of motion	• Torticollis (wry neck)
	• Nuchal rigidity	• Meningitis
	• Enlarged thyroid	• Hyperthyroidism
	• Crepitus over clavicle	• Fractured clavicle
CHEST • Symmetrical excursion • Breath sounds clear and equal • Transient rales at birth • Round • Breast engorgement (hormonal) • Transient murmurs	• Persistent murmur	• Patent ductus arteriosus
	• Visible activity over precordium	• Congenital heart anomaly • Congestive heart failure
	• Retractions	• Respiratory distress
	• Asymmetrical chest	• Pneumothorax
BACK, HIPS, BUTTOCKS, AND ANUS • Spine intact • Symmetrical gluteal folds • Equal limb lengths • Patent anus	• Pilonidal dimple or sinus (at base of sacrum)	• CNS anomaly • Covert spina bifida
	• Hip click • Unequal limb lengths • Asymmetrical gluteal folds	• Congenital hip dislocation
	• Absence of stools after 24 hours	• Imperforate anus • GI obstruction
ABDOMEN • Full, rounded, soft • Present bowel sounds • Palpable liver 1 to 2 cm below right costal margin • 2 arteries, 1 vein in cord; white cord with Wharton's jelly	• Scaphoid	• Diaphragmatic hernia
	• Distention	• Meconium ileus • GI obstruction • Hirschsprung's disease
	• Hepatosplenomegaly	• Sepsis
	• Purulent discharge at base of cord, foul odor	• Omphalitis (cord infection)
	• One artery	• Renal/heart anomalies
	• Omphalocele	• Abdominal contents in umbilicus (anomaly)
	• Gastroschisis	• Abdominal contents outside of abdomen (anomaly)
GENITALS Female: • Slightly edematous labia covering clitoris and labia minora • Pseudomenstruation • Visible hymenal tag Male: • Penis with foreskin intact • Meatus in middle at tip of penis • Descended testes • Slight edema of scrotum • Rugae on scrotum	• Labia minora and clitoris visible	• Prematurity
	• Undescended testes	• Prematurity
	• Meatus on dorsal surface penis	• Epispadias
	• Meatus on ventral surface penis	• Hypospadias
	• Fluid in testes	• Hydrocele
	• Intestine in inguinal canal	• Inguinal hernia

Figure 5-33 (continued)

MATERNITY NURSING

PHYSICAL EXAM OF THE NEWBORN (CONTINUED)

NORMAL	ABNORMAL	RATIONALE
EXTREMITIES Arms, hands, fingers, legs, feet, toes • Flexion • Symmetrical movement • Palpable brachial and radial pulses • Strong grasp reflex • Multiple palmar and plantar creases • Slightly bowed legs • Femoral pulses present • Positive Babinski's reflex	• Incurving little finger	• Down syndrome
	• Simian crease	• Down syndrome
	• Flapping tremors	• Drug withdrawal
	• Polydactyly	• Extra digit (family trait)
	• Syndactyly	• Webbed digit (family trait)
	• Difference in pulses between upper and lower extremities	• Coarctation of aorta
	• Absence of plantar creases	• Prematurity
	• Rigid fixation of ankle	• Clubfeet (talipes)
	• Absent Babinski's	• CNS injury

Figure 5-33 (continued)

HESI HINT: These neurological reflexes are transient, and, as such, disappear usually within the first year of life. In the pediatric client, prolonged presence of these reflexes can indicate CNS defects. Anticipate NCLEX-RN® questions regarding normal newborn reflexes. Physical assessment questions focus on normal characteristics of the newborn and the differentiation of conditions such as caput succedaneum and cephalhematoma.

NEUROMUSCULAR ASSESSMENT

REFLEX	NORMAL RESPONSE	LASTS UNTIL
ROOTING	• Turns toward stimuli when cheek or corner of lip is touched	3 to 4 months (possibly 1 year)
MORO	• When startled, baby symmetrically extends and abducts all extremities • Forefingers form "C"	3 to 4 months
TONIC NECK	• When neck is turned to side, baby assumes fencing posture	3 to 4 months
BABINSKI'S	• Stroke sole of foot from heel to ball and toes will hyperextend and fan apart from big toe	1 year to 18 months
PLANTAR	• Finger in base of toes causes curling downward	8 months
STEPPING	• Infant is held in upright position with feet touching a hard surface - makes walking motions	3 to 4 months

Figure 5-34

MATERNITY NURSING

HESI HINT: The umbilical cord should always be checked at birth. It should contain 3 vessels, 1 vein which carries oxygenated blood to the fetus and 2 arteries which carry unoxygenated blood back to the placenta. This is the opposite of normal circulation in the adult. Cord abnormalities usually indicate cardiovascular or renal anomalies

HESI HINT: Postnatally, the fetal structures of foramen ovale, ductus arteriosus and ductus venosus should close. If they do not, cardiac and pulmonary compromise will develop.

GESTATIONAL AGE ASSESSMENT

BY DATE	BY WEIGHT
PRETERM: 20 to 37 weeks gestation	**Small for Gestational Age (SGA):** Weight below the 10th percentile for estimated weeks of gestation
TERM INFANT: 38 to 42 weeks gestation	**Average for Gestational Age (AGA):** Weight between the 10th and 90th percentile for estimated weeks of gestation
POSTERM: >42 weeks gestation	**Large for Gestational Age (LGA):** Weight above the 90th percentile for estimated weeks of gestation

Figure 5-35

NURSING CARE OF THE NEWBORN

PREVENT	NURSING CARE
ASPIRATIONS	• Keep bulb syringe or suction immediately available: suction mouth and then nose. • Turn on side or stomach and pat firmly on the back holding head 10 to 15 degrees lower than feet.

HESI HINT: Suctioning the mouth first and then the nose. Stimulating the nares can initiate inspiration which could cause aspiration of mucus in oral pharynx.

INFECTION	• HANDWASHING!! This is the most effective preventive measure. • Scrupulous cord care: swab cord with alcohol at each diaper change or keep clean with mild soap and water (varies by hospital and provider). • Cover circumcision with petrolatum gauze; change gauze at each diaper change. • Do not allow visitors or personnel to attend to newborn if: active infection present, diarrhea, open wounds, infectious skin rash, and herpes virus. • Encourage breastfeeding for immunologic factors.

HESI HINT: Circumcision has become controversial since there is no real medical indication for the procedure and it does cause trauma and pain to the newborn. It was once thought to decrease the incidence of penile and cervical cancer, but some researchers say this is unfounded.

HYPOTHERMIA	• Keep dry and warm. • Place stockinette cap on head (greatest heat loss is through scalp). • Take temperature at admission and every 4 to 6 hours. • If temperature falls below 97°F (36.4°C), place radiant warmer and apply skin temperature probe to regulate isolette temperature. May also double wrap or put skin to skin with mother.

HESI HINT: HYPOTHERMIA (heat loss) leads to depletion of glucose and, therefore, the use of brown fat (special fat deposits fetus puts on in last trimester which are important to thermoregulation) for energy, resulting in ketoacidosis and possible shock. *Prevent by keeping neonate warm!*

HYPOGLYCEMIA	• Perform a heel-stick blood glucose assessment on all SGA or LGA babies, infants of diabetic mothers (IDM), jittery babies, or babies with high-pitched cry. *(See figure 5-37, Heel-Stick for Newborns)* • Report any blood glucose levels under 40 mg/dl in the full-term infant, under 30 mg/dl in the preterm infant. Normal serum glucose 40 to 80 mg/dl • Feed the baby early (5% Dextrose water, breastmilk, or formula) if a low glucose level is detected. • Prevent cold stress which leads to hypoglycemia.
HEMMORHAGIC DISORDERS	• Administer vitamin K to prevent hemmorhagic disorders. *(See figure 5-38, Vitamin K)*

Figure 5-36

NURSING CARE OF THE NEWBORN (CONTINUED)

HYPER-BILIRUBINEMIA	• Evaluate for Rh isoimmunization (Rh+ newborn, Rh-mother; maternal Rh+ antibodies are passed to the fetus and cause RBC hemolysis); or ABO incompatibility (mother blood type O, newborn blood type A or B, maternal anti-A or anti-B antibodies are passed to newborn and cause less severe hemolysis).
	• Bilirubin (byproduct of RBC destruction) binds to protein for excretion or metabolism.
	• Promote stooling by early feedings of MILK (protein binds bilirubin for excretion).
	• Assess birth and daily for presence of jaundice:
	  → Yellowish skin color, sclera, and mucous membranes.
	  → Proceeds cephalocaudally (relationship between the head and the base of the spine).
	• Give adequate fluids.
	• Monitor bilirubin levels.
	• Institute phototherapy if >12 mg/dl (varies by healthcare provider).

Figure 5-36 (continued)

HESI HINT: Physiologic jaundice (normal inability of the immature liver to keep up with normal RBC destruction) occurs at 2 to 3 days of life. If it occurs before 24 hours or persists beyond 7 days, it becomes pathologic. Typically, NCLEX-RN® questions ask about normal problem of physiologic jaundice which occurs 2 to 3 days after birth due to the liver's inability to keep up with RBC destruction and bind bilirubin. Remember, unconjugated bilirubin is the culprit.

HEEL-STICK FOR NEWBORNS

SKILL	PROCEDURE
HEEL STICK FOR BLOOD	• Wash hands and put on gloves. • Clean heel with alcohol and dry with a gauze pad. • Choose a site for puncture that avoids the plantar artery in the middle of the heel. • Use only the lateral surfaces of the heel. • Puncture deep enough to trigger a free flow of blood. Wipe away first drop with sterile gauze pad. • Collect blood in appropriate tube, on card, or glucose "stick."

Figure 5-37

VITAMIN K

DRUGS	INDICATIONS	ADVERSE REACTIONS	NURSING IMPLICATIONS
VITAMIN K (Aquamephyton Phytonadione)	• Prevention of hemorrhagic disorder in newborn • Infants are born with sterile gut, and have no enteric bacteria present for synthesis of vitamin K	• Inflammation at the injection site	• Usual order is 0.5 to 1 mg of vitamin K given IM in the first hour after birth • Use the vastus lateralis muscle of the thigh (never the gluteus until walking for at least 1 year) • Hold knee secure during procedure as neonate will try to move during injection

Figure 5-38

NURSING PLANS AND INTERVENTIONS

1. The nurse is responsible for monitoring the newborn whether rooming-in or in the nursery!
2. Facilitate parent/infant attachment.
3. Document daily the elimination patters:
   A. Stool progression: meconium (black, tarry, sticky) stool within the first 24 hours to transitional (yellowish-green) to milk stool (yellow). Report if no stool within 24 hrs.
   B. Should void within 4 to 6 hrs., then 1 deaper for each day of life, minimum until day 6. Day 6 and beyond should have a minimum of 6 to 8 diapers per day. Report if no urination within 24 hrs. May see brick-red "dust" in the first voidings (uric acid crystals).
4. Screen for PKU (phenylketonuria) after 2 to 3 days of milk ingestion. State laws differ regarding newborn screening. Many also screen

for hypothyroidism, sickle cell, and galactosemia.
5. Document nutritional intake and calculate nutritional needs:

> **HESI HINT:** DO NOT feed a newborn when the respiratory rate is over 60. Inform the physician and anticipate gavage feedings in order to prevent further energy utilization and possible aspiration.

   A. Demand feeding (bottle or breast) is preferred.
   B. Most bottle-fed newborns eat every 3 to 4 hours; breastfed infants every 2 to 3 hours (digested more quickly).
   C. After initial weight loss period, should gain approximately 1 ounce (30 grams) per day.
   D. Needs about 50 calories/lb or 108 calories/kg of body weight for the first 6 months.

> **HESI HINT:** A 7lb. 8oz. baby would need 50 calories x 7 pounds = 350 calories plus 25 calories (1/2 pound or 8 ounces) = 375 calories per day. Most infant formulas contain 20 calories/ounce. Dividing 375 by 20 = 18.75 ounces of formula needed per day.

6. Monitor lab values for anemia, infection, and polycythemia. *(See Appendix A for Normal Lab Values)*
   A. Hct.
   B. Hgb.
   C. Platelets.
   D. WBC.
7. Provide parent/family teaching on newborn care:
   A. Bathing: DO NOT submerge in water until cord falls off (7 to 10 days); continue cord care and keep diaper off cord.
   B. Diapering: use warm water to clean after voiding; soap and water with stools. (Remember, cleanse female perineum front to back); may use A&D cream for rashes.
   C. Crying: may cry 2 hours per day when hungry, wet, or bored. Pick the baby up; it is difficult to "spoil" the baby in the first year of life. Identify "fussy" periods and change environment when they occur.

   D. Comfort: enjoy "swaddling" avoid startling when picking up; try to burp when "fussy" or crying (may be a gas bubble).
8. Recognize signs and symptoms of a sick newborn who needs medical attention:
   A. Lethargy or difficulty waking.
   B. Temp above 100°F (32.2°C).
   C. Vomiting (large emesis, NOT spitting up).
   D. Green, liquid stools.
   E. Refusal of two feedings in a row.

> **HESI HINT:** Teach parents to take infant's temperature BOTH axillary and rectally. While axillary is recommended, some pediatricians will request a rectal temperature (core).
> **AXILLARY:** Place thermometer under arm and hold thermometer in place 5 minutes.
> **RECTALLY:** Use thermometer with BLUNT end. Insert thermometer ¼ to ½ inch and hold in place for 5 minutes. Hold feet and legs firmly.

REVIEW QUESTIONS
NORMAL NEWBORN
1. The newborn transitional period consists of the first _____ of life.
2. The nurse anticipates which newborn will be more at risk for problems in the transitional period. State three predisposing factors to respiratory depression in the newborn.
3. What is the danger of heat loss to the newborn in the first few hours of life?
4. Normal newborn temperature is _____.
   Normal newborn heart rate is _____.
   Normal newborn respiratory rate is ___.
   Normal newborn blood pressure is ___.
5. The nurse records a temperature below 97°F on admission of the newborn. What nursing actions should be taken?
6. True or False: The newborn's head is usually smaller than the chest.
7. During the physical exam of the newborn, the nurse notes the cry is shrill, high-pitched, and weak. What are the possible causes?
8. The nurse notes a swelling over the back part of the newborn head. Is this normal newborn variation?
9. What symptoms are common to most newborns with Down syndrome?
10. Identify three ways to determine the

presence of congenital hip dislocation in the newborn.

11. **Should the normal newborn have a positive or negative Babinski's reflex?**

12. **A small-for-gestational age newborn is identified as one who _____.**

13. **When suctioning the newborn with a bulb syringe, which should be suctioned first, the mouth or nose?**

14. **A new mother asks the nurse if circumcision is medically indicated in the newborn. How should the nurse respond?**

15. **Normal blood glucose in the term neonate is _____.**

16. **Why does the newborn need vitamin K in the first hour after birth?**

17. **Physiologic jaundice in the newborn occurs _____. It is caused by _____.**

18. **When is the screening test for phenylketonuria done?**

19. **A term newborn needs to take in _____ calories per pound per day. After the initial weight loss is sustained, the newborn should gain _____ per day.**

20. **List five signs and symptoms new parents should be taught to report immediately to a doctor or clinic.**

ANSWERS TO REVIEW QUESTIONS

1. 6 to 8 hours.
2. Cesarean section delivery; Magnesium sulfate given to mother in labor; Aspyxia/fetal distress in labor.
3. Leads to depletion of glucose (very little glycogen storage in immature liver); begins to use brown fat for energy producing ketones causing subsequent ketoacidosis and shock.
4. 97.7 to 99.4ºF.; 110 to 160 BPM; 30 to 60; BP 80/50.
5. Place newborn in isolette or under radiant warmer and attach a temperature skin probe to regulate isolette or radiant warmer temperature. Wrap newborn double if no isolette or warmer available and put cap on head. Watch for signs of hypothermia and

hypoglycemia.

6. FALSE: head is usually 2 cm larger unless severe molding occurred.
7. CNS anomalies, brain damage, hypoglycemia, drug withdrawal.
8. It depends on the exam. If it crosses suture lines and is a caput (edema), it is normal. If it does not cross suture lines, it is a cephalhematoma with bleeding between the skull and periosteum. This could cause hyperbilirubinemia. This is an abnormal variation.
9. Low set ears, simian crease on palm, protruding tongue, Brushfield's spots in iris, epicanthal folds.
10. Hip click determination, asymmetrical gluteal folds, unequal limb lengths.
11. Positive. The transient reflex is present until 12 to 18 months of age.
12. Has a weight below the 10th percentile for estimated weeks of gestation.
13. Mouth; stimulating the nares can initiate inspiration which could cause aspiration of mucus in oral pharynx.
14. There is controversy concerning this issue, but we do know it causes pain and trauma to the newborn, and the medical indication may be unfounded (prevention of penile and cervical cancer).
15. 40 to 80 mg/dl.
16. Sterile gut at delivery lacks intestinal bacteria necessary for the synthesis of vitamin K; vitamin K is needed in the clotting cascade to prevent hemorrhagic disorders.
17. Jaundice occurs at 2 to 3 days of life and is caused by immature liver's inability to keep up with bilirubin production of normal RBC destruction.
18. At 2 to 3 days of life or after enough milk ingestion to determine body's ability to metabolize amino acid phenylalanine.
19. 50, 1 ounce or 30 gm.
20. Lethargy, temperature >100ºF, vomiting, green stools, refusal of 2 feeds in a row.

ANTEPARTUM HEMORRHAGE: SPONTANEOUS ABORTION

- Bleeding from conception to 20 weeks gestation.
- Seventy-five percent of spontaneous abortions occur between 8 and 13 weeks and are usually related to chromosomal defects.
- Considered a **MEDICAL EMERGENCY**.

ANALYSIS (NURSING DIAGNOSES)
- Fluid volume deficit related to…
- Anxiety related to…

ASSESSMENT	NURSING PLANS AND INTERVENTIONS

• Gestational age 20 weeks or less, fetal viability absent.
• Uterine cramping, backache, and pelvic pressure.
• Vaginal, bright red bleeding.
  → Note number of perineal pads/hour.
  → Note symptoms of shock.
    • Rapid, thready pulse.
    • Pallor.
    • Hypotension.
    • Cool, clammy skin.
• Assess client/family emotional status, needs, and support system.
	• Identify type of abortion and subsequent management.
	• Monitor vital signs, level of consciousness every hour until stable.
	• Save all peripads, linens.
	• Start an IV with at least an 18g. over-the-needle catheter.
	• Give RhoGAM if indicated (Rh negative mother).
	• Teach client to notify nurse if the following occurs:
	  → Temp above 100.4°F.
	  → Foul smelling vaginal discharge.
	  → Bright red bleeding with any tissue larger than a dime.
	• Implement grief protocol if fetus loss occurs.
	  → Provide a memory packet (footprints, bracelet).
	  → Give client/family opportunity to see fetus (sex of fetus).
	  → Explain the grief process and refer to community resources for grief/loss. (RESOLVE and SHARE are examples of national bereavement support groups.)

TYPE AND TREATMENT

TYPE/DESCRIPTION	TREATMENT
Threatened: spotting without cervical changes.	**Threatened:** bedrest for 24 to 48 hours; no sexual intercourse for 2 weeks.
Inevitable or incomplete: moderate/heavy bleeding with tissue/products of conception present; open cervical os.	**Inevitable:** hospitalization; dilatation and curettage (D&C).
Complete: all products of conception passed; cervix closed.	**Complete:** no need for treatment.
Septic: fever, abdominal pain and tenderness; foul smelling vaginal discharge/bleeding from scant to heavy.	**Septic:** termination of pregnancy; antibiotic therapy; monitor for septic shock.
Missed: fetus has died/placenta atrophied but passage of products of conception has NOT occurred; cervix closed.	**Missed:** watchful waiting; check clotting factors and possibly terminate pregnancy if DIC prevention considered necessary.
Recurrent: loss of 3 or more pre-viable pregnancies.	**Recurrent:** varies based on etiology; if premature cervical dilation (incompetent cervix) is cause, prophylactic cerclage may be done.

Figure 5-39

HESI HINT: Clients with prior traumatic delivery, history of D&C, multiple abortions (spontaneous or induced), or daughters of DES mothers may experience miscarriage or preterm labor related to INCOMPETENT CERVIX. The cervix may be surgically repaired prior to pregnancy, or DURING gestation. A CERCLAGE (McDonald's suture) is placed around the cervix to constrict the internal os. The cerclage may be removed prior to labor if labor is planned or left in place if cesarean birth is planned.

GESTATIONAL THROPHOBLASTIC DISEASE (HYDATIDIFORM MOLE)	
• Chorionic villi degenerate into a bunch of clear vesicle, grape-like clusters. • Hydatidiform mole is a developmental anomaly. • An embryo is rarely present. • Predisposes the client to choriocarcinoma.	
ANALYSIS (NURSING DIAGNOSES) • Grieving related to … • Knowledge deficit (specify) related to … • Anxiety related to …	

ASSESSMENT	NURSING PLANS AND INTERVENTIONS
• Vaginal bleeding usually in first trimester. • Size/date discrepancy (uterus larger than expected for gestational age. • Other common findings include: → Anemia. → Excessive nausea and vomiting. → Abdominal cramping → Early symptoms of preeclampsia.	• Provide preoperative and postoperative D&C care. • Assess the following: → Vital signs. → Vaginal discharge. → Uterine cramping. • Provide discharge instructions. → Prevent pregnancy for one year. → Obtain monthly serum HCG levels for one year. • Teach signs of complications to be reported immediately to healthcare provider/clinic. → Bright red, frank vaginal bleeding. → Temperature spike over 100.4°F. → Foul-smelling vaginal discharge. • Refer to community resource for grief/loss.

Figure 5-40

ECTOPIC PREGNANCY

- Fertilized ovum is implanted outside the uterine cavity, usually in the fallopian tube.
- Occurs in one out of 200 pregnancies.
- Often occurs as result of tubular obstruction or blockage which prevents normal transit of the fertilized ovum.
- Considered a **MEDICAL EMERGENCY**.

ANALYSIS (NURSING DIAGNOSES)
- Alteration in comfort: pain related to…
- Grieving related to…

ASSESSMENT	NURSING PLANS AND INTERVENTIONS
• Early symptoms of pregnancy may be absent. • Missed period; full feeling in lower abdomen, lower quadrant tenderness. • Positive pregnancy test. • Signs of acute rupture include: → Vaginal bleeding. → Adnexal or abdominal mass. → Sharp, unilateral or bilateral pelvic pain; abdominal pain. → Referred shoulder pain. → Syncope: shock.	• Provide admission care. → Assess vital signs STAT. → Check for vaginal bleeding. → Start IV to administer fluids. → Notify healthcare provider immediately. • Perform gentle, moderate abdominal palpation and percussion. • Explain procedures as interventions continue; allow family member to be present if possible. • Prepare client for abdominal ultrasound. • Prepare client for possible laparotomy; give preoperative and postoperative surgical instructions. • Type and crossmatch for two units packed red blood cells.

Figure 5-41

HESI HINT: Suspect ectopic pregnancy in any woman of childbearing age who presents at an emergency room, clinic, or office with unilateral or bilateral abdominal pain. Most are misdiagnosed as appendicitis.

HESI HINT: A client who is 32-weeks gestation calls the healthcare provider because she is experiencing dark, red vaginal bleeding. She is admitted to the emergency room where the nurse determines the FHR to be 100 BPM. The client's abdomen is rigid and board-like, and she is complaining of severe pain. What action should the nurse take first? First the nurse must use knowledge base to differentiate between abruptio placentae (this client) from placenta previa (painless bright red bleeding occurring in the third trimester). The nurse should immediately notify the healthcare provider and no abdominal or vaginal manipulation or exams should be done. Administer O_2 per facemask. Monitor for bleeding at IV sites and gums due to the increased risk for DIC. Emergency Cesarean section is required since uteroplacental perfusion to the fetus is being compromised by early separation of the placenta from the uterus.

HESI HINT: Clients with abruptio placentae or placenta previa (actual or suspected) should have NO abdominal or vaginal manipulation.
- NO Leopold's maneuvers.
- NO vaginal exams.
- NO rectal exams, enemas, or suppositories.
- NO internal monitoring.

COMPARISON OF ABRUPTIO PLACENTAE AND PLACENTA PREVIA

ABRUPTIO PLACENTAE	PLACENTA PREVIA

• Partial or complete premature detachment of the placenta from its site of implantation in the uterus.
• Occurs in 1 out of 200 pregnancies.
• Usually occurs in late third trimester or in labor.
• Is the cause of 15% of maternal deaths.
• One-third of infants, born to mothers with abruptio placentae, die.
• **A MEDICAL EMERGENCY**!
• Cause unknown but is related to:
  → Hypertensive disorders.
  → High gravidity.
  → Abdominal trauma (uncommon)
  → Short umbilical cord.
  → Cocaine abuse.
	• Abnormal implantation of placenta in lower uterine segment.
	• Occurs in 1 out of 250 pregnancies.
	• Bleeding usually begins in the third trimester.
	• Degrees of previa described as:
	  → Partial: placenta lies over part of cervical os.
	  → Complete: placenta lies over entire cervical os.
	  → Marginal: edge of placenta meets the rim of the cervical os.
	  → Low-lying: placenta implants in lower uterine segment with a placental edge lying near the cervical os.
	• Associated with previous uterine scars, surgery, or fibroid tumors.
	• **A MEDICAL EMERGENCY**!

ASSESSMENT

ABRUPTIO PLACENTAE	PLACENTA PREVIA
• Bleeding can be concealed or overt. (If overt, is dark red). • Uterine tenderness. • Persistent abdominal pain. • Rigid, board-like abdomen. • Fetal heart rate abnormalities.	• Painless, bright red vaginal bleeding in third trimester. • Soft uterus. • Possible signs of shock. • Placenta in lower uterine segment (indicated by ultrasound). • Fetal heart rate is usually normal.

NURSING PLANS AND INTERVENTIONS

ABRUPTIO PLACENTAE	PLACENTA PREVIA

• Institute bedrest with NO vaginal or rectal manipulation and notify healthcare provider immediately.
• Monitor BP and pulse q15 minutes; apply electric BP monitor if available.
• Apply external uterine and fetal monitor.
• Place client in side-lying position to increase uterine perfusion.
• Closely monitor contractions and FHR.
• Begin IV infusion with 16 to 18g. catheter.
• Draw blood for CBC, clotting studies, Rh factor and type/crossmatch STAT.
• Watch for signs of developing DIC.
  → Bleeding gums/nose.
  → Reduced lab values for platelets, fibrinogen, and prothrombin.
  → Bleeding from injection sites, IV sites.
  → Ecchymosis.
• Prepare for immediate emergency Cesarean section.
• Monitor blood loss: save pads, linens.
• Provide constant nurse surveillance and allow presence of family if available.
• Provide emotional support; teach regarding usual management and expected outcomes of abruption.
	• Manage with bedrest to extend the period of gestation until fetal lung maturity is achieved (determined by a L/S ratio of at least 2:1), then delivery is accomplished.
	• If determined during labor, institute bedrest immediately, and notify physician.
	• Monitor BP and pulse q15 minutes.
	• Start IV to administer fluids.
	• Obtain blood specimen for CBC, clotting studies, Rh factor, and type/crossmatch.
	• Monitor contractions and fetal heart rate; place external monitor on client immediately.
	• Position side-lying.
	• Continue monitoring blood loss; save pads/linen.
	• Prepare client for ultrasound diagnosis.
	• Prepare client/family for possible Cesarean birth if placenta previa is COMPLETE.
	• Provide emotional support and appropriate teaching regarding usual management and outcomes of placenta previa.

Figure 5-42

HESI HINT: Disseminated intravascular coagulation (DIC) is a syndrome of abnormal clotting that is systematic and pathologic. Large amounts of clotting factors, especially fibrinogen, are depleted causing widespread external and/or internal bleeding. DIC is related to fetal demise, infection/sepsis, pregnancy-induced hypertension (preeclampsia) and abruptio placentae (DIC is discussed in more detail in Advanced Clinical Concepts).

ANEMIA
• Decrease in oxygen-carrying capacity of blood often related to iron deficiency and reduced dietary intake.
• Occurs in 20% of pregnant women.
• Associated with increased incidence of abortion, preterm labor, preeclampsia, infection, postpartum hemorrhage, and intrauterine growth retardation.

ANALYSIS (NURSING DIAGNOSES)
- Alteration in tissue perfusion related to…
- Alteration in nutrition: less than body requirements related to…

ASSESSMENT	NURSING PLANS AND INTERVENTIONS

• Fatigue, pallor.
• Hgb and Hct signs of anemia.
  → Hgb <11g/dl, Hct <37% in FIRST trimester.
  → Hgb <10.5g/dl, Hct <35% in SECOND trimester
  → Hgb <10 g/dl, Hct <32% in THIRD trimester
• *See Pediatric section for description of sickle cell anemia.*
• Poor nutritional intake.
• Non-compliance with prenatal vitamin/iron supplement.
	• Analyze 24-hour dietary recall.
	• Review/teach nutritional requirements for pregnancy. *(See Appendices A, Normal Values)*
	• Teach about oral administration of iron. *(See figure 5-44, Iron)*

Figure 5-43

IRON			
DRUG	**INDICATIONS**	**ADVERSE REACTIONS**	**NURSING IMPLICATIONS**
ferrous sulfate (Feosol)	• Iron deficiency anemia	• Constipation • Diarrhea • Gastric irritation • Nausea or vomiting	• Iron is best absorbed on an empty stomach • Take with vitamin C source such as orange juice to increase absorption • Avoid taking with cereal, eggs, or milk which decreases absorption • Take in the evening if problem exists with morning sickness • Stools will turn dark green to black • Check lab values for increased reticulocytes and rising Hgb and Hct

Figure 5-44

INFECTIONS	
• Sexually-transmitted diseases (STDs) and general infections.	
• Infections can be harmful to mother and fetus during the antepartum period. *(See figure 5-46, Infections, Maternal/Fetal Effects)*	
• Simple viral infections in the first trimester can cause serious fetal teratogenic effects.	
• STDs have a predilection for genital and perigenital site manifestations.	

ANALYSIS (NURSING DIAGNOSES)
- Potential for injury to mother/fetus related to…
- Knowledge deficit (specify) related to…
- Disturbance in self-concept related to…

ASSESSMENT	NURSING PLANS AND INTERVENTIONS
• History of multiple sex partners.	• *See Nursing Plans and Interventions for STDs in Medical Surgical section*.
• Previous history of STD or vaginal infections.	• Advise regarding immunity to rubella; if client lacks immunity, advise against working with children in terms of risk for exposure.
• Employment with high exposure to infection, e.g., childcare worker, healthcare worker.	• If diagnosed with infection, teach/counsel regarding maternal/fetal effects and how/why to follow the prescribed medical regime.
• Non-specific symptoms: fever, malaise.	
• General symptoms of STDs: vaginal discharge, genital lesions, dysuria, and dyspareunia.	
• Specific symptoms, e.g., herpes simplex blisters.	
• Laboratory studies: antibody titers, TORCH, VDRL, (may be negative if drawn too early), RPR, gonorrhea screen, vaginal wet-mount.	

Figure 5-45

INFECTIONS, MATERNAL/FETAL EFFECTS			
INFECTION	MATERNAL EFFECT	FETAL EFFECTS	TREATMENT
CHLAMYDIA TRACHOMATIS	• Mucopurulent vaginal discharge • Dysuria • Acute salpingitis • Pelvic inflammatory disease (PID) • Sterility or infertility	• Stillbirth/neonatal death • Preterm birth • Ophthalmia neonatorum • Pneumonia	• Treat with erythromycin; may need to treat partner • azithromycin (Zithromax)
HESI HINT: Tetracyeline is contraindicated in pregnancy because it darkens the teeth of the newborn.			
HUMAN PAPILLOMAVIRUS (HPV)	• Small or large, dry, wart-like growth on vulva, vagina, cervix, and/or rectum (condylomata acuminata)	• Possible chronic respiratory papillomatosis	• Laser ablation or cryotherapy • When pregnant, lesions usually left alone, unless mild laser treatment needed • Explain need for possible abdominal delivery due to fetal effect
HESI HINT: Podophyllin, which is usually used to treat HPV, is contraindicated in pregnancy because it is associated with fetal death, preterm labor, and cervical carcinoma.			

Figure 5-46

INFECTIONS, MATERNAL/FETAL EFFECTS (CONTINUED)

INFECTION	MATERNAL EFFECT	FETAL EFFECT	TREATMENT
GONORRHEA	• Dysuria • Purulent vaginal discharge • PID	• Ophthalmia neonatorum • Sepsis	• Includes both partners • Penicillin and/or erythromycin and Ceftriaxone used in pregnancy • Have partner(s) use condoms until cultures negative two times
SYPHILIS	• Chancre • Late abortion (Syphilis is most common cause) • Positive antibody screen; will not show positive if tested too soon after exposure (usually positive 6 weeks after exposure) • Positive tests for Treponema pallidum (FTA-ABS)	• Stillbirth • Congenital syphilis, characterized by snuffles (rhinitis) if mother has latent or tertiary syphilis • Hydrocephaly • Congenital cataracts • Copper colored rash • Cracks around the mouth • Hypothermia (neonate may have difficulty with thermoregulation	• Treatment before 16 weeks prevents placental transmission to fetus • Penicillin G • Erythromycin
TOXOPLAMOSIS	• Effects are absent or manifest as flu-like symptoms	• Stillbirth • Microcephaly • Hydrocephalus • Blindness • Deafness	• Treatment during pregnancy by sulfa drugs • May consider therapeutic abortion if discovered before 20 weeks

HESI HINT: Toxoplasmosis is usually related to exposure to cats, gardening (where cat feces may be found), or eating raw meat.

HEPATITIS	• May result in preterm birth	• Baby is HBsAg positive, IgM positive	• Carriers of hepatitis B are given a series of hepatitis immunizations which may prevent carrier status and chronic liver disease in newborn
RUBELLA (TORCH disease)	• Most severe if contacted in FIRST trimester • Therapeutic abortion offered	• Congenital heart defects • IUGR • Congenital cataracts • Hearing or vision problems may arise in later childhood	• No maternal treatment for the virus is available

HESI HINT: Rubella is teratogenic to the fetus during the FIRST trimester, causing congenital heart disease and/or congenital cataracts. All women should have their titers checked during pregnancy. If a woman's titers are low, she should receive the vaccine AFTER delivery and be instructed not to get pregnant within 3 months. Breastfeeding mothers may take the vaccine.

Figure 5-46 (continued)

INFECTIONS, MATERNAL/FETAL EFFECTS (CONTINUED)			
INFECTION	**MATERNAL EFFECT**	**FETAL EFFECT**	**TREATMENT**
Cytomegalovirus (CMV) OR CYTOMEGALIC INCLUSION DISEASE (CID) (TORCH disease)	• Maternal effects are absent or mononucleosis-like	• Stillbirth • Congenital CMV • Microcephaly • IUGR • Cerebral palsy • Mental retardation • Rash, jaundice, hepatosplenomegaly	• No treatment is available for mother or infant
HERPES SIMPLEX VIRUS (HSV) (TORCH disease)	• A primary or recurrent infection • Painful vesicular genital lesions • Cesarean delivery recommended during active lesion breakout	• Disseminated or localized skin infection • CNS abnormalities	• Safety of systematic acyclovis (Zovirax) in pregnant clients has not been established; should be used only in pregnant clients with life-threatening infection.
HESI HINT: ACYCLOVIR (used to treat herpes simplex) is NOT RECOMMENDED during pregnancy.			
HUMAN IMMUNODEFICIENCY VIRUS (HIV) ACQUIRED IMMUNE DEFICIENCY SYNDROME (AIDS)	• Usually asymptomatic • Chronic vaginitis • Susceptible to opportunistic diseases and immunologic suppression	• Affects fetus through transplacental transfer, exposure to maternal blood/body fluids, or through breast milk	• *See Advanced Clinical Concepts section, HIV INFECTION for further discussion*
BACTERIAL VAGINOSIS (vaginal infection)	• Milk-like discharge with fish-like odor • Itching, burning, pain • Can cause premature rupture of membranes • Postpartum endometritis	• Neonatal sepsis and death	• Treated with clindamycin or ampicillin • metronidazole (Flagyl)
MONILIAL VAGINITIS (Candida albicans, yeast) (vaginal infection)	• Common in diabetes and clients on long-term antibiotic therapy • Odorless thick, cheesy vaginal discharge • Severe vaginal itching • Dyspareunia	• Oral thrush or perineal rash	• Treated with Miconazole nitrate cream or Nystatin cream in pregnancy • Teach client to wear cotton undergarments and to abstain from intercourse until cured
TRICHOMONIASIS VAGINITIS (Trichomonas protozoa)	• Profuse, frothy, yellowish discharge • Irritation, itching • Dysuria • Dyspareunia	• Usually no fetal effects	• Treat with vaginal suppositories to reduce symptoms during the first and second trimester of pregnancy
HESI HINT: Although Metronidazole (Flagyl) is the treatment of choice for some vaginal infections, its use is *contraindicated* in the first trimester of pregnancy, and its use during the second trimester is controversial.			

Figure 5-46 (continued)

MATERNITY NURSING

PSYCHOSOCIAL CONCERNS: TEENAGE (ADOLESCENT) PREGNANCY

Pregnancy occurring at age 19 or younger.
- One out of 11 adolescent females in the U.S. becomes pregnant each year (1 million).
- Adolescent pregnancy is highly associated with anemia, preeclampsia, CPD (cephalopelvic disproportion), STDs, IUGR, and ineffective parenting.

ANALYSIS (NURSING DIAGNOSES)
- Knowledge deficit (specify) related to …
- Alteration in nutrition: less than/more than body requirements related to …

ASSESSMENT	NURSING PLANS AND INTERVENTIONS
<ul><li>Age 12 to 19.</li><li>Assess factors which influence the outcome of pregnancy:<ul><li>→ Previous history of menstrual or obstetrical complications.</li><li>→ Nutritional status: 24-hour diet recall and analysis.</li><li>→ Attitude toward pregnancy and becoming a mother.</li><li>→ Social support system, i.e., family, spouse/boyfriend, friends, school.</li><li>→ Exposure to battering from boyfriend, spouse, father, or other male.</li><li>→ Peer activities regarding smoking, drugs, and unsafe behaviors.</li><li>→ Client's activities regarding smoking, drugs, unsafe behaviors.</li><li>→ Economic status.</li><li>→ Educational level, knowledge of pregnancy, childbearing, and childrearing.</li><li>→ Access to prenatal care.</li></ul></li></ul>	<ul><li>Establish trust and rapport through interview first, and then proceed to therapeutic relationship.</li><li>Avoid authoritative, punitive approach to counseling; use an information-sharing approach.</li><li>Provide information in private regarding options of pregnancy termination, adoption, and local agencies supporting pregnant adolescents.</li><li>Praise adolescent for all health-maintenance activities, i.e., coming for pregnancy testing, making prenatal visits, and well-thought-out questions.</li><li>Allow support person to attend prenatal visits.</li><li>Relate nutritional information to resumption of figure postpartum, skin health, hair integrity, and other normal adolescent concerns.</li><li>Teach dangers related to substance abuse in pregnancy.</li><li>Smoking: low birth weight infant.</li><li>Alcohol: fetal alcohol syndrome.</li><li>Cocaine: preterm labor and abruptio placentae; subtle neurological changes in the neonate.</li><li>Teratogenic fetal effects highest in first trimester.</li><li>Encourage normal activities to achieve early developmental task of identity versus role-confusion; late adolescent developmental task of intimacy versus isolation.</li><li>Encourage to stay in school, continue identity as student.</li><li>Prevent social isolation by encouraging adolescent to continue normal activities, e.g., attendance at school functions, games, and family activities.</li><li>Provide information regarding childbirth classes, peer support groups.</li><li>Teach major milestones in fetal development (major fetal growth in 3rd trimester).</li><li>Monitor carefully for development of preeclampsia, nutritional disorders (anemia, IUGR).</li></ul>

Figure 5-47

MATERNITY NURSING

PRETERM LABOR

DESCRIPTION	ANALYSIS/ASSESSMENT
Onset of labor between 20 to 37 weeks gestation. Predisposing factors to preterm labor include: • Diabetes, cardiac disease, preeclampsia, and placenta previa. • Infection, especially urinary tract. • Over distention of uterus due to multiple pregnancy, hydramnios, large-for-gestational-age baby. Psychosocial factors. • Working outside home, if stressful. • Two or more children under age 5. • Financial stress. • No social support system. • Smoking >10 cigarettes/day. Preterm labor is responsible for 2 out of 3 neonatal deaths. Neonates over 2000 gm (4.5 pounds) or 32-weeks gestation have best chance of survival.	**ANALYSIS (NURSING DIAGNOSES)** • Anxiety related to… • Knowledge deficit related to… • Potential for injury to mother or fetus related to **NURSING ASSESSMENT** • True labor present, i.e., contractions with cervical change is occurring, e.g., more than 5 contractions/ hour, cervix <4 cm, <50% effaced, membranes intact and not bulging. • FHR 110 to 160 BPM with no distress. • No medical or obstetric disorder contraindicating continuance of pregnancy. • Fetal fibronectin is a test obtained from a cervical swab. Detection of fetal fibronectin is an indicator that preterm labor has begun.

NURSING PLANS AND INTERVENTIONS
PREMATURE LABOR NURSING CARE

ANTEPARTUM

• Use fetal development chart to show client when baby has mature lungs (36 weeks).
• Teach warning signs of labor:
   → Uterine contractions every 10 minutes or more often.
   → Menstrual-like cramps. Low, dull backache and pelvic pressure.
   → Increase or change in vaginal discharge.
   → Rupture of membranes.
• Teach self-assessment of uterine contractions.
   → Lying on left side, place fingers on top of uterus.
   → Note a periodic hardening or tightening with or without pain (contraction).
   → More than 5 contractions in an hour should be reported immediately to healthcare provider or clinic.
• Follow up teaching with written instructions about warning signs of labor.

INTRAPARTUM

HOME MANAGEMENT	HOSPITAL MANAGEMENT
• Teach need for bedrest with fetus OFF of the cervix, i.e., no sitting or kneeling. • Teach side-lying position and elevation of foot of bed to increase uterine perfusion and decrease uterine irritability. • Teach side effects and warning signs of medications. (May be taking oral tocolytic drugs (ritodrine or terbutaline*). (See figure 5-49, Medications for Intrapartal Complications)* • Avoid sexual stimulation: no sexual intercourse, nipple stimulation, or orgasm. • Increase oral fluid (2 to 3 l/day). • Empty bladder q2 hours. • Review what to do if membranes rupture or if signs of infection occur (fever, foul-smelling vaginal discharge).	• Place on bedrest in side-lying position with continuous fetal monitoring (external). • Notify healthcare provider **IMMEDIATELY**. • Magnesium Sulfate: decreases uterine activity through relaxation of smooth muscle secondary to magnesium replacing calcium in the cells. • Terbutaline (Brethine) and ritodrine (Yutopar): beta-adrenergic agent that acts on B_2 receptors causing uterine muscle relaxation. • Administer tocolytics as prescribed. *(See figure 5-49, Medications for Intrapartal Complications)* • Administer glucocorticoids (betamethasone) if prescribed to enhance fetal lung maturation or surfactant production if fetus is <35 weeks gestation. • Prepare for birth or low-birth-weight infant if preterm labor is not arrested. • Continuously monitor fetal heart rate.

Figure 5-48

MEDICATIONS FOR INTRAPARTAL COMPLICATIONS

DRUGS	INDICATIONS	ADVERSE REACTIONS	NURSING IMPLICATIONS
ritodrine HCL (Yutopar) Beta-sympathomimetic agent **terbutaline sulfate** (Brethine) Beta-sympathomimetic agent, Bronchodilator	• Stops preterm labor contractions	• CNS effects: → Severe nervousness → Tremulousness → Headache • CV effects: → Severe palpitations → Tachycardia → Chest pain → Pulmonary edema • GI effects: → Nausea → Vomiting → Diarrhea → Epigastric pain • Lab value distortions → Low K+ → Hyperglycemia	• Administer IV • Increase infusion rate q15 minutes depending on uterine response and maternal side effects • Get maternal EKG and lab values prior to beginning infusion • Place mother on bedside cardiac monitor • Monitor fetus continuously • Monitor vital signs q15 min. • Maternal pulse **SHOULD NOT EXCEED 140 BPM** • **FHR SHOULD NOT EXCEED 180 BPM** • I&O; weigh daily • Prepare woman for side effects • Notify healthcare provider of → High pulse, FHR changes, abnormal lab values → Signs of CHF: dyspnea, jugular vein distention, dry cough, rales in lung bases → Have antidote available, i.e., a beta blocking agent such as Propranolol (Inderal)
magnesium sulfate	• Central nervous system depressant administered to preeclamptic client to prevent seizures • May be used as a tocolytic to stop preterm labor contractions	• CNS depression manifested by: → Depressed respirations → Depressed DTRs • Decreased urine output • Pulmonary edema	• Hold if respiration <12/min, urine output <100 cc/4 hrs • DTRs absent • Monitor magnesium levels as prescribed and report values outside therapeutic range (5 to 8 mq/dl) • Remind client of warm, flushed feeling with IV administration • Keep calcium gluconate at bedside (antidote)

Figure 5-49

HESI HINT: Although the toxic side effects of magnesium sulfate are well known and watched for, it is just as important to get serum blood levels of magnesium sulfate above 4 mg/dl in order to prevent convulsions and reach therapeutic range.

HESI HINT: Hold next dose of magnesium sulfate and notify healthcare provider if any toxic symptoms occur (<12 respirations/ minute, urine output <100 cc/4 hours, absent DTRs, Magnesium Sulfate$_4$ >8 mg/dl).

HESI HINT: When administering magnesium sulfate. ALWAYS have antidote available (calcium gluconate, 20 ml vial of a 10% solution).

DYSTOCIA

- Difficult birth resulting from any cause.
- Can result from any one or all of the "5 Ps":
  - → Powers: primary uterine contractions and secondary abdominal bearing down efforts.
  - → Passage: maternal pelvis, uterus, cervix, vagina, perineum.
  - → Passenger: fetus and placenta.
  - → Psyche: response to labor by woman.
  - → Position: of the laboring woman.
- Dystocia is suspected when there is:
  - → A lack of progress in cervical dilatation.
  - → A lack of fetal descent.
  - → A lack of change in uterine contraction characteristics (frequency, strength, and duration).
- Dystocia, dysfunctional labor, and uterine inertia are terms used interchangeably.

ANALYSIS (NURSING DIAGNOSES)	NURSING ASSESSMENT
• Alteration in comfort: acute pain related to… • Anxiety related to… • Potential injury to mother/fetus related to…	• Hypertonic or Hypotonic uterine contractions. • Inability to bear down or push efficiently. • See below for Prolonged Labor Patterns.

NURSING PLANS AND INTERVENTIONS

- Notify healthcare provider if prolonged labor patterns occur on Friedman's curve.
- Assist with diagnostic procedures (ultrasound, pelvimetry, vaginal exam) to rule out cephalopelvic disproportion (CPD).
- Assist with amniotomy performed by healthcare provider: artificial rupture of membranes (AROM) may enhance labor forces.
  - → Explain procedure (it is painless).
  - → FHR assessed **IMMEDIATELY** after rupture to determine cord prolapse.
  - → Assess fluid for color, odor, and consistency (blood, meconium, or vernix particles).
- Initiate **OXYTOCIN INFUSION FOR INDUCTION** (initiation) or augmentation (stimulation) of labor and manage infusion delivery. *(See figure 5-51, Nursing Protocol for Administration of Oxytocin)*

PROLONGED LABOR PATTERNS

PATTERN	NULLIPARA	MULTIPARA
Prolonged latent phase	>20 hours	>14 hours
Prolonged active phase	<1.2 cm/hour	<1.5 cm/hour
Secondary arrest	No change for >2 hours	No change for >2 hours
Prolonged deceleration phase	>3 hours	>1 hour
Protracted descent	Descent of fetus <1 cm/hour	Descent of fetus <2 cm/hour
Arrest of descent	>1 hour	>1/2 hour

Figure 5-50

MATERNITY NURSING

303

HESI HINT: Dystocia frequently requires the use of oxytocin for augmentation or induction of labor. Uterine tetany is a harmful complication and careful monitoring is required. The desired effect is contractions q2 to 3 minutes, with duration of contractions no longer than 90 seconds. Continuously monitor FHR and uterine resting tone. If tetany occurs, turn off Pitocin, turn client to a side-lying position, and administer O_2 by facemask. Check output (should be at least 100 cc/4 hours). Oxytocin's most important side effect is its antidiuretic (ADH) effect, which can cause water intoxication. Using IV fluids containing electrolytes decreases the risk of water intoxication.

HESI HINT: The uterus is most sensitive to becoming tetanic at the beginning of the infusion. The client must ALWAYS be attended and contractions monitored. Contractions should last NO longer than 90 seconds to prevent fetal hypoxia.

HESI HINT: Women with previous uterine scars are prone to uterine rupture especially if oxytocin or forceps are used. If a woman complains of a sharp pain accompanied by the abrupt cessation of contractions, suspect uterine rupture, a MEDICAL EMERGENCY. Immediate surgical delivery is indicated to save the fetus and mother.

NURSING PROTOCOL FOR ADMINISTRATION OF OXYTOCIN

- Determine any contraindications to use of oxytocin.
  - → Known cephalopelvic Disproportion (CPD)
  - → Fetal stress.
  - → Placenta previa.
  - → Prior classical incision into uterus.
  - → Active genital herpes infection.
  - → Floating fetus.
  - → Unripe cervix.
- Add 10 units of oxytocin (1 cc Pitocin, Syntocinon) to 1 liter of IV fluid.
  - → Piggyback at the lowest port on the primary IV line.
    - Using the lowest port ensures that very little Pitocin will be in the primary line if an emergency requires discontinuing the drug.
    - Begin infusion slowly and increase at 20 to 30 minute increments until contractions occur every 2 to 3 minutes, are 40 to 60 seconds in duration and firm.
- Using external or internal fetal monitoring continuously monitor the following:
  - → FHR.
  - → Uterine resting tone.
  - → Contraction frequency, duration, and strength.

Figure 5-51

HYPERTENSIVE DISORDERS OF PREGNANCY	
GESTATIONAL HYPERTENSION	• B/P elevation occurs for the first time after mid-pregnancy. • No proteinuria.
TRANSIENT HYPERTENSION	• Gestational hypertension with no other signs of preeclampsia present at time of birth. • Resolves by 12 weeks gestation.
PREECLAMPSIA	• Pregnancy-specific syndrome that usually occurs after 20 weeks gestation (except with hydatidiform mole). • Gestational hypertension plus proteinuria.
HELLP SYNDROME	• While not technically classified as a separate hypertensive disorder of pregnancy, HELLP syndrome is a variant of severe preeclampsia with often very different risk factors and s/s.
ECLAMPSIA	• Seizures (with no known etiology, like epilepsy) in a woman with preeclampsia.
CHRONIC HYPERTENSION	• Hypertension that is observable before pregnancy or that is diagnosed before the 20th week of gestation (with the exception of hydatidiform mole).
PREECLAMPSIA SUPER-IMPOSED ON CHRONIC HYPERTENSION	• Chronic hypertension with new onset proteinuria and/or a worsening of the already present hypertension, thrombocytopenia, or increased liver enzyme values.

Figure 5-52

PREECLAMPSIA/ECLAMPSIA
• Most common hypertensive disorder, which develops during pregnancy characterized by elevated blood pressure, edema, and proteinuria. • Preeclampsia is characterized by an increase in BP of 30 mmHg systolic and/or 15 mmHg diastolic over previous/usual baseline with concomitant evidence of preeclampsia. • Usually develops during last 10 weeks of gestation or up to 48 hours post delivery. • Occurs in 6 to 7% of all pregnancies. • Occurs predominately in primigravidas. • Preeclampsia is a major cause of maternal death and fetal hypoxia/death. • Differentiated into three types: → Preeclampsia. → Eclampsia: preeclampsia with seizures/coma. → HELLP Syndrome. • There is NO known cause of preeclampsia. Pathophysiology is characterized by: → Generalized vasospasm and vasoconstriction leading to vascular damage over time. → Loss of plasma protein into the interstitial space (fluid is drawn into the extravascular spaces and results in hypovolemia). → Hypovolemia results in decreased perfusion to major organs including the uterus.
ANALYSIS (NURSING DIAGNOSES) • Potential for injury to fetus/mother related to… • Potential alteration in tissue perfusion related to… • Knowledge deficit (specify) related to…

Figure 5-53

MATERNITY NURSING

ASSESSMENT

- Obtain baseline BP at first prenatal visit.
- Risk factors associated with Preeclampsia:
  → Age below 17 years or above 35 years.
  → Low socioeconomic status.
  → Poor protein intake.
  → Previous hypertension.
  → Diabetes (gestational or preexisting).
  → Multiple gestation.
  → Hydatidiform mole.
  → Family history (mothers or sisters with Preeclampsia).
- Mild Preeclampsia
  → BP rises 30 mmHg systolic/15 mmHg diastolic over previous baseline or 140/90 or greater.
  → Abnormal rollover test; see below for BP Assessment of Antepartum Client: Rollover Test.
  → Presence of associated conditions (outlined above).
  → Weight gain >2 lbs/week.
  → Proteinuria ≥ 1+.
  → Edema especially around eyes, face, and fingers.
  → Hyperreflexia 3+.
  → CNS symptoms: possible mild headache, slight irritability.
  → Intrauterine growth retardation (IUGR), evidenced by size/date discrepancy.
- SEVERE Preeclampsia consists of all of the above symptoms PLUS any two of the following:
  → BP rises to 160 mmHg/110 mmHg on two or more occasions.
  → Proteinuria 3+ to 4+.
  → Generalized edema (very puffy face and/or hands).
  → DTRs 3+ or greater, plus clonus.
  → Oliguria (less than 100 cc/4 hours.
  → CNS symptoms: severe headache, visual disturbances (blurred vision, photophobia, blind spots), and possibly epigastric pain.
  → Elevate serum creatinine, thrombocytopenia, and marked liver enzyme elevation (SGOT).
- Severe IUGR; late decelerations of the FHR.
- Eclampsia:
  → Presence of seizure in the woman with pre-eclampsia
  → Tonic-clonic type seizures
- HELLP Syndrome
  → Characterized by hemolysis (H), elevated liver enzymes (EL), and low platelets (LP).
  → Increased risk for abruption, acute renal failure, hepatic rupture, preterm birth, and fetal and/or maternal death.
  → Etiology arises out of changes that occur with preeclampsia.
  → More commonly seen in older, Caucasian, multiperous women.
  → S/S include history of malaise, epigastric or right upper quadrant pain, nausea and vomiting.
  → Many women are normotensive and do not have proteinuria.
  → Should still be treated prophylactically with Magnesium Sulfate (because of increased CNS irritability that is part of the disease) even if hypertension is not present.
  → Women with HELLP are at high risk for developing the syndrome again in future pregnancies as well as for developing preeclampsia in other pregnancies not complicated by HELLP.

Figure 5-53 (continued)

NURSING CARE FOR CLIENT WITH PREECLAMPSIA ANTRAPARTUM	
HOME MANAGEMENT	**HOSPITAL MANAGEMENT**

• Inform client that absolute bedrest with bathroom privileges is necessary (except for regularly scheduled prenatal visits).
• Have client weigh daily and report greater than 2 lbs/wk gain.
• Teach client to test urine daily for protein.
• Provide client with list of signs to report immediately to caregiver.
  → CNS symptoms: visual disturbances, headache, nausea and vomiting, hyperreflexia, convulsions.
  → Hepatic sign: epigastric pain.
  → Renal signs: oliguria, proteinuria.
  → Fetal distress signs: decreased or absent fetal activity, unusual or extremely active fetus.
  → Signs of abruptio placentae: vaginal bleeding, abdominal pain.
• Teach prescribed diet.
  → High protein diet.
  → Limit salt intake (no longer completely restricted).
  → Maintain minimum of 35 cal/kg of body weight.
• Teach client therapeutic rationale of bedrest in left side-lying position (to increase uterine perfusion and prevent fetal distress).
• Reinforce need for stress reduction and home help in order to prevent further vascular constriction from circulating stress hormones/catecholamines.
	• If preeclampsia progresses to severe preeclampsia, hospitalization will be necessary.
	• Monitor level of consciousness, BP, and vital signs every 4 hours or more often if elevated/ abnormal.
	• Obtain fetal assessment continuously; apply external fetal monitor.
	• Assess for vaginal bleeding/abdominal pain.
	• Provide bedrest in left side-lying position.
	• Start intravenous infusion with 16 to 18g. venocatheter.
	• Insert indwelling urinary catheter with urine meter.
	• Monitor I&O hourly.
	• Maintain quiet, slightly-darkened environment with limited visitors.
	• Administer magnesium sulfate and anti-hypertensive drugs (rare unless diastolic BP consistently over 110), and possibly Pitocin for initiation/augmentation of labor. *(See figure 5-49, Medications for Intrapartal Complications)*
	• Assess daily for signs of coagulopathy.
	  → Petechiae under BP cuff.
	  → Platelet decrease or increase.
	  → Fibrinogen increase or decrease.
	• Assess deep tendon reflexes (DTR) and assess for clonus once each shift or more often if prescribed or abnormal.
	• Transfer to labor/delivery if necessary.
	  → Signs of pulmonary edema occur.
	  → HELLP syndrome occurs (Hemolysis, Elevated Liver enzymes, Low Platelets).
	  → Late decelerations of the fetal heart rate occur.
	  → Preterm labor begins.

Figure 5-53 (continued)

HESI HINT: Rarely are antihypertensive drugs used in the preeclamptic client. They are given only in the event of diastolic blood pressure over 110 mmHg. (CVA danger). Drug of choice is hydralazine HCL (Apresoline).

HESI HINT: Although delivery is often described as the "cure" for preeclampsia, the client can convulse up to 48 hours after delivery.

MATERNITY NURSING

- When the client with preeclampsia begins labor, control the amount of stimulation in the labor room.
  - → Keep nurse/client ratio at 1:1.
  - → If possible, put client in darkened, quiet, private room.
  - → Keep client on absolute bedrest, side-lying with bedrails up.
  - → Disturb client as little as possible with nursing interventions.
- Have client choose support person to stay with her and limit other visitors.
- Constantly explain rationale for procedures and care.
- Maintain intravenous line with 16 to 18 gauge venocatheter.
- Monitor blood pressure every 15 to 30 minutes keeping blood pressure cuff on or using electronic blood pressure monitor if available.
- Check urine for protein every hour and report increase.
- Determine deep tendon reflexes every hour and report increases.
- Administration of magnesium sulfate: *(See figure 5-49, Medications for Intrapartal Complications)*
  - → Usually given IV with a loading dose of 4 grams in 100 ml to 250 ml of solution give over 20 to 30 minutes to get the blood level up to therapeutic serum levels (5 to 8 mg/dl).
  - → Serum blood levels are usually maintained by infusing 2 gm/hour after loading dose.
- Monitor for toxicity during magnesium sulfate administration.
  - → Urinary output <30 ml/hour.
  - → Respirations <12/min.
  - → DTRs absent.
  - → Deceleration of the FHR, bradycardia.
- When magnesium sulfate is prescribed to be given IM:
  - → Give 10 grams (5 grams in each buttock) with 1 cc 1% lidocaine to decrease pain.
  - → Give deep in dorsal gluteal site with 3 inch, 20 gauge needle; give z-track or with rotation method.
  - → Expect onset within 30 minutes/1 hour, lasting 3 to 4 hours.
- If convulsions/seizures do occur:
  - → Stay with client and use call button to summon help. Have someone get healthcare provider STAT!
  - → Turn client on side to prevent aspiration.
  - → **DO NOT ATTEMPT TO FORCE OBJECTS INSIDE MOUTH OR PUT FINGERS INTO WOMAN'S MOUTH.**
  - → Administer O_2 at 10 l/min. by facemask and have suction available.
  - → Give magnesium sulfate as prescribed. *(See figure 5-49, Medications for Intrapartal Complications)*
  - → Assess labor/delivery status.
- During the post-delivery period:
  - → Assess blood pressure, respirations, DTRs, and urine output every 4 hours for 48 hours.
  - → Carefully assess uterine tone/fundal height for uterine atony resulting from magnesium sulfate administration.
  - → Monitor for blood loss: preexisting hypovolemia makes these women sensitive to even normal blood loss.
  - → Instruct client to report headache, visual disturbances, or epigastric pain.
  - → Check with the healthcare provider before administration of ANY ERGOT derivatives.

Figure 5-53 (continued)

HESI HINT: The major goal of nursing care for a client with preeclampsia is to maintain uteroplacental perfusion and prevent seizures. This requires the administration of magnesium sulfate. Withhold administration of magnesium sulfate if signs of toxicity exist: respirations <12/minute, absence of DTRs, and/or urine output <30 ml/hour.

MATERNAL/INFANT CARDIAC DISEASE

- Impaired cardiac function usually results from congenital defect or history of rheumatic heart disease with valve prolapse or stenosis.
- More commonly seen in women today due to surgical correction techniques in infancy enabling them to live to childbearing age.
- Dangerous due to plasma volume increase that accompanies pregnancy.
- Type and extent of disease:
  → Class I: Unrestricted physical activity. Ordinary physical activity does not cause cardiac symptomatology.
  → Class II: Ordinary activity causes fatigue, palpitations, dyspnea, and angina. Physical activity limited.
  → Class III: With less than ordinary activity, cardiac decompensation symptoms ensue. Moderate to marked limitation of activity.
  → Class IV: Symptoms of cardiac insufficiency occur even at rest. No activity allowed.

ANALYSIS (NURSING DIAGNOSES)
- Knowledge deficit related to…
- Anxiety related to…
- Ineffective family coping related to…

ASSESSMENT

- History of preexisting cardiac disease.
- Cardiac decompensation.
  → Subjective symptoms determined by client.
    - Increasing fatigue.
    - Dyspnea.
    - Feeling of smothering.
    - Dry, hacky cough.
    - "Racing" heart.
    - Swelling of feet, legs, and fingers.
  → Objective symptoms determined by health professional.
    - Pulse >100 BPM.
    - Crackles at lung bases even after deep breathing.
    - Orthopnea/dyspnea.
    - Respirations >25/min.
- Anemia possible (Hct <32%, Hgb <10 mg/dl).

NURSING CARE FOR THE CARDIAC MATERNITY CLIENT

ANTEPARTUM	INTRAPARTUM
<ul><li>Teach client to report any symptoms of cardiac decompensation (listed on previous page).</li><li>Encourage 8 to 10 hours sleep each night with daily rest periods.</li><li>Teach self-administration of heparin if prescribed. *(See Medical Surgical Nursing)*</li><li>Give diet plan, which includes high iron, high protein, and adequate calorie intake.</li><li>Inform client of anticipated difficult period for control at 28 to 32 weeks when plasma volume peaks in pregnancy.</li><li>Teach client to notify health care provider at first sign of infection.</li></ul>	<ul><li>Maintain a calm atmosphere allowing presence of support persons, and keep family informed at all times.</li><li>Maintain cardiac perfusion.<ul><li>→ Put client in semi-Fowler's, side-lying position.</li><li>→ Prevent Valsalva's maneuvers even during 2nd stage (obstructs left ventricular outflow).</li><li>→ Avoid hypotension if epidural anesthesia used.</li><li>→ Avoid use of stirrups in delivery room (can cause Popliteal vein compression and decreased venous return).</li></ul></li><li>Provide pain relief and supportive measures since pain can contribute to cardiac distress.</li><li>Monitor forceps delivery and episiotomy (will likely be performed to decrease the time of the 2nd stage).</li></ul>

Figure 5-54

MATERNITY NURSING

MATERNAL/INFANT CARDIAC DISEASE (CONTINUED)

NURSING CARE FOR THE CARDIAC MATERNITY CLIENT

POSTPARTUM

- Tailor care to the woman's functional classification.
- Continue semi or high-Fowler's position (head of bed raised) with side-lying maintained.
- Progress ambulation: dangling, sitting, standing, short to long ambulation according to tolerance and no symptoms of cardiac decompensation.
- Administer stool softeners as prescribed to prevent straining during bowel movement.
- Watch for symptoms of urinary infection: dysuria, white cells in urine, and pus in urine.
- Report ANY symptoms of cardiac decompensation to healthcare provider immediately.
  - → Tachycardia (pulse >100).
  - → Tachypnea (respirations >25).
  - → Dry cough.
  - → Rales in the lung bases.
- Report immediately ANY temperature spike over 100.4°F.
- Plan with the mother and family for support when returning home. If necessary, refer to community resource for homemaking services.

HESI HINT: Nursing care during labor and delivery for the client with cardiac disease is focused on prevention of cardiac embarrassment, maintenance of uterine perfusion, and alleviation of anxiety.

HESI HINT: Should these clients experience preterm labor, the use of beta-adrenergic agents such as terbutaline (Brethine) and ritodrine HCL (Yutopar) are contraindicated due to the chance of myocardial ischemia.

HESI HINT: Normal diuresis, which occurs in the postpartum period, can pose serious problems to the new mother with cardiac disease because of the increased cardiac output.

CONGENITAL HEART DISEASE IN NEWBORN

ASSESSMENT	NURSING PLANS AND INTERVENTIONS
• Weak cry, cyanosis worsening with crying. • Lethargy, hypotonia, and flaccidity. • Persistent bradycardia or tachycardia. • Tachypnea or other signs of respiratory distress. • Decreased/absent femoral or pedal pulses.	• Decrease energy utilization immediately. → No nippling (no pacifiers, no excessive stimulation). • Notify healthcare provider STAT of findings. • Transfer neonate to NICU for diagnostic workup.

HESI HINT: Coumadin may NOT be taken during pregnancy due to its ability to cross the placenta and affect the fetus. HEPARIN is the drug of choice; it does NOT cross the placental membrane.

Figure 5-54 (continued)

MATERNITY NURSING

HYPEREMESIS GRAVIDARUM

- Inability to control nausea and vomiting during pregnancy.
- Hyperemesis gravidarum is characterized by the inability to keep down solid food/fluids for 24 hours.
- It is linked to maternal hormones and possible psychological reaction to pregnancy.

ANALYSIS (NURSING DIAGNOSES)
- Risk for fluid volume deficit related to…
- Anxiety related to…

ASSESSMENT	NURSING PLANS AND INTERVENTIONS

Altered nutrition related to …
• Weight loss in pregnancy.
• Signs of dehydration.
   → Increased urine specific gravity.
   → Oliguria.
• Psychological distress (different from normal ambivalence in pregnancy).
• Fluid and electrolyte imbalance; potential metabolic acidosis.
	• Weigh daily at same time with like clothing.
	• Check urine 3x daily for ketones.
	• Monitor electrolytes and hydration status. Report abnormal lab values STAT to healthcare provider.
	• Progress diet from clear liquids to full liquids to bland, to full diet.
	• Check fetal heart rate (if possible, auscultate by Doppler) q8 hrs.
	• Provide psychological support to offset client's concerns.

Figure 5-55

HESI HINT: Recent research has found that *Helicobacter pylori,* (the bacterium that causes stomach ulcers) infection is another possible causative factor in hyperemesis. Other pregnancy and non-pregnancy risk factors for hyperemesis gravidarum include first pregnancy, multiple fetuses, age under 24, history of this condition in other pregnancies, obesity, and high fat diets.

HESI HINT: In severe cases of hyperemesis gravidarum, the healthcare provider may prescribe antihistamines, Vitamin B6, or phenothiazines to relieve nausea. The provider may also prescribe metoclopramide (Reglan) to increase the rate the stomach moves food into the intestines, or antacids to absorb stomach acid and help prevent acid reflux.

HESI HINT: Women who suffer from hyperemesis gravidarum are often deficient in thiamin, riboflavin, vitamin B6, vitamin A, and retinol-binding proteins.

DIABETES MELLITUS

- May manifest for the first time in pregnancy as the diabetogenic effects of pregnancy increase.
- Hormonal changes during pregnancy act to increase maternal cell resistance to insulin so that an abundant supply of glucose is available to the fetus.
- A preexisting reduction in insulin and the glucose-sparing effects of pregnancy compromise health of the mother/fetus.
- If insulin cannot move glucose into maternal cells, the mother will begin to metabolize fat and protein for energy producing ketones and fatty acids which result in ketoacidosis.

ANALYSIS (NURSING DIAGNOSES)
- Knowledge deficit about diabetes mellitus during pregnancy related to…
- Potential for injury to fetus/mother related to…

ASSESSMENT

- Predisposing factors include:
  - → Family history of diabetes.
  - → History of more than 2 spontaneous abortions.
  - → Hydramnios.
  - → Previous baby with a weight over 4,000 gm (8lb. 13.5 oz.).
  - → Previous baby with congenital anomalies.
  - → High parity.
  - → Obesity.
  - → Recurrent monilial vaginitis.
  - → Glycosuria.
- Abnormal glucose screen. A 1-hour glucose screen is routinely done on all pregnant women between 24 to 26 weeks gestation.
- Elevated Glycosylated hemoglobin (used to evaluate diabetic control by reflecting blood glucose level during the previous 6 to 8 weeks) indicates uncontrolled diabetes.
- Types of diabetes mellitus include:
  - → Type I (insulin dependent): schedule for Hemoglobin A1C test (glycosolated hemoglobin reflects glucose control for the life-span of the red blood cell, 120 days). Prone to ketosis.
  - → Type II (non-insulin dependent): in pregnancy, insulin is required to control maternal blood glucose levels.
  - → Type III (gestational diabetes): onset during pregnancy with return to normal glucose tolerance after delivery.
- Symptoms include the "three Ps": polyphagia, polydipsia, and polyuria.
- Hypoglycemia (usually in first trimester); insulin need may decrease.
- Hyperglycemia (2nd and 3rd trimester); amount of insulin needed increases.
- Increased incidence of preeclampsia, infection, and hydramnios.

NURSING PLANS AND INTERVENTIONS

- At diagnosis, implement the following:
  - → Review pathophysiology of disease.
  - → Teach home glucose monitoring (urine and blood).
  - → Demonstrate insulin administration.
  - → Identify signs of hypo and hyperglycemia and the immediate actions to be taken if signs are noted. *(See Diabetes Mellitus in Medical Surgical Nursing)*
  - → Stress importance of regular prenatal visits.
  - → Encourage verbalization of concerns regarding diagnosis.
- Refer client to dietician for individualized diet management.
  - → Calories: 35 to 50 cal/kg of ideal body weight.
  - → Complex carbohydrates: 50% of diet.
  - → Proteins: 20% of diet.
  - → Fat: less than 30% of diet.
  - → Distribute calories between 3 meals and 4 snacks.
  - → Review relationship between exercise and diet. Hyperglycemia can be prevented by consistent utilization of calories through exercise.

Figure 5-56

DIABETES MELLITUS (CONTINUED)

- Remind client of expected increased insulin needs in second and third trimester related to increasing diabetogenic effects of pregnancy.
- Review situations, which will complicate diabetic control: illness, diarrhea, and vomiting.
- Teach client to drink orange juice followed by glass of low-fat milk for hypoglycemic reaction or insulin reaction.
- Teach client s/s of ketoacidosis (fruity odor to breath, nausea and vomiting, exaggerated respiratory effort, altered mental state) and to come to hospital immediately if any of these symptoms occur.
- Remind client of need for scheduled delivery date, usually around 37 to 38 weeks gestation, when control becomes more difficult.
- See below for Nursing Care for the Diabetic Maternity Client.
- Provide care for the infant. *(See Nursing Care for Infant of Diabetic Mother)*

HESI HINT: GLUCOSE SCREEN
Client does NOT have to fast for this test. 50 gm of glucose is given and blood is drawn after one hour. If the blood glucose is greater than 135 mg/dl, then a three-hour glucose tolerance test (GTT) is done.

HESI HINT: High incidence of fetal anomalies occurs in pregnant diabetic women. Therefore, fetal surveillance is very important.
- Ultrasound exam.
- Alpha-fetoprotein (to determine neural tube anomalies).
- Non-stress and contraction stress tests.

HESI HINT: Oral hypoglycemics are not taken in pregnancy due to potential teratogenic effects on fetus. Insulin is used for therapeutic management.

HESI HINT: When a woman is admitted in labor with diagnosis of diabetes mellitus:
- She is more prone to preeclampsia, hemorrhage, and infection.
- Delivery is often scheduled between 37 to 38 weeks gestation to avoid the end of the 3rd trimester of pregnancy because this is a VERY difficult time to maintain diabetic control.

NURSING CARE FOR THE DIABETIC MATERNITY CLIENT

PREDELIVERY PERIOD	POSTDELIVERY PERIOD

• Insert an intravenous line for infusion of insulin and a glucose containing solution. Insulin does not cross placental barrier.
• On the day of delivery, carefully assess client for insulin administration.
• Regular insulin and glucose containing solution are titrated to maintain blood glucose levels between 60 and 100 in labor.
• Hourly determinations of blood glucose are done by finger stick.
• Position on left side to avoid pressure on vena cava from large fetus or hydramnios.
• Check urine for ketones hourly. Report any over 2+.
• Monitor fetus continuously using electronic fetal monitoring system.
	• Use a sliding-scale approach to insulin administration due to the precipitous fall in insulin requirements postdelivery.
	• Continue a 5% glucose infusion at 100 to 125 cc/hr.
	• Check urine each shift for ketones (sign of hyperglycemia, utilization of fat/protein for energy).
	• Monitor for complications:
	  → Preeclampsia.
	  → Postpartum uterine atony associated with uterine over distension.
	  → Infection.
	• Encourage breastfeeding, which decreases insulin requirements. Insulin DOES NOT cross into breast milk.
	• Contraception: Diaphragm with spermicide.

HESI HINT: It is useful to discontinue long-acting insulin administration on the day before the delivery is planned since insulin requirements are less in labor and drop precipitously after delivery.

Figure 5-56 (continued)

DIABETES MELLITUS (CONTINUED)	
NURSING CARE FOR INFANT OF DIABETIC MOTHER	
ASSESSMENT	**NURSING PLANS AND INTERVENTIONS**
• Macrosomia. • IUGR. • Hypoglycemia, hypocalcemia. • Hyperbilirubinemia, polycythemia. • Congenital anomalies. • Infection. • Prematurity.	• Observe for birth trauma: clavicle fracture or cerebral trauma. • Perform heel sticks for glucose assessment at 30 minutes of age, 1 hour, and as prescribed. • Observe for hypoglycemia: jitteriness. • Observe for hypocalcemia: jitteriness. • Begin small, frequent feedings at 1 hour of age.

Figure 5-56 (continued)

EMERGENCY DELIVERY
Emergency delivery (rapid, uncontrolled delivery) is an unsterile or an unassisted delivery that can be managed without complications to mother or fetus.
ANALYSIS (NURSING DIAGNOSES) • Potential for injury to mother/fetus related to… • Anxiety related to…
ASSESSMENT
• Bulging perineum. • Woman screaming that the baby is coming. • Presenting part visible at introitus.
NURSING PLANS AND INTERVENTIONS
• Do not, at any time, leave the client alone. • If possible, get precip basin from E.R. or closet if occurring in labor room (precip basin includes towels, scissors, cord clamps, bulb syringe and placenta basin). • Place clean towel under mother's buttocks. • Have client use hee-blow or blow-blow breathing technique to slow expulsion of head over perineum. • If amnion is still present, rupture with fingers or clean implement when head crowns. • Apply gentle counterpressure against presenting part (vertex) to prevent the fetus from "popping" over the perineum, which can lacerate tissue and cause fetal cerebral trauma. • Check for cord around neck and remove if loose; cut if tight. • Deliver anterior shoulder first by gently pressing downward under symphysis. • Apply upward pressure over perineum to deliver posterior shoulder. • Deliver entire body, holding baby in slightly head down position to facilitate mucus drainage. • Suction baby with bulb syringe quickly (mouth and nares). • Dry infant and cover with blanket or towel. • If equipment is available, clamp cord in two places and cut in between. If sterile supplies are not available, leave cord intact. • Do not milk the cord. • When signs of placental separation are seen (gush of blood, lengthening of cord), ask woman to gently push placenta out. • Put baby to mother's breast to contract uterus.

Figure 5-57

MATERNITY NURSING

CESAREAN BIRTH

Delivery of a fetus/fetuses through the abdomen.
- Whether planned (elective) or unplanned (emergency), the client is prone to complications.
  - → Anesthesia complications.
  - → Usual abdominal surgery complications.
  - → Sepsis.
  - → Thromboembolism.
  - → Injury to the urinary tract.
- Rate of Cesarean section births is approaching 25% in the U.S.
- Trend is to allow VBAC (vaginal birth after Cesarean) if a low transverse incision was performed and if the original complications for which a cesarean birth was indicated do not recur.

ANALYSIS (NURSING DIAGNOSES)
- Anxiety related to…
- Potential for injury to mother related to…
- Potential alteration in urinary elimination related to…

ASSESSMENT

- Elective or repeat cesarean birth scheduled.
- Emergency cesarean birth performed to prevent harm to mother/fetus.

NURSING CARE FOR CLIENT WITH CESAREAN BIRTH

PRE-CESAREAN BIRTH

- If surgery is planned, encourage couple to attend cesarean birth class.
  - → Tour of surgical area is usually provided.
  - → Film of cesarean birth is shown.
  - → Discussion is led by staff member.
- If emergency cesarean is necessary, obtain informed consent including healthcare provider's explanation of risks, benefits, and alternatives to surgery.
- Inform anesthesiologist of need for preoperative assessment.
- Assist with anesthesia, usually epidural.
- Administer pre-op medications if prescribed.
  - → Usually, due to fetus in utero, no analgesia or sedative is prescribed preoperative.
    - May receive antacid to alkalize stomach contents (if aspiration occurs, less damage will be done to lung tissue) or drug such as a histamine receptor antagonist, which is a gastric antisecretory drug to reduce production of gastric secretions.
- Shave abdomen from xiphoid to ¼ way down thigh, including pubic area (varies by institution).
- Insert Foley catheter.
- Lab studies: type and crossmatch for 2 units packed red blood cells, CBC, and chemistry.
- Catheterized or clean-catch urinalysis.
- Remove dentures, contact lenses, rings, and fingernail polish and give to support person.
- Notify nursery, neonatologist, and/or pediatrician of impending cesarean birth.
- Allow presence of support person in operative suite unless hospital policy contraindicates.
- Maintain safety during transfer to operative suite.

INTRAOPERATIVE CARE

- Prior to abdominal prep:
  - → Place wedge under one hip to displace uterus laterally.
  - → Keep client warm via warm blankets.
  - → Monitor and document fetal heart tones continually.
- Apply grounding pad to leg.
- Perform abdominal scrub (prep).
- Perform circulating nurse duties per institutional protocol.
- If client is awake, assess and meet psychosocial needs.

Figure 5-58

MATERNITY NURSING

CESAREAN BIRTH (CONTINUED)

POST-CESAREAN BIRTH

- Receive complete report including the type of uterine incision performed.
- Fundal height and consistency assessment may be difficult due to abdominal bandage and pain. Note on chart if unable to determine, but gentle attempts should be made.
- Assess temperature every hour in recovery room, then q4 hrs x 24 hrs., q8 hrs. thereafter if within normal limits.
- Assess heart rate, respirations, breath sounds, bowel sounds, and SaO_2 per unit protocol.
- Begin I&O assessment q8 hours.
- Administer pain medication as prescribed. The trend is toward patient-controlled analgesia (PCA pumps) and postoperative epidural analgesia with morphine sulfate (Duramorph), fentanyl citrate (Sublimaze) or meperidine (Demerol). *(See figure 5-59, Narcotic Analgesics)*
- Encourage participation in infant care ASAP and take mother/couple to nursery often.
- Demonstrate splinting of abdomen, coughing, deep breathing, and incentive spirometer use to prevent respiratory complications from stasis of lung secretions.
- Maintain aseptic technique to prevent sepsis:
  - → Teach handwashing technique.
  - → Assess incisional healing q8 hours.
  - → Scrupulous peri care/pad changes.
  - → Assessment of lochia for foul odor (indicative of infection).

HESI HINT: If a woman is medicated, the responsible adult accompanying her must sign the necessary consent forms. State laws differ as to the acceptability of a friend signing the consent form rather than a relative.

HESI HINT: Babies delivered abdominally miss out on the vaginal squeeze and are born with more fluid in the lungs, predisposing the newborn to transient tachypnea (TTN) and respiratory distress.

HESI HINT: The preferable low-transverse uterine incision usually results in less postoperative pain, less bleeding, and less incidents of ruptured uterus. The classical, vertical incision on the uterus may involve part of the fundus, resulting in more postoperative pain, bleeding, and an increased chance of uterine rupture.

HESI HINT: Due to the exploration and cleansing of the uterus just after delivery of the placenta, the amount of lochia may be scant in the recovery room. However, pooling in the vagina and uterus while on bedrest may result in blood running down the client's leg when she first ambulates. Cesarean birth clients have the same lochial changes, placental site healing, and aseptic needs as do vaginal birth clients.

HESI HINT: A laparotomy of any kind, including cesarean birth, predisposes the client to postoperative paralytic ileus. When the bowel is manipulated in surgery, it ceases peristalsis, which may persist. Symptoms include: absent bowel sounds, abdominal distension, tympany on percussion, nausea and vomiting, and of course, obstipation (intractable constipation). Early ambulation is an effective nursing intervention.

Figure 5-58 (continued)

MATERNITY NURSING

NARCOTIC ANALGESICS			
DRUGS	**INDICATIONS**	**ADVERSE REACTIONS**	**NURSING IMPLICATIONS**
fentanyl citrate (Sublimaze)	• Used as an adjunct to anesthesia	• Respiratory depression, apnea • Bradycardia, hypotension	• Have resuscitation equipment readily available • Do not mix with IV barbiturates
morphine sulfate (Astramorph Pf, Duramorh, MS Contin) *(See figure 2-30 for more narcotic information)*	• Often first choice for severe pain	• Nausea, vomiting, constipation • Respiratory depression, depression of cough reflexes • Hypotension	• Check respirations and BP prior to administration; hold administration if respirations <12 or if hypotension exists • Have antagonist, naloxone HCL (Narcan), available in case of respiratory depression

Figure 5-59

REVIEW QUESTIONS

HIGH-RISK DISORDERS

1. What instructions should the nurse give the woman with a threatened abortion?
2. Identify the nursing plans and interventions for a woman hospitalized with hyperemesis gravidarum.
3. Describe discharge counseling for a woman after hydatidiform mole evacuation by D&C.
4. What condition should the nurse suspect if a woman of childbearing age presents to an emergency room with bilateral or unilateral abdominal pain with or without bleeding?
5. List three symptoms of abruptio placentae and three symptoms of placenta previa.
6. What specific information should the nurse include when teaching human papillomavirus detection and treatment?
7. State three principles pertinent to counseling and/or teaching a pregnant adolescent.
8. What complications are pregnant adolescents more prone to develop?
9. All pregnant women should be taught preterm labor recognition. Describe the warning symptoms of preterm labor.
10. List the predisposing factors to preterm labor.
11. When is preterm labor able to be arrested?
12. What is the major side effect of beta-adrenergic (Terbutaline, Ritodrine) tocolytic drugs?
13. What special actions should the nurse take in the intrapartum period if preterm labor is unable to be arrested?
14. A prolonged latent phase for a multipara is _____ and for a nullipara is _____. Multiparas average cervical dilatation is _____ cm/hr in the active phase and nulliparas average cervical dilatation is _____ cm/hr

in the active phase.
15. What are the major goals of nursing care related to pregnancy-induced hypertension with preeclampsia?
16. Magnesium sulfate is used to treat Preeclampsia.
    A. What is the purpose for administration of magnesium sulfate?
    B. What is the main action of magnesium sulfate?
    C. The antidote for magnesium sulfate?
    D. List the three main assessment findings indicating toxic effects of magnesium sulfate.
17. What are the major symptoms of preeclampsia?
18. What is the priority nursing action after spontaneous or artificial rupture of membranes?
19. What is the most common complication of oxytocin augmentation or induction of labor? List three actions the nurse should take if such a complication occurs.
20. List the symptoms of water intoxication from the antidiuretic hormone (ADH) effect of Pitocin (oxytocin).
21. State three nursing interventions during FORCEPS delivery.
22. What is the cause of preeclampsia?
23. What interventions should the nurse implement to prevent further CNS irritability in the preeclampsia client?
24. A woman on Orinase (oral hypoglycemic) asks the nurse if she can continue this medication in pregnancy. How should the nurse respond?
25. Name three maternal and three fetal complications of gestational diabetes.

26. When should the nurse hold the dose of magnesium sulfate and call the physician?
27. State three priority nursing actions in the postdelivery period for the client with preeclampsia.
28. When are the two most difficult times for control for the pregnant diabetic?
29. Why is regular insulin used in labor?
30. List three conditions clients with diabetes mellitus are more prone to develop.
31. When is cardiac disease in pregnancy most dangerous?
32. Does insulin cross the placental/breast barrier?
33. The goal for diabetic management during labor is euglycemia. How is it defined?
34. What contraceptive technique is recommended for diabetic women?
35. List the symptoms of cardiac decompensation in the laboring client with cardiac disease.
36. What interventions can the nurse implement to maintain cardiac perfusion in a laboring cardiac client?
37. Gentle counterpressure against the perineum during an emergency delivery prevents ____ and _____.
38. When may a vaginal birth after Cesarean (VBAC) be considered by a woman with a previous Cesarean section?
39. Prior to anesthesia for Cesarean section delivery, the mother may be given an antacid OR a gastric antisecretory drug (histamine receptor antagonist). State the reasons why these drugs are given.
40. Clients who have had a Cesarean section are prone to what postoperative complications?

ANSWERS TO REVIEW QUESTIONS

1. Maintain strict bedrest for 24 to 48 hours. Avoid sexual intercourse for two weeks.
2. Weigh daily; urine ketone checks 3x daily; progressive diet; check FHR q8 hours; monitor for electrolyte imbalances.
3. Prevent pregnancy for one year. Return to clinic/MD for monthly hCG levels for one year. Postoperative D&C instructions: call if bright red vaginal bleeding or foul smelling vaginal discharge occurs, or temperature spike over 100.4°F.
4. Ectopic pregnancy.
5. Abruption: fetal distress; rigid, board-like abdomen; pain; dark red or absent bleeding.

Previa: painless, bright red vaginal bleeding; fetal heart rate normal; soft uterus.
6. Detection of dry, wart-like growths on vulva or rectum. Need for pap smear in the prenatal period. Treatment with laser ablation (CANNOT USE PODOPHYLLIN in pregnancy). Associated with cervical carcinoma in mother and respiratory papillomatosis in neonate.
7. Nurse must establish trust/rapport before counseling/teaching begins. Adolescents do not respond to an authoritarian approach. Consider the developmental tasks of identity and social/ individual intimacy.
8. Preeclampsia, IUGR, CPD, STDs, Anemia.
9. More than 5 contractions/hour, cramps, low, dull backache; pelvic pressure; change in vaginal discharge.
10. Urinary tract infection; over distension of uterus; diabetes; Preeclampsia; cardiac disease; placenta previa, psychosocial factors, i.e., stress.
11. Cervix is <4 cm dilated, <50% effacement, and membranes intact and not bulging out of the cervical os.
12. Tachycardia.
13. Monitor the FHR continuously and limit drugs, which cross placental barriers to prevent fetal depression or further compromise.
14. >14 hours, >20 hours, 1.5, 1.2.
15. Maintenance of uteroplacental perfusion; prevention of seizures; prevention of complications such as HELLP syndrome, DIC, and abruption.
16. Answers areas follows:
    A. Prevent seizures by decreasing CNS irritability.
    B. Central nervous system depression (seizure prevention).
    C. Calcium gluconate.
    D. Reduced urinary output, reduced respiratory rate, and decreased reflexes.
17. Increase in BP of 30 mmHg systolic and 15 mmHg diastolic over previous baseline; hyperflexia; proteinuria (albuminuria); CNS disturbances; headache, and visual disturbances; epigastric pain.
18. Assessment of the fetal heart rate.
19. Tetany. Turn off Pitocin. Turn pregnant woman to side. Administer O$_2$ by mask.
20. Nausea and vomiting, headache, and hypotension.
21. Ensure empty bladder. Auscultate FHR

before application, during, and between traction periods. Observe for maternal lacerations and newborn cerebral/facial trauma.

22. The person who determines the exact cause will be our next NOBEL prize winner! However, the underlying pathophysiology appears to be generalized vasospasm with increased peripheral resistance and vascular damage. This decreased perfusion results in damage to numerous organs.

23. Darken room, limit visitors, maintain close 1:1 nurse/client ratio, place in private room, plan nursing interventions all together so client is disturbed as little as possible.

24. No, oral hypoglycemic medications are teratogenic to the fetus. Insulin will be used.

25. Maternal: hypoglycemia, hyperglycemia, ketoacidosis.
Fetal: macrosomia, hypoglycemia at birth, fetal anomalies.

26. When the client's respirations are <12/ minute, DTRs are absent, or urinary output is <100 cc/4 hours.

27. Monitor for signs of blood loss. Continue to assess BP and DTRs q4 hours. Monitor for uterine atony.

28. Late in the 3rd trimester and in the postpartum period when insulin needs to drop sharply (the diabetogenic effects of pregnancy drop precipitously).

29. It is short-acting, predictable, can be infused intravenously and discontinued quickly if necessary.

30. Preeclampsia, hydramnios; infection.

31. At peak plasma volume increase, 28 to 32 weeks gestation and during Stage II labor.

32. No, therefore insulin-dependent women may breastfeed.

33. 60 to 100 mg/dl.

34. Diaphragm with spermicide. Avoid birth control pills that contain estrogen and IUDs, which are an infection risk.

35. Tachycardia, tachypnea, dry cough, rales in lung bases, dyspnea, and orthopnea.

36. Position client in a semi or high-Fowler's position. Prevent Valsalva's maneuvers. Position client in a supine or R/T for regional anesthesia. Avoid stirrups because of possible popliteal vein compression and decreased venous return.

37. Maternal lacerations, fetal cerebral trauma.

38. If a low uterine transverse incision was performed and can be documented AND if the original complication does not recur, i.e., CPD.

39. Antacid buffers alkalize the stomach secretions. If aspiration occurs, less lung damage ensues. An antisecretory drug reduces gastric acid, reducing the risk of gastric aspiration.

40. Paralytic ileus, infection, thromboembolism, respiratory complications, and impaired maternal infant bonding.

Postpartum High-Risk Disorders

Postpartum Infections

Any clinical infection of the genital canal that occurs within 28 days of delivery.

ANALYSIS (NURSING DIAGNOSES)

- Potential for injury related to….
- Knowledge deficit (specify) related to…
- Alteration in comfort: pain related to…

NURSING ASSESSMENT

- Women predisposed to infection include those with:
  - → Rupture of membranes >24 hours.
  - → Any lacerations or operative incisions (forceps, episiotomy, or Cesarean section).
  - → Hemorrhage.
  - → Hematomas.
  - → Lapses in aseptic technique before or after delivery, e.g., faulty perineal care.
  - → Anemia or poor physical health prior to delivery.
  - → Intrauterine manipulation, manual removal of placenta, retained placental fragments.
- Puerperal morbidity:
  - → Temperature of 100.4°F or higher.
  - → Occurs within the first 24 hours after delivery.
  - → Temperature elevation on two successive days or two successive 4-hour assessments.
- Signs of infection: *(See Assessment Data for Puerperal Infections)*
- Most common organisms are streptococcal and anaerobic organisms; least common organism is staphylococcus.

ASSESSMENT DATA FOR PUERPERAL INFECTION

INFECTION	ASSESSMENT DATA
PERINEAL INFECTION	• Temperature 101 to 104°F (38.3 to 40°C) • Red, swollen, very tender perineum (episiotomy site) • Purulent drainage, induration
ENDOMETRITIS (Infection of Lining of Uterus)	• Temperature 101 to 102°F (38.3 to 39.9°C) • Pulse >100 • Malaise. anorexia • Excess fundal tenderness long after expected • Uterine subinvolution • Lochia return to rubra from serosa • Foul-smelling lochia
PARAMETRITIS (Pelvic Cellulites)	• Temperature 103 to 104°F (39.4 to 40°C) • Tachycardia, tachypnea • Severe uterine and cervical tenderness • WBC >25,000 • Palpable pelvic abscess
PERITONITIS	• Chills and temperature to 105°F • Rapid, thready pulse to 140 BPM • Decreased urinary output • Paralytic ileus, abdominal distension, absence of bowel sounds
THROMBOPHLEBITIS (Deep Vein)	• Minimal if any fever • Positive Homan's sign • Pain in calf or dull ache in leg • Swelling in extremity below pain
URINARY TRACT INFECTION CYSTITIS (Bladder)	• Slight or no temperature • Dysuria, frequency, urgency, suprapubic tenderness • Hematuria, bacteriuria • Cloudy urine

Figure 5-60

POSTPARTUM INFECTIONS (CONTINUED)

ASSESSMENT DATA FOR PUERPERAL INFECTIONS

INFECTIONS	ASSESSMENT DATA
PYELONEPHRITIS (Kidney)	• Temperature 102°F and higher, chills • Flank pain and costovertebral angle tenderness • Nausea and vomiting • Dysuria, urgency, cloudy urine, hematuria, bacteriuria
MASTITIS (Breast)	• Sore, cracked nipple • Flu-like symptoms: malaise, chills, and fever • Red, warm lump in breast

NURSING PLANS AND INTERVENTIONS

• Implement general care pertinent to any client with a diagnosed infection:
  → Use and teach good handwashing technique (HWT).
  → Assess and record vital signs, especially temperature, q4 hours or more often if indicated.
  → Manage fever by increasing fluids, cool baths, administration of acetaminophen (Tylenol) p.o. or by suppository.
  → Assess for signs of dehydration: inelastic skin turgor, dry mucous membranes, increased urine specific gravity.
  → Maintain hydration: increase fluid intake to 2 to 3 l/day.
  → Promote nutrition: basic 4 food groups and increase intake of vitamin C foods (for healing) and protein (for tissue repair).
  → Emphasize need for adherence to medication regime (take entire antibiotic series).
  → Maintain cleanliness, personal hygiene.
  → Implement medical and nursing interventions for specific diagnosed infections.

Perineal infection
• Keep warm; may use hot water bottle in bed if chilled.
• Assess site daily for decrease in redness, pain, and discharge.
• Assist with sitz bath and peri lamp 2 to 3 x daily; encourage meticulous peri care.
• Administer antibiotics and analgesics as prescribed.

Endometritis
• Usually maintain bedrest with bathroom privileges (Fowler's or Semi-Fowlers position).
• Palpate fundus and abdomen q8 hours to assess pain and involution.
• Antibiotics usually administered IV, often using a heparin lock. *(See figure 5-61, Antibiotics)*

Parametritis
• Promote lochial/uterine drainage by semi-Fowler's position.
• Determine amount and odor of lochia (heavy, foul-smelling usually indicates anaerobic bacteria).
• Monitor for development of pelvic thrombophlebitis: clot in ovarian vein will cause acute abdominal pain.
• Administer IV antibiotics.

Peritonitis	**Mastitis**
• Client usually transferred to Intensive Care: MEDICAL EMERGENCY. • O₂ by mask. • IV antibiotics. • Insertion of nasogastric tube for gastric decompression, prevention of vomiting from paralytic ileus. • Assess abdomen 3 x daily for tympany, distension, and bowel sounds. • Monitor and document I&O.	• Obtain culture and sensitivity on breast milk. • Breastfeed every 2 to 3 hours and make sure breasts are emptied with each feed. • Do not abruptly cease breastfeeding unless healthcare provider prescribes. • May have to discontinue breastfeeding if pus is in breast milk, or if antibiotic is contraindicated in breastfeeding. Mother should manually empty the breasts and discard the milk to maintain milk production and reduce congestion. • If newborn develops diarrhea, contact healthcare provider regarding changing antibiotic. • Usually treated at home by PO antibiotics. • Bedrest for 48 hours. • Monitor for abscess formation, need for incision and drainage.

Figure 5-60 (continued)

321

MATERNITY NURSING

POSTPARTUM INFECTIONS (CONTINUED)

NURSING PLANS AND INTERVENTIONS

Deep vein thrombophlebitis • **See Medical Surgical Nursing for Interventions.** • Administer anticoagulant therapy (heparin for 6 weeks). **(See Medical Surgical Nursing figure 3-19, Anticoagulants)**	Cystitis and pyelonephritis • Collect urine for analysis and culture. • Avoid catheterization if at all possible.	Sexually transmitted disease (STDs) • **See Medical Surgical Nursing for Interventions.** • Breastfeeding and rooming-in are affected when the mother has a STD.

HESI HINT: Nurse must be especially supportive of postpartum client with infection because it usually implies isolation from newborn until organism is identified and treatment begun. Arrange phone calls to nursery and window viewing. Involve family, spouse, significant others in teaching, and encourage other family members to continue neonatal attachment activities.

HESI HINT: Most common iatrogenic cause of UTI is urinary catheterization.
• Encourage clients to void frequently and not ignore the urge.
• IV antibiotics are usually administered to clients with pyelonephritis.

HESI HINT: Remember, the risk of postpartum infections increases for clients who experienced problems during pregnancy (e.g., anemia, diabetes) or experienced trauma during labor and delivery.

BREASTFEEDING/ROOMING-IN PROCEDURES FOR MOTHERS WITH STDS

STDs	ROOMING-IN	BREASTFEEDING
AIDS/HIV POSITIVE	YES	NO
CYTOMEGALOVIRUS (CMV	YES	NO
CHLAMYDIA	YES	YES
GONORRHEA (Untreated) **Medication x 24 hours**	NO YES	NO YES
HEPATITIS	YES	YES
HERPES	YES	YES
SYPHILIS (Untreated) **Medication x 24 hours**	NO YES	NO YES
TRICHOMONIASIS	YES	YES

HESI HINT: Clients taking anticoagulants can usually expect to have heavy menstrual periods.

HESI HINT: In most cases, a mother who is on antibiotic therapy can continue to breastfeed unless the healthcare provider thinks the neonate is at risk for sepsis by maternal contact. Sulfa drugs are used cautiously in lactating mothers because they can be transferred to the infant in breast milk.

HESI HINT: Many times mastitis can be confused with a blocked milk sinus, which is treated by nursing closer to the lump and by rotating the baby on the breast. Breastfeeding is not contraindicated for women with mastitis, unless pus is in the breast milk, or the antibiotic of choice is harmful to the infant. If either of these occurs, milk production can still be fostered by manual expression.

Figure 5-60 (continued)

MATERNITY NURSING

ANTIBIOTICS			
DRUGS	**INDICATIONS**	**ADVERSE REACTIONS**	**NURSING IMPLICATIONS**
ampicillin (Ampicin, Ampilean)	• Broad-spectrum antibiotic used to treat postpartum endometritis, mastitis	• Rash, dermatitis • Nausea, vomiting • GI irritation	• Do not administer to clients with penicillin sensitivity • Does appear in breast milk, but may not cause neonate any discomfort
gentamicin sulfate (Garamycin)	• Aminoglycoside antibiotic used for serious puerperal infections	• GI irritation • Nephrotoxicity • Ototoxicity • Neurotoxicity • Possible hypersensitivity	• Do not mix with any other drug • Observe for ototoxicity: ataxia, tinnitus, headache • Observe for nephrotoxicity: elevated BUN and creatinine • Observe for neurotoxicity: parasthesia, muscle weakness • Monitor I&O closely

Figure 5-61

POSTPARTUM HEMORRHAGE

• A leading cause of maternal mortality that demands prompt recognition and intervention.
• Hemorrhage can be caused by:
  → Uterine atony (poor muscle tone).
  → Lacerations of the vagina.
  → Cervix, perineum, or labia hematomas development.
  → Retained placental fragments.
  → Full bladder.
• Predisposing factors include:
  → High parity.
  → Dystocia, prolonged labor.
  → Operative delivery: Cesarean or forceps delivery, intrauterine manipulation.
  → Over distension of the uterus: polyhydramnios, multiple gestation, large neonate.
  → Abruptio placentae.
  → Previous history of postpartum hemorrhage.
  → Infection.
  → Placenta previa.

Figure 5-62

POSTPARTUM HEMORRHAGE (CONTINUED)

ANALYSIS (NURSING DIAGNOSES)
- Potential fluid volume deficit related to…
- Anxiety related to…
- Potential for infection related to…

ASSESSMENT

- Excessive uterine bleeding during the first hour following delivery (more than one saturated pad/15 minutes).
- Excessive uterine bleeding during the postpartum period (more than one saturated pad/hour).
- Blood loss of more than 500 ml. during delivery; or loss of 1% or more of body weight (1 ml = 1 gm).
- Signs of hypovolemic shock:
  - → Decreased blood pressure.
  - → Weak, rapid pulse.
  - → Cool, clammy skin, color ashen or gray.

- Signs of hematomas developing in perineum:
  - → Intense perineal pain.
  - → Swelling and blue-black discoloration on perineum.
  - → Pallor, tachycardia, and hypotension (great blood loss). Feeling of pressure in vagina, urethra, and bladder.
  - → Possible urinary retention, uterine displacement.
- Signs of bleeding from unrepaired laceration:
  - → Continuous trickle from vagina.
  - → Bleeding in spurts.
  - → Bleeding in presence of contracted fundus.
- Signs of bleeding from uterine atony:
  - → Soft, boggy uterus usually above umbilicus.
  - → Fundus does not firm up with massage.

NURSING PLANS AND INTERVENTIONS
NURSING CARE FOR MATERNITY CLIENT WITH HEMORRHAGE

EARLY POSTPARTUM	LATE POSTPARTUM	HEMATOMA DEVELOPMENT
• Review chart for predisposing factors. • Monitor vital signs, fundus, lochia q 1 hour. • Monitor level of consciousness. • Keep the bladder empty. • Call MD if atony/bleeding continues despite massage. • Anticipate increasing Pitocin (oxytocin) IV infusion and/or administering ergot preparation IM. • Count pads saturated and time required to saturate. • Monitor I&O (at least 30 cc/hr output); be sure to maintain fluid replacement.	• Anticipate quick hospitalization and determination of cause of bleeding. • Type and crossmatch for possible blood transfusion. • Administer oxytocic drugs and possibly ergot preparations as prescribed. • Administer antibiotics as prescribed. • Keep the client warm and be alert to symptoms of shock. • Possibly prepare client for surgical repair of laceration, evacuation of hematomas, or curettage for removal of placental fragments (most common reason for late postpartum hemorrhage).	• Apply ice pack to perineum to decrease swelling and pain. • Prepare client for surgical incision if hematoma is large. • Monitor vital signs closely. Since hemorrhage is covert, hypovolemia and anemia can occur unknowingly. • Administer analgesics and antibiotics as prescribed. • If severe hemorrhage and hypovolemic shock occur, notify physician immediately and: → Increase IV infusion quickly to wide open. → Give O_2 by mask at 10 liters → Monitor vital signs q5 to 15 minutes. → Lower head of bed, position client supine. → Assist with insertion of CVP (central venous pressure) line or hemodynamic catheter. → Insert Foley catheter.

Figure 5-62 (continued)

MATERNITY NURSING

324

> **HESI HINT:** During medical emergencies such as bleeding episodes, clients need calm, direct explanations and assurance that all is being done that can be done. If possible, allow support person at bedside. Risk-management principles state that the suit-prone client is one who feels things are being hidden from her or that adequate attention is NOT being given to HER problem.

> **HESI HINT:** Risk factors for hemorrhage include: dystocia, prolonged labor, over distended uterus, abruptio placentae, and infection.

> **HESI HINT:** What immediate nursing actions should be taken when a postpartum hemorrhage is detected?
> - Perform fundal massage.
> - Notify the healthcare provider if the fundus does not become firm with massage.
> - Count pads to estimate blood loss.
> - Assess and record vital signs.
> - Increase IV fluids (additional IV line may be indicated).
> - Administer oxytocin infusion as prescribed.

REVIEW QUESTIONS

POSTPARTUM HIGH-RISK DISORDERS

1. May women with a positive HIV antibody test breastfeed?
2. What are the common side effects of antibiotics used to treat puerperal infection?
3. How does the nurse differentiate symptomatology of cystitis from pyclonephritis?
4. What are the signs of endometritis?
5. What are the nursing actions for endometritis and parametritis?
6. State four risk factors or predisposing factors to postpartum infection.
7. State four risk factors or predisposing factors to postpartum hemorrhage.
8. What immediate nursing actions should be taken when a postpartum hemorrhage is detected?
9. Must women diagnosed with mastitis stop breastfeeding?

ANSWERS TO REVIEW QUESTIONS

1. No, HIV has been found in breast milk. (New England Journal of Medicine, August 1991).
2. GI adverse reactions: nausea, vomiting, diarrhea, and cramping. Hypersensitivity reactions: rashes, urticaria, and hives.
3. Pyelonephritis has the same symptoms as cystitis (dysuria, frequency, and urgency) with the addition of flank pain, fever, and pain at costovertebral angle.
4. Subinvolution (boggy, high uterus), lochia returns to rubra with possible foul smell, temperature 100.4°F or higher, unusual fundal tenderness.
5. Measures to promote lochial drainage; antipyretic measures (acetaminophen, cool baths); administration of analgesics and antibiotics as prescribed; increase fluids with attention to high-protein/high-vitamin C diet.
6. Operative delivery, intrauterine manipulation, anemia or poor physical health, traumatic delivery, and hemorrhage.
7. Dystocia or prolonged labor, over distension of the uterus, abruptio placentae, and infection.
8. Fundal massage. Notify healthcare provider if massage does NOT firm fundus. Count pads to estimate blood loss. Assess/record vital signs. Increase IV fluids and administer oxytocin infusion as prescribed.
9. No, women who abruptly stop breastfeeding may make the situation worse by increasing congestion/engorgement and providing further media for bacterial growth. Client may HAVE to discontinue breastfeeding if pus is present or if antibiotics are contraindicated for neonate.

MATERNITY NURSING

MAJOR DANGER SIGNALS IN THE NEWBORN

- Sixty percent of neonates requiring special care at birth can be identified through the prenatal history and another 20% through a review of intrapartal risk factors.
- Infants with Apgar scores of 7 to 10 rarely need resuscitative efforts, scores of 4 to 6 indicate mild to moderate asphyxia, and scores of 0 to 3 indicate severe asphyxia.
- The family experiences extreme challenges in adapting to the crisis of a sick baby.

DANGER SIGNS BY SYSTEM

SYSTEM	DESCRIPTION
CENTRAL NERVOUS SYSTEM	• Lethargy, high-pitched cry, jitteriness, seizures and bulging fontanels
RESPIRATORY SYSTEM	• Apnea (lack of breathing for 15 to 20 seconds), tachypnea, flaring nares, retractions, seesaw breathing, grunting, abnormal blood gases
CARDIOVASCULAR SYSTEM	• Abnormal rate and rhythm, persistent murmurs, differentials in pulse, dusky skin color, and circumoral cyanosis
GASTROINTESTINAL SYSTEM	• Absent feeding reflexes, vomiting, abdominal distention, changes in stool patterns, and no stool
METABOLIC SYSTEM	• Hypoglycemia, hypocalcemia, hyperbilirubinemia, labile temperature
Newborn weight is a major variable in determining survival	• Low birth weight (LBW): 2500 gm or less • Very low birth weight (VLBW): 1500 gm or less

Figure 5-63

HESI HINT: "Jitteriness" is a clinical manifestation of hypoglycemia and hypocalcemia. Laboratory analysis is indicated to differentiate between the two etiologies.

HESI HINT: To avoid metabolic problems brought on by cold stress, the first step, and number one priority, in management of the newborn is to prevent loss of body heat, followed by ABCs. Neonates produce heat by non-shivering thermogenesis, by burning brown fat. The neonate is easily stressed by hypothermia and develops acidosis from hypoxia. Prevent chilling (keep under radiant warmer or in isolette). If cold, the first signs exhibited are prolonged acrocyanosis, skin mottling, tachycardia, and tachypnea. If cold stressed, warm slowly over 2 to 4 hours since rapid warming may produce apnea. The neonate needs glucose, he/she has little glycogen storage and needs to be fed.

MANAGEMENT OF NEWBORN RESUSCITATION

NURSING PLANS AND INTERVENTIONS

- Bag and mask ventilations are done at 30 to 50 breaths/minute.
- Chest massage done at rate of 100 to 120/minute.
- Start IV fluids (usually umbilical vein, may use peripheral vein).
- Administer sodium bicarbonate and/or epinephrine as prescribed. *(See figure 5-65, Newborn Resuscitation)*
- Administer glucose as prescribed (stress rapidly causes hypoglycemia).
- Assign someone to support parents during resuscitation.
- Resuscitative efforts may be evaluated by the Silverman-Anderson Index of Respiratory Distress.
Five criteria are graded:
    - → Upper chest synchronization.
    - → Lower chest retractions.
    - → Xiphoid retractions.
    - → Nares dilation (flaring).
    - → Expiratory grunt.

Figure 5-64

MATERNITY NURSING

NEWBORN RESUSCITATION

DRUGS	INDICATIONS	ADVERSE REACTIONS	NURSING IMPLICATIONS
sodium bicarbonate	• Correction of severe metabolic acidosis in asphyxiated infants after adequate ventilation begun	• Fluid overload • Hypernatremia • Intracranial hemorrhage	• Do not mix with calcium solutions, causes precipitate • Use PEDIATRIC concentration of the drug • Infuse slowly and monitor I&O
epinephrine	• Asystole or severe bradycardia	• Tachyarrhythmias	• Make sure ventilation of newborn is adequate • Do not inject directly into artery • Monitor apical pulse or connect to ECG before use

Figure 5-65

OXYGEN THERAPY FOR THE NEWBORN

NURSING PLANS AND INTERVENTIONS

- PRINCIPLE: always administer O_2 at the lowest concentration possible to correct hypoxia. Use an O_2 analyzer to determine exact O_2 concentration. Oxygen is a "drug." Hypoxia and hyperoxia are both dangerous.
- O_2 toxicity results in:
  - → Retinopathy of prematurity (retrolental fibroplasias, RLF).
  - → Bronchopulmonary dysplasia (BPD).
- O_2 is prescribed in percent and represents the FiO_2 (fraction of inspired O_2 in the "air"). Room air has a FiO_2 of 21% (O_2 can be prescribed from 21 to 199%).
- Administer O_2 to the newborn via:
  - → Oxyhood: concentrations up to 100%.
  - → Nasal prongs: low concentrations.
  - → CPAP: continuous positive airway pressure.
    - • Reduces work of breathing; keeps alveoli open to prevent Atelectasis (works like the expiratory grunt).
    - • By nasal prong or mechanical ventilator.
- ECMO (extracorporeal membrane oxygenation: blood oxygenated outside body through bypass procedure).
- Monitor for problems associated with neonatal hypoxia:
  - → Respiratory acidosis.
  - → Organ damage.
    - • Necrotizing Enterocolitis (NEC): hypoxic-ischemic injury to the mucosa of the intestinal tract resulting in abdominal distension, sepsis, and nutritional impairment.
    - • Patent ductus arteriosis (PDA): return to fetal circulation to provide O_2 to brain and large organs. Results in worsening respiratory distress and pulmonary edema due to increased blood flow to lungs.
    - • Intraventricular hemorrhage (IVH): hypoxia causes vessel damage in the tiny periventricular capillaries resulting in symptoms of increased intracranial pressure (ICP), i.e., seizures, decreased or absent reflexes, hypotonia, bulging fontanels, enlarged head circumference, setting sun eyes, shrill cry, hypothermia, apnea or bradycardia.

Figure 5-66

MATERNITY NURSING

OXYGEN THERAPY FOR THE NEWBORN (CONTINUED)
NURSING PLANS AND INTERVENTIONS

- Closely monitor the partial pressure of O_2 in the newborn's arterial blood, i.e., Po_2.
- Monitor oxygenation status:
  - → Monitor arterial oxygen saturation level using pulse oximetry. It has a direct relationship to the partial pressure of O_2 in the arterial blood. Oxygen saturation should NOT fall below 90.
  - → Monitor O_2 levels by placing a $TcPo_2$ (transcutaneous oxygen pressure monitor) on the newborn. $TcPo_2$ levels should range 60 to 80 mmHg.
  - → Draw blood gas determinations from an arterial line every 3 to 4 hours. ALWAYS correlate O_2 saturation (svO_2) and $TcPo_2$ readings with blood gases.
- Criteria for mechanical ventilation: oxygen administration by other means does NOT reverse respiratory acidosis: pH <7.2, Po_2 <50, Pco_2 >60.

Figure 5-66 (continued)

HESI HINT: The Po_2 should be maintained between 50 to 90 mmHg. Po_2 <50 signifies hypoxia, Po_2 >90 signifies oxygen toxicity problems.

NEONATE WITH SEPSIS
Infections, especially in the preterm infant, can be overwhelming due to the immaturity of the immune system

ANALYSIS (NURSING DIAGNOSES)
- Potential alteration in thermoregulation related to…
- Potential for injury related to…

ASSESSMENT	NURSING PLANS AND INTERVENTIONS

• Lethargy.
• Temperature instability.
• Difficulty feeding.
• Subtle color changes; mottling, duskiness.
• "Just acts funny"; subtle changes in behavior.
• Respiratory distress, apnea.
• Hyperbilirubinemia.
	• Prevent infection in the high-risk newborn by:
	  → Meticulous handwashing: 3 minutes before day begins, 1 minute in between each baby.
	  → Apply Triple-dye antimicrobial to cord.
	  → Maintain sterile technique during procedures.
	  → Avoid rings and other jewelry in nursery.
	  → During contact with body secretions, use **UNIVERSAL PRECAUTIONS! WEAR GLOVES!**
	  → Document IV site appearance every 30 min. to one hour.
	  → Watch SKIN INTEGRITY: use little tape; use sheepskin, waterbed, and ROM.
	  → Staff member with ANY herpes lesion that has NOT reached the crusting stage should not be in the nursery.
	  → Maintain adequate nutrition: calculate calorie, protein and fluid needs according to weight.
	• If neonate develops signs of sepsis:
	  → Place in incubator/isolette and put in isolation room if possible.
	  → Assist healthcare provider with a sepsis workup: blood cultures, spinal tap (CSF), urine collection, chest x-ray, chemistry, and CBC with differential.
	  → Administer antibiotics as prescribed.

Figure 5-67

HESI HINT: Antibiotic dosage is based on the neonate's weight in kilograms. Peak and trough drug levels are drawn to evaluate if therapeutic drug levels have been achieved. Closely monitor the neonate for adverse effects of ALL drugs.

MATERNITY NURSING

PRETERM NEWBORN CARE

Supportive care for the neonate born at less than 38-weeks gestation is based on the level of immaturity identified by gestational/physical assessment.

ANALYSIS (NURSING DIAGNOSES)

- Impaired gas exchange related to…
- Ineffective thermoregulation related to…
- Alteration in nutrition: less than body requirements related to…
- Infection related to…

ASSESSMENT

Respiratory distress due to:
- Lung immaturity.
- Lack of surfactant lining alveoli (air sacs).
- Immaturity of respiratory center in brain causing apnea and bradycardia.
- Patent ductus arteriosis (PDA), usually related to hypoxia.
- Results in RDS (hypoxia and hypercarbia).

Temperature instability related to:
- Insufficient subcutaneous fat.
- Larger ratio of body surface area to body weight.
- Extended, open body position.
- Immature hypothalamus.

Nutrition problems related to:
- Poorly developed suck.
- Small stomach.
- Immature digestion process: lacks some gastric and pancreatic enzymes (no bile salts).
- Hypoglycemia: decreased glycogen storage in liver.
- Anemia: lack of fetal iron.
- Hyperbilirubinemia: immature ability of liver to handle bilirubin metabolism.

Fluid and electrolyte problems related to:
- Limited concentration/excretion ability of kidneys.
- Metabolic acidosis: decrease buffering capacity.
- Hypocalcemia (<7 mg/dl): inability to store and absorb calcium.

Immunologic immaturity due to:
- No IgM antibodies.
- No phagocytosis.
- Thin skin barrier.
- Intraventricular hemorrhage (IVH): weak, fragile capillaries in ventricles of brain.

HESI HINT: Sepsis can be indicated by both a temperature *increase* and a temperature *decrease*.

HESI HINT: Drugs used to treat neonatal infections can be ototoxic and nephrotoxic. *Close* monitoring of therapeutic levels and observation for side effects are required.

HESI HINT: Renal immaturity in the preterm infant makes the monitoring of IV fluid administration and drug therapy crucial. Closely monitor BUN and creatinine levels when administering the "mycin" antibiotics to treat infections in the neonate.

Figure 5-68

NURSING PLANS AND INTERVENTIONS

- Provide and monitor O_2 therapy.
- Monitor thermoregulation:
  → Place under radiant warmer.
  → Cover with plastic wrap to reduce insensible water loss.
  → Warm all things that touch newborn: hands, equipment, O_2, and surfaces.
  → Maintain abdominal skin temperature at 98 to 98.9°F (skin temperature probe taped over liver); and report any temperature under 97°F or over 99°F (both increase energy expenditure).
- Monitor fluid and electrolytes: observe for signs of:
  → Hypoglycemia: jitteriness, tremors, lethargy, hypotonia, apnea, weak or high-pitched cry, eye-rolling, and seizures.
  → Hypocalcemia: jitteriness, apnea, increased muscle tone, edema, abdominal distension, feeding intolerance, and Chvostek's sign (twitching over tapped parotid gland).
  → Fluid volume excess: edema, tachycardia, bulging fontanels, and rales in lungs.
  → Fluid volume deficit: sunken fontanels, poor skin turgor, and dry mucous membranes.
- If under 1500 gm., report weight loss >12% in first few days of life (180 gm.).
- Weigh diapers daily:
  → Record diaper weight before putting on infant.
  → Weigh diaper after voiding (1 cc urine = 1 gram of weight).
- Maintain urine output of 1 ml/kg/hour and specific gravity of 1.005 to 1.012.
- Prevent intracranial hemorrhage (increased risk in VLBW).
  → Monitor vital signs, fontanels, muscle tone, and activity.
  → Monitor Hct level.
  → Follow minimal stimulation protocol.
- Maintain nutrition: Breast milk is best.
  → 110 to 150 calories/kg/day. 140 to 160 ml/kg/day.
  → Give oral nipple feedings if neonate:
    - Can suck well, has gag reflex, and has a coordinated suck-swallow ability.
    - >34 weeks gestation and gaining 20 to 30 gm/day.
    - Consumes feeding for 20 minutes or longer, without signs of fatigue, and tachycardia.
- Uses modified "preemie" formulas, provide 24 calories/ounce (increase calories without increasing fluid).
- GAVAGE feeding: indicated to avoid aspiration from a weak suck, uncoordinated suck, and respiratory distress. *(See figure 5-69, Gavage Feeding)*
- Total parenteral nutrition (TPN): for preterm or post surgical neonate who cannot handle/metabolize enteral feedings.
  → Monitor glucose, serum and urine.
  → Administer any IV fluid with a dextrose content above 12.5% through a central line.
  → Monitor lab values daily. May include: Hct, and serum electrolytes.
  → Administer calcium supplement and vitamin D to prevent rickets.
  → Vitamin E (Tocopherol) supplement is given as antioxidant to enhance cellular integrity, i.e., prevent oxygen toxicity and red cell destruction.
- Prevent injury from hyperbilirubinemia. *(See Nursing Care of Newborn With Hyperbilirubinemia)*
- Support family/parental adjustment:
  → *See Emotional Aspects/High-Risk Neonates.*
  → Initiate early visitation and accompany parents on first visit to ICU.
  → Provide information to parents daily.
  → Teach care-giving skills.
  → Continue to enhance parent/infant bonding.
  → Plan for discharge using multidisciplinary approach.

Figure 5-68 (continued)

MATERNITY NURSING

PRETERM NEWBORN CARE

EMOTIONAL ASPECTS RELATED TO CARE OF HIGH-RISK NEONATES

- Without adequate attention to the emotional and developmental needs of the "sick" neonate, the following may occur:
  - → Failure-to-thrive (slow or absent growth).
  - → Avoidance of eye contact with people.
  - → Absent, weak crying, i.e., is trying to say, "I give up."
- A baby who has been over stimulated with procedures or activities will need time out from interaction.
- Sick neonates need developmentally-appropriate stimulation and may need services of occupational and physical therapists for developmental assessment and intervention.
- Nurses may cuddle, swaddle, sing to, offer pacifiers, and put mobiles/decals in crib (assuming baby is not on minimal stimulation protocol to prevent intraventricular hemorrhage IVH).

Figure 5-68 (continued)

GAVAGE FEEDING

NEWBORN CLIENT

- Gather equipment: sterile feeding tube (5 to 8 Fr.); calibrated syringe for formula; stethoscope; sterile syringe without needle; paper tape; formula/medications if prescribed.
- Position newborn with head slightly elevated and towel under shoulders.
- Measure distance from bridge of the infant's nose to the earlobe to a point halfway between the xiphoid process and the umbilicus.
- Pass tube along back of tongue, advancing as newborn swallows.
- Test placement:
  - → Inject .5ml. air using a sterile syringe while simultaneously listening for air "bubble" into stomach with stethoscope over epigastrium.
  - → Aspirate small amount stomach contents and check pH to verify gastric contents (<3).

HESI HINT: If tube passes into trachea, newborn can make NO noise, i.e., no crying. Newborn may gag, cough, or become cyanotic.

- Aspirate and measure any residual stomach contents and reduce volume of feeding by amount residual obtained (if healthcare provider prescribes).
- Attach large feeding syringe to tube with plunger removed, pour in warmed formula or breast milk and allow to flow by gravity. Hold 6 to 8 inches above newborn head for slow feeding: 20 minutes or 1 ml/minute.
- Stop flow at neck of syringe by pinching tubing.
- Clear tubing with small amount of sterile water (1 to 2 cc).
- Pinch tubing and withdraw quickly to avoid administering the feeding nasopharyngeally.
- May burp infant.
- Position on right side to minimize possibility of regurgitation and aspiration.
- Postpone any treatments for one hour so feeding is retained.
- Record amount of residual, type and amount of feeding, the time the feeding was started and the time the feeding ended, and the newborn's response to the feeding.

TOTAL PARENTERAL NUTRITION

- Solutions administered via a central intravenous access site or peripherally inserted central venous catheter (PICC).
- Potential complications associated with total parenteral nutrition (TPN) include hyperglycemia, electrolyte imbalance, infection, and dehydration.

Figure 5-69

MATERNITY NURSING

331

HYPERBILIRUBINEMIA

Excessive accumulation of bilirubin (usually unconjugated) in the blood due to red blood cell hemolysis.

ANALYSIS (NURSING DIAGNOSES)
- Potential for injury related to…
- Impaired gas exchange related to…
- Parental anxiety related to…

ASSESSMENT	NURSING PLANS AND INTERVENTIONS
<ul><li>Predisposing risk factors:<ul><li>→ Rh incompatibility.</li><li>→ ABO incompatibility.</li><li>→ IUGR pitocin induction</li><li>→ Prematurity.</li><li>→ Sepsis.</li><li>→ Perinatal asphyxia.</li><li>→ Maternal diabetes mellitus or intrauterine infections. Cephalhematoma</li></ul></li><li>Jaundice: sclera, skin (if whole body is yellow OR palms are yellow, there is a danger of kernicterus, bilirubin encephalopathy, resulting from bilirubin deposition in brain).</li><li>Total bilirubin determinations:<ul><li>→ Level increases more than 5 mg/day.</li><li>→ Term: level >12 mg/dl.</li><li>→ LBW: level 10 to 12 mg/dl or >.</li><li>→ Preterm: level >5 mg. (more sensitive to kernicterus at lower bilirubin concentrations).</li></ul></li><li>Positive direct Coomb's test: indicates presence of maternal antibody on the fetal RBC (an indication of sensitization). If >1:64, an exchange transfusion is indicated.</li><li>Increased reticulocyte count usually indicates ABO incompatibility.</li><li>Anemia.</li><li>Urine/stools may be dark.</li></ul>	<ul><li>Notify healthcare provider of any abnormal assessment factors present.</li><li>Implement orders for phototherapy. **PHOTOTHERAPY DECOMPOSES BILIRUBIN IN THE SKIN THROUGH OXIDATION.**<ul><li>→ Place unclothed neonate 18" under a bank of lights for several hours or days until bilirubin levels fall below 12 mg/dl.</li><li>→ Place opaque mask over eyes to prevent retinal damage.</li><li>→ Monitor skin temperature.</li><li>→ Cover genitals with a small diaper or mask to catch urine/stool while leaving skin surface open to light.</li><li>→ Turn q2 hours to avoid skin breakdown.</li><li>→ Turn off the lights for 5 to 15 minutes q8 hours to assess for conjunctivitis.</li><li>→ Monitor for signs of dehydration.</li></ul></li><li>Maintain hydration: nipple, gavage feedings, and IV fluids.</li><li>Assist with exchange transfusion.</li><li>Promote excretion of bilirubin through feeding and stools.</li><li>Bilibed or blanket are frequently used to allow rooming in or home phototherapy (no need for eye patches).</li></ul>

Figure 5-70

MATERNITY NURSING

HESI HINT: To assess for skin jaundice, apply pressure with thumb over bony prominences to blanch skin. After removing thumb, area will look yellow before normal skin color reappears. The best areas for assessment are the nose, forehead, and sternum. In dark-skinned infants, observe conjunctival sac and oral mucosa.

HESI HINT: Lab tests measure total and direct (conjugated, excretable, non-fat soluble) bilirubin levels. The dangerous bilirubin is the unconjugated, indirect (fat-soluble), which is measured by subtracting the direct from the total bilirubin.

HESI HINT: Maintenance of hydration is crucial for all infants. The preterm infant is already at risk for fluid and electrolyte imbalances due to increased body surface area from extended body positioning and larger body area in related to body weight. Phototherapy treatment for hyperbilirubinemia (level >12 mg/dl) increases the risk for dehydration.

SUBSTANCE ABUSE EFFECTS ON THE NEONATE

Effects on the neonate from maternal substance abuse are related to the substance as well as the amount of the substance abused.

CIGARETTE SMOKING

ASSESSMENT	NURSING PLANS AND INTERVENTIONS
• Small neonate. • IUGR (increases with the number of cigarettes smoked). • Neonates of mothers who are exposed to smoke-filled environments are also at risk.	• Teach the antepartum client that IUGR can be minimized or eliminated when smoking is stopped early in pregnancy. • Treat infant as a small-for-gestational-age infant.

NARCOTIC USE

ASSESSMENT	NURSING PLANS AND INTERVENTIONS
• Neonatal Narcotic Withdrawal Syndrome: → Irritability, hyperactivity. → High-pitched cry. → Coarse, flapping tremors. → Poor feeding, frantic sucking, vomiting/diarrhea. → Nasal stuffiness.	• Swaddle and minimize handling. • Decreased environmental stimuli. • Provide pacifier. • Place in prone position with sheepskin. • Cover elbows, knees to prevent skin breakdown. • Keep bulb syringe close at hand.

ALCOHOL INTAKE

ASSESSMENT	NURSING PLANS AND INTERVENTIONS
• Fetal Alcohol Syndrome (FAS): → Microcephaly. → Growth retardation. → Short palpebral fissures. → Maxillary hypoplasia. • Long-term complications of FAS: → Mental retardation. → Poor coordination. → Facial abnormalities. → Behavioral deviations (irritability). → Cardiac and joint abnormalities. • The combined effects of cigarette smoking and alcohol consumption during pregnancy cause greater fetal anomalies than the sum of their individual effects.	• Determine how much and how often the mother drank alcoholic beverages during pregnancy and/or while breastfeeding (alcohol intake has serious harmful effects on the fetus, especially when consumed during the sixteenth to eighteenth week of pregnancy). • Decrease environmental stimuli. • Provide enteral feedings if neonate has incoordinate sucking and swallowing.

Figure 5-71

REVIEW QUESTIONS

NEWBORN HIGH-RISK DISORDERS

1. List the major CNS danger signals, which occur in the neonate.
2. A baby is delivered blue, limp, and with a heart rate <100. The nurse dries the infant, suctions the oropharynx and gently stimulates the infant while blowing O_2 over the face. The infant still does not respond. What is the next nursing action?
3. What does the Silverman-Anderson index measure?
4. What are the two major complications of O_2 toxicity?
5. Necrotizing enterocolitis results from _____ and is manifested by _____. Ischemia/hypoxia results in _____.
6. Intraventricular hemorrhage is more common in _____ and results in symptoms of ____.
7. What conditions make oxygenation of the newborn more difficult?
8. In order to prevent problems with oxygenating the newborn, what parameters can the nurse observe?
9. What are the cardinal symptoms of sepsis in a newborn?
10. A premature baby is born and develops hypothermia. State the major nursing

interventions to treat hypothermia.

11. Nurses often weigh diapers in order to determine exact urine output in the high-risk neonate. Explain this procedure.

12. What factors does the nurse look for in determining the newborn's ability to take in nourishment by nipple/mouth?

13. What complications are associated with total parenteral nutrition (TPN)?

14. In order to prevent rickets in the preterm newborn, what supplement is given?

15. List four nursing interventions to enhance family/parent adjustment to a high-risk newborn.

16. List risk factors for hyperbilirubinemia.

17. List symptoms of hyperbilirubinemia in the neonate.

18. Write one nursing diagnosis generated from the data pertinent to hyperbilirubinemia.

19. List three nursing interventions for the neonate undergoing phototherapy.

20. List the symptoms of neonatal narcotic withdrawal.

21. Neonates who are "sick" are prone to receive too much stimulation in the form of invasive procedures and handling and too little developmentally-appropriate stimulation and affection. How might such an infant respond?

22. How should the nurse determine the length of a tube needed for oral gavage feeding of a newborn?

23. What are the two best ways to test for correct placement of the gavage tube in the infant's stomach?

24. What characteristics would the nurse expect to see in a neonate with fetal alcohol syndrome?

Answers to Review Questions

1. Lethargy, high-pitched cry, jitteriness, seizures, and bulging fontanels.

2. Begin oxygenation by bag and mask at 30 to 50 breaths/minute. If heart rate is <60, start cardiac massage at 100 to 120/minute. Assist healthcare provider in setting up for intubation procedure.

3. Respiratory difficulty.

4. Retrolental fibroplasias and bronchopulmonary dysplasia.

5. Ischemic hypoxia, abdominal distention, sepsis, and a lack of absorption from intestines. Injury to the intestinal mucosa.

6. Premature neonates and VLBW babies; increased intracranial pressure.

7. Respiratory distress syndrome: alveolar prematurity/lack of surfactant, anemia, and polycythemia.

8. Po_2 50 to 90, svO_2 60 to 80 mmHg.

9. Lethargy, temperature instability, difficulty feeding, subtle color changes, subtle behavioral changes and hyperbilirubinemia.

10. Place under radiant warmer or in incubator with temperature skin probe over liver. Warm all items touching newborn. Place plastic wrap over neonate.

11. Diaper is weighed in grams before applying. Weigh diaper after wetting. Calculate and record each gram of added weight as one cc of urine.

12. Good suck, coordinated suck-swallow, takes less than 20 minutes to feed, gaining 20 to 30 gm/day.

13. Hyperglycemia, electrolyte imbalance, dehydration, and infection.

14. Calcium and vitamin D.

15. Initiate early visitation at ICU. Provide daily information to family. Encourage participation in support group for parents. Encourage all attempts at care-giving (enhances bonding).

16. Rh incompatibility, ABO incompatibility, prematurity, sepsis, perinatal asphyxia.

17. Bilirubin levels rising 5 mg/day, jaundice, dark urine, anemia, high reticulocyte (RBC) count, and dark stools.

18. Potential for injury related to predisposition of bilirubin for fat cells in brain.

19. Apply opaque mask over eyes. Leave diaper loose so stools/urine can be monitored. Turn every 2 hours. Watch for dehydration.

20. Irritability, hyperactivity, high-pitched cry, frantic sucking, coarse flapping tremors, and poor feeding.

21. Failure-to-thrive, lack of crying.

22. From the bridge of the nose, to the earlobe, to a point halfway between the xiphoid and the umbilicus.

23. Aspiration of stomach contents with pH testing, and auscultation of air bubble injected into stomach.

24. Microcephaly, growth retardation, short palpebral fissures, and maxillary hypoplasia.

THERAPEUTIC COMMUNICATION

DESCRIPTION: The exchange of verbal and non-verbal interactions between healthcare providers and clients for a goal-directed purpose.

1. Communication is the primary tool used in the delivery of psychiatric nursing care and all nurse-client interactions. *(See figure 6-1, Helpful Techniques)*

2. The focus of therapeutic interaction is to assist the client with gaining insight into thoughts, feelings, and behaviors. *(See figure 6-2, Useful Phrases; and Figure 6-3, Forbidden Phrases)*

HELPFUL TECHNIQUES

ACKNOWLEDGMENT	Recognizing the client's opinions and/or statements without imposing your own values and judgment.
CLARIFYING	The process of making sure you understood the meaning of what was said.
CONFRONTATION	Calling attention to inconsistent behavior, information shared or not shared.
FOCUSING	Assisting the client to explore a specific topic.
INFORMATION-GIVING	Feedback about client's observed behavior.
OPEN-ENDED QUESTIONS	Questions which require more than a "Yes" or "No" response.
REFLECTING/RESTATING	Paraphrasing/repeating what the client said. (Be careful not to overuse; client will feel as though you are not listening.)
SILENCE	Can be therapeutic or can be used to control interaction. Use carefully with paranoid client; may be misinterpreted or could be used to support paranoid ideation.
SUGGESTING	Offering alternatives, e.g., "Have you ever considered...?"

Figure 6-1

HESI HINT: The purpose of therapeutic interaction with clients is to allow them the autonomy to make choices when appropriate. Keep statements value free, advice free, and reassurance free. Remember, JUST THE FACTS! NO OPINIONS!

HESI HINT: What action should the nurse take in a "psychiatric situation" when the client describes a physical problem? Assess, assess, assess! If the client with paranoid schizophrenia on the psychiatric unit complains of chest pain, take his/her blood pressure. If the OB client who has delivered a dead fetus complains of perineal pain – look at the perineal area (she may have a hematoma). Just because the focus of the client's situation is on his/her psychological needs, it does not mean that the nurse can ignore physiological needs.

USEFUL PHRASES

DESCRIPTION	EXAMPLES
• These are phrases, which are useful in therapeutic interaction. • Keep the interaction open, genuine, and client-centered. • Keep the client as the focus. • Be aware of your own feelings and anxiety level.	• "Tell me about …" • "Go on …" • "I'd like to discuss what you're thinking …" • "What are your thoughts …" • "Are you saying that …" • "What are you feeling?" • "It seems as if …"

Figure 6-2

FORBIDDEN PHRASES	
DESCRIPTION	**EXAMPLES**
• These are phrases, which should NOT be used when interacting with clients. Avoid them at all costs (especially if they appear on an exam). • Avoid social interaction, clichés, and saying too much. • Avoid changing subjects. • Avoid words like "good," "bad," "right," "wrong," and "nice."	• "You should…" • "You'll have to…" • "You can't…" • "Let's…" • "If it was me, I'd…" • "Why don't you" • "I think you…" • "It's the policy on this unit." • "Don't worry." • "Everyone …" • "Why…?" • "Just a second…" • "I know…"

Figure 6-3

HESI HINT: Remember, nurses are "nice" people, but they are also *therapeutic*.

HESI HINT: Basic communication principles can be applied to all clients:
• Establish trust.
• Demonstrate a non-judgmental attitude.
• Offer self; be empathetic, NOT sympathetic.
• Use active listening.
• Accept and support client's feelings.
• Clarify and validate client's statement.
• Use matter-of-fact approach.

HESI HINT: Remember, a nurse's nonverbal communication may be more important than his/her *verbal* communication.

HESI HINT: A question concerning nurse-client confidentiality often appears on the NCLEX-RN®. For the nurse to tell a client that she/he will not tell anyone about their discussion, puts the nurse in a difficult position. Some information MUST be shared with other team members for the client's safety (e.g., suicide plan) and optimal therapy.

Coping Styles (Defense Mechanisms)

DESCRIPTION: Coping styles are automatic psychological processes that protect the individual against anxiety and from the awareness of internal and external dangers or stressors. The individual may or may not be aware of these processes. *(See figure 6-4, Coping Styles)*

COPING STYLES (DEFENSE MECHANISMS)		
STYLE	**DESCRIPTION**	**EXAMPLE**
DENIAL	Unconscious failure to acknowledge an event, thought, or feeling that is too painful for conscious awareness.	A woman diagnosed with cancer tells her family all the tests were negative.
DISPLACEMENT	The transference of feelings to another person or object.	After being scolded by his supervisor at work, a man comes home and kicks the dog for barking.
IDENTIFICATION	Attempt to be like someone or emulate the personality, traits, or behaviors of another person.	A teenage boy dresses and behaves like his favorite singer.
INTELLECTUALIZATION	Using reason to avoid emotional conflicts.	A wife of a substance abuser describes, in detail, the dynamics of enabling behavior, yet continues to call her husband's work to report his Monday morning absence as an "illness."
INTROJECTION	Incorporation of values or qualities of an admired person or group into one's own ego structure.	A young man deals with a business client in the same fashion his father deals with business clients.
ISOLATION	Separation of an unacceptable feeling, idea, or impulse from one's thought process.	A nurse working in an emergency room is able to care for the seriously injured by isolating or separating her feelings and emotions related to the clients' pain, injuries, or death.
PASSIVE-AGGRESSION	Indirectly expressing aggression toward others. A facade of overt compliance masks covert resentment.	An employee arrives late to a meeting and disrupts others after being reminded of the meeting earlier that day and promising to be on time.
PROJECTION	Attributing one's own thoughts or impulses to another person.	A student who has sexual feelings towards her teacher, tells her friends the teacher is "coming on to her."
RATIONALIZATION	Offering an acceptable, logical explanation to make unacceptable feelings and behavior acceptable.	A student who did not do well in a course says it was poorly taught and the course content was not important anyway.
REACTION FORMATION	Development of conscious attitudes and behaviors which are opposite of what is really felt.	A person who dislikes animals does volunteer work for the Humane Society.

Figure 6-4

COPING STYLES (CONTINUED)

STYLES	DESCRIPTION	EXAMPLE
REGRESSION	Reverting to an earlier level of development when anxious or highly stressed.	After moving to a new home, a 6-year-old starts wetting the bed.
REPRESSION	The INVOLUNTARY exclusion of a painful thought or memory from awareness.	A young man, whose mother died when he was twelve, cannot tell you how old he was or the year she died.
SUBLIMATION	Substitution of an unacceptable feeling with a more socially acceptable one.	A student who feels too small to play football becomes a champion marathon swimmer.
SUPPRESSION	The INTENTIONAL exclusion of feelings and ideas.	When about to lose Tara, Scarlet O'Hara says, "I'll think about it tomorrow."
UNDOING	Communication or behavior done to negate a previously unacceptable act.	A young man who used to hunt wild animals now chairs a committee for the protection of animals.

Figure 6-4 (continued)

TREATMENT MODALITIES

DESCRIPTION: Psychiatric/mental health treatment modalities used to promote mental health. *(See figure 6-5, Types of Treatment Modalities)*

TYPES OF TREATMENT MODALITIES
MILIEU THERAPY
• The planned use of people, resources, and activities in the environment to assist with improving interpersonal skills, social functioning, and activities of daily living. • "Here and Now" focus, e.g., assist the client in dealing with the realities of TODAY rather than focusing on situations and behaviors of the past. • Uses limit setting. • Involves client in making decisions about own care. • Uses activities, which support group sharing, cooperation, and compromise, e.g., unit government groups. • Nursing interventions support client privacy and autonomy, and give clear expectations.
BEHAVIOR MODIFICATION
• A process used to change ineffective behavior patterns that focuses on consequences for actions rather than peer pressure. • Positive reinforcement is used to strengthen desired behavior, e.g., a client is praised or given a token that can be exchanged for cigarettes or desired activity. • Negative reinforcement is used to decrease or eliminate inappropriate behavior, e.g., ignoring undesirable behavior, removing a token or privilege, "time out." • Role modeling and teaching new behaviors are important interventions.
FAMILY THERAPY
• A form of group therapy that identifies the entire family as the client. • Based on the concept of the family as a system of interrelated parts forming a whole. • The focus is on the patterns of interaction within the family and NOT on any individual member. • The therapist assists the family in identifying roles assigned to each member based on family rules. • Life scripts (living out parent's dreams) and self-fulfilling prophecies (unconsciously following what one thinks should happen, therefore, setting it up to happen) are identified. • Congruent and incongruent communication patterns and behaviors are identified. • Goal is to decrease family conflict and anxiety, and to develop appropriate role relationships.
CRISIS INTERVENTION
• A form of therapy that is directed at the resolution of an immediate crisis, which the individual is unable to handle alone. • A crisis may develop when previously learned coping mechanisms are ineffective in dealing with the current problem. • Individual is usually in a state of disequilibrium. • If client is in a panic state as a result of the disorganization, be very directive. • Focus on the problem, not the cause. • Identify support systems. • Identify fast coping patterns used in other stressful situations. • Goal is to return individual to pre-crisis level of functioning. • Crisis intervention is usually limited to six weeks.
COGNITIVE THERAPY
• Directed at dispelling clients' irrational beliefs and distorted attitudes. • Focused, problem solving therapy. • Therapist and client work together to identify and solve problems and overcome difficulties. • Short term of 2 to 3 months duration. • Cognitive restructuring. • Cognitive behavior.

TYPES OF TREATMENT MODALITIES (CONTINUED)

ELECTROCONVULSIVE THERAPY (ECT)

Description: Use of electrically-induced seizures for psychiatric purposes. Used with severely depressed clients who fail to respond to antidepressant medication and therapy. May be used with extremely suicidal clients because two weeks are needed for antidepressants to take effect.

NURSING CARE PRIOR TO ECT	NURSING CARE FOLLOWING ECT

• Prepare client by teaching what the treatment involves.
• Avoid the word "shock" when discussing treatment with client and family.
• Anticholinergic, i.e., atropine sulfate is usually given 30 minutes before treatment to dry oral secretions.
• A quick-acting barbiturate to induce anesthesia (e.g., Anectine) is given to client before the ECT. This helps prevent any bone or muscle damage.
• Have an emergency cart, suction equipment, and O_2 available in the room.
	• Maintain patent airway - client is in an unconscious state immediately following ECT.
	• Check vital signs every 15 minutes until client is alert.
	• Reorient client after ECT (they are usually confused upon awakening).
	• Common complaints after ECT include:
	   → Headache.
	   → Muscle soreness.
	   → Nausea.

HESI HINT: Nausea is a common complaint after ECT. Vomiting by the unconscious client can lead to aspiration. Because post-ECT clients are unconscious, the nurse must observe closely for the possibility of aspiration, i.e., MAINTAIN A PATENT AIRWAY!

GROUP INTERVENTIONS

Description: Process used with 2 or more clients who develop interactive relationships and share at least one common goal or issue.

TYPES	PHASES	ADVANTAGES
• May be closed (set group) or open (new members may join) • May be small or large (>10 members) • Multiple types (psychoeducation, supportive therapy, psychotherapy, self-help) • Common nurse-led intervention groups include medication, symptom management, anger management, & self-care.	**Initial/orientation phase characterized by:** • High anxiety. • Superficial interactions. • Testing the therapist to see if he/she can be trusted. **Middle/working phase characterized by:** • Problem identification. • Beginning of problem solving. • Beginning of the group sense of "we". **Termination phase characterized by:** • Evaluation of experience. • Feelings ranging from anger to joy are invoked.	• Develop socializing techniques • Provide the opportunity to try new behaviors. • Promote a feeling of universality, e.g., not being alone with problems. • Provide an opportunity for feedback from the group which may correct distorted perceptions. • Allows clients to look at alternate ways to analyze and deal with problems.

Figure 6-5 (continued)

PSYCHIATRIC NURSING

REVIEW QUESTIONS

THERAPEUTIC COMMUNICATION TREATMENT MODALITIES

1. After the fourth group meeting, the informal leader makes a statement that she believes she can help the group more than the assigned facilitator and has better credentials. Identify the group dynamics and stage of development.

2. On an in-patient psychiatric unit, clients are expected to get up at a certain time, attend breakfast at a certain time, and come for their medication at the correct time. What form of therapy is incorporated into this unit?

3. The wife of a man killed in a motor vehicle accident has just arrived at the emergency room and is told of her husband's death. What nursing actions are appropriate for dealing with this crisis?

4. A ten-year-old is admitted to the children's unit of the psychiatric facility after stabbing his sister. His behavior is extremely aggressive with the other children on the unit. Using a behavior modification approach with positive reinforcement, design a treatment plan for this child.

5. The ten-year-old, his sister, mother, and the mother's live in boyfriend are asked to attend a therapy meeting. Who is the "client" that will be treated during this session?

6. A 66-year-old woman is admitted to the psychiatric unit with agitated depression. She has not responded to antidepressants in the past. What would be the medical treatment of choice for this client?

7. Describe the nurse's role in preparing clients for electroconvulsive therapy (ECT).

8. Describe the nursing interventions used to care for a client during and after electroconvulsive therapy.

ANSWERS TO REVIEW QUESTIONS

1. The informal leader is "testing," which is a behavior indicative of a new group trying to establish trust. This group is still in the orientation phase of development.

2. Milieu.

3. Take her to a quiet room, ask her if there are family, friends, or clergy you can call for her. Assess her need for medication and discuss with healthcare provider. Stay with her, be firm and directive, and assess previous successful coping strategies.

4. Assess what activities he enjoys. Set up a token system – when he displays non-aggressive behavior, he earns a token good towards participating in the activity selected. He loses a token when he becomes aggressive.

5. The entire family.

6. Electroconvulsive therapy (ECT).

7. Give accurate, non-judgmental information about the treatment. Explore client's concerns. Administer the following as prescribed: Atropine sulfate to dry oral secretions, a quick-acting barbiturate to induce anesthesia such as Brevital Sodium, and a muscle relaxant such as Anectine. Check emergency equipment, be sure suction equipment and O_2 are available.

8. Maintain patent airway. Check vital signs every 15 minutes until alert. Remain with client following treatment until conscious. Reorient, if confused.

ANXIETY

DESCRIPTION: Anxiety is unexplained discomfort, tension, apprehension, or uneasiness, which occurs when a person feels a threat to self. The threat may be real or imagined and is a very subjective experience.

LEVELS OF ANXIETY	
LEVEL	**DESCRIPTION**
MILD	• Associated with daily life; motivates learning. • Increased level of sensory awareness, and alertness. • Thoughts are logical; able to concentrate and problem solve. • Appears calm and in control.
MODERATE	• Continues to motivate learning. • Attentive; able to focus and problem solve. • Dull perceptions of sensory stimuli; becomes hesitant. • Speech rate and volume increase; becomes wordy. • Restless (frequent body movements and gestures). • May be converted to physical symptoms such as headaches, nausea, or diarrhea.
SEVERE	• "Fight or flight" response. • Sensory stimuli input is disorganized. • Perceptions may be distorted. • Concentration and problem solving ability impaired. • Selective attention; focuses on only one detail. • Verbalizes emotional pain, e.g., "I need help; I can't stand this." • Tremors, increased motor activity, e.g., pacing, wringing hands.
PANIC	• Perceptions grossly distorted; unable to differentiate real and unreal. • Unable to concentrate or problem solve; loss of rational, logical thinking. • Feeling of being overwhelmed, helpless. • Loss of control; unable to function. • Behavior may be angry and aggressive, or withdrawn, clinging and crying. • Immediate intervention is needed at this level.

Figure 6-6

HESI HINT: Common physiological responses to anxiety include increased heart rate and blood pressure; rapid, shallow respirations; dry mouth, tight feeling in throat; tremors, muscle tension; anorexia; urinary frequency; palmar sweating.

HESI HINT: Anxiety is very contagious and is easily transferred from client to nurse AND from nurse to client. FIRST, the nurse must assess his/her own level of anxiety and remain calm. A calm nurse assists the client to gain control, decrease anxiety, and increase feelings of security.

PSYCHIATRIC NURSING

ANXIETY DISORDERS

GENERALIZED ANXIETY DISORDER

Unrealistic, excessive, and/or persistent (lasting 6 months or longer) anxiety and worry about two or more life circumstances. Previously-learned coping mechanisms are inadequate to deal with this level of anxiety. Multiple etiologic theories exist including (but not limited to) neurobiochemical and psychodynamic theories.

ANALYSIS (NURSING DIAGNOSES)
- Anxiety related to…
- Ineffective individual coping related to…

ASSESSMENT	NURSING PLANS AND INTERVENTIONS

• Severe anxiety.
• Motor tension:
  → Restlessness.
  → Easily fatigued.
  → Feeling "shaky".
  → Tense.
• Autonomic hyperactivity:
  → Shortness of breath.
  → Heart palpitations.
  → Dizziness.
  → Diaphoresis.
  → Frequent urination.
• Vigilance and scanning:
  → Difficulty concentrating.
  → Sleep disturbance.
  → Irritability, easily angered.
• "On edge," appearance of being nervous.
• Low self-esteem.
	• Assess client to recognize anxiety and label the feeling, e.g., "What are you feeling now?"
	• Help client identify the relationship between the stressor and the level of anxiety.
	• Provide opportunities to learn and test different adaptive coping responses.
	• Encourage exercise, deep breathing techniques, visualization, relaxation techniques, and biofeedback.
	• Decrease environmental stimuli.

PANIC DISORDERS/PHOBIAS

Discrete periods of intense fear or discomfort that are unexpected and may be incapacitating.
- Characterized by an irrational fear of an external object, activity, or situation.
- A chronic condition that has exacerbations and remissions.
- The client transfers anxiety or fear from its source to a symbolic object, idea, or situation.
- Recognizes that fear is excessive and unrealistic, but "can't help it."

ANALYSIS (NURSING DIAGNOSES)
- Ineffective individual coping related to …
- Impaired social interaction related to …

COMMON PHOBIAS

TYPE	DESCRIPTION
ACROPHOBIA	Fear of heights
Agoraphobia	Fear of crowds or open places
Claustrophobia	Fear of closed-in places
Hydrophobia	Fear of water
Nyctophobia	Fear of the dark
Thanatophobia	Fear of death

Figure 6-7

ANXIETY DISORDERS (CONTINUED)

HESI HINT: When a client describes a phobia or expresses an unreasonable fear, the nurse should acknowledge the feeling (fear) and refrain from exposing the client to the identified fear. After trust is established, a desensitization process may be prescribed. Desensitization is the nursing intervention for phobia disorders. The nurse should:
- Assist client to recognize factors associated with feared stimuli that precipitate a phobic response.
- Teach and practice with client alternative adaptive coping strategies such as the use of thought substitution (replacing a fearful thought with a pleasant thought), and relaxation techniques. Role-playing is useful when the client is in a calm state.
- Expose client progressively to feared stimuli, offering support with the nurse's presence.
- Provide positive reinforcement whenever a decrease in phobic reaction occurs.
- NOTE: In all likelihood, the desensitization process will be overseen by a mental health practioner (NP, psych CNS, or psychologist).

HESI HINT: The nurse should place an anxious client where there are reduced environmental stimuli – a quiet area of the unit, away from the nurse's station.

PANIC DISORDERS/PHOBIAS

ASSESSMENT	NURSING PLANS AND INTERVENTIONS

• Coping styles used: *(See figure 6-4, Coping Styles)*
  → Displacement.
  → Projection.
  → Repression.
  → Sublimation.
• Autonomic hyperactivity.
• Panic attacks usually peak at 10 minutes but can last up to 30 minutes with a gradual return to normal functioning.
• Disruption in personal life as well as work life.
• Possible use of alcohol and drugs to decrease anxiety.
	• Establish TRUST; listen, use calm approach, and direct, simple questions. Remain with client, do not leave alone.
	• Provide safe environment.
	• Draw client's attention away from feared object/situation.
	• Discuss with the client alternative coping strategies and encourage use of such alternatives.
	• Suggest substitution of positive thoughts for negative ones.
	• Assist in desensitizing client.
	• Gradually and systematically introduce the client to the anxiety-producing stimuli.
	• Pair the anxiety-producing stimuli with another response such as relaxation or exercise.
	• Encourage sharing of fears and feelings with others.
	• Administer antianxiety medications as indicated. *(See figure 6-8 Antianxiety Drugs)*
	• Administer selective seratonin reuptake inhibitors (SSRIs) or other medications as indicated. *(See figure 6-17, Antidepressant Drugs)*
	• Decrease intake of caffeine, nicotine.

OBSESSIVE-COMPULSIVE DISORDER

Anxiety associated with repetitive thoughts (obsession) or irresistible impulses (compulsion) to perform an action. Fear of losing control is a major symptom of this disorder.

ANALYSIS (NURSING DIAGNOSES)
- Impaired social interaction related to…
- Ineffective individual coping related to…

Figure 6-7 (continued)

ANXIETY DISORDERS (CONTINUED)

ASSESSMENT	NURSING PLANS AND INTERVENTIONS
• Use of coping styles to control anxiety: *(See figure 6-4,Coping Styles)* → Repression. → Isolation. → Undoing. • Magical thinking (belief that one's thoughts or wishes can control other people or events). • Evidence of destructive, hostile, aggressive, and delusional thought content. • Difficulty with interpersonal relationships. • Interference with normal activities, e.g., a client who "must" wash her hands all morning and cannot take her children to school. • Safety issues involved in repetitive performance of the ritualistic activity, e.g., dermatitis may occur as a result of the continuous washing of hands. • Recurring intrusive thoughts. • Recurring, repetitive behaviors that interfere with normal functioning.	• Provide for client's physical needs. • Allow performance of the compulsive activity with attention given to safety (e.g., skin integrity of a hand washer). • Explore meaning and purpose of the behavior with client. • Avoid punishment or criticism. • Establish routine to avoid anxiety-producing changes. • Assist client with learning alternative methods of dealing with stress. • Avoid reinforcing compulsive behavior. • Limit the amount of time for performance of ritual, and encourage client to gradually decrease the time. • Administer anti-anxiety medications as indicated. *(See figure 6-8 Antianxiety Drugs)* • Administer SSRIs and Tricyclic Antidepressants as indicated. *(See figure 6-17, Antidepressant Drugs)*

HESI HINT: The best time for interaction with a client is at the completion of the performed ritual. The client's anxiety is lowest at this time; therefore, it is an optimal time for learning.

HESI HINT: Compulsive acts are used in response to anxiety, which may or may not be related to the obsession. It is the nurse's responsibility to help alleviate anxiety. Interfering will increase anxiety. These acts should be allowed as long as the client's acts are free of violence. The nurse should:
• Actively listen to the client's obsessive themes.
• Acknowledge effects that ritualistic acts have on the client.
• Demonstrate empathy.
• Avoid being judgmental.

POSTTRAUMATIC STRESS DISORDER

Severe anxiety, which results from a traumatic experience (war, earthquake, rape, incest).

ANALYSIS (NURSING DIAGNOSES)
• Post-traumatic response related to…
• Ineffective individual coping related to…

ASSESSMENT	NURSING PLANS AND INTERVENTIONS
• Anxiety; level is proportional to the perceived degree of threat experienced by the client. • Anxiety manifested in symptomatic behaviors: → Intrusive thoughts. → Flashbacks of the experience. → Nightmares. → Emotional detachment. • Responses to anxiety include: → Shock. → Anger. → Panic. → Denial. • Self-destructive behavior such as suicidal ideation and substance abuse. • Visible reminders of trauma, e.g., scars, physical disabilities.	• Provide consistent, non-threatening environment. • Implement suicidal/homicidal precautions if assessment indicates risk. • Listen to client's details of events to identify MOST troubling aspect of event. • Assist client to develop objectivity in perception of event and identify areas of no control. • Assist client to regain control by identifying past situations which have been handled successfully. • Administer antianxiety and antipsychotic medications to decrease anxiety, manage behavior, and provide rest. *(See figure 6-8 Antianxiety Drugs, See figure 6-23, Antipsychotic Drugs/Phenothiazines; and figure 6-24, Antipsychotic Drugs/Non-Phenothiazines)*

Figure 6-7 (continued)

345

PSYCHIATRIC NURSING

ANTIANXIETY DRUGS

DRUGS	INDICATIONS	ADVERSE REACTIONS	NURSING IMPLICATIONS
BENZODIAZEPINES • chlordiazepoxide HCL (Librium) • diazepam (Valium) • prazepam (Centrax) • oxazepam (Serax) • alprazolam (Xanax) • clorazepate dipotassium (Tranxene) • Lorazepam (Ativan)	• Reduce anxiety • Induce sedation, relax muscles, inhibit convulsions • Treatment of alcohol/drug withdrawal symptoms • Safer than sedative-hypnotics	• Sedation • Drowsiness • Ataxia • Dizziness • Irritability • Blood dyscrasias • Habituation and increased tolerance	• Administer at bedtime to alleviate daytime sedation. • Greatest harm occurs when combined with alcohol or other CNS depressants. • Avoid driving or working around equipment. • Gradually taper drug therapy due to withdrawal effects – do not stop suddenly. • Used only as short term and as supplemental to other meds.
NONBENZODIAZEPINES • buspirone (Buspar)	• Does not exhibit muscle relaxant or anticonvulsant activity • Is not effective for management of substance use	• Dizziness	• Takes several weeks for antianxiety effects to become apparent. • Intended for short-term use.
zolpidem (Ambien)	• Used for short-term treatment of insomnia		

Figure 6-8

REVIEW QUESTIONS

ANXIETY DISORDERS

1. State five autonomic responses to anxiety.
2. Identify the coping style used by a person who feels guilty about masturbating as a child, and develops a hand-washing compulsion as an adult?
3. Identify anxiety-reducing strategies the nurse can teach.
4. Which levels of anxiety facilitate learning?
5. A Vietnam veteran is plagued by nightmares and is found trying to strangle his roommate one night. List, in order of priority, the appropriate nursing interventions.
6. A client displays a phobic response to flying. Describe the desensitization process that would probably be implemented.
7. A client is in the middle of an extensive ritual, which focuses on food during lunch. However, the client is scheduled for group therapy, which is about to start. What action should the nurse take?

ANSWERS TO REVIEW QUESTIONS

1. Shortness of breath, heart palpitations, dizziness, diaphoresis, frequent urination.
2. Undoing.
3. Deep breathing techniques, visualization, relaxation techniques, exercise, biofeedback.
4. Mild to moderate.
5. Protect roommate from harm. Stay with client. If the client is agitated, administer anti-anxiety medications as prescribed. Arrange for private room. Place client on homicidal precautions at night.
6. Talk about planes. Look at pictures of planes. Make plans to accompany client during a visit to airport. Accompany client into a plane. Allow the client to board a plane alone. Accompany the client on a short flight while listening to a relaxation tape.
7. Allow client to complete the ritual. Discuss with the group leader the possibility of allowing the client to enter the group late. Arrange for client to begin lunch earlier so that the ritual can be completed prior to scheduled activities.

PSYCHIATRIC NURSING

SOMATOFORM DISORDERS

A group of disorders characterized by the expression of unexplained physical symptoms that have no physical basis.
- The physical symptom is thought to be an unconscious expression of an internal conflict.
- Somatoform disorders occurs more often in women and begin before 30 years of age.
- Children may learn that physical complaints are an acceptable coping strategy and are rewarded by receiving attention for this behavior. This is referred to as secondary gain
- These clients may abuse analgesics without relief from pain and/or discomfort. Accumulate prescriptions from "doctor shopping" to relieve physical symptoms.

ANALYSIS (NURSING DIAGNOSES)
- Alteration in comfort: chronic pain related to…
- Ineffective individual coping related to…
- Disturbance in self-concept related to…

ASSESSMENT	NURSING PLANS AND INTERVENTIONS
• Preoccupation with pain or bodily function for at least six months duration. • History of frequent "doctor shopping." • Absence of emotional concern regarding the physical impairment. • May report excessive dysmenorrhea. • Vital signs may be elevated similar to a panic attack. • Fear of having a serious disease. • Excessive use of analgesics. • Rumination about physical symptoms. • Drug abuse; drug screening needed to determine presence of abuse and, if present, the level of abuse. • Depression and presence of suicidal ideation. • Social or occupational impairment. • Presence of blindness, deafness, paralysis, or seizures suggestive of a neurologic disease.	• Convey a non-judgmental attitude. • Record duration and intensity of pain with attention to factors that precipitate onset. • Encourage expression of angry feelings. • Implement suicide precautions if indicated. • No one medication is particularly recommended. Co-morbid disorders such as anxiety or depression are treated with disorder specific medications. • Focus interactions and activities away from self and pain. • Help client identify connection between pain and anxiety. • Increase time and attention given to client as reward for not focusing on self or physical symptoms. • Help client identify needs met by the sick role, e.g., attention, and freedom from responsibility. *(See figure 6-11, Terms Associated With Somatoform Disorders)* • Encourage use of anxiety-reducing techniques such as deep breathing, visualization, meditation, exercise, and relaxation.

Figure 6-9

TYPES OF SOMATOFORM DISORDERS

DISORDER	DESCRIPTION	EXAMPLE
SOMATIZATION DISORDER	Recurrent somatic complaints for which frequent medical attention is sought. There is no medical pathology present.	A client, who complains of chest pains, but has a normal EKG and normal cardiac enzymes.
HYPOCHONDRIASIS	The belief and fear of having a disease, which includes misinterpretation of physical signs as "proof" of the presence of the disease.	A client has a rash, which is quite minor, but insists that he has a serious disease such as lupus.
CONVERSION DISORDER	A disorder characterized by transferring a mental conflict into a physical symptom for which there is no organic cause.	Blindness, paralysis, seizures, deafness, or pseudocyesis (false pregnancy).

Figure 6-10

HESI HINT: Be aware of your own feelings when dealing with this type of client. It is a challenge to be non-judgmental. The pain is real to the person experiencing it. These disorders cannot be explained medically: they result from internal conflict. The nurse should:
- Acknowledge the symptom or complaint.
- Reaffirm that diagnostic test results reveal no organic pathology.
- Determine the secondary gains acquired by the client.

PSYCHIATRIC NURSING

TERMS ASSOCIATED WITH SOMATOFORM DISORDERS	
TERM	**DEFINITION**
LA BELLE INDIFFERENCE	Term used to describe the lack of concern over physical illness. Seen in conversion reactions.
PRIMARY GAIN	A decrease in anxiety resulting from the ability to deal with a stressful situation.
SECONDARY GAIN	The rewards obtained from the sick role, e.g., freedom from certain responsibilities, sympathy.

Figure 6-11

REVIEW QUESTIONS
SOMATOFORM DISORDERS
1. Describe the difference between primary and secondary gains.
2. Explain the difference between somatization and hypochondriasis.
3. An air traffic controller suddenly develops blindness. All physical findings are negative. The client's history reveals an increased anxiety about job performance and fear about job security. What type of disorder is this? What purpose is the blindness serving? What nursing interventions are indicated?
4. A 29-year-old secretary has visited seven different doctors in the last year with a complaint of chest pain, heart palpitations, and shortness of breath. She is certain she is having a heart attack in spite of the healthcare provider's reassurance that all tests are normal. What type of disorder is this? What nursing actions are indicated?
5. Five years ago, a woman was involved in a motor vehicle accident that killed her friend who was a passenger in the car she was driving. Since that time, she has been unable to work because of severe back pain. The pain is unrelieved by prescribed medications. What type of disorder is this? What are the contributing causes? Describe the nursing care.

1. Primary gain is a decrease in anxiety, which results from some effort made to deal with stress. Secondary gain is the advantage, other than reduced anxiety, which occurs from the sick role.
2. Somatization is used to describe a person who has many recurrent complaints with no organic basis as opposed to someone with hypochondriasis who has unrealistic or exaggerated physical complaints. The concerns of those who are experiencing somatization, as well as those who are hypochondriacal, are so exaggerated that they interfere with social and occupational functioning.
3. Conversion reaction. Decreases the anxiety about job. Assist with ADL, encourage expression of anger, teach relaxation techniques, and assist with the identification of anxiety related to job security and performance.
4. Hypochondriacal disorder. Decrease anxiety, teach relaxation techniques, explore relationship between the symptoms and past experiences with heart disease. Focus interactions away from bodily concerns.
5. Somatization disorder. Unresolved grief, anxiety. Evaluate pain medication use and/or abuse. Document duration and intensity of pain. Assist client to identify precipitating factors related to request for medication.

PSYCHIATRIC NURSING

348

DISSOCIATIVE DISORDERS

- An alteration in the function of consciousness, personality, memory, or identity.
- Dissociative disorders may be sudden and temporary or gradual and chronic.
- Persons afflicted with these types of disorders handle stressful situations by "splitting" from the situation into a fantasy state.

ANALYSIS (NURSING DIAGNOSES)
- Ineffective individual coping related to…
- Potential for violence directed at self/others related to…

ASSESSMENT	NURSING PLANS AND INTERVENTIONS
<ul><li>Depression, mood swings, insomnia, potential for suicide.</li><li>Varying degrees of orientation.</li><li>Varying levels of anxiety.</li><li>Impairment of social and occupational functioning.</li><li>Alcohol and/or drug abuse. (Drug screening is necessary to determine presence and level of abuse).</li></ul>	<ul><li>Reduce environmental stimulation to decrease anxiety.</li><li>Stay with client during periods of depersonalization (client is often fearful, and the nurse's presence will assist in providing support/comfort during fearful episode).</li><li>Demonstrate acceptance of client's behavior during various experiences and personalities.</li><li>Document emergence of different personalities if present.</li><li>Implement suicide precautions if assessment indicates risk.</li><li>Encourage client to identify stressful situations that cause a transition from one personality to another.</li><li>Help client to identify effective coping patterns used in other stressful situations.</li><li>Assist client to use new alternative coping methods.</li></ul>

TYPES OF DISSOCIATIVE DISORDERS

TYPE	DESCRIPTION
PSYCHOGENIC AMNESIA	<ul><li>The sudden, temporary inability to recall extensive personal information.</li><li>Usually occurs after a traumatic event such as a threat of death or injury, an intolerable life situation, or a natural disaster.</li><li>The most common dissociative disorder.</li></ul>
PSYCHOGENIC FUGUE	<ul><li>Characterized by a person suddenly leaving home or work with the inability to recall their identity and behavior when he/she is unable to recall their past identity.</li><li>This disorder rarely occurs.</li><li>Excessive use of alcohol may contribute to a fugue state.</li></ul>
DISSOCIATIVE IDENTITY DISORDER	<ul><li>Presence of two or more distinct personalities within an individual.</li><li>The personalities emerge during stress.</li></ul>
DEPERSONALIZATION	<ul><li>Characterized by a temporary loss of one's reality and/or the ability to feel and express emotions.</li><li>Client expresses a fear of "going crazy."</li><li>Client describes a sense of "strangeness" in the surrounding environment.</li></ul>

Figure 6-12

HESI HINT: The nurse should be aware that ALL behavior has meaning.

HESI HINT: Avoid giving clients with dissociative disorders too much information about past events at one time. The various types of amnesia, which accompany dissociative disorders, provide protection from pain. Too much, too soon, may cause decompensation.

REVIEW QUESTIONS

DISSOCIATIVE DISORDERS

1. Describe the difference between psychogenic amnesia and a psychogenic fugue.
2. What is a multiple personality disorder?
3. List three possible causes of psychogenic amnesia.
4. Describe depersonalization disorder.

1. Psychogenic amnesia is the sudden inability to recall certain events in one's life. A psychogenic fugue state is characterized by the individual leaving home and being unable to recall their identity or their past.
2. Presence of two or more distinct personalities within an individual. The personalities emerge during stress.
3. Traumatic event such as a threat of death or injury, an intolerable life situation, or a natural disaster.
4. A temporary loss of one's reality, a loss of the ability to feel and express emotions, or a sense of "strangeness" in the surrounding environment. These individuals express a fear of "going crazy."

PERSONALITY DISORDERS

PERSONALITY DISORDERS		
CLUSTER A: ODD-ECCENTRIC		
NAME	DESCRIPTION	EXAMPLE
PARANOID PERSONALITY	• Displays pervasive and long-standing suspiciousness. • Mistrusts others, suspicious, fearful. • Projects blame for own problems onto others. • Is in touch with reality. • Verbally: Hostile, accusatory dialogue, which is reality based. • Nonverbally: Appears suspicious, tense, distant, watchful, and angry.	Teacher always suspects students of cheating during an exam or obtaining test questions prior to the exam.
SCHIZOID PERSONALITY	• Socially detached, shy, introverted. • Avoids interpersonal relationships, lacks social skills. • Cold, quiet, and aloof, has few friends. • Emotionally detached, introverted, unresponsive, with autistic thinking. • Verbally: Says little, appears withdrawn and seclusive. • Nonverbally: Dull, humorless, with little expression.	Computer programmer who works day and night; his only "relationship" is with his computer.
SCHIZOTYPAL PERSONALITY	• Interpersonal deficits • Eccentricities and odd beliefs • Social isolation	A person who spends hours walking on the street, wears a hat with all kinds of things hanging from it, and all sorts of mismatched clothes.

Figure 6-13

PERSONALITY DISORDERS (CONTINUED)		
CLUSTER B: DRAMATIC EMOTIONAL		
NAME	**DESCRIPTION**	**EXAMPLE**
ANTISOCIAL PERSONALITY	• Aggressive "acting out" behavior pattern, without ANY remorse. • Clever and manipulative in order to meet own self-centered needs. • Lacks social conscience and ability to feel remorse; is emotionally immature and impulsive. • Ineffective interpersonal skills impair forming close and lasting relationships. • Verbally: Disparaging, humiliating, belligerent toward those perceived as a threat. • Nonverbally: Cold, callous, and insensitive to others, can display socially gracious behaviors in order to meet own needs.	A prison inmate tries to get special privileges by bribing the guards, i.e., he acts out the role of a "con-artist."
BORDERLINE PERSONALITY	• Disturbances regarding self-image, sexual, social, and occupational roles. • Impulsive, self-damaging behavior, suicidal gestures. • "Other directed," overly dependent on others. • Unable to problem solve or learn from experiences. • Tend to view others as either "all good" or "all bad" (e.g., "splitting" behavior). • Verbally: Self-critical, demanding, whiny, manipulative, argumentative, can become verbally abusive. • Nonverbally: Highly-changeable and intense affect, impulsive behaviors.	Teenage girl who threatens to commit suicide when her boyfriend leaves, but in six weeks has new boyfriend and is "clinging" to him.
HISTRIONIC PERSONALITY	• Seeks attention by overreacting and exhibiting hyperexcitable emotions. • Overly dramatic, seeks attention, and tends to exaggerate. • Chaotic relationships, demonstrating angry outbursts or tantrums. • Verbally: Loud, excitable, overreactive, attempts to draw attention to self. • Nonverbally: Immature, self-centered, dependent on attention and care from others, seductive and flirty.	Hostess at a party who is overly excited to see the guests and welcomes them in a loud, "showy" manner that draws attention to herself.
NARCISSISTIC PERSONALITY	• Perceives self as all-powerful and important, critical of others, arrogant. • Exaggerated feeling of self-importance and self-love. • Needs attention and admiration. • Preoccupied with power and appearance. • Exploits others. • Verbally: Talks about self incessantly and does whatever necessary to draw attention to self. • Nonverbally: Inattentive and indifferent to others, appears only concerned with self.	Star football player whose success has "gone to his head."

Figure 6-13 (continued)

PSYCHIATRIC NURSING

PERSONALITY DISORDERS (CONTINUED)		
CLUSTER C: ANXIOUS - FEARFUL		
NAME	**DESCRIPTION**	**EXAMPLE**
AVOIDANT PERSONALITY	• Socially inhibited • Inadequacy • Hypersensitive to negative criticism, rejection • Longs for relationships	A man who refuses to play on the work softball team because he is afraid his teammates will make fun of him.
DEPENDENT PERSONALITY	• Unreasonable wishes, wants, and needs are expressed in a demanding, whining manner while professing independence and denying dependent behavior. • Passive, without accepting responsibility for consequences of his/her own behavior. • Low self-esteem, sees self as stupid, unable to make decisions. • Dependent on others to meet his/her needs. • Verbally: Self-depreciating, demanding others to meet needs. • Nonverbally: Appears dull, uninterested in others, dissatisfied with self.	Adult who exhibits adolescent type behavior – wants others to take care of him/her while at the same time declares independence.
OBSESSIVE COMPULSIVE PERSONALITY	• Attempt to control self through the control of others. • Inattention to new facts or different viewpoints. • Cold and rigid toward others. • Perfectionistic, inflexible, and stubborn. • Blind conformity and obedience toward rules. • Excessive neatness and cleanliness. • Preoccupation with work efficiency and productivity. • Verbally and nonverbally expresses disapproval of those whose behaviors/standards are different from theirs.	Nurse who insists that all staff on his/her unit wear a freshly starched uniform every day and has no tolerance for those who are not as "professional" as he/she is.

Figure 6-13 (continued)

> **HESI HINT:** Personality disorders are long-standing behavioral traits that are maladaptive responses to anxiety and cause difficulty in relating and working with other individuals. NCLEX-RN® questions sometimes test personality disorder content by describing management situations.

ANALYSIS (NURSING DIAGNOSES)
1. Disturbance in self-concept related to…
2. Ineffective individual coping related to…
3. Impaired social interactions related to…
4. Alteration in thought processes related to…

NURSING PLANS AND INTERVENTIONS
1. Establish trust; use straightforward approach.
2. Protect client from injury to self/others.
3. Assist client to recognize manipulative behavior.
4. Focus on client's strengths and accomplishments.
5. Set limits on manipulative behaviors when necessary.
6. Reinforce independent, responsible behaviors.
7. Assist client to recognize the need to respect the needs and rights of others.
8. Encourage socialization with others to improve skills.

REVIEW QUESTIONS
PERSONALITY DISORDERS

Give an example of a behavior or a description of an individual who exhibits each of the following personality disorders:

1. **Obsessive-Compulsive:**
2. **Antisocial:**
3. **Borderline:**
4. **Dependent:**
5. **Narcissistic:**
6. **Histrionic:**
7. **Paranoid:**
8. **Schizoid:**
9. **Maladaptive:**

ANSWERS TO REVIEW QUESTIONS

1. Orderliness, rigid.
2. Inability to conform to social norms.
3. Needy, always in a crisis, self-mutilating, unable to sustain relationships, splitting behavior.
4. Unable to make decisions for self, allows others to assume responsibility for his/her life.
5. Feelings of self-importance and entitlement. May exploit others to get own needs met.
6. Dramatic, flamboyant, needs to be the center of attention.
7. Suspicious, shows mistrust of others, is watchful and secretive.
8. Isolated and introverted, has no close friends.
9. Does not think anything he/she does is wrong, e.g., authorities are "out to get them."

PSYCHIATRIC NURSING

EATING DISORDERS

ANOREXIA NERVOSA

- A psychiatric disorder involving a voluntary refusal to eat and maintain minimal weight for height and age.
- A distorted body image and fear of becoming obese drives the excessive dieting and exercise.
- A reported 15-20% of those diagnosed die.
- More common in females than males.
- Occurs in adolescents and young adults.
- Often associated with parent-child conflicts about dependency issues. The child often feels as though her body and weight are her only areas of control.
- Possible etiological factors:
  → A dysfunctional family system.
  → Unrealistic expectations of perfection.
  → Ambivalence about maturation and the assumption of independence.

ANALYSIS (NURSING DIAGNOSES)
- Alteration in nutrition: less than body requirements related to …
- Disturbance in self-concept related to …
- Alteration in family process related to …

ASSESSMENT

- Weight loss of at least 15% of ideal/original body weight.
- Excessive exercise.
- Apathy about physical condition and inordinate pleasure in weight loss.
- Skeletal appearance (usually hidden by baggy clothes).
- Distorted body image (usually sees self as fat).
- Has low self-esteem.
- Hair loss and dry skin.
- Irregular heart beat, decreased pulse and BP resulting from decreased fluid volume.
- Amenorrhea for at least three months.
- Delayed psychosexual development (adolescents) or disinterest in sex (adults).
- Dehydration and electrolyte imbalance (decreased potassium, sodium, and chloride) resulting from:
  → Diet pill abuse.
  → Enema and laxative abuse.
  → Diuretic abuse.
  → Self-induced vomiting.

NURSING PLANS AND INTERVENTIONS

- Monitor weight, vital signs, and electrolytes (especially potassium, thyroid levels, and calcium/phosphorus for osteoporosis).
- Provide a structured, supportive environment, especially during mealtimes.
- Set a time limit for eating.
- Carefully monitor food and fluid intake.
- Be alert to client choosing low-calorie foods.
- Be alert to possible discarding of food through others or in pockets, wastebaskets, or drawers.
- Monitor client after meals for possible vomiting.
- Monitor activity level to prevent excessive exercise.
- Use positive reinforcement to build self-esteem and develop a realistic body image.
- Devise a behavior modification treatment program if indicated.
  → Include an established weight goal and weigh on a regular schedule.
  → Weigh in same clothes with back to scale; this prevents manipulation & arguing about exact weight.
  → Praise weight gain versus food intake.
- Focus interactions away from food and eating.
- Implement suicide precautions if assessment indicates risk.
- Administer antidepressant medications as indicated. *(See figure 6-17, Antidepressant Drugs)*
- Encourage family therapy.
- Provide snacks in between meals
- Monitor activity and assess for weakness, fatigue, and pathological fractures .
- Provide safe environment and assess for suicide ideation. Implement suicide precautions, if necessary
- Assess for water loading prior to weighing.

Figure 6-14

PSYCHIATRIC NURSING

HESI HINT: People with Anorexia gain pleasure from providing others with food and watching them eat. These behaviors reinforce their perception of self-control. Do not allow these clients to plan or prepare food for unit-based activities.

BULIMIA NERVOSA

An eating disorder characterized by eating excessive amounts of food followed by self-induced vomiting. Bulimic clients usually report a loss of control over eating during the binging.

ANALYSIS (NURSING DIAGNOSES)
- Disturbance in self-concept related to…
- Alteration in family process related to…

ASSESSMENT	NURSING PLANS AND INTERVENTIONS
• *See Nursing Assessment for Anorexia.* • Diarrhea or constipation, abdominal pain, and bloating. • Dental damage due to excessive vomiting (gastric hydrochloric acid erodes dental enamel). • Sore throat and chronic inflammation of the esophageal lining, with possible ulceration. • Financial stressors related to food budget. • Concerns with body shape and weight; bulimics usually are not underweight.	• Monitor weight, vital signs, and electrolytes (especially potassium). • Provide a structured supportive environment, especially around mealtime. • Monitor client after meals for possible vomiting. • Assist client to learn strategies, other than eating, to deal with feelings. • Encourage client to express feelings of anger. • Discuss strategies to stop vomiting and laxative use. • Use positive reinforcement to build self-esteem and develop a realistic body image. • Administer antidepressant medications as indicated. *(See figure 6-17, Antidepressant Drugs)* • Promote family therapy.

HESI HINT: Individual with Bulimia often use syrup of ipecac to induce vomiting. If ipecac is not vomited and is absorbed, cardiotoxicity may occur and can cause conduction disturbances, cardiac dysrhythmias, fatal myocarditis, and circulatory failure. Because heart failure is not usually seen in this age group, it is often overlooked. Assess for edema and listen to breath sounds.

HESI HINT: Physical assessment and nutritional support are a priority; the physiological implications are great. Nursing interventions should increase self-esteem and develop a positive body image. Behavior modification is useful and effective. Family therapy is most effective since issues of control are common in these disorders. (Therapy is usually long term.)

Figure 6-14 (continued)

REVIEW QUESTIONS

EATING DISORDERS

1. Describe the clinical symptoms of anorexia nervosa.
2. State two psychodynamic differences between anorexia and bulimia.
3. A client with anorexia has her friend bring her several cookbooks so she can plan a party when she is discharged. What nursing intervention is appropriate in addressing this behavior?
4. Anorexia nervosa may be precipitated by what factors?
5. What might the initial treatment include for a client admitted to the hospital with a diagnosis of bulimia nervosa?

ANSWERS TO REVIEW QUESTIONS

1. Weight loss of at least 15% of ideal/original body weight; hair loss; dry skin; irregular heart rate; decreased pulse; decreased blood pressure; Amenorrhea; dehydration; electrolyte imbalance.
2. Anorexia nervosa deals with issues of control and a struggle between dependence and independence. Bulimia deals with loss of control ("binge" eating) and guilt (purging).
3. Discuss activities that don't involve food, which may take place after discharge. Discuss the cookbooks with the treatment team and, if the treatment plan indicates, take books from client.
4. Mother-daughter conflicts usually focusing on independence/dependence issues; discomfort with maturation; need for control; desire for perfection.
5. Blood work to evaluate electrolyte status; replenish electrolytes and fluids as indicated; carefully monitor for evidence of vomiting.

PSYCHIATRIC NURSING

MOOD DISORDERS

Disturbances in mood manifested by extreme sadness or extreme elation.

DEPRESSIVE DISORDERS

Pathological grief reactions ranging from mild to severe states. *(See figure 6-15, Symptoms of Varying Degrees of Depression)*

ANALYSIS (NURSING DIAGNOSES)
- Potential for self-directed violence related to…
- Disturbance in self-concept related to…
- Self-care deficit related to…

ASSESSMENT	NURSING PLANS AND INTERVENTIONS

• Determine type of depression.
  → Exogenous: caused by a reaction to environmental or external factors.
  → Endogenous: caused by an internal biological deficiency (biogenic amines at receptor sites in the brain).
• Determine the degree of depression.
• Determine current suicide risk. *(See figure 6-16, Care of the Suicidal Client)*
• Lab tests and values:
  → Dexamethasone-suppression test (DST).
    • Indirect marker of depression.
    • Considered positive/abnormal if postdexamethasone cortisol level is greater than 5 mg/dl.
  → Biogenic amines:
    • Decreased serotonin indicative of depression.
    • Decreased norepinephrine indicative of depression.
	• Directly ask client about feelings/plans of harming self.
	• Implement suicide precautions if assessment indicates risk. *(See figure 6-16, Care of the Suicidal Client)*
	• Monitor sleep, nutrition, and elimination patterns.
	• Assist client with activities of daily living.
	• Initiate interaction with client (use non-demanding approach).
	• Insist on participation in activities. Do not give the client a choice about participating in activities, e.g., "It's time to go to the gym for basketball."
	• Observe for **sudden elevation in mood**. May indicate increased potential for **suicide risk**.
	• Assist client in the identification of a support system.
	• Encourage discussion of feelings of helplessness, hopelessness, loneliness, or anger.
	• Administer antidepressant medication as indicated.
	• Sit in silence with client if non-talkative.
	• Spend time with client and return when promised.

HESI HINT: Depressed clients have difficulty hearing and accepting compliments because of their lowered self-concept. Comment on signs of improvement by noting the behavior, e.g., "I noticed you combed your hair today" NOT, "You look nice today."

Symptoms of Varying Degrees of Depression

Mild	Moderate	Severe
• Feelings of sadness. • Difficulty concentrating and performing usual activities. • Difficulty maintaining usual activity level.	• Feelings of helplessness/ powerlessness. • Decreased energy. • Sleep pattern disturbances. • Appetite/weight changes. • Slowed speech, thought, movement (may also be agitated and hyperactive). • Rumination of negative feelings.	• Feelings of hopelessness, worthlessness, guilt, shame. • Despair. • Flat affect. • Indecisiveness. • Lack of motivation. • Change in physical appearance (slumped posture, unkempt). • Suicidal thoughts. • Possible delusions and/or hallucinations. • Sleep and appetite disturbances. • Loss of interest in sexual activity. • Constipation.

Figure 6-15

HESI HINT: The most important signs and symptoms of depression are a depressed mood with a loss of interest or pleasure in life. The client has sustained a loss. Other symptoms include:
- Significant change in appetite often accompanied by a change in weight – either weight loss or gain.
- Insomnia or hypersomnia (usually sleeping during the day – often because the client is not sleeping at night due to anxiety).
- Fatigue or a lack of energy.
- Feelings of hopelessness, worthlessness, guilt, or over-responsibility.
- Loss of ability to concentrate or think clearly.
- Preoccupation with death or suicide.

HESI HINT: The nurse knows depressed clients are improving when they begin to take an interest in their appearance or begin to perform self-care activities, which were previously of little or no interest.

CARE OF THE SUICIDAL CLIENT
SUICIDE PRECAUTIONS
• Obtain history; a previous suicide attempt is a most significant risk factor. Other risk groups include those with biologic/organic causes of depression such as substance abuse, organic brain disorders, or other medical problems. • Be aware of the major warning signs of an impending suicide attempt: → A client begins giving away his/her possessions. → A previously depressed client becomes happy. They have made the decision to commit suicide, are no longer debating the possibility, and have figured out how they can accomplish the suicide.
EVALUATE INTENT
Directly ask the client about his/her intent. **Example**: "Do you ever think about harming yourself?"
If a client is currently contemplating suicide, ask about his/her plans for carrying out the attempt. **Example**: "Do you have a plan for harming yourself?"
Identify the method chosen – the more lethal the method the higher the probability that an attempt is imminent. "What is your plan for harming yourself?" **Example**: A client mentions a shotgun and plans to put it to his head and pull the trigger.
EVALUATE INTENT
Determine the availability of the method chosen. If the method is readily available, the attempt is more likely. **Example**: The client has a loaded shotgun in his room – readily available.
NURSING INTERVENTIONS
Express concern for the client. **Example**: "I am very concerned that you are feeling so bad that you want to harm yourself."
Tell the client that you will share this information with the staff. **Example**: "I need to share this with the staff so that we can provide for your safety until you are feeling better."
Offer the client hope. **Example**: "You're feeling bad at this moment, but these feelings will pass. We have medications and treatments that can help you through the bad times."
Stay with the client – never leave a suicidal client alone. Legally, the nurse should follow the policy of the institution regarding suicidal clients and should be able to demonstrate that these policies were carried out. Follow the agency policy regarding the removal of potentially hazardous objects such as razors, etc.

Figure 6-16

HESI HINT: The nurse should suspect an imminent suicide attempt if a depressed client becomes "better," e.g., happy or even elated. Be aware – a happy affect may signify that the client feels relieved that a plan has been made and he/she is ready for the suicide attempt.

HESI HINT: When dealing with a depressed client, the nurse should assist with personal hygiene tasks and encourage the client to initiate grooming activities even when he/she does not feel like doing so. This helps promote self-esteem and a sense of control.

HESI HINT: An important nursing intervention for the depressed client is to sit quietly with the client. When answering NCLEX-RN® questions, remember that you are working at Utopia General and there is plenty of time and staff to provide ideal nursing care. Do not let the realities of clinical situations deter you from choosing the best nursing intervention. The best intervention is to sit quietly with the client, offering support with your presence.

HESI HINT: There are always drug questions on the NCLEX-RN®. Here are some tips: Know common side effects for drug groups. For example:
- Anti-Anxiety Drugs = sedation, drowsiness.
- Antidepressant Drugs = anticholinergic effects, postural hypotension.
- MAO inhibitors = hypertensive crisis.

Know specific problems or concerns for drug therapy. For example:
- Lithium requires renal function assessment and monitoring.
- Phenothiazines cause extrapyramidal effects (EPS); tardive dyskinesia can be permanent if client is not assessed regularly for signs of tardive dyskinesia!

Know specific client teaching for drug therapy. For example:
- Phenothiazines = photosensitivity, need to wear protective clothing, sunglasses.
- MAO inhibitors = dietary restrictions to prevent hypertensive crisis.

ANTIDEPRESSANT DRUGS

DRUGS	INDICATIONS	ADVERSE REACTIONS	NURSING IMPLICATIONS
TRICYCLICS • **amitriptyline HCL** (Elavil) • **desipramine HCL** (Norpramin) • **imipramine HCL** (Tofranil) • **nortriptyline HCL** (Aventyl) • **protriptyline HCL** (Vivactil)	• Depression • Clients with morbid fantasies do not respond well to these drugs	• Anticholinergic effects: dry mouth, blurred vision, constipation, and urinary retention • CNS effects: sedation, psychomotor slowing, and poor concentration • Cardiovascular effects: tachycardia, orthostatic, hypotension, quinidine-like effect on the heart (assess history of MI) • GI effects: nausea and vomiting • Narrow therapeutic index (can be lethal in overdose)	• Administer at bedtime to minimize sedative effect • Takes 2 to 6 weeks to achieve therapeutic effects • 1 to 3 weeks should elapse between discontinuing tricyclics and initiating MAO inhibitors • Teach client to avoid alcohol • Avoid concurrent use of antihypertensive drugs • Carefully evaluate suicide risk
MAO-INHIBITORS (Monoamine Oxidase Inhibitors) • **isocarboxazid** (Marplan) • **phenelzine sulfate** (Nardil) • **tranylcypromine sulfate** (Parnate)	• Depression • Phobias • Anxiety	• Tachycardia • Urinary hesitancy, constipation • Impotence • Dizziness • Insomnia • Muscle twitching • Drowsiness • Dry mouth • Fluid retention • ***Hypertensive crisis***: severe hypertension, severe headache, chest pain, fever, sweating, nausea and vomiting	• Must ***not*** be used with tricyclics (causes ***hypertensive crisis***) • Major concern is need for dietary restrictions – ***certain drug and food interactions can cause hypertensive crisis*** • Instruct client ***not*** to eat foods with high tyramine content: aged cheese, red wine, beer, beef/chicken, liver, yeast, yogurt, soy sauce, chocolate, bananas • Teach client: ***not*** to take over-the-counter drugs without physician approval; the warning signs of hypertensive crisis (headaches, palpitations, increased BP); and to use caution around machinery

Figure 6-17

ANTIDEPRESSANT DRUGS (CONTINUED)

DRUGS	INDICATIONS	ADVERSE REACTIONS	NURSING IMPLICATIONS
SSRIs • **fluoxetine HCL** (Prozac) • **paroxefine** (Paxil) • **sertraline** (Zoloft) • **fluvoxamine** (Luvox) • **citalopram** (Celexa)	• Depression • Anxiety • Panic disorder • Aggression • Anorexia nervosa • OCD	• Drowsiness • Dizziness, light-headedness • Headache • Insomnia • Depressed appetite • Serotonin syndrome • Sexual disfunction • Allergic reaction or rash – withhold drug if occurs	• Effective 2 to 4 weeks after treatment is initiated • Should **NOT** be used with MAO inhibitors: cause hypertensive crisis (violent reaction) • Wait at least 14 days between discontinuing MAO inhibitor and starting Prozac • At least 5 weeks should lapse between discontinuing Prozac and initiating an MAO inhibitor • May be given in evening if sedation occurs. • Monitor for serotonin syndrome (defined by at least 3 symptoms) → rapid onset of altered mental states → agitation → myoclonus → hyper reflexia → fever → shivering → diaphoresis → ataxia → diarrhea • Caution client about OTC use of St. John's Wort
NEWER ANTIDEPRESSANT DRUGS • **trazadone** (Desyrel) • **mitrazapine** (Remeron) • **maprotiline** (Ludiomil) • **buproprian** (Wellbutrin) • **amoxapine** (Asendin) • **nefazodone** (Serzone) • **venlafaxine** (Effexor)	• Depression • Trazadone: insomnia, dementia with agitation	• Safer than tricyclics and MAO inhibitors in terms of side effects	• Effective 2 to 4 weeks after treatment is initiated

Figure 6-17 (continued)

BIPOLAR DISORDER OR MANIC DEPRESSIVE ILLNESS

An affective disorder, which is manifested by mood swings of euphoria, grandiosity, and an inflated sense of self-worth. This disorder may or may not include sudden swings to depression. In order to be diagnosed with a bipolar disorder, according to the DSM-IV-TR classification, a client must have at least one episode of major depression. Client may cycle, going from elevation to depression with normal periods of activity in between.

ANALYSIS (NURSING DIAGNOSES)
- Potential for violence related to…
- Alteration in thought processes related to…
- Self-care deficit related to…

ASSESSMENT	NURSING PLANS AND INTERVENTIONS
• Determine level of depression exhibited. *(See figure 6-15, Symptoms of Varying Degrees of Depression)* • Determine level of mania exhibited. *(See figure 6-19, Characteristics of Varying Degrees of Mania)* • Assess nutrition and hydration status. • Assess level of fatigue. • Assess danger to self and others in relation to level of impulse impairment present.	• Maintain client's physical health: provide nutrition, rest, and hygiene. • Provide safe environment (grandiose thinking and poor impulse control can result in accidents and/or altercations with other clients). • Decrease environmental stimulation, e.g., place in private room or seclusion room. • Implement suicide precautions if assessment indicates risk. • Use consistent approach to minimize manipulative behavior. • Use frequent, brief contacts to decrease anxiety. • Implement constructive limit-setting. • Avoid giving attention to bizarre behavior, e.g., dress and language. • Try to meet needs as soon as possible to keep client from becoming aggressive. • Provide small, frequent feedings of food that can be carried e.g., small finger sandwiches. • Engage in simple, active, non-competitive activities. • Avoid distracting or stimulating activities in the evening to help promote sleep/rest. • Praise self-control, acceptable behavior. • Promote family involvement in therapy, teaching, and medication compliance. • Administer lithium, sedatives, and anti-psychotics as prescribed. *(See figure 6-20, Antimanic/Mood Stabilizing Drugs)*

HESI HINT: Monitor serum lithium levels carefully. The therapeutic range is between 0.5 and 1.5 mEq/L. The therapeutic and toxic levels are very close in reading. Signs of toxicity are evident when lithium levels are more than 1.5 mEq/L. Blood levels should be drawn 12 hours after LAST dose.

HESI HINT: Manic clients can be very caustic toward authority figures. Be prepared for personal "put downs." Avoid arguing or becoming defensive.

Figure 6-18

PSYCHIATRIC NURSING

CHARACTERISTICS OF VARYING DEGREES OF MANIA	
DEGREE	**CHARACTERISTICS**
MILD	• Feeling of being on a "high" • Feelings of well-being • Minor alterations in habits • Usually does not seek treatment because of pleasurable effect
MODERATE	• Grandiosity • Talkative • Pressured speech • Impulsiveness • Excessive spending • Bizarre dress and grooming
SEVERE	• Extreme hyper-activity • Flight of ideas • Non-stop activity, e.g., running, pacing • Sexual acting out; explicit language • Talkative • Overly responsive to external stimuli • Easily distracted • Agitated and possibly explosive • Severe sleep disturbance • Delusions of grandeur or persecution

Figure 6-19

HESI HINT: What activities are appropriate for a manic client?
• **Noncompetitive physical activities, which require the use of large muscle groups.**

HESI HINT: Where should a manic client be placed on the unit?
• **Make every attempt to reduce stimuli in the environment. Place the client in a quiet part of the unit.**

HESI HINT: What interventions should the nurse use if a client becomes abusive?
• Redirect negative behavior or verbal abuse in a calm, firm, non-judgmental, non-defensive manner.
• Suggest a walk or physical activity.
• Set limits on intrusive behavior. For example, "When you interrupt, I cannot explain the procedure to the others; please wait your turn."
• If necessary, seclude or administer medication if client becomes totally out of control. Always remember to use compassion because nurses are "nice" people.

Antimanic/Mood Stabilizing Drugs

Drugs	Indications	Adverse Reactions	Nursing Implications
• **lithium carbonate** (Carbolith)	• Bipolar disorders, especially the manic phase	• Nausea, fatigue, thirst, polyuria, and fine hand tremors • Weight gain • Hypothyroidism • **EARLY** signs of toxicity: diarrhea, vomiting, drowsiness, muscle weakness, lack of coordination	• Lithium is excreted by the kidney. Maintain serum levels 0.5 to 1.5 mEq/l.. Assess electrolytes, especially sodium. • Baseline studies of renal, cardiac and thyroid status must be obtained before lithium therapy is begun. • Teach client **EARLY** symptoms of lithium toxicity. If drug is continued, coma, convulsions, and death may occur. • Instruct client to keep salt usage consistent. • Use with diuretics is contraindicated. Diuretic-induced sodium depletion can increase lithium levels causing toxicity.

Anticonvulsant Mood Stabilizers

Drugs	Indications	Adverse Reactions	Nursing Implications
• **valproic acid** (Depakene)	• Used in bipolar disorder alone or with lithium	• GI distress, i.e., nausea, anorexia, vomiting • Hepatotoxicity • Neurological symptoms, i.e. tremor, sedation, headache, dizziness	• Administer with food • Monitor blood levels • Maintain serum levels 50 to 125 mcg/ml
• **carbamazepine** (Tegretol)	• Used in bipolar disorders • Used as alternative to lithium	• Dizziness • Ataxia • Blood dyscrasias	• Maintain serum levels at 8 to 12 g/ml • Stop drug if WBC drops below 3000/mm^3 or neutrophil count goes below 1500/mm^3 • Monitor hepatic and renal function

PSYCHIATRIC NURSING

HESI HINT: Two atypical antipsychotic drugs are also indicated for mania (risperidone and olanzapine; *see figure 6-25 Atypical Antipsychotic Drugs*).

REVIEW QUESTIONS

MOOD DISORDERS

1. Identify physiologic changes, which often occur with depression.
2. A client, who has been withdrawn and tearful, comes to breakfast one morning smiling and interacting with her peers. Prior to breakfast she gave her roommate her favorite necklace. What actions should the nurse take and why?
3. Name the components of a suicide assessment.
4. A client on your unit refuses to go to group therapy. What is the most appropriate nursing intervention?
5. A client is standing on a table loudly singing the "Star Spangled Banner" encircled by sheets, which have been set afire. In order of priority, describe appropriate nursing actions.

ANSWERS TO REVIEW QUESTIONS

1. Weight change (loss or gain), constipation, fatigue, lack of sexual interest, somatic complaints, and sleep disturbances.
2. Assess for suicidal ideation, plan, and means to carry out plan. Place on precautions as indicated. A sudden change in mood and giving away possessions are two possible signs that a suicide plan has been developed.
3. Existence of a plan, method, availability of method chosen, lethality of method chosen, identified support system, and history of previous attempts.
4. Accompany client to the group; do not give client option. Client needs to be mobilized.
5. Remove client and other persons in the vicinity to a safe area and activate hospital fire plan. When area is safe, place client in quiet environment with low stimulation and medicate as indicated.

THOUGHT DISORDERS:

SCHIZOPHRENIA

DESCRIPTION: A psychiatric disorder characterized by thought disturbance, altered affect, withdrawal from reality, regressive behavior, difficulty with communication, and impaired interpersonal relationships. *(See figure 6-22, Types of Schizophrenia)*

> **HESI HINT:** There are five types of schizophrenia specified under the DSM-IV-TR. The DSM-IV-R is a diagnostic manual prepared by the American Psychiatric Association that provides diagnostic criteria for all psychiatric disorders.

NURSING ASSESSMENT

1. Assess for disturbance in thought process.
   A. Interpret content of internal and external stimuli.
      1) Symbolism: meaning given to words by client to screen thoughts and feelings that would be difficult to handle if stated directly.
      2) Delusions: fixed false beliefs that may be persecutory, grandiose, religious, or somatic in nature.
      3) Ideas of reference: belief that conversations or actions of others have reference to the client.
   B. Form: construction of verbal communication.
      1) Looseness of association: lack of clear connection from one thought to the next.
      2) Tangential or circumstantial speech: fails to address the original point, gives many nonessential details.
      3) Echolalia: constantly repeats what is heard.
      4) Neologism: creates a new word.
      5) Preservation: repeats same word or phrase in response to different questions.
      6) Word salad: jumbled mixture of real and made up words.
   C. Process: flow of thoughts.
      1) Blocking: gap or interruption in speech due to absent thoughts.
      2) Concrete thinking: thinking based on fact versus abstract and intellectual points.
2. Assess for disturbance in perception.
   A. Hallucinations: false sensory perception, usually auditory or visual in nature.
   B. Illusions: misinterpretation of external environment.
   C. Depersonalization: perceives self as alienated or detached from real body.
3. Assess for disturbance in affect (feelings or mood).
   A. Blunted or flat.

B. Inappropriate.

C. Incongruent to context of situation or event.

4. Assess for disturbance in behavior.

   A. Incoherent and disorganized.

   B. Impulsive, uninhibited.

   C. Posturing, unusual mannerisms.

   D. Social withdrawal, neglects personal hygiene.

   E. Exhibits echopraxia: repetition of another person's movements.

5. Assess for disturbance in interpersonal relationships.

   A. Difficulty establishing trust.

   B. Difficulty with intimacy.

   C. Fear and ambivalence toward others.

ANALYSIS (NURSING DIAGNOSES)

1. Alteration in thought process related to…

2. Sensory-perceptual alteration (auditory/visual related to…

NURSING PLANS AND INTERVENTIONS

1. Establish trust.

2. Sit with mute clients.

3. Provide safe and secure environment.

4. Assist with physical hygiene and ADL.

5. Use matter-of-fact, non-judgmental approach.

6. Use clear, simple, concrete terms when talking with client.

7. Accept and support client's feelings; use clarification.

8. Reinforce congruent thinking. Stress reality.

9. Avoid arguing or agreeing with inaccurate communication.

10. Set limits on behavior.

11. Avoid stressful situations.

12. Structure time for activities to limit time for withdrawal.

13. Encourage client to identify positive characteristics related to self.

14. Praise socially acceptable behavior.

15. Avoid fostering a dependent relationship.

16. Promote family involvement in therapy, teaching, and medication compliance.

NURSING INTERVENTIONS FOR THE DELUSIONAL/HALLUCINATING CLIENT	
CLIENT IS DELUSIONAL	**CLIENT IS HALLUCINATING**
• Encourage recognition of distorted reality. • Divert focus from delusional thought to reality; do not permit rumination of false ideas. • Do not agree with or support delusions. • Avoid arguing about the delusion, be very matter-of-fact. • Avoid physically touching client, especially if delusions are persecutional. • Administer anti-psychotic drugs. *(See figure 6-23, Antipsychotic Drugs/Phenothiazines and figure 6-24, Antipsychotic Drugs/Non-Phenothiazines)* • Monitor and treat side effects of psychotropic drugs. *(See figure 6-26, Side Effects of Psychotropic Drugs and Nursing Interventions)* • Administer antiparkinsonian drugs. *(See figure 6-27, Antiparkinsonian drugs)*	• Protect client from injury that might result from responding to commands of the voices; pay attention to the content. • Avoid denying or arguing with client about the hallucination. • Discuss your observations with client, e.g., "You appear to be listening to something." • Make frequent, but brief remarks to interrupt the hallucinations. • Administer antipsychotic drugs. *(See figure 6-23, Antipsychotic Drugs/Phenothiazines and figure 6-24, Antipsychotic Drugs/Non-Phenothiazines)* • Monitor and treat side effects of psychotropic drugs. *(See figure 6-26, Side Effects of Psychotropic Drugs and Nursing Interventions)* • Administer antiparkinsonian drugs. *(See figure 6-27, Antiparkinsonian drugs)*

Figure 6-21

TYPES OF SCHIZOPHRENIA	
TYPE	**BEHAVIORAL CHARACTERISTICS**
CATATONIC	• Stupor (decrease in reaction to the environment) or mutism • Rigidity (maintenance of a posture against efforts to be moved) • Posturing (waxy flexibility) • Negativism (resistance to instructions) • Excitement (severely agitated, out of control) • Potential for violence to self/others during stupor or excitement
DISORGANIZED	• Incoherence • Flat or inappropriate affect • Disorganized, uninhibited behavior • Unusual mannerisms • Socially withdrawn • NO delusions present
PARANOID	• Systematized delusions and/or hallucinations related to a single theme • Ideas of reference • Potential for violence if delusions are acted upon
RESIDUAL	• Socially withdrawn • Inappropriate affect • Eccentric or peculiar behavior • Absence of prominent delusions and/or hallucinations • No current psychotic behavior exhibited
UNDIFFERENTIATED	• Prominent delusions/hallucinations • Incoherence and grossly disorganized behaviors • Does not meet any of the criteria for the other types

Figure 6-22

PERSONALITY DISORDERS, CLUSTER A (PARANOID)

DESCRIPTION: Characterized by suspicious, strange behavior, which may be precipitated by a stressful event. May manifest as intense hypochondriasis.

NURSING ASSESSMENT
1. Determine degree of suspiciousness and mistrust of others.
2. Assess degree of anxiety.
3. Determine if delusions are present.
   A. Reference or control.
   B. Persecution.
   C. Grandeur.
   D. Somatic.
4. Assess degree of insecurity.

ANALYSIS (NURSING DIAGNOSES)
1. Potential for violence related to…
2. Alteration in thought process related to…
3. Social isolation related to…

NURSING PLANS AND INTERVENTIONS
1. Establish trust.
2. Be truthful and honest; follow through on commitments.
3. Assist client to identify situations that provoke anxiety and aggressive behaviors.
4. Avoid confrontation with the client over delusions.
5. Help client to focus on feelings, which cause the delusions.
6. Assist in identifying thoughts, perceptions, and own conclusions of reality.
7. Avoid talking and laughing where client can see

but not hear you.

8. Engage in noncompetitive activities that require concentration.
9. Involve client in treatment plan.
10. Promote family involvement in therapy, teaching, and medication compliance.
11. Avoid stepping into client's personal space or touching client!

HESI HINT: Do not argue with a client about their delusions. Logic does NOT work, it only increases the client's anxiety. Be matter-of-fact and divert delusional thought to reality. Trust is the basis for all interactions with these clients. Be supportive and non-judgmental. Stress increases anxiety and the need for delusions and hallucinations. Do not agree you hear voices (you should be the client's contact with reality), but acknowledge your observation of the client, for example, "You look like you're listening to something."

HESI HINT: Use Bleuler's four As to help remember the important characteristics of schizophrenia:
- Autism (preoccupied with self)
- Affect (flat)
- Associations (loose)
- Ambivalence (difficulty making decisions)

ANTIPSYCHOTIC DRUGS/PHENOTHIAZINES			
TRADITIONAL DRUGS	**INDICATIONS**	**ADVERSE REACTIONS**	**NURSING IMPLICATIONS**

• **chlorpromazine HCL** (Thorazine)
• **trifluoperazine HCL** (Stelazine)
• **thioridazine HCL** (Mellaril)
• **perphenazine** (Trilafon)
• **triflupromazine** (Vesprin)
	• To control psychotic behavior: hallucinations, delusions, and bizarre behavior	• Drowsiness
		• Orthostatic hypotension
		• Weight gain
		• Anticholinergic effects
		• Extrapyramidal effects
		  → Pseudo-parkinsonism
		  → Akathisia
		  → Dystonia
		  → Tardive dyskinesia
		• Photosensitivity
		• Blood dyscrasias: granulocytosis, leukopenia
		• Neuroleptic malignant syndrome
			• Extrapyramidal effects are MAJOR concern
			• Monitor elderly clients closely
			• Takes 2 to 3 weeks to achieve therapeutic effect
			• Keep client supine for 1 hour after administration and advise to change positions slowly because of effects of orthostatic hypotension
			• Teach client to avoid:
			  → Alcohol
			  → Sedatives (potentiate effect of CNS depressants)
			  → Antacids (reduce absorption of drug)

• **fluphenazine HCL** (Prolixin)	• To control psychotic behavior • Useful in treatment of psychomotor agitation associated with thought disorders	• Same as other phenothiazines	• Absorbed slowly • Used with noncompliant clients because it can be administered IM once every 14 days

Figure 6-23

PSYCHIATRIC NURSING

ANTIPSYCHOTIC DRUGS/NON-PHENOTHIAZINES

TRADITIONAL DRUGS	INDICATIONS	ADVERSE REACTIONS	NURSING IMPLICATIONS
• **haloperidol** (Haldol) • **chlorprothixene** (Taractan) • **thiothixene** HCL (Navane)	• To control psychotic behavior • Less sedative than phenothiazines	• Severe extrapyramidal reactions • Leukocytosis • Blurred vision • Dry mouth • Urinary retention	• Teach client to avoid alcohol
LONG ACTING • **fluphenazine decanoate** (Prolixin Decanoate) • **haloperidol decanoate** (Haldol Decanoate)	• Clients who require supervision with medication regimes	• Similar to Prolixin and Haldol	• Similar to Haldol and Prolixin • Prolixin can be given every 7 to 28 days • Haldol can be given every 4 weeks • Requires several months to reach steady-state drug levels

Figure 6-24

ATYPICAL ANTIPSYCHOTIC DRUGS

DRUGS	INDICATIONS	ADVERSE REACTIONS	NURSING IMPLICATIONS
• **risperidone** (Risperdal) • **olanzapine** (Zyprexa) • **quetiapine** (Seroquel) • **aripaprazole** (Abilify) • **ziprasidone** (Geodon) • **clozapine** (Clozaril))	• Treat positive and negative symptoms of schizophrenia without significant EPS • Clients who have not responded well to typical antipsychotics or have side effects from typical antipsychotics • Fewer side effects • Clozapine has superior efficacy in clients who have been treatment resistant.	• Risperdal: Neuroleptic Malignant Syndrome(NMS), EPS, dizziness, GI symptoms (nausea, constipation), anxiety. • Zyprexa: drowsiness, dizziness, weight gain, EPS, agitation. • Seroquel: drowsiness, dizziness, headache, EPS, anticholinergic effects. • Clozaril: agranulcytosis, drowsiness, dizziness, GI symptoms, Neuroleptic Malignant Syndrome	• Monitor WBC weekly for first 6 months, then biweekly • Baseline VS and ECG, report abnormal VS • Monitor for symptoms of NMS and EPS • Change positions slowly

Figure 6-25

SIDE EFFECTS OF PSYCHOTROPIC DRUGS AND NURSING INTERVENTIONS

SIDE EFFECT	CHARACTERISTICS	NURSING INTERVENTIONS
BLOOD DYSCRASIAS • **Agranulocytosis: occurs in first weeks of treatment** • **Thrombocytopenia: decreased platelets**	Sore throat, fever, chills	• Protect from infections • Provide comfort measures: gargle for sore throat, use of lozenges and analgesics
	Bruises carefully, petechia	• Teach client safety measures
EXTRAPYRAMIDAL EFFECTS • **Parkinsonism: occurs within 1 to 4 weeks after initiation of treatment**	Rigidity, shuffling gait, pill rolling hand movements, tremors, dyskinesia, mask-like face	• Administer anticholinergics drugs, i.e., Cogentin, Artane. Other drugs for EPS include Benadryl, Symmetrel, Ativan, Klonopin. Inderal for akathisia and Vitimin E for tardive dyskinesia
• **Akathisia: occurs within 1 to 6 weeks after initiation of treatment**	Restlessness, agitation, and pacing. Sudden difficulty sitting still (can be confused with tardive dyskinesia).	• Rule out anxiety. Can ask client, "Are you feeling so restless that you can't sit still?"
• **Dystonia: occurs within 1 to 2 days after initiation of treatment**	Limb and neck spasms, uncoordinated, jerky movements, difficulty speaking and swallowing, rigidity and muscle spasms	• Emergency treatment is with IM anticholinergics drug • *Have respiratory emergency equipment available*
• **Tardive Dyskinesia: develops late in treatment**	Involuntary tongue and lip movements, blinking, choreiform movements of limbs and trunk.	• Permanent side effect; antiparkinsonian drugs are of no help in decreasing symptoms • Teach client/family to report side effects **EARLY**
PHOTOSENSITIVITY	Sunlight: exposed skin turns blue and color changes occur in eyes but does not cause vision impairment	• Teach client to stay out of sun, wear protective clothing and sunglasses • Skin discoloration will disappear within 6 months after drug is discontinued
NEUROLEPTIC MALIGNANT SYNDROME	Life Threatening Emergency High fever, tachycardia, stupor, increased respirations, severe muscle rigidity	• Increased risk with phenothiazines • Early recognition is important, transfer to medical facility for hydration, nutritional support and treatment of possible respiratory failure and renal failure
SEROTONIN SYNDROME	Confusion, disorientation, autonomic dysfunction.	• Notify healthcare provider STAT • Provide systems support
ANTICHOLINERGIC EFFECTS	Dry mouth, blurred vision, tachycardia, nasal congestion, constipation, urinary retention, orthostatic hypotension	• Encourage sips of water, chewing sugarless gum, or hard candy • Increase fiber in diet • Change positions slowly for dizziness • Report urinary retention to physician • Tolerance to these side effects will usually occur

Figure 6-26

PSYCHIATRIC NURSING

ANTIPARKINSONIAN DRUGS			
DRUGS	**INDICATIONS**	**ADVERSE REACTIONS**	**NURSING IMPLICATIONS**
• **trihexyphenidyl HCL** (Artane) • **benztropine mesylate** (Cogentin)	• Acts on the extrapyramidal system to reduce disturbing symptoms	• Anticholinergic effects • Drowsiness • Headaches • Urinary hesitancy • Memory impairment	• Usually given in conjunction with antipsychotic drugs

Figure 6-27

REVIEW QUESTIONS

SCHIZOPHRENIC/PARANOID DISORDERS

1. A client is sitting alone talking quietly. There is no one around. What nursing action should be taken?
2. A client dials 222-2222 and asks for his fiance, Candice Bergen. This is an example of what type of thought disorder?
3. A client has been sitting in the same position for two hours. He is mute. What type of schizophrenia is this client experiencing? Describe appropriate nursing interventions for this client.
4. A client is very agitated. He believes that the CIA has tapped the phone, is sending messages through the television, and that you are an agent who has been planted by the agency. In order of priority, list the appropriate nursing actions to intervene in this situation. What type of delusion is this client experiencing?
5. The nurse asks the client, "What brought you to the hospital?" The client's response is, "The bus." What type of thinking is this client exhibiting?

ANSWERS TO REVIEW QUESTIONS

1. Quietly approach client and note the behavior. Assess content of the hallucinations, e.g., "I noticed you talking. Are you hearing voices? Can you tell me about the voices you are hearing?"
2. Delusion of grandeur.
3. Catatonic: Spend time with client; assist with ADL; be alert to potential for violence toward self/others; be aware of fluid and nutrition needs.
4. Approach client and offer solitary activity to distract. Assess need for medication. Encourage verbalization of feelings and promote outlet for expression. Paranoid disorder with delusions of

reference (CIA).
5. Concrete.

SUBSTANCE ABUSE

DESCRIPTION: Regular use of substances that affect the central nervous system resulting in behavioral changes. Chemicals produce physiological and/or psychological dependence.

ALCOHOLISM

Drinking pattern that interferes with physical, social, familial, vocational, and emotional functioning.

NURSING ASSESSMENT

1. Patterns indicative of alcoholism:
   A. Episodic drinking (binges).
   B. Continuous drinking.
   C. Morning drinking.
   D. Increase in family fighting about drinking.
   E. Increase in absences from work or school, especially Monday.
   F. Blackouts.
   G. Hiding drinking pattern.
   H. Legal problems (DWIs).
   I. Health problems such as gastritis.
2. Family history of alcoholism or substance abuse.
3. Dependent, yet resentful toward authority.
4. Impulsive, abusive behavior.
5. Impaired judgment, memory loss.
6. Incoordination, slurred speech.
7. Mood varies between euphoria and depression.
8. Intoxication as determined by blood alcohol level (BAL); 0.10% or greater is considered intoxicated.
9. Previous experience with treatment centers or Alcoholics Anonymous (AA).
10. Alcohol withdrawal symptoms:
    A. Begins shortly after drinking stops, as soon as 4 to 6 hours.

B.   Anxiety, nausea, insomnia, tremors, hyper alertness, and restlessness.

C.   Sudden or gradual increase in all vital signs.

D.   Delirium tremens (DTs) may appear 12 to 36 hours after last drink.

    1)   Tachycardia, tachypnea, diaphoresis.

    2)   Marked tremors.

    3)   Hallucinations.

    4)   Paranoia.

E.   Grand mal seizures possible.

11.   Assess health status for chronic, alcohol-related illness.

A.   Chronic gastritis.

B.   Cirrhosis and hepatitis.

C.   Korsakoff's syndrome: organic syndrome which frequently follows delirium tremens, associated with chronic alcoholism.

D.   Wernicke's syndrome: a severe disorder (encephalopathy) occurring in chronic alcoholics probably due to a deficiency in vitamin B_1 (thiamin). May escalate Korsakoff's syndrome. Treat with thiamine chloride.

E.   Malnutrition and dehydration.

F.   Pancreatitis.

G.   Peripheral neuropathy.

ANALYSIS (NURSING DIAGNOSES)

1.   Potential for injury related to…

2.   Ineffective family coping related to…

3.   Alteration in nutrition: less than body requirements related to…

NURSING PLANS AND INTERVENTIONS

1.   Maintain safety, nutrition, hygiene, and rest.

2.   Implement suicide precautions if assessment indicates risk.

3.   Provide care during withdrawal:

A.   Monitor vital signs, I&O, electrolytes.

B.   Observe for impending delirium tremens.

C.   Prevent aspiration; implement seizure precautions.

D.   Reduce environmental stimuli.

E.   Medicate with anti-anxiety medication, usually Librium, or Ativan. *(See figure 6-8, Antianxiety Drugs)*

F.   Provide high-protein diet and adequate fluid intake (limit caffeine).

G.   Provide vitamin supplements, especially B_1 and B complex.

H.   Provide emotional support.

4.   Rehabilitation

A.   Use direct, matter-of-fact, non-judgmental attitude.

B.   Confront denial and rationalization (main coping styles used by alcoholics).

C.   Confront manipulations; set firm limits on behavior.

D.   Set short-term, realistic goals.

E.   Help increase self-esteem.

F.   Explore ways to increase frustration tolerance without alcohol.

G.   Identify ways to decrease loneliness.

H.   Encourage client to accept responsibility for own behavior.

I.   Identify availability of support systems (family, friends, church, AA).

J.   Identify activities and friendships not related to drinking.

K.   Provide group and family therapy; refer family to Alanon.

5.   Provide client/family teaching regarding the side effects of Antabuse if used as a deterrent to drinking. *(See figure 6-29, Alcohol Deterrent)*

DRUG ABUSE

DESCRIPTION: State of dependency produced by repeated use of a substance, which involves altered perception and/or mood.

DRUG ABUSE	
ASSESSMENT	**NURSING PLANS AND INTERVENTIONS**
<ul><li>Determine pattern of drug use.<ul><li>→ What drugs are used?</li><li>→ What the drug of choice is.</li><li>→ How much is used and how often?</li><li>→ How long has drug/s been used?</li></ul></li><li>Physical evidence of drug usage:<ul><li>→ Needle track marks.</li><li>→ Cellulitis at puncture site.</li><li>→ Poor nutritional status. Inflammation of nasal passages.</li></ul></li><li>Possible causes of drug dependency:<ul><li>→ Desire to escape reality and problems.</li><li>→ Low self-esteem.</li><li>→ Peer or cultural pressure.</li><li>→ Inherent susceptibility to drug dependence.</li></ul></li><li>Symptoms of withdrawal and overdose are particular for the drug used. *(See figure 6-30, Drug Withdrawal and Overdose Symptoms)*</li></ul>	<ul><li>Assess level of consciousness and vital signs. (Rapid withdrawal can be fatal for persons addicted to barbiturates, anti-anxiety medications, and hypnotics.)</li><li>Monitor I&O and electrolytes.</li><li>Implement suicide precautions if assessment indicates risk.</li><li>Provide adequate nutrition, hydration, and rest.</li><li>Administer medications according to detoxification protocol of medical unit.</li><li>Phenothiazines may be used to decrease the discomfort of withdrawal.</li><li>Confront denial (main coping style used by substance abusers).<ul><li>→ Focus on substance abuse problem.</li><li>→ Confront placing blame on external problems.</li></ul></li><li>Reinforce reality with simple, concrete terms.</li><li>Encourage verbal expression of anger and depression.</li><li>Assist with identification of stressors and areas of conflict.</li><li>Encourage exploration of alternate coping strategies.</li><li>Positively reinforce insight into behavior patterns.</li><li>Help identify an appropriate support system.</li><li>Provide support to significant others.</li><li>Teach danger of AIDS and blood-related diseases.</li></ul>

ANALYSIS (NURSING DIAGNOSES)
1. Potential for injury related to…
2. Potential for infection related to…
3. Disturbance in self-concept related to…

Figure 6-28

HESI HINT: Know what defense mechanisms are used by chemically dependent clients. Denial and rationalization are the two most common coping styles used – their use must be confronted so accountability for the client's own behavior can be developed.

HESI HINT: What basic needs have priority when working with chemically dependent clients? Nutrition is a priority. Alcohol and drug intake has superseded the intake of food for these clients.

HESI HINT: What behaviors are expected during withdrawal?
In the alcoholic, delirium tremens (DTs) occurs 12 to 36 hours after the last intake of alcohol. Know the symptoms. In drug abuse, withdrawal symptoms are specific to the type of drug.

ALCOHOL DETERRENT			
DRUG	**INDICATIONS**	**ADVERSE REACTIONS**	**NURSING IMPLICATIONS**
disulfiram (Antabuse)	• Treatment of alcoholism; aversion therapy • Interferes with breakdown of alcohol causing an accumulation of acetaldehyde (a by-product of alcohol in the body)	*Severe* side effects occur if alcohol is consumed: • Nausea and vomiting • Hypotension, headaches • Rapid pulse and respirations • Flushed face and bloodshot eyes • Confusion • Chest pain • Weakness, dizziness	• Teach client what to expect if alcohol is consumed while taking the drug. • Be aware that some alcoholic clients use the "side effects" as a means of "punishing" themselves or as a form of masochism and, if a client repeatedly consumes alcohol while taking the drug, the healthcare provider should be notified. • Persons with serious heart disease, diabetes, epilepsy, liver impairment, or mental illness should ***not*** take Antabuse.

Figure 6-29

HESI HINT: What medications can the nurse expect to administer to chemically dependent clients? In treating alcohol withdrawal, Librium or Ativan are commonly used. Antabuse is often used as a deterrent to drinking alcohol. Client teaching should include the effects of consuming any alcohol while on Antabuse. Encourage client to read all labels of over-the-counter medications and food products, which may contain small amounts of alcohol.

DRUG WITHDRAWAL AND OVERDOSE SYMPTOMS			
DRUGS	**WITHDRAWAL**	**OVERDOSE**	**EFFECT**
OPIATES • heroin • morphine • meperidine • codeine • opium • methadone	• Watery eyes, runny nose, dilated pupils • Anxiety • Diaphoresis, fever • Nausea, vomiting, and diarrhea • Achiness • Abdominal cramps • Insomnia • Tachycardia	• Respiratory depression leading to respiratory arrest • Circulatory depression leading to cardiac arrest • Unconscious leading to coma • Death	• General physical and mental deterioration • Rapid tolerance • Impaired judgment
Cocaine	• Depression • Fatigue • Disturbed sleep • Anxiety • Psychomotor agitation	• Tachycardia • Pupillary dilatation • Increased BP • Cardiac arrhythmias • Perspiration, chills • Nausea, vomiting	• Psychological dependence • Tolerance within hours or days
Amphetamines	• Depression • Fatigue • Disturbed sleep	• Restlessness • Tremors • Rapid respiration • Confusion • Assaultive behavior • Hallucinations • Panic	• Paranoid delusions
Hallucinogenics	• No withdrawal	• Panic • Psychosis	• Flashbacks • Impaired judgment
ANTIANXIETY DRUGS benzodiazepines: • Valium • Serax • Ativan	• Tremors • Agitation • Anxiety • Abdominal cramps • Grand mal seizures	• Drowsiness • Confusion • Hypotension • Coma → death	• Withdrawal occurs if there is abrupt cessation • Temporary psychosis

Figure 6-30

HESI HINT: What type of therapy is used with chemically dependent clients? Group therapy is effective as well as support groups such as Alcoholics Anonymous, Narcotics Anonymous, etc.

HESI HINT: Harm reduction is a community health strategy designed to reduce the harm of substance abuse to families, individuals, community, and society.
Eamples:
• More compassionate drug treatment options including abstinence and drug substitution models.
• HIV related interventions such as needle exchanges.
• Directed drug use management should the client wish to continue use.
• Changes in laws concerning possession of paraphernalia and drug use.

REVIEW QUESTIONS

SUBSTANCE ABUSE

1. Three days ago, a client was admitted to the medical unit for a GI bleed. His BP and pulse rate gradually increased, and he developed a low-grade fever. What assessment data should the nurse obtain? What kind of anticipatory planning should the nurse develop?
2. What physical signs might indicate that a client is abusing intravenous medications?
3. What behaviors would indicate to the nurse manager that an employee has a possible substance abuse problem?
4. A client becomes extremely agitated, abusive, and very suspicious. He is currently undergoing detoxification from alcohol with Librium 25 mg q6 hours. What nursing actions are indicated?
5. A client, in the third week of a cocaine rehabilitation program, returns from an unsupervised pass. The nurse notices that he is euphoric and is socializing with the other clients more than he has in the past. What nursing actions are indicated?

1. Obtain a drug and alcohol consumption assessment including type, frequency, and time of last dose/drink. Call the healthcare provider and report findings. Anticipate withdrawal/delirium tremens. Provide a quiet, safe environment. Place on seizure precautions. Anticipate giving a medication like Librium.
2. Needle track marks; cellulitis at puncture site; poor nutritional status.
3. Change in work performance, withdrawal, increase in absences (especially Monday or Friday), increase in number of times tardy, long breaks, late returning from lunch.
4. Notify the healthcare provider immediately and anticipate an increase in dose or frequency of Librium. Provide a quiet, safe environment. Approach in a quiet, calm manner. Avoid touching client.
5. Notify healthcare provider of observed behavior change. Get a urine drug screen as prescribed. Confront client with observed behavior change.

PSYCHIATRIC NURSING

ABUSE	
CHILD ABUSE	

Includes physical and mental injury, sexual abuse, and neglect.

ANALYSIS (NURSING DIAGNOSES)
- Fear related to…
- Alteration in parenting related to…

ASSESSMENT	NURSING PLANS AND INTERVENTIONS

• Most important indicators of child abuse:
  → Injuries are NOT congruent with the child's developmental age or skills.
  → Injuries do NOT correlate with the stated cause.
  → Delay in seeking medical care.
• Bruises in unusual places and in various stages of healing.
• Bruises, welts from belts, cords, etc.
• Burns (cigarette, iron); immersion burns (symmetrical in shape).
• Whiplash injuries from being shaken.
• Bald patches where hair has been pulled out.
• Fractures in various stages of healing.
• Failure to thrive, unattended physical problems.
• Torn, stained, bloody underclothes.
• Lacerations of external genitalia.
• Bedwetting, soiling.
• Sexually-transmitted diseases.
• Parent sees child as "different" from other children.
• Parent uses child to meet own needs.
• Parent seldom touches or responds to child; may be very critical of child.
• Child appears frightened and withdrawn in the presence of parent or adult.
• Family history of frequent moves, unstable employment, marital discord, and family violence.
• One parent answers all the questions.
	• ***Nurses are legally required to report all cases of suspected child abuse*** to the appropriate local/state agency.
	• Take color photographs of injuries.
	• Document factual, objective statements of child's physical condition, child-family interaction, and interviews with family.
	• Establish trust, and care for the child's physical problems. These are the PRIMARY and IMMEDIATE needs of these children.
	• Recognize own feelings of disgust and contempt for the parents.
	• Utilize principles of crisis intervention.
	• Assist child/family to develop self-esteem.
	• Teach basic child development and parenting skills to family.
	• Support need for family therapy.

HESI HINT: Select only one nurse to care for an abused child. Abused children have difficulty establishing trust. The child will be less anxious with one consistent caregiver.

Figure 6-31

PSYCHIATRIC NURSING

	ABUSE (CONTINUED)

INTIMATE PARTNER VIOLENCE

- A criminal act of physical, emotional, economic, or sexual abuse between an assailant and victim, who most commonly are, or were in an intimate relationship (may be marital or dating).
- Abuse is usually a tension-releasing action as well as a lack of impulse control.
- Assailant may come from a family where battering and physical violence were present.
- Persons act more violently when drinking or using drugs.
- The relationship is usually characterized by extreme jealousy and issues of power and control.
- Women in a battering relationship may lack self-confidence and feel trapped. They may be embarrassed about their situation, which results in isolation and dependency on the abuser.
- Often begins during pregnancy and/or occurs more frequently during pregnancy.

ANALYSIS (NURSING DIAGNOSES)
- Disturbance in self-concept related to…
- Ineffective family coping related to…

ASSESSMENT	NURSING PLANS AND INTERVENTIONS
• Delay between time of injury and time of treatment. • Anxious when answering questions about injury. • Abdominal injuries during pregnancy. • Looks to abuser for answers to questions related to injuries. • Depression and/or suicidal ideation. • Feeling of responsibility for "provoking" partner. • Low self-esteem. • Abrasions, cuts, lacerations, sprains, black eyes. • Psychosomatic/somatoform complaints. • Concurrent use of alcohol, drugs.	• Establish trust; use non-judgmental approach. • Treat physical wounds and injuries. • Document factual, objective statements of client's physical condition, injuries, and interaction with partner/family. • Determine potential for further violence. • Provide crisis intervention. • Refer to shelter if necessary and/or desired with adult's consent. • Assist client with contacting authorities if charges are to be pressed.

HESI HINT: Women who are abused may rationalize the spouse's behavior and unnecessarily accept the blame for his actions. The woman may or may not choose to press charges. Be sure to give her the number of a shelter or "help line" for future occurrences, as well as develop a safety plan.

Figure 6-31 (continued)

PSYCHIATRIC NURSING

ABUSE (CONTINUED)	
ELDERLY ABUSE	

- An act, which causes physical, verbal, or psychosocial injury or exploitation as well as the physical neglect of an aged adult.
- Abuse of the elderly is under reported; estimated number varies from 1% to 10% of the elderly population.
- The majority of abuse is committed by spouses and children but also includes other caregivers.

ANALYSIS (NURSING DIAGNOSES)
- Fear related to…
- Alteration in family process related to…

ASSESSMENT	NURSING PLANS AND INTERVENTIONS
• Bruises on the upper arms (bilaterally, from being shaken). • Broken bones from falls (resulting from being pushed). • Dehydration or malnourishment. • Overmedication. • Poor physical hygiene, improper medical care. • Withdrawn behavior, feels hopeless, helpless. • May be demanding, belligerent, and aggressive. • Repeated visits to health care agency for injuries/ falls. • Injuries do not correlate with stated cause. • Misuse of money by children or legal guardians.	• Establish trust; use non-judgmental approach. • Meet physical needs, treat wounds and injuries. • Document factual, objective statements of client's physical condition, injuries, and interaction with significant other/family. • Report suspected abuse to appropriate local/ state authorities. • Arrange community resources to provide "respite care" for the caregiver. • Arrange visiting nurses, nutrition services, or adult day care if possible.

HESI HINT: It is difficult for an elderly person to admit abuse for fear of being placed in a nursing home or being abandoned. Therefore, it is imperative to establish a trusting relationship with the elderly client.

Figure 6-31 (continued)

RAPE AND SEXUAL ASSAULT

A crime involving lack of consent, force, and sexual penetration. An act of aggression, NOT passion.

ANALYSIS (NURSING DIAGNOSES)
- Rape trauma syndrome related to…
- Powerlessness related to…

ASSESSMENT	NURSING PLANS AND INTERVENTIONS
• Physical assessment with careful documentation of injuries. • Emotional status: self-blame, anxious, fear, humiliation, disbelief, and anger. • Coping behaviors. • Identify support system. • Obtain details of the assault.	• Communicate non-judgmental acceptance. • Provide physical care to treat injuries. • Give clear, concise explanations of all procedures to be performed. • Document factual, objective statements of physical assessment; record client's EXACT WORDS in describing the assault. • Notify police, encourage victim to prosecute. • Collect and label evidence carefully in the presence of a witness. • Notify Rape Crisis Team or counselor if available in the community. • Allow discussion of feelings about the assault. • Advise of potential for venereal disease, pregnancy, and HIV. • Provide information about medical care available. • Support client, family, and friends.

Figure 6-31 (continued)

HESI HINT: Rape victims are at high risk for Post Traumatic Stress Disorder (PTSD). Immediate intervention to diminish distress is vital. The nurse should also assess for and intervene for sequallae such as unwanted pregnancy, sexually transmitted diseases, and HIV risk.

HESI HINT: Questions on the NCLEX-RN® regarding physical/sexual abuse usually focus on three aspects:
- **Physical manifestations of abuse.**
- **Client safety.**
- **Legal responsibilities of the nurse** – In children, the nurse is legally responsible to report all suspected cases of abuse. In intimate partner abuse, it is the adult's decision; the nurse should be supportive of their decision. Remember to document objective factual assessment data and the client's exact words in cases of sexual abuse/rape.

REVIEW QUESTIONS

ABUSE

1. What family dynamics are often seen in child abuse cases?
2. What behavior might the nurse observe in a child who is abused?
3. Identify nursing interventions for dealing with an abused child.
4. When does battering of women often begin or escalate?
5. What dynamics prevent a battered spouse from leaving the battering situation?
6. Why is elder abuse so under reported?
7. What types of abuse are seen in the elderly?
8. Identify nursing interventions for working with a rape survivor.

ANSWERS TO REVIEW QUESTIONS

1. Parent sees child as "different" from other children. Parent uses child to meet their own needs. Parent seldom touches or responds to child. Parent may be very critical of child. Family history of frequent moves, unstable employment, marital discord, and family violence. One parent answers all the questions.
2. Child may appear frightened and withdrawn in the presence of parent or adult.
3. Must report all cases of suspected abuse to appropriate local/state agency. Take color photographs of injuries. Document factual, objective statements of child's physical condition, child-family interactions, and interviews with family. Establish trust, and care for the child's physical problems. These are the PRIMARY and

PSYCHIATRIC NURSING

379

IMMEDIATE needs of these children. Recognize own feelings of disgust and contempt for the parents. Teach basic child development and parenting skills to family.

4. During pregnancy.
5. A woman in a battering relationship may lack self-confidence and feel trapped. She is often embarrassed to tell friends and family, so she becomes isolated and dependent upon the abuser.
6. It is difficult for an elderly person to admit abuse for fear of being placed in a nursing home or being abandoned.
7. Abuse can be physical, verbal, psychosocial, exploitive, or physical neglect.

8. Communicate non-judgmental acceptance. Provide physical care to treat injuries. Give clear, concise explanations of all procedures to be performed. Notify police, encourage victim to prosecute. Collect and label evidence carefully in the presence of a witness. Document factual, objective statements of physical condition; record client's EXACT WORDS in describing the assault. Notify Rape Crisis Team or counselor if available in the community. Allow discussion of feelings about the assault. Advise of potential for venereal disease, HIV, or pregnancy and describe medical care available.

ORGANIC DISORDERS

DELIRIUM AND DEMENTIA	
Abnormal psychological or behavioral signs and symptoms, which occur as a result of cerebral disease, systemic dysfunction, or use/exposure to exogenous substances. *(See figure 6-33, Description of Delirium/Dementia)*	
ANALYSIS (NURSING DIAGNOSES) • Alteration in thought processes related to… • Self-care deficit (dressing and grooming) related to…	
ASSESSMENT	**NURSING PLANS AND INTERVENTIONS**
• Limited attention span, easily distracted. • Confusion and disorientation, impaired judgment. • Delusions, visual hallucinations, or sensory illusions. • Labile affect; sudden anger. • Anxiety and/or depression. • Loss of recent and remote memory. • Confabulation (making up responses, stories to fill in lost memory). • Impaired coordination. • Increased psychomotor activity. • Slurring of speech. • Decreased personal hygiene. • Sleep deprivation, day/night reversal. • Incontinence/constipation.	• Provide safe, consistent environment. • Maintain health, nutrition, safety, hygiene, and rest. • Assist with ADL. • Provide support to client/family. • Provide routine in daily activities. • Clearly mark the bathroom. • *See Dementia in Gerontological Nursing for Additional Interventions.* • Reorient the client as needed. • Use simple, direct statements

HESI HINT: Confusion in the elderly is often "accepted" as part of growing old. This confusion may be due to dehydration with resulting electrolyte imbalance. Think "sudden change" when obtaining a history. Such changes are usually due to a specific stressor, and treatment for the causative stressor will usually result in correcting the confusion.

Figure 6-32

HESI HINT: Confabulation is not lying. It is used by the client to decrease anxiety and protect the ego.

HESI HINT: Nursing interventions for the confused elderly should focus on:
• Maintaining the client's health and safety.
• Encouraging self-care.
• Reinforcing reality orientation (e.g., "Today is Monday," and call the client by name).
• Providing a consistent, safe environment – engage client in simple tasks, activities to build self-esteem.

PSYCHIATRIC NURSING

DESCRIPTION OF DELIRIUM/DEMENTIA

DELIRIUM	DEMENTIA
DESCRIPTION: An acute process, which, if treated, is usually reversible. It is recognized by its SUDDEN onset.	**DESCRIPTION:** Cognitive impairments characterized by gradual, progressive onset; it is irreversible. Judgment, memory, abstract thinking, and social behavior are affected.
Occurs in response to a specific stressor such as: • Infection • Drug reaction • Substance intoxication or withdrawal • Electrolyte imbalance • Head trauma • Sleep deprivation Treatment of choice is the correction of the causative disorder.	**Most frequently seen in:** • Alzheimer's disease • Multi-infarcts (brain) **Also occurs in:** • Huntington's chorea • Parkinson's disease • Multiple sclerosis and brain tumors • Wernicke-Korsakoff Syndrome (chronic alcoholics)

Figure 6-33

ALZHEIMER'S MEDICATIONS

DRUGS	ADVERSE REACTIONS	NURSING IMPLICATIONS
acetyl cholinesterase inhibitors • **tacrine hydrochloride** (Cognex) • **donepezil HCI** (Aricept) • **rivastigmine** (Exelon) • **galantamine** (Reminyl)	• Overall - nausea and diarrhea • Cognex: considerable GI distress elevated liver enzymes	• Teach clients that they should take NO anticholinergic medication • Medications should not be used in cases of severe liver impairment • Take with meals to avoid GI upset • Do not discontinue abruptly

Figure 6-34

REVIEW QUESTIONS
ORGANIC MENTAL DISORDERS
1. **List five causes of delirium.**
2. **Describe the nursing care for a client with Alzheimer's disease.**
3. **Identify three or more causes of dementia.**

ANSWERS TO REVIEW QUESTIONS
1. Infection, alcohol withdrawal, electrolyte imbalance, sleep deprivation, brain injury, i.e., subdural hematomas.
2. Provide a safe, consistent environment. (Do not make changes if possible. Change increases anxiety and confusion.) Stick to routines. If client wanders, make sure they have a nametag. Provide assistance as needed with ADL. Make sure bathroom is clearly labeled.
3. Alzheimer's disease, multi-infarcts (brain), Huntington's chorea, multiple sclerosis, Parkinson's disease.

PSYCHIATRIC NURSING

CHILDHOOD AND ADOLESCENT DISORDERS	
ATTENTION DEFICIT (HYPERACTIVITY) DISORDER (ADD/ADHD)	
Developmentally inappropriate attention, impulsiveness, and hyperactivity.	
ANALYSIS (NURSING DIAGNOSES) • Potential for injury: trauma related to… • Impaired social interaction related to…	
ASSESSMENT	**NURSING PLANS AND INTERVENTIONS**
Perform complete physical assessment. • More prevalent in boys. • Failure to listen and follow instructions. • Difficulty playing quietly or sitting still. • Disruptive, impulsive behavior. • Distractibility to external stimuli. • Excessive talking. • Shifts from one unfinished task to another. • Underachievement in school performance.	• Decrease environmental stimuli. • Set limits on behavior when indicated. • Provide a safe, comfortable environment. • Initiate a behavior contract to help child manage own behavior. • Administer medications as prescribed. *(See figure 6-36, Stimulants)*
CONDUCT DISORDER	**OPPOSITIONAL DEFIANT DISORDER**
Antisocial behavior in a child or adolescent characterized by violation of laws, societal norms, and the basic rights of others without feelings of remorse or guilt.	Behavior, which fails to adhere to established norms, but does NOT violate the rights of others.
ANALYSIS (NURSING DIAGNOSES) CONDUCT AND DEFIANT DISORDERS • Potential for violence related to… • Disturbance in self-esteem related to… • Ineffective family coping related to…	
ASSESSMENT	**ASSESSMENT**
• Physical fighting • Running away from home • Lying, stealing • Cruelty to animals • Frequent truancy • Vandalism, arson • Use of alcohol, drugs	• Argumentative • Blaming others for their problems • Defies rules and authority • Uses obscene language • Resentful, vindictive
NURSING PLANS AND INTERVENTIONS – CONDUCT AND DEFIANT DISORDERS	
• Assess verbal/nonverbal cues for escalating behavior to decrease outbursts. • Use a non-authoritarian approach. • Avoid asking "why" questions. • Initiate a "show of force" for child who is out of control. • Use "quiet room" when external control is needed. • Clarify expressions or jargon if meaning is unclear. • Redirect angry feelings to "safe" alternative such as a pillow or punching bag. • Implement behavior modification therapy if indicated. • Role-play new coping strategies with client.	
HESI HINT: Children also experience depression, which often presents as headaches, stomachaches, and other somatic complaints. Be sure to assess suicidal risk, especially in the adolescent.	

Figure 6-35

PSYCHIATRIC NURSING

STIMULANTS			
DRUGS	**INDICATIONS**	**ADVERSE REACTIONS**	**NURSING IMPLICATIONS**
• **dextroamphetamine sulfate** (Dexedrine) • **methylphenidate HCL** (Ritalin) • **pemoline** (Cylert)	• Treat ADD/ADHD • Methylphenidate is also used to treat narcolepsy	• May interact with MAO inhibitors producing fever and hypertensive crisis • Nervousness, and insomnia; dizziness • Tourette's syndrome • Tachycardia, palpitations, angina, dysrhythmias • Anorexia, weight loss, nausea, and abdominal pain	• Short acting, 2 to 4 hours • Teach to take last dose at least 6 hours before bedtime if insomnia occurs • Administer 1 to 3 doses daily • Administer with or after meals to avoid appetite suppression • Monitor heart rate, rhythm, and BP • Monitor height and weight to detect growth suppression

Figure 6-36

REVIEW QUESTIONS
CHILDHOOD AND ADOLESCENT DISORDERS

1. A 7-year-old boy is disruptive in the classroom and is described by his parents as "hyperactive." What is the most probable psychiatric disorder? What are the signs and symptoms of this disorder? What drug is usually prescribed for this disorder?

2. A 15-year-old boy is threatening to drop out of school. His parents, both alcoholics, say they can't stop him. He has just been arrested for stealing a car and breaking into a house. What is the most probable disorder? Develop nursing diagnoses and interventions for this disorder.

ANSWERS TO REVIEW QUESTIONS

1. Attention deficit disorder (ADD/ADHD). More prevalent in boys, failure to listen or follow instructions. Difficulty playing quietly, disruptive, impulsive behavior, difficulty sitting still, distractibility to external stimuli, excessive talking, shifts from one unfinished task to another, and underachievement in school performance. Ritalin.

2. Conduct Disorder.
   A. Potential for violence related to … depending on client.
   B. Disturbance in self-esteem related to … depending on client.
   C. Ineffective family coping related to … depending on client.
   D. Assess verbal/nonverbal cues for escalating behavior to decrease outbursts. Use a non-authoritarian approach. Avoid asking "why" questions. Initiate a "show of force" for child who is out of control. Initiate suicide precautions when assessment indicates risk. Use "quiet room" when external control is needed. Clarify expressions or jargon if meaning is unclear. Redirect angry feelings to "safe" alternative such as a pillow or punching bag. Implement behavior modification therapy if indicated. Role-play new coping strategies.

PSYCHIATRIC NURSING

Gerontological Nursing

1. Aging is an individual process, which affects people differently.
2. For the purpose of data collection, those 65 years of age and older are considered older adults.
3. The number of elderly is increasing in the U.S.; by the year 2020 it is expected that 20% of the population will be over the age of 65.
4. Eighty percent of the elderly have one or more chronic illnesses, and 50% have two or more chronic illnesses.
5. The elderly are the greatest users of health care.
6. Only 5% of the elderly live in institutional settings.

Theories of Aging

Sociological Theories

1. Disengagement theory: progressive social disengagement occurs with aging.
2. Activity theory: successful aging (as measured by the individual's satisfaction with life) depends on maintaining a high level of activity and involvement.

Biological Theories

1. Wear and tear theory: after repeated use and damage, body structures and functions wear out from stress.
2. Free radical theory: oxidation releases chemicals that affect the cell membrane and DNA replication; relates aging to environmental pollutants.
3. Immune Theory: the aging process affects the immune system causing ↓T cells, ↑incidence of infection.

Psychological Theories

1. Short-term memory suffers an age-related decline.
2. Long-term memory undergoes minimal change.
3. Memory is affected by changes in the environment, e.g., moving, changes in caregivers, etc.

> **HESI HINT:** Either a lack of stimulation or an overload of changes can result in confusion. Provide as much consistency and routine as possible when caring for the elderly in order to reduce the possibility of creating confusion.

Physiological Changes

Physiological Changes in the Elderly

DESCRIPTION: The aged are vulnerable to disease because of decreased physiologic reserve, less flexible homeostatic processes, and less effective body defenses.

Aging is characterized by the concept of LOSS.

- Physiological and psychosocial losses occur even in "healthy" aging.
- Increased longevity contributes to the demand placed on the health care system.
- Diseases in the elderly do not always present classic signs and symptoms.
- Chronic illness becomes more prevalent as one ages.
- Resistance to stressors diminishes as one ages.
- The frail elderly (those over 75 years of age) are the fastest growing segment of the population and the highest users of health care.

> **HESI HINT:** Changes in the heart and lungs result in less efficient utilization of O_2, which reduces an individual's capacity to maintain physical activity for long periods of time. Physical training for older persons can significantly reduce blood pressure and increase aerobic capacity. NCLEX-RN® questions ask about teaching and designing rehab programs for the elderly – they should contain something about exercise and nutrition.

> **HESI HINT:** Older persons often complain that they cannot get to sleep at night and do not sleep soundly even after they fall asleep. This is because they have shorter stages of sleep, particularly shorter cycles from stages 1 to 4 and REM sleep (stage 4 is deep sleep). They are easily awakened by environmental stimuli. They often compensate by napping during the day, which leads to further disruptions of night sleep. A common response is use of prescription sleeping pills which can create still further problems of disorientation, etc.

Figure 7-1

PHYSIOLOGICAL CHANGES IN THE ELDERLY
CARDIOVASCULAR SYSTEM

DESCRIPTION: Age-related changes in the cardiovascular system predispose the older person to developing dysrhythmias and other cardiac problems.

- Cardiac output decreases as a result of a decrease in heart rate and stroke volume (heart rate slows with age, resting heart rate remains unchanged).
- Cardiac output decreases because vessels lose elasticity. The heart's contractility decreases in response to increased demands.
- Diastolic murmurs are present in over one-half of the elderly due to mitral and aortic valves becoming thick and rigid.
- Dysrhythmias (bradycardia, tachycardia, atrial fibrillation and heart block) increase as one ages, in part R/T ↑ systolic B/P and ↑size of the atriums.
- Significant increases in systolic BP occur as a result of altered distribution of blood flow and increased peripheral resistance.
- Arteriosclerosis increases with age and can cause cardiovascular problems:
  - → Peripheral vascular disease.
  - → Edema.
  - → Coronary artery disease: acute coronary insufficiency, MI, dysrhythmias, congestive heart failure (CHF).

HESI HINT: Both systolic and diastolic blood pressure tend to increase with normal aging, but the elevation of the systolic is greater. REMEMBER the physiology of blood pressure, which is expressed as a ratio of systolic to diastolic pressure. Systolic refers to the level of blood pressure during the contraction phase whereas diastolic refers to the stage when the chambers of the heart are filling with blood.

ANALYSIS (NURSING DIAGNOSES)
- Activity intolerance related to…
- Alteration in tissue perfusion related to…
- Alteration in comfort related to…
- Decreased cardiac output related to…

ASSESSMENT	NURSING PLANS AND INTERVENTIONS
- Dizziness or blackouts with sudden position change (orthostatic hypotension). - Diuresis after lying down.	- Monitor blood pressure in lying, sitting, and standing positions. - Teach to avoid fatigue. - Encourage regular, low-level exercise. - Teach to change positions slowly to avoid injury/falls.
- Feelings of heart palpitations	- Take apical/radial pulse; note deficits or rhythm abnormalities.
- Swelling in hands and feet. (Rings and shoes have become tight). - Weight gain without changes in eating pattern.	- Teach to avoid extreme hot and cold because of decreased peripheral sensation. - Teach to avoid sitting with feet in a dependent position. - Weigh daily if indicated. - Encourage frequent rest periods.
- Difficulty breathing at night. (Ask older person if they are using an increased number of pillows at night). - Confusion, personality changes resulting from O$_2$ deficit.	- Encourage strict adherence to medication regime; no over-the-counter drugs (may interfere with digitalis). - Determine support system for follow-up.

HESI HINT: Dysrhythmias in the elderly are particularly serious since older persons cannot tolerate decreased cardiac output, which can result in syncope, falls, and transient ischemic attacks (TIAs). Pulse may be rapid, slow, or irregular.

HESI HINT: Angina symptoms may be absent in the elderly or they may be confused with GI symptoms.

Figure 7-2

PHYSIOLOGICAL CHANGES IN THE ELDERLY	
RESPIRATORY SYSTEM	

Many older adults, along with the normal changes brought on by increased age, have respiratory diseases.
- Respiratory muscles become rigid and lose strength, thereby restricting ventilation and decreasing vital capacity.
- Lessened ability to cough and deep breathe.
- Lungs lose elasticity, become rigid (greatest change occurs in persons 70 years and older), decreasing pulmonary circulation.
- Although total lung capacity and tidal volume are unaffected by age, gas exchange is reduced. Po_2 decreases to 75 mmHg at age 70, Pco_2 is unchanged by age.

HESI HINT: With aging, the muscles that operate the lungs lose elasticity so that respiratory efficiency is reduced. Vital capacity (the amount of air brought into the lungs at one time) decreases. Breathing may become more difficult after strenuous exercise or after climbing up several flights of stairs. The rate of decline has been found to be slower in more active persons. The nurse should encourage older persons to remain physically active for as long as possible.
Declining muscle strength may impair cough efficiency. This fact makes older persons more susceptible to chronic bronchitis, emphysema, and pneumonia.

ANALYSIS (NURSING DIAGNOSES)
- Ineffective breathing pattern related to…
- Impaired gas exchange related to…
- Ineffective airway clearance related to…
- Activity intolerance related to…

ASSESSMENT	NURSING PLANS AND INTERVENTIONS
• Confusion may be the first sign of respiratory infection. • Respiratory infection in an older person is an acute emergency. • Pneumonia is a major cause of death in the older generation.	• Encourage clients to receive pneumonia vaccine and an influenza vaccine yearly. • Remember that hypoxia can be manifested as confusion. Encourage client to get assistance with medication regimen to prevent hypoxia.
• Breathlessness. • Dyspnea and fatigue (COPD).	• If client is a smoker, encourage him/her to **STOP**. (Regardless of age, cardiovascular and respiratory status does improve with smoking cessation and exercise). • For elderly postoperative clients, turning, deep breathing, and use of incentive spirometer is imperative to prevent complications.

HESI HINT: COPD is the major cause of respiratory disability in the elderly.	

• Cough present and sputum produced.	• Encourage deep breathing. Teach breathing techniques, such as pursed lip breathing to facilitate respirations. • Some ventilatory assistance techniques, such as postural drainage, pose hazards for the elderly.

Figure 7-3

PHYSIOLOGICAL CHANGES IN THE ELDERLY

GASTROINTESTINAL SYSTEM

- Age-related changes are bothersome but are rarely a direct cause of death.
- Relaxation of the lower esophageal sphincter results in delayed emptying and an increased **RISK OF ASPIRATION**.
- Decreased peristalsis and impaired absorption contribute to constipation problems.
- Hiatal hernia incidence increases with age.
- Delayed gastric emptying makes digestion of large amounts of food difficult.
- Decreased hunger sensations.
- Decreased production of pepsin and hydrochloric acid.
- Decreased absorption of calcium.
- Decreased absorption of vitamins B_1 and B_2.
- Diverticulosis of the sigmoid colon occurs in one-third of those over age 60.
- Decreased enzyme production in the liver affects drug metabolism and detoxification processes.
- Decrease in the amount of bile in the gall bladder causes an increased difficulty with emptying.
- Loss of teeth is common, resulting in decreased ability to chew food adequately.

HESI HINT: Aging changes that contribute to chronic constipation:
- **The number of enzymes in the small intestine is reduced and simple sugars are absorbed more slowly, resulting in decreased efficiency of the digestive process.**
- **The smooth muscle content and muscle tone of the wall of the colon decrease. Anatomical changes in the large intestine result in decreased intestinal motility.**
- **Psychological factors, as well as abuse of over-the-counter laxatives.**
- **Decreases in fluid intake and mobility contribute to constipation.**

ANALYSIS (NURSING DIAGNOSES)
- Alteration in bowel elimination: constipation related to…
- Potential alteration in fluid balance related to…
- Alteration in oral tissue mucous membrane related to…

ASSESSMENT	NURSING PLANS AND INTERVENTIONS
• Brittle teeth due to thinning enamel.	• Encourage good oral hygiene. Use soft toothbrush.
• Receding gums resulting from periodontal disease (the major cause of tooth loss after the age of 30).	• Assess dentures for proper fit.

HESI HINT: Tooth loss is NOT a normal aging process. Good dental hygiene, good nutrition, and dental care can prevent tooth loss.

• Decrease in taste sensation.
• Dry mouth due to a decrease in saliva production.
• Poor tolerance of high-fat meals and poor absorption of fat-soluble vitamins.
• Decreased glucose tolerance.
	• Promote adequate bowel functioning:
	  → Determine what is "normal" GI functioning for each individual.
	  → Increase fiber and bulk in the diet.
	  → Provide adequate hydration.
	  → Encourage regular exercise.
	  → Encourage eating small, frequent meals.
	  → Discourage the use of laxatives and enemas.
	• Encourage use of different spices to increase taste sensation.
	• Educate elderly clients about hidden sodium (canned soup, antacids, over-the-counter medications).

HESI HINT: Older people appear to eat small quantities of food at mealtimes. This is because the digestive system of older persons features a decrease in contraction time of the muscles and more time is needed for the cardiac sphincter to open. Therefore, it takes more time for the food to be transmitted to the stomach. Thus, the sensation of fullness may occur before the entire meal is consumed.

Figure 7-4

PHYSIOLOGICAL CHANGES IN THE ELDERLY	
GENITOURINARY SYSTEM	
Normal aging does not impact continence or sexual functioning, but mental, physical, and cognitive changes can have a significant impact.	

ANALYSIS (NURSING DIAGNOSES)
- Alteration in acid-base balance related to…
- Alteration in self-concept related to…
- Alteration in patterns of urinary elimination related to…
- Sexual dysfunction related to…

HESI HINT: Older persons have a higher risk of developing renal failure because normal age-related changes result in compromised renal functioning. The nurse should pay careful attention to urinary output in older clients because it is the first sign of loss of renal integrity.

ASSESSMENT	NURSING PLANS AND INTERVENTIONS

KIDNEY
 • Size decreases due to reduced renal tissue growth.
 • Glomerular filtration rate is decreased due to a decrease in renal blood flow because of decreased cardiac output. Decreased renal clearance of drugs results.
 • Tubular function diminishes.
   → Lower specific gravity occurs because the tubulars are less capable of concentrating urine.
   → Proteinuria of 1+ is common.
   → BUN increases to 30 mg/dl.
 • Glucose reabsorption decreases.
   → Classic symptoms of diabetes mellitus may not appear in the elderly client.
   → Symptoms of diabetes mellitus in the elderly client may include fatigue, infection, and sensory changes caused by neuropathy.
 • Chronic diseases such as atherosclerosis also decrease renal functioning in the elderly.
	• Observe for signs of dehydration or electrolyte imbalance.
	 • Encourage an intake of at least 2 to 3 liters of fluid daily.
	 • Instruct client about importance of completing antibiotics until entire prescription is gone, even if symptoms go away.
	 • Write out antibiotic schedule with any special instructions. Print in large letters.

BLADDER • The capacity of the bladder decreases by one-half resulting in urinary frequency and nocturia. • Emptying the bladder becomes difficult because of a weakening of the bladder and perineal muscles and because of a decrease in sensation or urge to void (this sets up a propensity for UTIs due to residual urine in the bladder). • Increased frequency and dribbling occur in men because of a weakened bladder and enlarged prostate. • Prostatic enlargement may cause urinary retention and bladder infection in males. • Women may experience stress incontinence.	• Initiate a bladder-training program if indicated. • Encourage elderly women to void at first urge when possible. • Initiate a skin care program if incontinence is present. • Provide methods of dealing with incontinence. Kegel exercises can help. • Avoid sleeping pills and sedation, which may cause nocturnal incontinence. • Avoid caffeine as it promotes diuresis.

HESI HINT: Kegal exercises consist of tightening and relaxing the vaginal and urinary meatus muscles. These exercises have been very successful in reducing the incidence of incontinence. They must be done consistently, and they can be done unobtrusively at home.

HESI HINT: The elderly with incontinence may seek isolation, thereby predisposing themselves to loneliness.

Figure 7-5

HESI HINT: 15 to 30% of community-based elderly and almost 50% of elderly living in nursing homes suffer from difficulties with bladder control. Older persons may be more sensitive to alcohol and caffeine since these substances inhibit the production of antidiuretic hormone (ADH). An assessment of sensitivity to bladder problems is essential when planning nursing care.

HESI HINT: *MEDICATION ALERT:*
As one ages, the total number of functioning glomeruli decreases until renal function has been reduced by nearly 50%. This decrease in the filtration efficiency of the kidneys has grave implications for persons who are taking medication. Of particular importance are penicillin, tetracycline, and digoxin, which are primarily cleared from the blood stream by the kidneys. These drugs remain active longer in an older person's system. Therefore, they may be more potent, indicating a need to adjust the dosage and frequency of administration.

PHYSIOLOGICAL CHANGES IN THE ELDERLY	
REPRODUCTIVE SYSTEM	
ASSESSMENT	NURSING PLANS AND INTERVENTIONS
FEMALE REPRODUCTIVE ORGANS • Perineal muscle weakness and atrophy of the vulva occurs with age. • Estrogen production decreases when menopause occurs. • Vaginal mucous membrane becomes dry, elasticity of tissue decreases, surface becomes smooth, and secretions become reduced and more alkaline. • Incidence of vaginitis increases. • Libido does not change.	• Observe for signs of vaginitis; report and treat if present. • Perineal care should be promoted. • Note. Elderly rape victims sustain particularly extensive penetration trauma. • Prescription creams can help with vaginal dryness.
MALE REPRODUCTION ORGANS • Testosterone production decreases. • Testicular size decreases. • Libido does not change.	• Encourage annual digital examination for early identification of prostate cancer.

Figure 7-6

PHYSIOLOGICAL CHANGES IN THE ELDERLY

NEUROLOGICAL SYSTEM

Neurologic disease is the major cause of disability in the elderly. Alzheimer's disease, cerebral vascular accidents, and Parkinson's disease are the major disorders in this category. *(See Medical Surgical Nursing)*

- Brain
  - → Cerebral blood flow and oxygen utilization are decreased.
  - → Neurons do not regenerate, therefore neurological losses are permanent.
- Peripheral nerves:
  - → Decreased ability to respond to multiple stimuli because of a decrease in both autonomic and sympathetic nervous system functioning.

HESI HINT: Alzheimer's disease is the most common irreversible dementia of old age. It is characterized by deficits in attention, learning, memory, and language skills. Discuss the problems family members have in dealing with Alzheimer's clients in relation to the following disease manifestations:
- **Depression**
- **Night wandering**
- **Aggressive or passiveness**
- **Failure to recognize family members**

ANALYSIS (NURSING DIAGNOSES)
- Alteration in cerebral tissue perfusion related to…
- Alteration in sensory perceptions related to…
- Impaired communication related to…
- Impaired social interaction related to…

ASSESSMENT	NURSING PLANS AND INTERVENTIONS
• Headache; determine type and difference from previous headaches.	• Perform a complete mental status exam and test cognitive thinking. • Record level of consciousness.

• Transient ischemic attacks (TIAs) manifested as:
  → Weakness.
  → Difficulty speaking.
  → "Blackouts."
• Tremors in hands while at rest.
• Decrease of arm swing while walking.
	• Record sensory awareness (vision, hot and cold sensations, pain).
	• Place food within visual field.
	• Provide alternate method of communication if indicated.
	• Arrange environment for optimum SAFE self-care. Reorient older person to environment as needed.
	• Provide activities based on cognitive level of functioning.
	• Keep precautionary respiratory equipment at bedside (higher risk for choking aspiration).
	• Decrease noise and clutter in environment; keep environment as consistent as possible.

• Gait disturbances resulting from less efficient kinesthetic senses. • Delay in reflex response to noxious stimuli (hot surfaces, bumping into objects, etc.).	• Orientation is enhanced by windows, calendars, and clocks. Reorient by asking specific questions in a calm, direct way. • Life history events are a good way to begin the reorientation process. • Allow as much autonomy as possible. • Provide assistive devices as needed for ambulation. • Minimize potential sources of injury in environment.

HESI HINT: Strokes from cerebral thrombosis are more common in older persons than are strokes from cerebral hemorrhage. Clots tend to develop when patient is awake or just arousing.

Figure 7-7

PHYSIOLOGICAL CHANGES IN THE ELDERLY

ENDOCRINE SYSTEM

ANALYSIS (NURSING DIAGNOSES)
- Activity intolerance related to…
- Fatigue related to…

ASSESSMENT	NURSING PLANS AND INTERVENTIONS
Reduced thyroid activity *(See Medical Surgical Nursing, Hypothyroidism)*. Often symptoms go undiagnosed in the older adult being attributed to "normal for age." • T_3 level decreases. • Metabolic rate slows.	• Encourage thyroid testing for older clients who seem depressed. Hypothyroidism is often "dismissed" as depression. • *See Medical Surgical Nursing, Hypothyroidism.*
• Aldosterone blood level and urinary excretion decrease. • Estrogen production ceases with menopause; ovaries, uterus, and vaginal tissue atrophy. • Gonadal secretion of progesterone and testosterone decreases.	• Elderly clients may have difficulty with "lifelong" medication regimen. Develop memory cues for medications and caution against abrupt withdrawal.
• Glucose intolerance may occur with aging.	• *See Medical Surgical Nursing, Diabetes*.

Figure 7-8

PHYSIOLOGICAL CHANGES IN THE ELDERLY

MUSCULOSKELETAL SYSTEM

DESCRIPTION: Age-related changes in the musculoskeletal system are gradual but have significant impact on levels of mobility, which put the elderly at risk for falls and fractures.

ANALYSIS (NURSING DIAGNOSES)
- Pain related to…
- Potential disuse syndrome related to…
- Potential for injury related to…

ASSESSMENT	NURSING PLANS AND INTERVENTIONS
BONE: • Bone loss begins at about age 40. • Bone loss is more common in women than men. • Osteoporosis occurs most often in women. *(See Medical Surgical Nursing)*	• *See Medical Surgical Nursing, Osteoporosis* • Adequate calcium intake may help lessen osteoporosis changes (recommend 1000 mg daily). • Establish muscle strengthening program (small weights, aquatic therapy).
MUSCLE: • Muscle cells are lost and not replaced. • Older persons fatigue more easily because of changes in enzyme activity. • Lean body mass decreases with increased body fat.	• Prevent accidents by ensuring a safe environment. • Remove all hazards so that pathways are clear. • Provide adequate lighting day and night to prevent falls. • Teach client not to back up, but to turn around to move in the direction they wish to go. • Encourage regular exercise.
JOINTS: • Cartilage erosion occurs. • Range of motion of joints decreases.	• Multiple medications, especially diuretics and sedatives, contribute to falls. • Older persons should change positions slowly to prevent orthostatic hypotension.

Figure 7-9

GERONTOLOGICAL NURSING

HESI HINT: Impaired mobility, impaired skin integrity, decreased peripheral circulation, and a lack of physical activity place the elderly at risk for developing decubitus ulcers.

HESI HINT: Ways to help prevent/decrease the occurrence of falls:
• Adequate lighting.
• Paint the edges of stairs a bright color.
• Place a bell on elderly person's cat (since cats move quickly and get underfoot).
• Wear proper footwear that supports the foot and contributes to balance (made of non-slippery materials).

HESI HINT: Fractured hip and hip replacement are common in elderly persons. Teach the proper way to sit and rise after hip replacement so that the body-to-lap angle is not less than 90 degrees. They should not lean forward while sitting (can cause dislocation of the prosthesis).

PHYSIOLOGICAL CHANGES IN THE ELDERLY	
INTEGUMENTARY SYSTEM	
DESCRIPTION: Skin, hair, and nail changes occur with aging and can cause problems with discomfort and self-esteem.	
ANALYSIS (NURSING DIAGNOSES) • Skin integrity impairment related to… • Potential for injury related to…	

ASSESSMENT	NURSING PLANS AND INTERVENTIONS

• Thin skin provides a less effective barrier from trauma. Varicosities (brown or blue discolorations) indicate poor circulation.
  → Less effective in retaining water.
  → Decreased ability for the skin to detect and regulate temperature.
  → Skin dries because of a decrease in endocrine secretion.
  → Loss of elastin and increased vascular fragility.
• Hair loss, increased facial hair in women.
• Decrease in number and size of sweat glands.
• Brittle and thick nails.
	• Encourage use of oils or lubricants on skin at least twice a day.
	• Discourage use of powder, which can be drying.
	• Avoid over-exposure to sunlight.
	• Encourage good nutrition and increased fluid intake.
	• Maintain adequate humidity in the environment.
	• Avoid temperature extremes.
	• Teach good foot care.
	• Observe bony prominences for signs of pressure.
	• Poor peripheral circulation may retard the healing of foot and hand lesions.

HESI HINT: Peripheral circulation decreases as one ages. Regular assessment of the feet is very important because it increases the opportunity to discover and treat skin care problems early. These problems could become more serious because of decreased circulation.

HESI HINT: Older persons have dry, wrinkled skin because they lose subcutaneous fat and the second layer of skin, the dermis, becomes less elastic.

Figure 7-10

PHYSIOLOGICAL CHANGES IN THE ELDERLY

SENSORY SYSTEM

DESCRIPTION: Changes in the sensory system which affect sight, hearing, taste, touch, smell, and balance occur gradually and are often unnoticed.

ANALYSIS (NURSING DIAGNOSES)
- Alteration in sensory perception related to…
- Potential for injury related to…
- Potential for social isolation related to…

ASSESSMENT	NURSING PLANS AND INTERVENTIONS
VISION • Reduce tear production. • Presbyopia: age-related decrease in the ability of the eye to accommodate for near vision. • Arcus senilis: glossy white ring encircling the periphery of the cornea (appears either partially or completely). • Cataracts: an abnormal progressive clouding or opacity of the lens of the eye (a common vision problem affecting the elderly). • Glaucoma incidence increases.	• Provide interventions to supplement loss of sensory input. • Encourage social interaction. • Use bright colors and large print for written materials. • Describe environment verbally to the visually impaired to increase orientation and decrease confusion. • Arrange for glasses if appropriate. • Maximize visual and non-visual aids such as large print books, recorded books, and lighted mirror. • Encourage use of artificial tears; avoid rubbing, picking at eyes – infection risk. • Encourage regular eye exams; assist with administering eye drops.

HESI HINT: Diminished eyesight results in:
- **A loss of independence (ADL and driving).**
- **A lack of stimulation.**
- **The inability to read.**
- **A fear of blindness.**

HEARING: • Presbycusis: age-related decrease in hearing acuity, auditory threshold, pitch and tone discrimination, and speech intelligibility (ability to understand another person's speech). • High-pitched hearing diminishes first. • Ability to discriminate tones is lost.	• Provide auditory cues to supplement loss of sensory input. • Supply written materials to the hearing impaired to reinforce what may not have been heard. • Directly face the hearing-impaired individual when talking to them so they can read lips and interpret facial expressions (also lessens suspicion). • Decrease background noises. • Arrange for hearing aids if appropriate.

HESI HINT: Lower the tone of your voice when talking to an older person who is hearing-impaired. High-pitched tones, (i.e., women's voices) are the first hearing to go, therefore, lowering the pitch of your voice increases the likelihood that an older person with a hearing loss will be able to hear you speak.

HESI HINT: Presbycusis (age-related hearing loss) can result in decreased socialization, avoidance of friends and family, decreased sensory stimulation, and hazardous conditions when driving.

GUSTATION (TASTE) AND OLFACTION (SMELL): • Taste buds decrease and atrophy resulting in decreased sensitivity for taste. • It is not known if the sense of smell is affected by aging.	• Use stronger spices if tolerated to increase taste of foods. Use substitutes for salt and sugar. • Adapt ethnic favorites to dietary and taste limitations.

HESI HINT: Use frequent touch to decrease the sense of isolation and to compensate for visual and auditory sensory loss.

Figure 7-11

GERONTOLOGICAL NURSING

PSYCHOSOCIAL CHANGES

NURSING ASSESSMENT
1. Loss of spouse, children, friends.
2. Loss of role in the work place and in the family.
   A. Affects status and prestige; can produce feelings of uselessness and nonparticipation.
   B. Withdrawal or disengagement from the mainstream of life may occur after retirement.
3. Loss of socioeconomic status.
   A. Decreased income usually occurs.
   B. Those on fixed incomes experience the effects of inflation more profoundly than the rest of the population.
   C. Loss of income affects the quality of health care available to the individual.
4. Loss of physical capacity.
5. Evaluate level of depression and suicidal risk.
6. Determine alcohol usage.

> **HESI HINT:** Older persons undergo a great many changes, which are usually associated with LOSS (loss of spouse, friends, career, home, health, etc.). Therefore, older persons are extremely vulnerable to emotional and mental stress.

ANALYSIS (NURSING DIAGNOSES)
1. Self-esteem disturbance related to…
2. Powerlessness related to…

NURSING PLANS AND INTERVENTIONS
1. Determine the losses the older client is currently having and has had in the past 2 years.
2. Promote activities that allow the individuals to use past experiences and knowledge, thereby promoting a feeling of self-worth and increasing self-esteem.
3. Promote reminiscing about significant life experiences.

> **HESI HINT:** INTEGRITY vs. DESPAIR is Erikson's final stage of growth and development. Reminiscing is a means of setting one's life in order (accepting life and self), which is the task of this stage of Erikson's development theory. The goal of this stage is to feel a sense of meaning in one's life, rather than to feel despair or bitterness that life was wasted. The major task of old age is to redefine self in relation to a changed role. Those persons who had been in charge of situations most of their lives may now find themselves in dependent positions. The role adjustment is a major task of old age.

> **HESI HINT:** Think about the following situations and discuss the nursing care for each.
> - A nursing supervisor who has had a stroke and is sent to a long-term facility for rehabilitation.
> - An oil company executive retires after 42 years with the company to travel in his recreational vehicle with his wife and dog.
> - Shortly after their 53rd wedding anniversary, a woman who has never worked outside the home loses her husband to brain cancer.

DEMENTIA

> **HESI HINT:** There are many conditions that can imitate dementia in the older adult. A key role for the nurse is to complete assessment to rule out other possible causes.

DESCRIPTION: Permanent, progressive impairment in cognitive functioning manifested by memory loss (both long-term and short-term), accompanied by an impairment in judgment, abstract thinking, and social behavior.
1. The two most common types of dementia are multiinfarct dementia and Alzheimer's disease.
   A. Multi-infarct dementia results from repeated strokes, which can cause complete deterioration of the cerebral tissue.
   B. Alzheimer's disease is characterized by brain atrophy, a progressive physical and mental deterioration lasting 5 to 14 years before death occurs.
2. Incidence:
   A. 1.2 million in the U.S. over the age of 65.
   B. 10 to 20% of the elderly population.
3. Leading cause of institutionalization

of the elderly (nearly two-thirds of the institutionalized elderly have some form of cognitive impairment).
4. Approximately 20% of those diagnosed with dementia are actually pseudo-dementias and are reversible. Possible causes of false dementias include:
    A. Drug side effects, interactions, and adverse reactions. Lithium, barbiturates, atropine, and bromides are known to have dementia as a side effect.
    B. Depression.
    C. Nutritional deficits.
    D. Metabolic disorders, hypothyroidism, anemia, hypoglycemia.
5. Irreversible dementia has a gradual onset with a progressive downward course. (Alzheimer's disease is the most common type.)

NURSING ASSESSMENT
1. Slow, insidious onset, which is unrelated to a specific etiology, condition, or situation.
2. Personality changes often accompanied by withdrawal.
3. Confusion, often unnoticed by the client.
4. Memory loss.
    A. Client is usually aware of memory loss.
    B. Memory loss begins with recent memory loss and progresses to total memory loss.
5. Risk factors.
    A. Family history of dementia.
    B. Family history of Down syndrome.
    C. Enzyme deficiency.
    D. Immune system deficiency.
    E. Aluminum toxicity.
    F. Acetylcholine deficiency (neurotransmitter).

ANALYSIS (NURSING DIAGNOSES)
1. Self-care deficit related to…
2. Alteration in thought process due to…
3. Risk for injury related to…

NURSING PLANS AND INTERVENTIONS
1. Keep client functioning and actively involved in social and family activities as long as possible.
2. Maintain an orderly, almost ritualistic schedule to promote a sense of security.
3. Assign to a regularly scheduled reality orientation on a daily basis.
    A. Keep client oriented as to time, place, and person (repeatedly).
    B. Keep a calendar and clock within sight at all times.
        1) Display a calendar and clock that can be read by older persons, i.e., a clock with large numbers and a calendar that can be read by those with deteriorating vision.
        2) Be sure the date and time are **ACCURATE**, i.e., keep the calendar current and the clock in working order.
4. Encourage family to bring pictures of family members from home. Familiar objects promote a sense of continuity and security.
5. Administer prescribed drugs to reduce emotional lability, agitation, and irritability or prescribed antidepressant as indicated.
6. Speak in a slow, calm voice; avoid excitement.
7. Provide support and education to family and long-term caregivers.

HEALTH MAINTENANCE AND PREVENTIVE CARE FOR THE ELDERLY
NURSING PLANS AND INTERVENTIONS
1. Encourage periodic health appraisal and counseling to prevent illness.
    A. EKG to detect subtle heart abnormalities.
    B. Chest x-ray to detect TB or lung cancer.
    C. Pulmonary function tests to detect chronic bronchitis and emphysema.
    D. Tonometer test to measure intraocular pressure as a test for glaucoma.
    E. Blood glucose to detect diabetes mellitus.
    F. Pap smear to detect cancer of cervix.
    G. Hearing and vision testing to detect sensory deprivation.
    H. Breast self-examination monthly.
2. Promote accident prevention.
    A. Prevent falls.
    B. Maintain physical and mental activities to improve confidence and mobility.
    C. Rise to upright position slowly because of the possibility of postural hypotension (orthostatic hypotension).
    D. Encourage regular exercise.

3. Protect against infectious diseases.
   A. Teach to avoid individuals who are ill.
   B. Encourage immunization against influenza and pneumonia.
   C. Encourage nutritious diet and plenty of fluids.
4. Avoid temperature extremes, prevent hypothermia.
5. Encourage elderly to stop smoking – it is NEVER too late.
6. Educate about proper foot care.
7. Encourage proper nutrition and weight control.
8. Encourage use of support services (Meals-on-Wheels) and support groups (church).
9. Discourage over-the-counter medication use. Review all medications yearly and encourage the client to throw away outdated drugs and prescriptions.

Disease and conditions that affect the elderly are the same ones that affect younger adults. *(See **Medical and Surgical Nursing**)*
However, in the elderly, signs and symptoms of pathology may be subtle, slow to develop, and quite different from those seen in younger persons. *(See figure 7-12, Diseases and Conditions in Terms of the Elderly)*

Diseases and Conditions in Terms of the Elderly

Disease/Condition	Description in Terms of the Elderly	Nursing Implications
Delirium	• Confused states develop over short periods of time if caused by systemic illness or medications. • Usually develops suddenly.	• Establish a meaningful environment. • Help maintain body awareness. • Help client cope with confusion, delusions and illusions. • ***See Nursing Interventions for Dementia***
Cardiac Dysrhythmias	• Incidence increases with age. • More serious in elderly because of lower tolerance of decreased cardiac output (can result in syncope, falls, TIAs, and confusion). • Symptoms result from compromised circulation and O_2 deficit.	• Assess, prevent, and manage dysrhythmias. • Advise smoking cessation. • Encourage exercise and weight control.
Cataracts	• Often a result of normal aging changes. • Most common pathologic problem affecting elderly's eyesight. • Treated with surgical removal.	• Teach instillation of eye drops. • Reduce glare in environment. • Assistance required post-op because affected eye is covered – disorientation may occur.
Glaucoma	• Risk of acquiring increases with age.	• Loss of sensory input can result in confusion.
Cerebrovascular Accident (CVA)	• Interruption of cerebral circulation caused by occlusion or hemorrhage in the brain. • Risk increases with age.	• Prevent deterioration of client's conditions. • Maximize functional abilities (occupational therapy). • Assist client in accepting physical deficits. • Check gag reflex before client receives food or fluids. • Prevent injuries to paralyzed limbs.
Decubitus Ulcer	• Immobility puts elderly at risk for developing decubitus ulcers.	• Reposition frequently. • Massage bony prominences. • Provide adequate nutrition.
Hypothyroidism	• Usually occurs after age 50. • Symptoms are often similar to normal aging changes, and they have an insidious onset making it difficult to detect in the elderly. • Elderly are at greater risk developing myxedema coma (life threatening).	• Often diagnosed as depression. With treatment, signs of depression disappear. • Caution against abruptly discontinuing medication.
Thyrotoxicosis (Graves' Disease)	• Symptoms may be absent or attributed to other more common diseases in the elderly. • Weight loss and CHF may be predominant symptoms.	• Precipitated by stressful events such as trauma, surgery or infection. Be alert for signs and symptoms. • Can be fatal if untreated.

Figure 7-12

GERONTOLOGICAL NURSING

DISEASES AND CONDITIONS IN TERMS OF THE ELDERLY (CONTINUED)

DISEASE/CONDITION	DESCRIPTION IN TERMS OF THE ELDERLY	NURSING IMPLICATIONS
COPD	• Major cause of respiratory disability in the elderly. • Most elderly persons exhibit both chronic bronchitis and chronic emphysema. • Fatigue is a frequent result because of the increased work required to breathe (dyspnea).	• Encourage to stop smoking. • Keep in mind older person's state of confusion when teaching about treatment regimen. • Plan rest periods to allow patient to maintain oxygen levels.
URINARY TRACT INFECTIONS (UTI)	• Incidence increases with age. • Older persons are often asymptomatic or exhibit vague, ill-defined symptoms. • With infections, older persons often become confused.	• Suspect UTI when client's voiding habits change.

Figure 7-12 (continued)

REVIEW QUESTIONS

GERONTOLOGICAL NURSING

1. What are normal memory changes that occur as one ages?
2. What symptoms might the nurse expect to see in an older person who has had an overload of changes as well as a respiratory infection?
3. Why can the BP of older adults be expected to increase?
4. What is the major cause of respiratory disability in the elderly?
5. List five nursing interventions to promote adequate bowel functioning for older persons.
6. How can a female nurse increase the older client's ability to hear her speak?
7. What is the most common visual problem occurring in the elderly?
8. Describe the following conditions which occur in the elderly:
   * Presbyopia
   * Arcus senilis
   * Presbycusis
9. Describe the onset of Alzheimer's disease.
10. What is the purpose of a reality orientation group?
11. What are 2 factors that cause decrease in excretion of drugs by the kidneys?

ANSWERS TO REVIEW QUESTIONS

1. Short-term memory declines while long-term memory undergoes minimal change.
2. Confusion.
3. Heart work increases in response to increased peripheral resistance.
4. COPD.
5. Determine what is "normal" GI functioning for each individual, increase fiber and bulk in the diet, provide adequate hydration, encourage regular exercise, and encourage eating, small, frequent meals.
6. Lower the pitch or tone of her voice.
7. Cataracts.
8. Describe:
   A. Decreased ability of the eye to accommodate for close work.
   B. Glossy white ring encircling the periphery of the cornea.
   C. Decrease in hearing acuity, auditory threshold, pitch and tone discrimination, and speech intelligibility.
9. Slow, insidious onset with a progressive downward course.
10. To keep the client oriented to time, place, and person.
11. Decrease in glomerular filtration and slowed organ functioning.

NORMAL VALUES

HEMATOLOGIC

TEST	ADULT	CHILD	INFANT/NEWBORN	ELDERLY	NURSING IMPLICATIONS
Hgb Hemoglobin g/dl	Male: 13.0 to 17.0 Female: 12.0 to 15.0 Pregnant: > 11.0	11.0 to 16.0	Infant: 10.0 to 15.0 Newborn: Term 14.0 to 24.0 Preterm 15.0 to 17.0	Both Sexes 10.0 to 17.0	• Capillary blood values are 2 to 3 g/dl greater than venous blood values, for neonates, otherwise capillary values do not difer • High altitude living increases values • Drug therapy can alter values • Values are usually decreased during pregnancy, 10 to 14% (<12%, further assess)
Hct Hematocrit %	Male: 39 to 51 Female: 36 to 45 Pregnant: > 33	31 to 43	Infant: 30 to 40 Newborn: Term 44 to 64 Preterm 45 to 55	Male: 36 to 56 Female: 30 to 54	• Prolonged stasis from vasoconstriction secondary to the tourniquet can alter values • Pregnancy values are usually decreased 32 to 42%
RBC Red Blood Cell Count million/mm³	Male: 4.4 to 5.7 Female: 4.0 to 5.3 Pregnant: 5.0 to 6.25	3.8 to 5.5	Infant: 3.8 to 5.5 Newborn: Term 4.8 to 7.1 Preterm 4.8 to 7.1	Both Sexes 3.0 to 5.0	• Never draw specimen from arm with infusing IV • Exercise and high altitudes can cause an increase in values • Pregnancy values are usually decreased • Drug therapy can alter values
WBC White Blood Cell Count 1000/mm³	Both Sexes: 4.0 to 10.0 Pregnant: 5.0 to 15.0	5.0 to 10.0	Infant: 5.0 to 17.5 Newborn: Term 9.0 to 30.0 Preterm 10.0 to 20.0	Male: 4.25 to 14.0 Female: 3.1 to 12.0	• Anesthetics, stress, exercise, and/or convulsions can caused increased values • Drug therapy can decrease values • 24 to 48 hours postpartum, normal to have as high as 25.0

HESI CLINICAL TIP: Laboratory values that are MOST important to know for the NCLEX-RN® are Hgb, Hct, WBCs, Na, K, BUN, Blood glucose, ABGs or blood gases, bilirubin for newborn, therapeutic range for PT and PTT.

NORMAL VALUES
HEMATOLOGIC

TEST	ADULT	CHILD	INFANT/NEONATE	ELDERLY	NURSING IMPLICATIONS
SED Rate Erythrocyte Sedimentation Rate (ESR) mm/hr	Male: 1 to 10 Female: 1 to 20 Pregnant: ↑ 2nd and 3rd trimesters	3 to 13	Infant: 3 to 13 Newborn: 0 to 2	Male: 15 to 20 Female: 20 to 30	• Elevated in first trimester of pregnancy
PT Prothrombin Time	12 to 14 Slight ↓ in pregnancy	12 ro 14	Neborn/Neonate 12 to 20	Same as adult	• Used in regulating Coumadin therapy • Therapeutic range is 1.5 to 2.5 times normal/control
PTT Partial Thromboplastin Time Seconds	30 to 45 Slight ↓ in pregnancy	< 60	Newborn: <90	Same as adult	• Used in regulating heparin therapy • Therapeutic range is 1.5 to 2.5 times normal/control
APTT Activated Partial Thromboplastin Time Seconds	35 to 45	Same as adult	Infant: <90	Same as adult	• Therapeutic range is 2 times normal/control • Used in regulating heparin therapy

NORMAL VALUES
BLOOD CHEMISTRY

TEST	ADULT	CHILD	INFANT/NEWBORN	ELDERLY	NURSING IMPLICATIONS
Alkaline Phosphatase IU/L	Male: 19 to 74 Female: 12 to 63 Pregnant: ↑ week 12 to 6 weeks postpartum	Child: 90 to 230 Adolescent: 100 to 250	Infant: 100 to 330 Newborn: 50 275	Male: 19 to 74 Female: 12 to 64	• Hemolysis of specimen can cause a false elevation in values
Albumin g/dl	3.5 to 5.0 Pregnant: Slight ↑	4.0 to 5.8	Infant: 4.4 to 5/3 Newborn: 3/6 to 5.4	3.2 to 4.5	• No special preparation

Normal Values
Blood Chemistry

Test	Adult	Child	Infant/Newborn	Elderly	Nursing Implications
Bilirubin Total mg/dl	0.1 to 1.2 Pregnant: Unchanged	Same as adult	0 to 1 day: < 6 1 to 2 day: < 8 3 to 5 day: <12 After 5 days < 1	0.2 to 1.2	• NPO except for water 8 to 12 hours prior to testing • Prevent hemolysis of blood during venipuncture • Do NOT shake tube; can cause inaccurate values • Protect blood sample from bright light
Bilirubin Direct mg/dl	0.1 to 0.4	Same as adult	0 to 1.0	0.1 to 0.4	• Same as for bilirubin total
Calcium mg/dl	9.0 to 10.5	Same as adult	Infant: 9.0 to 11.0 Newborn: 7.0 to 12.0	8.5 to 10.5	• No special preparation • Use of Thiazide diuretics can cause increased calcium values
Chloride mEq/L	95 to 105	101 to 105	Infant: 95 to 110 Newborn: 93 to 112	94 to 106	• Do not collect from arm with infusing IV solution
Cholesterol mg/dl	Male: 150 to 190 Female: 160 to 195 Pregnant: ↑ from 16 to 32weeks, then stabilizes	120 to 240	Infant: 70 to 175 Newborn: 45 to 170	Over 40: 200 to 210 Over 65: 150 to 250	• NPO except for water 8 hours prior to testing
CPK Creatine Phosphokiinase U/L	Male: 17 to 148 Female: 10 to 79	> 100	Newborn: 10 to 300	Same as adult	• Specimen must not be stored prior to running test
Creatinine mg/dl	0.7 to 1.5	Same as adult	Up to 1 yr. 0.3 to 1.1	0.6 to 1.8	• Preferred but not necessary to be NPO 8 hours prior to testing • Ratio of 1:20, Creatinine to BUN indicates adequate kidney functioning
Glucose mg/dl	60 to 110	60 to 100	Infant: 60 to 100 Newborn: 30 to 80	52 to 135	• NPO except for water 8 hours prior to testing • Caffeine can cause increased values
Hco₃	22 to 28	Same as adult	Same as adult	Same as adult	• None

APPENDICES

NORMAL VALUES
BLOOD CHEMISTRY

TEST	ADULT	CHILD	INFANT/NEWBORN	ELDERLY	NURSING IMPLICATIONS
Iron mcg/dl	65 to 175	50 to 120	Infant: 40 to 100 Newborn: 100 to 250	Same as adult	• Preferred but not necessary to be NPO 8 hours prior to testing
TIBC Total iron Binding Capacity mcg/dl	250 to 450	350 to 450	Infant: 100 to 400 Newborn: 60 to 175	Same as adult	• None
LDH Lactic Dehydrogenase IU/L	60 to 220	Male: 50 to 150 Female: 40 to 140	Newborn: 300 to 1500 Then same as child	71 to 207	• No IM injections 8 to 12 hours prior to testing • Hemolysis of blood will cause false positive
Potassium mEq/L	3.5 to 5.5	3.5 to 4.7	Infant: 4.1 to 5.3 Newborn: 5.0 to 7.7 Neonate: (cord) 5.6 to 12.0	3.5 to 5.6	• Hemolysis of specimen can result in falsely elevated values • Exercise of the forearm with tourniquet in place may cause an increased potassium value
Protein Total g/dl	6.0 to 8.2	6.2 to 8.0	Newborn: 4.6 to 7.6	6.0 to 7.8	• Preferred but not necessary to be NPO 8 hours prior to testing
AST/SGOT aspartate aminotransferase IU/L	AST/SGOT: 5 to 40	AST/SGOT 5 to 40	AST/SGOT 20 to 160	AST, SGOT: Slightly higher than adult	• Hemolysis of specimen can result in falsely elevated values • Exercise may cause an increased value
ALT/SGPT alanine aminotransferase U/ml	ALT/SGPT: 5 to 35	ALT/SGPT 5 to 35	ALT/SGPT 5 to 70	ALT, SGPT: Slightly higher than adult	
Sodium mEq/L	135 to 145	138 to 145	Infant: 139 to 146 Newborn: 139 to 162	Male: 134 to 147 Female: 135 to 145	• Do not collect from arm with infusing IV solution
Triglycerides mg/dl	Male: 40 to 150 Female: 30 to 140	30 to 150	Infant/Newborn 5 to 40	160 to 190	• NPO 12 hours before testing • No alcohol for 24 hours before test
Urea Nitrogen mg/dl	4 to 22	> 20	Infant/Newborn: 5 to 15	8 to 18	• None

Appendix A

ARTERIAL BLOOD CHEMISTRY

Test	Adult	Child	Infant/Newborn	Elderly	Nursing Implications
pH	7.35 to 7.45 Pregnant: 7.40 to 7.45	Same as adult	Newborn: 7.32 to 7.49 Infant:	Same as adult	• Specimen must be heparinized • Specimen must be iced for transport • All air bubbles must be expelled from sample • Direct pressure to puncture site must be maintained
Pco_2 mmHg	35 to 45 Pregnant: 27 to 32	Same as adult	Newborn: 26 to 41 Infant: 27 to 41	Same as adult	• Specimen must be heparinized • Specimen must be iced for transport • All air bubbles must be expelled from sample • Direct pressure to puncture site must be maintained
Po_2 mmHg	80 to 100 Pregnant: 104 to 108	Same as adult	Newborn: 60 to 70 Infant: 83 to 108	Same as adult	• Specimen must be heparinized • Specimen must be iced for transport • All air bubbles must be expelled from sample • Direct pressure to puncture site must be maintained
HCO_3 mEq/L	21 to 28 Pregnant: 18 to 31	Same as adult	Newborn: 16 to 24 Infant: 21 to 28	Same as adult	• Specimen must be heparinized • Specimen must be iced for transport • All air bubbles must be expelled from sample • Direct pressure to puncture site must be maintained
O_2 saturation %	95 to 100	Same as adult	Newborn: 85 to 90 Infant: 95 to 99	95	• Specimen must be heparinized • Specimen must be iced for transport • All air bubbles must be expelled from sample • Direct pressure to puncture site must be maintained

APPENDICES

Food Groups and Servings Per Day

Food Group	Child	Adult	Pregnant	Lactating
Dairy	Under 9 years: 2 to 3 servings; 9 to 12 years: 3 or more servings; Teenager: 4 or more servings	2 or more servings	4 or more servings	4 or more servings
Protein	2 or more servings	2 or more servings	3 servings	2 servings
Vegetable and Fruits	4 or more servings; At least 1 serving of vitamin A and 1 of vitamin C	4 or more servings (same as child's recommendations)	2 servings vegetables; 2 servings fruit	2 servings vegetables; 2 servings fruit
Bread and Cereal	4 or more servings	4 or more servings	4 servings	4 servings

Daily Requirements for Fat Soluble Vitamins

Vitamin	Food Source
A	• Liver, fish oils • Whole milk, egg yolk, fortified margarine, and butter • Dark green and deep orange fruits and vegetables, i.e., apricots, broccoli, cantaloupe, carrots, pumpkin, winter squash, sweet potatoes, and spinach
D	• Fortified and full-fat dairy products • Egg yolks • Can be synthesized in the skin when exposed to sunlight
E	• Vegetable oils and their products such as salad oils, margarine and peanuts. Baby food such as peaches, apricots, and spinach
K	• Green leafy vegetables such as lettuce, cabbage, spinach, peas, asparagus, and meat

Foods High in Sodium

Vegetables	Condiments	Mischellaneous
• Canned vegetables • Carrots, particularly canned • Tomatoes, particularly canned • Tomato catsup • Tomato juice	• Bouillon cubes • Mustard, prepared • Olives, pickled; canned or bottled • Pickles, cucumber, dill • Salad dressings, commercially prepared • Soy sauce	• Bacon • Cheeses • Ready-to-eat breakfast cereals • Peanut butters • Soups, commercially prepared, canned • Corned beef

Daily Requirements for Water Soluble Vitamins

Vitamin	Food Sources
C	• Citrus fruits, cantaloupes, strawberries, tomatoes, potatoes, broccoli, green peppers and spinach
B_1 (thiamine)	• Pork, liver, whole grains, peas, eggs, milk, peanuts, oatmeal, and pasta
B_2 (riboflavin)	• Milk, and milk products, eggs, cheddar cheese, organ meats, and whole grains
B_e (nicotinic acid)	• Dairy products, beef, pork, fish, liver, whole grains, peanuts, and green vegetables
B_6 (pyridoxine)	• Meat, liver, tuna, poultry, potatoes, wheat, and corn
Folic Acid	• Green leafy vegetables, broccoli, green beans, whole grains, and nuts
B_{12}	• Glandular meats (such as liver), yeast, green leafy vegetables, milk and cheese

Daily Requirements for Some Minerals

Mineral	Food Sources
Calcium	• Milk, cheese, dark green vegetables, and legumes
Phosphorus	• Milk, cheese, poultry, and whole grains
Magnesium	• Whole grains and green leafy vegetables
Iron	• Meats, eggs, legumes, whole grains, green leafy vegetables, and dried fruits
Iodine	• Marine fish, shellfish, dairy products, iodized salt, and some breads
Potassium	• Citrus fruits and dried fruits, bananas, watermelon, potatoes, legumes, tea, and peanut butter
Zinc	• Meats, seafood, and whole grains

APPENDICES

APPENDICES

INDEX

Chronic renal failure, 84, 90, 171

Cirrhosis, 41, 48, 120, 125, 371

Cleft lip and/or cleft palate, 227, 228, 230, 267, 285

Client needs, 2, 5, 6, 137, 189, 364

Coarctation of the aorta, 208, 209, 287

Communicable diseases, 108, 194, 198

Computer adaptive testing (CAT), 7

Computed axial tomography (CAT) scan, 152,

Congenital dislocated hip, 216, 239, 242

Congenital heart disorders, 208

Congenital megacolon, 229

Congestive heart failure (CHF), 31, 41, 53, 109, 111, 112, 120, 208, 212, 214, 222, 286, 355, 386

Consent, 11, 13, 14, 54, 193, 253, 281, 315, 316, 377, 379

Contraception, 279-281, 313

Coping styles, 66, 67, 337, 338, 344-346, 371, 372

Corticosteroids, 74-76, 113, 115, 128, 129, 136, 137, 143, 154, 155, 170, 241

Crime, 9, 10, 379

Cushing's syndrome, 42, 129, 135, 225

Cyanotic heart defects/disease, 210, 212

Cystic fibrosis, 82, 204, 207, 232

Cystocele, 175, 182

D

Death and grief, 66, 67

Defense mechanism, (see Coping styles)

Degenerative joint disease, 138, 142, 143

Delirium, 152, 371, 372, 375, 380, 381, 398

Dementia, 360, 380, 381, 391, 395, 396, 398

Diabetes insipidus, 43

Diabetes Mellitus, 48, 53, 91, 101, 123, 124, 130-133, 135, 144, 159, 162, 188, 235, 236, 249, 252, 256, 259, 280, 299, 301, 306, 312-314, 317, 318, 322, 332, 373, 389 392, 396

Diarrhea, 3, 22, 23, 26, 41, 42, 48, 58-60, 62, 65, 70-72, 84, 88, 93, 99, 106, 107, 114-116, 119, 121, 123, 125, 126, 130, 133-135, 145, 151, 157, 166, 169-171, 201, 202, 206, 213, 214, 223, 229, 235, 261, 288, 296, 302, 313, 321, 325, 333, 344, 357, 362, 265, 374, 381

Digitalis preparations, 33, 36, 85, 109, 110, 112

Disaster nursing, 19, 27

Disseminated intravascular coagulation (DIC), 29, 296.

Dissociative disorders, 351, 352

Diuretics, 40-43, 53, 61, 98, 99, 109, 112, 153, 155, 161, 163, 174, 212, 221, 222, 363, 392

Diverticular diseases, 116

Down syndrome, 215, 222, 253, 285, 287, 290, 396

Drug abuse (see Abuse)

Dysrhythmias, 42, 43, 75, 91, 95, 96, 99, 105-107, 109, 110, 112, 128, 208, 383, 398

Dystocia, 252, 265, 303, 304, 323, 325

E

Eating disorders, 354, 355

Ectopic pregnancy, 295, 318

Elder abuse (see Abuse)

Electrocardiogram (ECG) or (EKG), 42, 49-52, 54, 61, 84, 91, 95, 105-107, 212, 302, 327, 347, 368, 396

Electrolyte imbalance, 40, 42, 43, 49, 53, 59, 86, 89, 105, 172, 229, 311, 318, 331, 332, 334, 354, 355 380, 381, 389

Endocrine, 75, 125, 128, 135, 170, 234, 235, 236, 392, 393

Epiglottitis, 197, 205, 207

Esophageal atresia, 227, 230, 285

Eye drop administration, 144, 146

Eye trauma, 146

F

Fertilization, 243, 244

Fetal monitoring, 252, 254, 263, 271, 301, 304, 313

Fluid and electrolyte balance, 29, 40, 48, 90, 204, 229

Fracture, 2, 35, 92, 139, 140-143, 152, 219, 237, 238, 242, 286, 314, 376, 392, 393

G

Gavage feeding, 214, 290, 330-332, 334

Gerontological nursing, 380, 385, 399

Glasgow coma scale, 148, 149, 152, 161

Glaucoma, 107, 143-146, 158, 226, 394, 396, 398

Glomerulonephritis, acute (AGN), 83, 206, 222, 223, 226

Goiter, 125-127

Good Samaritan Act, 11, 12, 14

Graves' disease, 125, 126, 398

Growth and development, 4-6, 61, 191, 192, 205, 211, 215, 217, 222, 231, 234, 235, 395

Guillain-Barré syndrome, 159

H

Hashimoto's disease, 127

Head injury, 152, 153, 155

Health Insurance Portability and Accountability Act of 1996 (HIPAA), 13

NOTES

NOTES

NOTES

NOTES

NOTES

NOTES

NOTES

NOTES

NOTES

NOTES

NOTES

NOTES

NOTES